Clinical Guide to Oral Diseases

Clinical Guide to Oral Diseases

Dimitris Malamos
DDS, MSC, PhD, Dip. O.M
Oral Medicine Specialist
Diplomat of the European Association of Oral Medicine
Head of the Oral Medicine Clinic at the National Organization for the Provision of Health Services
1st Health Region and at Iatrokosmos
Athens, Greece

Crispian Scully
CBE, DSc, DChD, DMed (HC), Dhc (Multi), MD, PhD, PhD (HC), FMedSci, MDS,
MRCS, BSc, FDSRCS, FDSRCPS, FFDRCSI, FDSRCSEd FRCPath, FHEA
Emeritus Professor
University College
London, UK

Content Editor
Márcio Diniz Freitas
Special Care Dentistry Unit
University of Santiago de Compostela
Spain

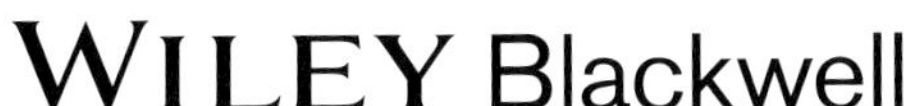

This edition first published 2021

Registered Offices
John Wiley & Sons, Inc., 111 River Street, Hoboken, NJ 07030, USA
John Wiley & Sons Ltd, The Atrium, Southern Gate, Chichester, West Sussex, PO19 8SQ, UK

Editorial Office
9600 Garsington Road, Oxford, OX4 2DQ, UK

For details of our global editorial offices, customer services, and more information about Wiley products visit us at www.wiley.com.

Wiley also publishes its books in a variety of electronic formats and by print-on-demand. Some content that appears in standard print versions of this book may not be available in other formats.

Library of Congress Cataloging-in-Publication Data

Names: Malamos, Dimitris, author. | Scully, Crispian, author.
Title: Clinical guide to oral diseases / Dimitris Malamos, Crispian Scully.
Description: Hoboken, NJ : Wiley-Blackwell, 2021. | Includes index.
Identifiers: LCCN 2020032170 (print) | LCCN 2020032171 (ebook) | ISBN 9781119328117 (paperback) | ISBN 9781119328131 (adobe pdf) | ISBN 9781119328155 (epub)
Subjects: MESH: Mouth Diseases–diagnosis | Diagnosis, Oral | Case Reports
Classification: LCC RK60.7 (print) | LCC RK60.7 (ebook) | NLM WU 140 | DDC 617.6/01–dc23
LC record available at https://lccn.loc.gov/2020032170
LC ebook record available at https://lccn.loc.gov/2020032171

Cover Design: Wiley
Cover Image: courtesy of Dimitris Malamos

Set in 9.5/12.5pt STIXTwoText by SPi Global, Pondicherry, India

Printed and bound in Singapore by Markono Print Media Pte Ltd

10 9 8 7 6 5 4 3 2 1

Contents

Preface

The idea of writing this book was born one Sunday afternoon three years ago, when Professor Scully and I discussed some interesting and intriguing clinical cases for diagnosis. We thought it would be a good idea to provide various clinical photos, and respond to relevant questions in a way that the readers could be led to the proper diagnosis. Professor Scully wanted this new book to be reader-friendly and hoped to approach the common oral diseases in a different way. This book would not be compared to any of the other outstanding and well-written textbooks on oral medicine, as it would not be a complete review of oral diseases or rare syndromes.

This guide aims to present a large selection of clinical cases that are representative of the majority of oral common diseases that are seen in a daily clinical practice, and it is recommended to all physicians and oral health providers, including dental and medical undergraduate and postgraduate students, dentists and medical practitioners, especially dermatologists, as well as ear, nose and throat specialists, internists, and oncologists.

Despite Professor Scully's sudden death, the composition of the book writing took place as an effort to follow his idea. The book is designed to provide a short revision of oral medicine by using three different groups of multiple choice questions (MCQs) and answers based on clinical colored photos. Each group of questions has different degrees of difficulty in answering. The first group of questions is adequate for undergraduate students and is related to diagnosis; the second is addressed to medical and dental practitioners; while the last and more difficult is for postgraduate students.

This book is divided into three parts. The first part includes Chapters 1–14 and refers to the classification of oral lesions by appearance and symptomatology; the second part comprises Chapters 15–24 and encompasses the most common oral lesions by location; while the third part consists of Chapters 25–27 and refers to the oral lesions that are normal variations, or have an age predilection, or are part of various clinical phenomena. Parts I and III are composed of 10 cases in each chapter, while the Part II has five cases in each chapter. Additionally, a concise table and a short text relevant to each chapter and containing a list of the common oral lesions/conditions is provided before cases presentation.

This book is based on more than 260 good quality, colored clinical photos, making this guide a brief practical atlas of common oral diseases. These clinical images come from my personal records, and I am deeply grateful to my patients who gave their permission, and to my publication team for plotting these images carefully. Their help was unique, and without it, this book would not be feasible.

Dimitris Malamos
Athens, 2020

Foreword

It is an honor and an immense satisfaction for me to provide the prologue for this book for two main reasons: the experience of its authors and the originality of this proposed editorial. When reviewing this ''Clinical Guide to Oral Diseases", one is surprised by the practical perspective with which its authors have imbued it, combining basic principles of problem-based learning with excellent images and an accurate and essential critical overview for arguing the differential diagnosis of each injury. Throughout the 27 chapters, the authors conduct an exhaustive review of the most common oral injuries based on the discussion of case studies. This approach perfectly combines Dimitris Malamos' clinical experience and Crispian Scully's academic rigor.

All of these features make this book a cross-sectional work, which can be useful both for undergraduate students, general dentists and specialists in the setting of medical-surgical dentistry. In the end, the success of the clinical activity is not based on academic titles but rather on the knowledge and expertise of the observer. In some manner, Professor Scully had already promulgated this idea during his final years, because he tended to end his emails with a phrase attributed to Goethe, "One only sees what one looks for. One only looks for what one knows."

Pedro Diz Dios
MD, DDS, PHD, EDOM, FRCSEd ad hominem
Professor of Special Care Dentistry
Santiago de Compostela University, Spain

Acknowledgment

I would like to thank the individuals whose help made this Clinical Guide possible; particularly Mrs J. Saiprasad for being so helpful and co-operative in determination to overcome delays in publication Mrs Carolyn Holleyman for checking the flowcharts and webcases, Mrs Susan Engelken for the cover of the book and especially Mr Vincent Rajan as Production Editor organizing and resolving problems before the publication and Mrs A. Argyropouloy for revising the text. I am grateful to my mentors Professor G. Laskaris (Greece) and Professor C. Scully (United Kingdom) as I truly appreciated their teaching and encouragement to me, to become seriously involved in Oral Medicine. Professor Scully's friendship, advice and expertise is still a part that I miss, and this book was written in his memory.

I wish also to express my sincere gratitude to Dr Pedro Diz Dios and to Dr Marcio Diniz Freitas for their help and advice throughout the preparation of this book. The participation of Dr Marcio Diniz Freitas as Content editor is precious.

Finally, I am especially indebted to my wife Vasiliki and my children Panagiotis and Katerina for their continuous love and support for all those years of my involvement in Oral Medicine, and during the preparation of this guide.

About the Companion Website

Don't forget to visit the companion website for this book:

www.wiley.com/go/malamos/clinical_guide 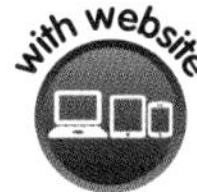

There you will find valuable material designed to enhance your learning, including:

- Clinical cases
- Further reading

Scan this QR code to visit the companion website

Section I

1

Bleeding

Bleeding in the mouth may be a sign of various conditions related to the structure of blood vessels, the number or function of white blood cells and especially platelets, the deficiency or dysfunction of clotting factors or even interaction of various drugs. Some of these bleeding disorders appear at a very young age; some are also found among close relatives (inherited) while others are noticed later with a negative family history (acquired). The severity of the bleeding ranges from minor hemorrhages from gingivae and other parts of the oral mucosa with the formation of petechiae or ecchymosis (Figure 1.0), to extensive bleeding in other parts of the body, causing severe blood loss, even jeopardizing the patient's life.

The more important causes of oral bleeding are seen in Table 1.

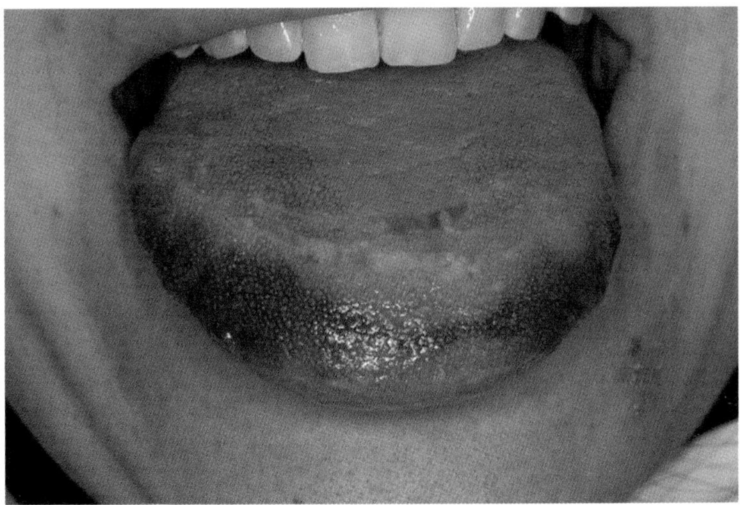

Figure 1.0 Tongue hematoma in a woman with seizures.

Clinical Guide to Oral Diseases, First Edition. Dimitris Malamos and Crispian Scully.

Companion website: www.wiley.com/go/malamos/clinical_guide

Table 1 Conditions related to oral bleeding.

Common and important conditions
• Local conditions ■ Gingivitis/periodontitis ■ Granuloma pyogenic/giant cell ■ Jaw fracture ■ Trauma ■ Tumors invading blood vessels • Systemic conditions ○ Congenital ■ Hemophilia A or B ■ Von Willebrand's disease ■ Other factor deficiencies ■ Glanzman thrombasthenia ○ Acquired - related to coagulation ■ Liver disease ■ Vit. K deficiency, warfarin drug use ■ Disseminated intravascular coagulation - related to thrombocytopenia ■ Idiopathic ■ Drug-induced ■ Collagen vascular disease ■ Sarcoidosis ■ Hemolytic anemia ■ Leukemia ■ Myeloma ■ Waldestmom - related to platelet dysregulation ■ Alcoholism ■ Chronic renal failure ■ Drugs ■ Liver disease - related to vascular disorders ■ Angina bullosa hemorrhagica ■ Angiomas ■ Ehrler-Danlos syndrome ■ Hereditary hemorrhagic telangiectasia ■ Infections from Ebola, HIV, HSV; EBV, Rubella ■ Marfan syndrome ■ Purpura ■ Scurvy - related to fibrinolysis ■ Amyloidosis ■ Streptokinase treatment

Case 1.1

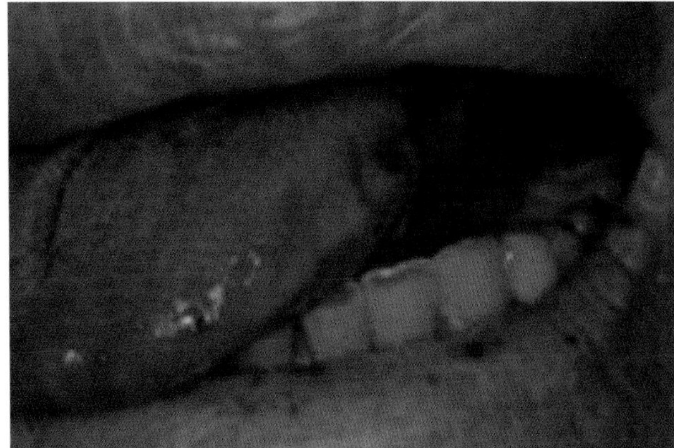

Figure 1.1a

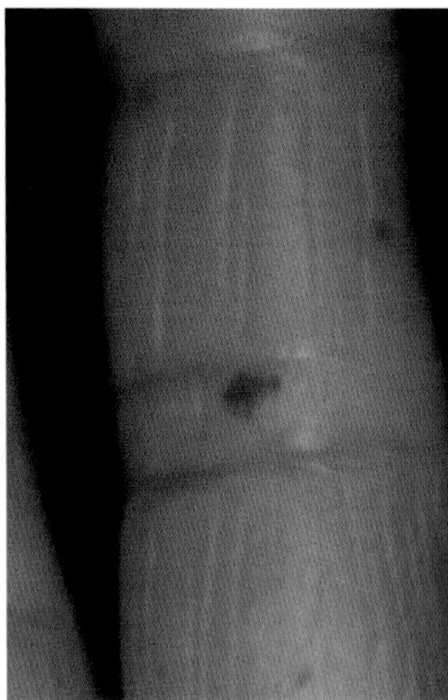

Figure 1.1b

CO: A 62-year-old woman was referred by her family doctor for evaluation of several red spots on her lips, mouth, and the skin of her fingers.

HPC: The red spots had been present since childhood, but had become greater on the surface of her face over the last five years causing cosmetic problems and patient's concern.

PMH: Her medical history revealed a chronic iron deficiency anemia which still remained despite the fact that

The following abbreviations are used throughout the book – CO: Complains of; HPC: History of present complaint; PMH: Past medical history; OE: oral examination.

the patient was in the post-menopause phase and had been treated occasionally with iron tablets. No other serious medical problems were recorded except for a few episodes of nose and gut bleeding which had caused her to ask for medical advice. She was a non-smoker and non-drinker.

OE: The examination revealed numerous red vascular papules, variable in size, ranging from pin head-like lesions to small red plaques at the vermilion border of her lips, and on the tongue and buccal mucosae (Figure 1.1a). A few asteroid-like red lesions, were also seen on the skin of her fingers (Figure 1.1b) and inside her nose which were responsible for her episodes of epistaxis.

Q1 Which is the possible cause of her red spots?

A Crest syndrome
B Sjogren syndrome
C Rendu-Osler-Weber syndrome
D Rosacea
E Ataxia-telangiectasia

Answers:

A No
B No
C Rendu-Osler-Weber syndrome or hereditary hemorrhagic telangiectasia (HHT) is a rare autosomal dominant condition that affects blood vessels throughout the body (telangiectasia; arteriovenous malformations) with a tendency for bleeding. This vascular dysplasia is commonly seen in oral, nasopharynx, lung, liver, spleen, gastrointestinal and urinary tracts, conjunctiva and the skin of arms and fingers.
D No
E No

Comments: Skin telangiectasias are also seen in patients with ataxia telangiectasia, Crest and Sjogren syndromes. In rosacea, main vascular lesions are the broken vessels that are located exclusively on the skin predominantly on the middle of the face, as in ataxia telangiectasia. In ataxia telangectasia, the vascular lesions are associated with poor coordination, and in Crest syndrome with calcinosis and sclerodactyly and Raynaud phenomenon. Sjogren's syndrome affects the mouth, eyes, nose and other organs causing dryness, swelling of the salivary glands and facial telangiectases.

Q2 Which are the main complications of this condition?

A Anemia
B Pulmonary hemorrhage
C Ischemic stroke
D Skin photosensitivity
E Mental retardation

Answers:

A Iron deficiency anemia is a very common complication induced by a series of episodes of blood loss through the nose (epistaxis) and gastrointestinal tract (melena stools) from telangiectic lesions.
B Pulmonary hemorrhage is mainly found in patients older than 40 years old and with multiple visceral involvements, causing breathing problems, portal hypertension and liver cirrhosis.
C Ischemic stroke is a rare yet serious complication in patients with HHT, and requires special care.
D No
E No

Comments: The vascular lesions on facial skin sometimes cause cosmetic problems, but never skin photosensitivity, while the brain lesions of HHT may cause neuro-psychiatric complications with various pathways which have not been related to mental illness before.

Q3 Which genes are linked with this condition?

A Endoglin gene (ENG)
B Fibroblast growth factor receptor 3 (FGFR3)
C Activin receptor like kinase (ALK-1)
D Collagen type I alpha 1 chain(COL1A1)
E Dentin sialophosphoprotein (DSPP)

Answers:

A Engoglin gene mutations have been isolated in HHT families (type 1)
B No
C Activin receptor like kinase (ALK-1)mutations have been found in HHT (type 2)

Comments: Mutations in the COL1A1 and COL1A2 genes are related to the development of the majority of osteogenesis imperfecta (>90%), while FGFR3 is associated with fibrous dysplasia and DSPP with dentinogenesis imperfecta.

Case 1.2

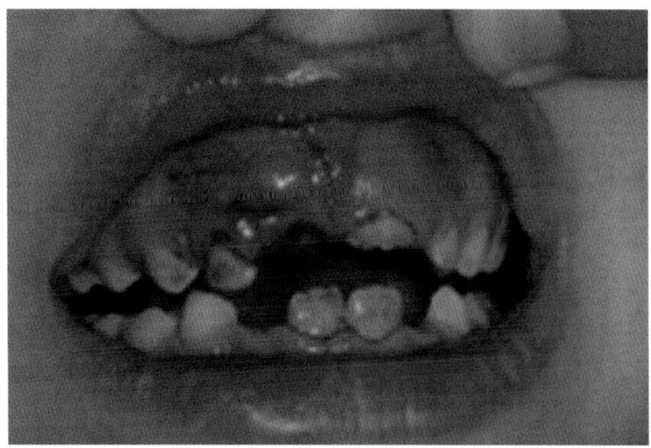

Figure 1.2

CO: A six-year-old boy was admitted with bleeding of his mouth.

HPC: The patient sustained a facial injury during a football match half an hour before the bleeding.

PMH: He was a healthy child with no serious medical problems. He was very sociable, and used to take part in all activities at his kindergarten.

OE: He is a very young child, feeling stress and fear because of the bleeding in his mouth, especially from the area of deciduous central right incisor. This tooth had been pushed into its hemorrhagic and swollen gingivae (Figure 1.2). No other problems with the rest of his teeth, jaws, and oral mucosa were noticed.

Q1 What is the possible cause of the hemorrhage of this child?

- **A** Trauma
- **B** Self-induced
- **C** Infections
- **D** Children abuse
- **E** Bleeding disorders

Answers:

- **A** Facial trauma is commonly noticed among children and characterized by soft tissue injuries (lips, oral mucosae, face) or deep ones into the maxilla or mandibular bone and their associated teeth. Facial trauma is responsible for the "impressive" bleeding due to the high vascularity of this area.
- **B** No
- **C** No
- **D** No
- **E** No

Comments: The absence of multiple bruises and hematomas alone, or with the different ages of lesions combined with the history of the accident and type of injuries in a child's body is an easy way to exclude bleeding disorders or child abuse from the diagnosis. The absence of fever, swelling and erythema in the lesion rules out infections (bacterial, viral, or fungal). In addition to this, the lack of similar lesions in the past together with the child's good healthy social life reinforces the idea that the lesion was not self-induced.

Q2 Which is/are the difference(s) of facial trauma between children and adolescents?

- **A** Etiology
- **B** Bone involvement
- **C** Symptomatology
- **D** Complications
- **E** Recovery rate

Answers:

- **A** Facial trauma is caused by falling in children and by assault or altercation in adolescents.
- **B** Fractures of nose bones or jaws are more common in adolescents rather than in children.
- **C** The symptomatology in children does not fit with the severity of the lesions and is more remarkable than in adolescents.
- **D** The facial trauma in children is more superficial than in adolescents and their complications seem to be minimal.
- **E** The younger the children, the easier their recovery.

Q3 Which is the clinician's first priority when faced with a patient with facial injury?

- **A** Calm patient and his parents
- **B** Retain the airway open
- **C** Check for broken or dislocated teeth
- **D** Stop bleeding
- **E** Treat facial wound (cleaning and suturing)

Answers:

- **A** No
- **B** Retaining child's airway open is the first priority as the mucosal edema is disproportional with the patient's airway tract. The clinician should remove obstacles like debris, clots and foreign bodies

from the oropharynx, control the location of patient's tongue while in severe cases an orotracheal intubation could be mandatory.
- **C** No
- **D** No
- **E** No

Comments: The second priority for the clinicians is to control bleeding by putting direct pressure on the facial injury. Having bleeding under control, clinicians are then able to properly examine the soft tissue injury, investigate for possible teeth and jaws fractures and then go further to cleanse and suture the wound, as well as reassuring the patient and his parents.

Case 1.3

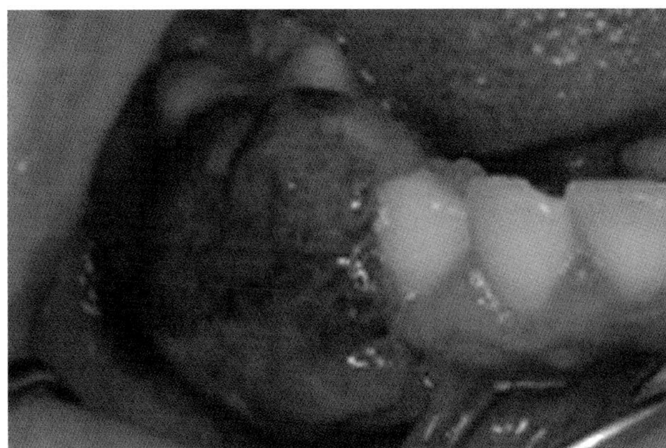

Figure 1.3

CO: A 32-year-old woman presented with a soft hemorrhagic lump on her lower left gingivae.

HPC: The lump appeared three months ago and became gradually bigger, covering the whole crown of the second premolar, thus causing eating difficulties and phobias to the patient of being a malignant neoplasm.

PMH: A healthy woman at the third month after baby delivery, with no serious medical problems and drug use apart from iron and calcium tablets prescribed by her gynecologist during her pregnancy. Smoking or drinking habits were plentiful.

OE: A very soft penduculated mass on the gingivae from the distal part of the 1st lower right premolar to the 1st molar. It was very soft, vascular and sensitive, and was bleeding easily with slight probing and caused eating problems (Figure 1.3). The lesion developed gradually and reaching its biggest site at the last month of pregnancy and began to decrease slowly within the next three months after her delivery. No other similar lesions were found within her mouth, other mucosae or skin. Regional or systemic lymphadenopathy was not recorded.

Q1 What is this lesion?
- **A** Kaposi's sarcoma
- **B** Pregnancy epulis
- **C** Peripheral giant cell granuloma
- **D** Gingival hemangioma
- **E** Peripheral ossifying fibroma

Answers:
- **A** No
- **B** Pregnancy epulis is a localized hyperplastic hemorrhagic soft lesion on the upper and lower gingivae of pregnant women with decayed teeth and poor oral hygiene. The lesion grows slowly and reaches its largest size during the last trimester of pregnancy.
- **C** No
- **D** No
- **E** No

Comments: In contrary to pregnancy epulis the gingival hemangiomas are found earlier (at childhood); sarcoma Kaposi are usually associated with lymphadenopathy and have an aggressive course. The peripheral odontogenic fibroma has a firmer feel on palpation, while the peripheral giant cell epulis does not improve with the baby's birth and is associated with endocrinopathies.

Q2 Which are the other oral conditions seen during pregnancy?
- **A** Melasma
- **B** Pregnancy gingivitis
- **C** Increased risk of caries
- **D** Erosions of teeth
- **E** Sialorrhea

Answers:
- **A** No
- **B** Pregnancy gingivitis is the commonest complication of pregnancy and can start even from the second month, reaching its peak on the eight

month of pregnancy. This type of gingivitis is due rather to the action of increased female hormones on their gingival receptors rather than to microbial plaque.

C Pregnant women tend to be at increased risk of caries as the number of cariogenic bacteria in the mouth, and the frequency of eating, especially sweet food as a means of coping with nausea, are increased.

D Erosions on the palatal tooth surface and especially on the upper anterior teeth are common and are also attributed to the acidity of gastric juice that reaches the mouth during vomiting.

E Sialorrhea is a common finding in pregnant women and caused by the increased nausea and vomiting recorded during their pregnancy.

Comments: Melasma or pregnancy mask as it is known, is characterized by a brown discoloration of the facial skin and lips, but is never seen within the mouth of pregnant women and those taking contraceptives or hormone replacement medications.

Q3 Which conditions have been detected in babies, related to the periodontal status of their mothers?

A Premature birth
B Low weight
C Vision or hearing deficits
D Mental retardation
E Dental anomalies

Answers:

A Women with chronic inflammation of their gingivae seem to produce a number of inflammatory cytokines, some of which are responsible for the uterine muscle contractions which finally induce early labor.

B Premature babies show incomplete growth and low weight.

C Vision or hearing deficits are commonly seen in premature babies whose early birth may be associated with the periodontal problems of their mother.

D No

E No

Comments: The mental status of pregnant women may worsen their periodontal problems by increased secretion of cortisol and refusal of tooth brushing, while the periodontitis per se does not affect the mental status or dentition of their children.

Case 1.4

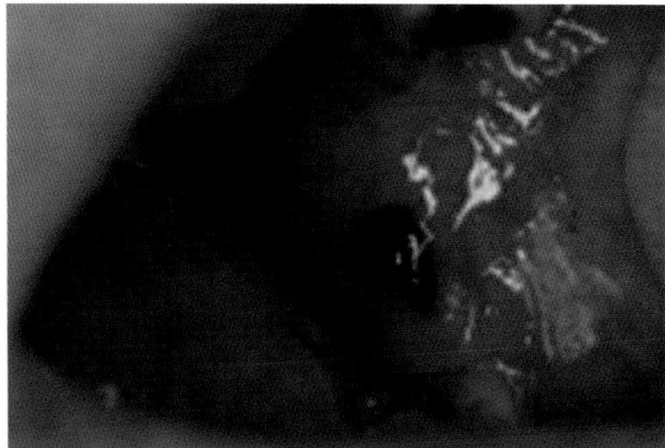

Figure 1.4

CO: A 42-year-old woman came in with a hemorrhagic bulla inside her cheek.

HPC: The bulla appeared three hours ago after eating a sandwich. No similar bullae were recorded in her or her close relatives in the past.

PMH: From her medical records a few episodes of allergic rhinitis controlled with antihistamine and steroids in crisis were recorded. No blood and other systemic diseases, other allergies or drug uptakes were recorded.

OE: Examination revealed a large bulla with hemorrhagic content on the left buccal mucosa at the occlusion level (Figure 1.4). The bulla appeared during mastication and was easily broken during the examination's manipulations, leaving a painful superficial ulceration. No other bullae, ulcerations or petechiae and ecchymoses were seen on the oral and other mucosae or skin. Cervical lymphadenopathy was not seen.

Q1 Which is the disease responsible for this bulla?

A Thrombocytopenia
B Burns
C Mucous membrane pemphigoid
D Angina bullosa hemorrhagica
E Hemorrhagic mucocele

Answers:

- **A** No
- **B** No
- **C** No
- **D** Angina bullosa hemorrhagica (ABH) is an acute, benign condition characterized by the development of subepithelial bullae filled with blood that are not attributed to any systemic disorders. A chronic trauma, consumption of hot and spicy or abrasive foods, or difficulties in restorative or periodontal treatment are considered to be the commonest causes.
- **E** No

Comments: Hemorrhagic bullae are often seen in other conditions such as thrombocytopenia, mucous pemphigoids and burns, but the presence of specific elements indicated the diagnosis. The appearance of low platelets and ecchymoses, epistaxis, and gingival bleeding in thrombocytopenia, the presence of numerous bullae with clear fluid in mucous pemphigoid, and the lack of close contact with thermal, chemical, or electrical elements in burns help to exclude these conditions from the diagnosis. Mucoceles are thicker and more resistant, while the bullae in angina are thinner and more easily break.

Q2 Which of the drugs below are usually related to the development of this condition?

- **A** NSAIDs
- **B** Antibiotics
- **C** Steroids
- **D** Anti-diabetics
- **E** Bronchodilators

Answers:

- **A** No
- **B** No
- **C** Chronic use of steroids, especially inhalers, causes oral mucosa atrophy and decreases the submucosa's elastic fiber content, resulting in capillary breakdown locally, finally forming the characteristic hemorrhagic bullae.
- **D** No
- **E** No

Comments: Diabetes mellitus has also been associated with hemorrhagic bulla formation due to increased vascular fragility in these patients, and not to the drug for blood sugar reduction. Similar bullae could also be seen in patients who take antibiotics or bronchodilators and have various autoimmune diseases. As for NSAIDs, these drugs are responsible for peptic ulcers and bleeding from the intestine, but more rarely for skin bullous rash and fever.

Q3 Which of the histopathological finding(s) is/or are characteristics of this condition?

- **A** Subepithelial bulla
- **B** Intra-epithelial abscess of neutrophils
- **C** Mononuclear inflammatory infiltration of submucosa deep to the muscles
- **D** Direct immunofluorescence negative
- **E** Eosinophils accumulation in the corium

Answers:

- **A** The breakage of the epithelial–connective tissue junction due to topical agents leads to local capillary hemorrhage and subepithelial bulla formation.
- **B** No
- **C** No
- **D** Direct immune-fluorescence is always negative. DI is always positivein pemphigus and other intra-epithelial blistering diseases.
- **E** No

Comments: The inflammatory response in ABH is intense and located only at the superficial parts of submucosa, often containing neutrophils but not eosinophils and mast cells.

Case 1.5

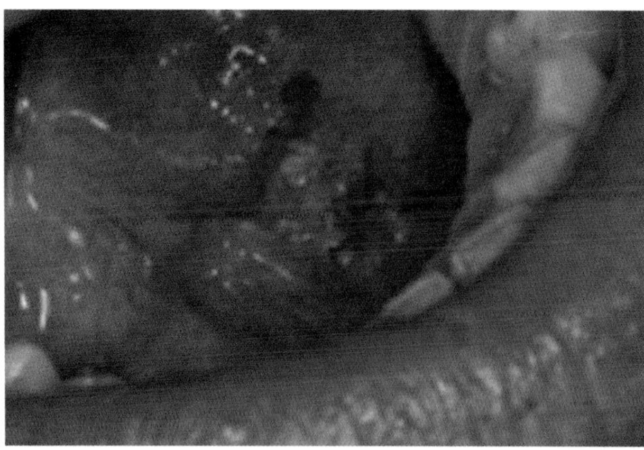

Figure 1.5

CO: A 48-year old man was presented with a hemorrhagic lesion on the floor of his mouth.

HPC: The lesion appeared sixmonths ago while the bleeding was noticed during eating three days ago.

PMH: No serious medical problems were recorded apart from an episode of severe pneumonia which was diagnosed last December and was treated with a strong course of antibiotics. No other drugs were taken, but the patient was a smoker (>40 cigarettes, daily) and a drinker (4–5 glasses of wine or relevant spirit per meal).

OE: The examination revealed an asymptomatic white lesion on the floor of mouth extended from the left lower premolar to the molar region. The lesion was fixed in palpation and had a warty-like surface with two to three bleeding areas (Figure 1.5). Smoking-induced lesions such as increased gingival pigmentation, nicotinic stomatitis and brown teeth discoloration were also found, together with ipsilateral, fixed, enlarged cervical lymph nodes where oral or skin petechiae and ecchymoses were not seen.

Q1 What is the cause of bleeding?

- **A** Traumatic ulceration
- **B** Pemphigus vegetans
- **C** Verrucous leukoplakia
- **D** Giant verruca vulgaris
- **E** Squamous carcinoma

Answers:

- **A** No
- **B** No
- **C** No
- **D** No
- **E** Squamous cell carcinoma is the cause of his oral bleeding. This tumor is a locally aggressive, tumor which appears as an indurated swelling , ulceration or plaque of various cellular differentiation and risk of metastasis. This lesion grows either slowly and superficially, but in majority of cases grows fast and invades deep tissues such as muscles and blood vessels causing muscle dysfunction and bleeding.

Comments: This tumor differs from other vegetating oral lesions such as hyperplastic traumatic ulcerations, pemphigus vegetans, verrucous leucoplakia, and verrucous vulgaris. The lack of local trauma or other vegetating lesions in the flexures of the patient rules out traumatic ulceration and pemphigus vegetans from the diagnosis, while the hard consistency and strong fixation of the lesion with the underling tissues is not an indication of verrucous vulgaris and leukoplakia where biopsy is required.

Q2 Although the verrucous carcinoma is a variation of oral carcinomas, it differs from the other types in the following histological characteristics:

- **A** Evidence of dysplasia in adjacent epithelium
- **B** Shape of the rete pegs
- **C** Absence of keratinization
- **D** Location of mitosis
- **E** Basal basement membrane status

Answers:

- **A** Dysplastic epithelium is often seen close to the oral squamous, but not to verrucous carcinomas.
- **B** The shape of rete pegs entering the corium is variable in the majority of oral carcinomas, but is bulbous, like elephant feet in verrucous carcinoma.
- **C** No
- **D** In oral carcinomas, the mitoses are scattered in the basal and spinous layer, while in verrucous carcinoma they are located mainly in the basal layer.
- **E** In oral carcinomas the basal membrane is invaded by tumor islands, but in verrucous carcinoma it is intact and the tumor grows superficially as well.

Comments: Keratinization is commonly seen in both tumors; however keratin pearls are mainly found in squamous carcinoma, while keratin plugs are found in verrucous carcinomas.

Q3 Which of the measures below is/are not amenable to control bleeding from an oral carcinoma?

- **A** Identification of the underlying cause of oral bleeding
- **B** Blood investigations
- **C** Packing-dressing
- **D** Suturing
- **E** Radiotherapy

Answers:

- **A** No
- **B** No
- **C** No
- **D** No
- **E** Radiotherapy is sometimes useful to the control of excessive bleeding that may arise from lung but not oral carcinomas. Patients with oral carcinomas and other head and neck tumors have already received the maximum dose of radiotherapy when bleeding begins, and therefore other aggressive measures such as arterial embolization should be undertaken.

Comments: Clinicians must control oral bleeding by following some basic steps such as the identification of the causative factor by taking a comprehensive history and careful clinical examination; excluding bleeding diseases by checking white blood count and clotting profiles as well as packing or dressing with hemostatic agents, while in more severe cases with cauterization, suturing, or embolization should be used.

Case 1.6

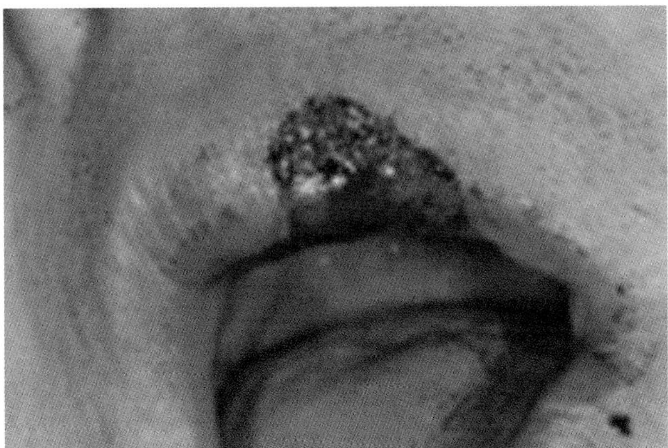

Figure 1.6a

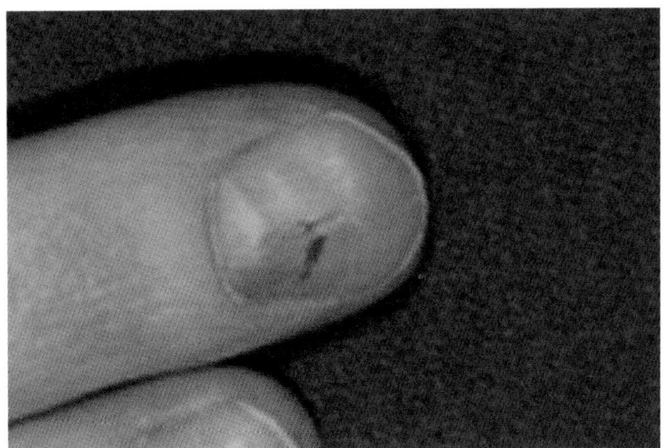

Figure 1.6b

CO: A 24-year-old male was referred for an evaluation of bleeding from his upper lip.

HPC: The hemorrhage appeared on his upper lip during eating from a broken bulla three hours ago.

PMH: This young man suffers from Down syndrome and over the last two years he has been complaining about multiple bullae on the skin of his legs, mouth, and genitals. He had a short course of steroid cream for skin bullae which was not effective, causing him to refuse any other medications since then.

OE: An anxious young man, showing numerous ulcerations inside his mouth, lips, and legs as a result of ruptured bullae due to friction. A hemorrhagic ulceration on his upper lip (Figure 1.6a) together with a tiny hemorrhage of the nail bed of his middle finger was found (Figure 1.6b). No other hemorrhagic lesions (petechiae or ecchymoses) were seen inside his mouth, skin or other mucosae. On the other hand, epistaxis was not referred and general symptomatology was absent. The patient was admitted to an examination, and blood results revealed no clotting disorders while biopsy of the skin revealed a subepithelial bulla with positive immunofluorescence of IgG and C3 along the basement membrane zone (BMZ).

Q1 What is the cause of his lip bleeding?
- **A** Self-induced lip trauma
- **B** Pemphigoid disorders
- **C** Clotting disorder
- **D** Erythema multiforme
- **E** Herpetic stomatitis

Answers:
- **A** No
- **B** Pemphigoid bullous diseases (mucous and bullous) are a group of subepithelial bullous disorders which affect mainly the mouth (mucous type; or less frequently bullous type) or the skin. They have a characteristic immunofluorescence profile. Their bullae break easily and leave painful hemorrhagic ulcerations covered with hemorrhagic crusts as seen in this patient.
- **C** No
- **D** No
- **E** No

Comments: Clotting disorders are easily excluded from the diagnosis as the blood tests were negative. Herpetic stomatitis causes similar hemorrhagic oral lesions but is ruled out as this condition lacks chronic skin lesions and its severe mouth lesions occur only once and not constantly, as seen in this patient. Erythema multiforme shows similar findings with the patient's lesions, but is also excluded due to the short duration of its lesions and presence of fibrin instead of IgG and C_3 with BMZ. Factitious illness is a problem in the disabled but not in Down syndrome patients, as these are less likely to develop maladaptive behavior and the patient did not show any aggressive behavior capable of causing self-induced lesions in his body.

Q2 Which of the bullous disorders is/or are initiated with urticarial skin lesions?
- **A** Pemphigus vulgaris
- **B** Bullous pemphigoid
- **C** Cicatricial pemphigoid
- **D** Paraneoplastic pemphigus
- **E** Dermatitis herpetiformis

Answers:
- **A** No
- **B** Bullous pemphigoid is a chronic subepithelial blistering disease that starts as an urticarial eruption which develops large firm bullae, especially in flexor skin areas over a course of weeks to months.
- **C** No
- **D** No
- **E** Dermatitis herpetiformis is a chronic pruritic papulovesicular eruption which is associated with urticarial wheals and located symmetrically on the extensor surfaces of skin.

Comments: Although paraneoplastic pemphigus and cicatricial pemphigoid are chronic bullous disorders affecting oral and other mucosae and appear either as fragile intra-epithelial bullae associated with a neoplasm (leukemia or lymphoma) or subepithelial bullae, they are never associated with pruritic rash and scarring.

Q3 Which lip conditions are presented with lip bleeding?
- **A** Exfoliate cheilitis
- **B** Erythema multiforme
- **C** Actinic prurigo
- **D** Granulomatous cheilitis
- **E** Perioral dermatitis

Answers:
- **A** Exfoliate cheilitis is a common cheilitis characterized by the production of keratin scales in the vermilion border of lips in young women with anxiety, who have the habit of removing the scales by rubbing them against their teeth thus leaving ulcerated hemorrhagic lesions.
- **B** Erythema multiforme is an acute mucocutaneous reaction characterized by erythematous plaques, painful hemorrhagic bullae and erosions in the skin (target like lesions), in the mouth and other mucosae. The presence of hemorrhagic crusts on the lips is pathognomonic for this condition.
- **C** Chronic exposure to solar radiation causes actinic prurigo, a photodermatosis affecting the skin, lips and conjunctiva. Lips are usually erythematous, scaly and in places bleed while the skin lesions appear as itchy, red papillae or nodules on cheeks, nose, forehead or arms, and eyes showing hyperemia, photophobia and pseudopterygium.
- **D** No
- **E** No

Comments: Perioral dermatitis is a chronic itchy papulopustular rash affecting the skin around the mouth while granulomatous cheilitis is a chronic, persistent swelling of lips due to granulomatous inflammations. Neither of them have a bleeding tendency.

Case 1.7

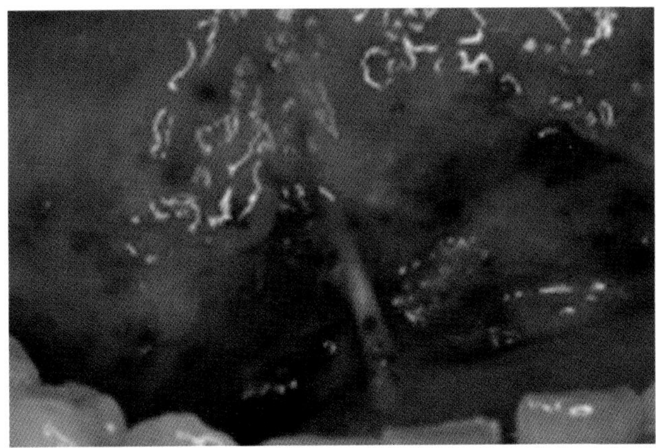

Figure 1.7

CO: A 36-year-old woman was presented with hemorrhage from her tongue.

HPC: Her tongue bleeding appeared one month ago when she gave birth to a baby girl. The bleeding had arisen from a superficial strawberry-like soft mass on the dorsum and inferior part of her tongue while it deteriorated with mastication movements.

PMH: Her medical history revealed no serious diseases such as bleeding disorders. A case of iron deficiency anemia was only recorded since puberty which was treated with iron supplements as well as a few tongue surgeries for the elimination of a vascular lesion of her tongue in the past. The patient was not a supporter of smoking or drinking habits, while she used to spend her free time painting.

OE. The oral examination revealed multiple small hemorrhagic dots on the dorsum and inferior part of tongue (Figure 1.7) which were similar to a mature strawberry. These dots are superficial and could easily bleed with touching, and were overlying a soft vascular mass. This mass was detected when she was one year old, and became larger during puberty, requiring surgery. It remained stable until her pregnancy when it became bigger and was occasionally bleeding. No other similar lesions, petechiae, or ecchymoses were found on her body.

Q1 What is the cause of bleeding?

- **A** Hemangioma
- **B** Vascular malformation
- **C** Kaposi sarcoma
- **D** Pregnancy pyogenic granuloma
- **E** Wegener granulomatosis

Answers:

- **A** No
- **B** Vascular malformations are characterized by abnormalities of the capillary, venous or arteriovenous vascular bed which appear at birth or a few months later, and grow gradually. Contrary to other vascular lesions though, they do not resolve; instead they can be exacerbated with various conditions such as pregnancy.
- **C** No
- **D** No
- **E** No

Comments: Based on the early onset and long duration of this single lesion,without resolution throughout the coming years hemangiomas are easily excluded while the long duration and slow progress without other similar lesions in patient's body or general symptomatolog rules out extensive pyogenic grannulomas or Wegener granulomatatosis from the diagnosis.

Q2 What are the differences between hemangiomas and vascular malformations?

- **A** Location
- **B** Course
- **C** Symptomatology
- **D** Pathogenesis
- **E** Complications

Answers:

- **A** No
- **B** Hemangiomas appear mostly at birth, grow rapidly and resolve during puberty while vascular malformation remain or even worsen.
- **C** No
- **D** Hemangiomas are characterized by endothelial hyperplasia while in vascular malformations the endothelial cell turnover is normal.
- **E** Both hemangiomas and vascular malformations cause a variety of complications from mild esthetic disfiguration to severe possibility of jeopardizing the patient's life dependent on the size and location of the lesion closely to vital organs.

Q3 Which of the syndromes below is/or are not associated with this condition?

- **A** Sturge-Weber syndrome
- **B** PHACE syndrome
- **C** Proteus syndrome
- **D** Maffucci syndrome
- **E** Blue rubber bleb nevus syndrome (BRBNS)

Answers:

A No

B PHACE syndrome is characterized by multi-organ lesions such as posterior fossa anomalies; facial hemangiomas, arterial and cardiac anomalies as well as eye problems

C No

D No

E No

Comments: Abnormal vascular malformations are often seen in a number of syndromes like Sturge-Weber; Maffucci, Proteus and blue rubber belb but all of them have different clinical presentation. Sturge-Weber syndrome is characterized by numerous facial (port-wine stain) and cerebral angiomas, glaucoma, seizures and mental retardation while in Maffucci syndrome, angioma is associated with numerous endochondromas. Proteus syndrome has characteristic skin, bone, muscle and vascular abnormal growths, while venous malformations of the gastrointestinal tract and skin are seen in blue rubber bleb nevus syndrome.

Case 1.8

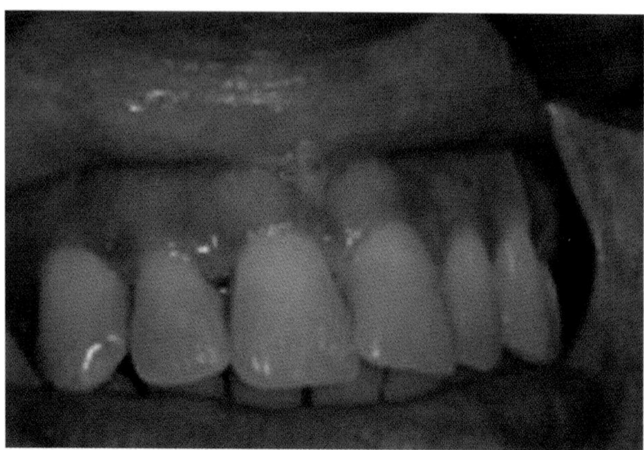

Figure 1.8

CO: A 68-year-old woman was presented with hemorrhagic gingivae over the last three months.

HPC: Her gingivae showed areas of hemorrhage over the last three months and was associated with generalized lymphadenopathy, fever, weight loss and sweating at night.

PMH: Hyperlipidemia and diabetes mellitus were the only serious diseases reported. A recent blood check-up revealed an increased number of eosinophils and lymphocytes as well as chronic sideropenic anemia, despite her proper diet. No smoking or drinking habits, but a chronic exposure to chemicals because of her job at a painting industry was reported.

OE: The examination revealed swollen, soft, edematous and hemorrhagic gingivae that were associated with a few scattered petechiae on buccal mucosae. The gingivae were pale and easily bled from the interdental papillae (Figure 1.8). A few ecchymoses were also found on her legs and associated with a generalized lymph node enlargement.

Q1 What is the cause of her gingival bleeding?

A Acute ulcerative gingivitis

B Scurvy

C Leukemia

D Plasma cell gingivitis

E Wegener disease

Answers:

A No

B No

C Leukemia is the cause. Leukemia is a malignant neoplasm of white blood cells characterized by an abnormal growth of a certain type of white cells, anemia, easy bruising or bleeding, susceptibility to infections, swollen lymph nodes, together with weight loss and night sweating, as was also observed in this patient who was finally diagnosed of having chronic lymphocytic leukemia

D No

E No

Comments: Gingival bleeding is a common finding in other local conditions such as in acute ulcerative and plasma cell gingivitis, or systemic diseases such as Wegener disease and scurvy. The lack of necrosis of interdental papillae (seen in acute ulcerative gingivitis) and the erythematous and edematous red attached gingivae (in plasma cell gingivitis) or the erythematous swollen-like-strawberries gingivae (in Wegener disease) and the ulcerated, swollen gingivae with deep pocketing (in scurvy) exclude the above diseases from the diagnosis.

Q2 Which laboratory tests are routinely used for the diagnosis of this condition?

A White blood count

B Immunophenotypic analysis with flow cytometry

C Bone marrow biopsy

D Urine analysis

E Cerebral fluid biochemical analysis

Answers:

A White blood count shows an increased number of lymphocytes (>10,000 cells/mm^3).

B The flow cytometric analysis of the bone marrow aspiration cells and peripheral blood cells with the use of a series of monoclonal antibodies allow the identification of hematologic malignancies including chronic lymphocytic leukemia (CLL).

C Bone marrow biopsy is used in undiagnosed cases of blood dyscrasias showing the replacement of bone marrow cells with pathologic lymphocytes.

D No

E No

Comments: Urinalysis and cerebrospinal fluid (CSF) analysis are useful only in a diagnosis of aggressive leukemias like CLL, involving bladder and brain respectively.

Q3 Which other conditions are associated with this disease?

A Anemia

B Thrombocytopenia

C Eosinophilia

D Complement deficiency

E Paraproteinemia

Answers:

A Anemia is a very common complication of CLL due to: (i) bone marrow accumulation of abnormal lymphocytes inducing the replacement of stem cells producing red cells; (ii) increased production of tumor necrosis factor (TNF) that suppresses red blood cell production; (iii) increased red cell destruction by circulated auto-antibodies; and (iv) medications used for treatment of CLL that suppress red cell production.

B Thrombocytopenia is responsible for the increased bleeding tendency among patients with CLL.

C Eosinophilia is sometimes a preclinical sign of various hematological malignancies including lymphomas and CLL.

D Complement deficiency is a common finding and seems to limit CD20 monoclonal cytotoxicity in treatment's efficacy for these patients.

E Monoclonal proteins are present in significant number of patients with CLL.

Case 1.9

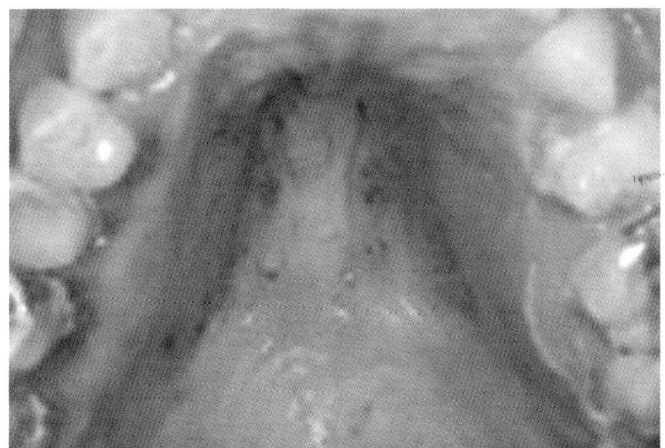

Figure 1.9

CO: A 32-year-old woman was presented with red spots on her palate.

HPC: The red palatal lesions were asymptomatic and discovered by her GDP during her regular dental check-up last week.

PMH: Her medical history revealed an asymptomatic HIV infection over the last 14 months and a few opportunist lung infections this winter. She was on no medication at the moment apart from a few broad antibiotics taken for her respiratory infections. Her HIV infection was probably caught after a blood transfusion given 10 years ago to recover after a car accident. She was non-smoker or drinker.

OE: A few scattered red spots on both parts of hard and occasionally soft palate and buccal mucosae. These lesions did not bleach with pressure, but were associated with severe periodontal disease regardless of her young age (Figure 1.9) and cervical lymphadenitis.

Q1 What is the cause of palatal petechiae?

A Fellatio

B Infectious mononucleosis

C Nicotinic stomatitis

D HIV-induced thrombocytopenia

E Rendu-Osler-Weber syndrome

Answers:

A No

B No

C No

D Palatal petechiae on this lady appear due to thrombocytopenia induced by HIV infection. This

is one of the early manifestations of the disease such as atypical oral ulcerations, infections like pseudo-membranous or erythematous candidiasis, reactivation of herpes zoster infection and acute ulcerative gingivitis/periodontitis.
E No

Comments: Rendu-Osler-Weber syndrome can be easily excluded, as this is about having scattered telangiectasia since childhood, in contrast with the hemorrhagic spots (petechiae) that were found in this young lady. Asymptomatic petechiae are also seen on the soft palate and on margins of the hard with the soft palate after orogenital sex, which this lady had not reported. Asymptomatic palatal red spots are characteristics in nicotinic stomatitis, but the red spots there represent the inflamed duct openings of minor salivary glands and not petechiae. Palatal petechiae associated with general lymphadenopathy are also seen in patients with infectious mononucleosis, but the typically increased number of monocytes in the blood test and positive mononucleosis (mono) test, excludes this condition from diagnosis.

Q2 Which is/are the difference/s between petechiae and purpura?
A Size
B Location
C Reaction to pressure
D Symptomatology
E Shape

Answers:
A Petechiae are hemorrhagic spots with a diameter of <5 mm while purpura have a 5–9 mm diameter.
B No
C No
D No
E Petechiae have round, regular lesions while the shape of purpura and ecchymoses may be irregular.

Comments: Both hemorrhagic lesions do not blanch with pressure, are usually asymptomatic and can be found anywhere in the body.

Q3 What are the causes of thrombocytopenia apart from an HIV infection?
A Leukemia
B Epilepsy
C Hepatitis C infection
D Heavy alcohol consumption
E Anorexia nervosa

Answers:
A Thrombocytopenia is very common sign of an acute myelogenous and lymphocytic leukemia, as well as in advanced chronic lymphocytic and in progressive myelogenous leukemia. The reduced number of platelets has been attributed to: (i) bone marrow replacement by leukemic cells; (ii) increased destruction of platelets by swollen spleen or cytotoxic drugs for leukemia treatment; and (iii) immune destruction of platelets in some CLL cases.
B No
C Thrombocytopenia is a major problem in HCV+ patients as it interferes with various measurements for its diagnosis and follow-up. The cause of thrombocytopenia is multifarious and is due to: (i) immunogenicity; (ii) direct bone marrow suppression; (iii) hypersplenism; (iv) decreased production of thrombopoeitin; and (v) drug reactions.
D The chronic use of alcohol affects the production, survival time and functions of platelets while it also increases their destruction rate by an enlarged spleen leading to thrombocytopenia. The cessation of drinking within the second week raises the number of platelets again.
E Anorexia nervosa causes thrombocytopenia. The reduced production of platelets is attributed mainly to low thrombopoietin rather than folic acid levels due to malnutrition.

Comments: Anti-epileptic drugs such as valproate and levetiracetam but not the disease per se cause thrombocytopenia.

Case 1.10

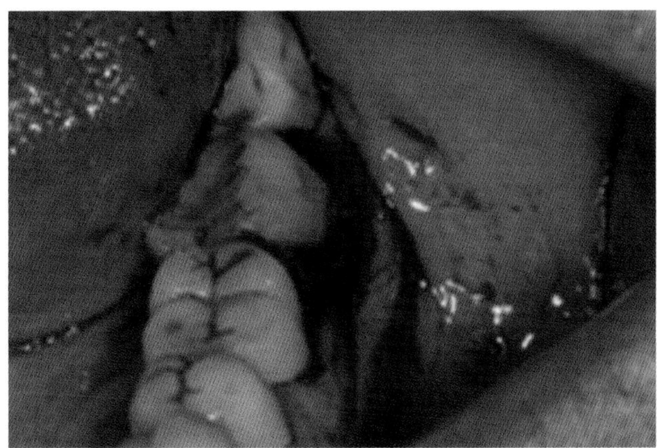

Figure 1.10

CO: A 42-year-old man was admitted with gingival bleeding since the previous night.

HPC: The bleeding started suddenly after eating a snack with potato chips and became more intense and constant on the lower molar gingivae. No similar bleeding episodes had been reported previously by him or his close relatives.

PMH: Mild hypertension and cardiological problems were reported and controlled with diet and a heart mitral valve replacement five years ago, which was followed by daily use of the drug warfarin since then. Allergies or other systemic diseases and smoking or drinking habits were not recorded, while his diet was poor in green vegetables only.

OE: Spontaneous bleeding from all his gingivae but mainly from his lower left molars with incomplete clot formation was noticed. The clot was very soft and there was constant bleeding arising from the interdental papillae (Figure 1.10). This did not end with pressure, rinses with cold saline mouthwashes or antiseptics. A few petechiae were also seen near the occlusal lines of the buccal mucosae, but also in other mucosae or the skin. Cervical or systemic lymphadenopathy was also missing.

Q1 What is the main cause of gingival bleeding?

- **A** Local trauma
- **B** Dental plaque
- **C** Warfarin-induced
- **D** Vitamin C deficiency
- **E** Liver cirrhosis

Answers:

- **A** Local trauma induced from hard foods such as potato chips could be a predisposing factor for gingival bleeding in patients regardless their oral hygiene status.
- **B** No
- **C** Warfarin is the main cause, as it blocks one of the enzymes that use vitamin K to produce clotting factors, thus causing incomplete clot formation similar to that was seen in this patient.
- **D** No
- **E** No

Comments: Dental plaque is responsible for gingival infection and bleeding in healthy and diseased patients, but it does not affect the clotting cascade. A vitamin C deficiency can cause alterations in collagen synthesis, making the small vessels of the gingivae weak and vulnerable to easy bleeding, either with a minor trauma or automatically. However, the patient's diet is correct, without any alcohol use and includes a great a number of foods that are rich in Vitamin C, apart from green fruits and vegetables which were excluded due to his warfarin uptake.

Q2 Which is/are the blood test/s used for checking a bleeding disorder?

- **A** WBC
- **B** D-dimers
- **C** PT
- **D** A PTT
- **E** Vitamin D levels

Answers:

- **A** White blood count (WBC) is required to check the number of platelets (thrombocytopenia) as well as the presence of anemia.
- **B** D-dimers measure a specific type of cross-linked fibrin degradation, while the elevated levels are indicators of recent clotting activity such as clotting dissemination or intravascular coagulation.
- **C** Prothrombin time (PT) is the time for blood to clot in a general screen that evaluates factors VII, X, II and II.
- **D** Activated partial thromboplastin time, also known as A PTT, is a sensitive indicator of coagulation and evaluates additionally to PT factors such as

prekallikrein, factors VII, IX and high molecular weight kininogen, and examines how both the intrinsic clotting pathway and the common final pathway are working.

E No

Comments: Vitamin D is required for regulation of calcium and phosphorus in the body. Its deficiency is common and related to osteoporosis in older patients and rickets in children but not with clotting diseases.

Q3 Which of the drugs below enhance the bleeding?

A Aspirin
B Fluconazole
C Metronidazole
D Phenytoin
E Omeprazole

Answers:

A Aspirin is often used together with warfarin in patients with valve replacement and increases the bleeding tendency, but it is always dependent on the intensity of the treatment.

B Fluconazole is the drug of choice for various fungal infections. In combination with warfarin, it can increase the hypoprothrombinemic effect of the second drug by interfering with its metabolism and inhibiting the liver enzymes CYP450 2C19 and 3A4.

C Metronidazole increases the plasma concentration of warfarin by inhibiting the action of CYP450 2CR enzyme that is responsible for the metabolic clearance of the active enantiomers of warfarin.

D No

E Omeprazole is sometimes related to an increased action of warfarin, but their interaction seems to have a minor, doubtful or limited clinical significance.

Comments: Phenytoin, a well-known antiepileptic drug, has a complex interaction with warfarin. It initially increases but later reduces INR after a prolonged application.

2

Blue and/or Black Lesions

Blue and black oral lesions have been characterized by increased pigmentation due to accumulation either of melanin (true) or hemosiderin, metals, chemical coloring agents and drug metabolites (non-true discoloration) within the oral mucosa and teeth. These lesions may be manifestations of a group of congenital or acquired diseases with traumatic, reactive, neoplasmatic, and infective origin (Figure 2.0a and b).

The most common causes of black or blue pigmentation are listed in Table 2.

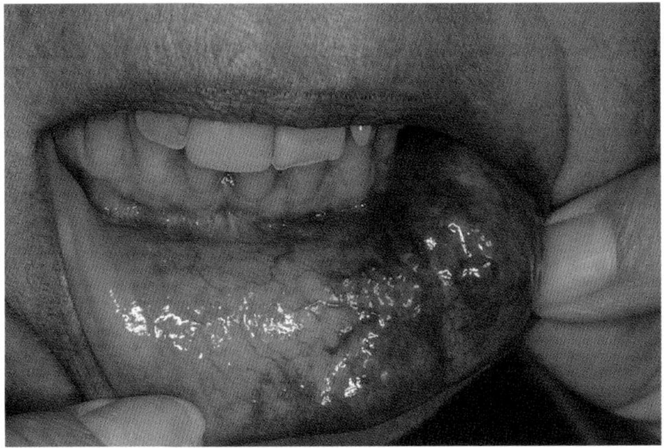

Figure 2.0a Blue lesion.

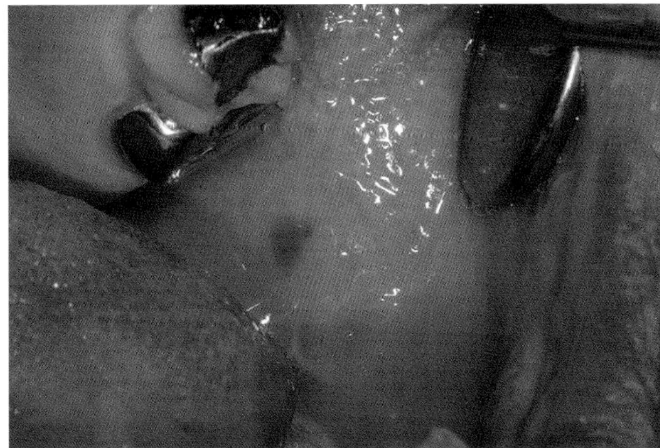

Figure 2.0b Black lesion.

Clinical Guide to Oral Diseases, First Edition. Dimitris Malamos and Crispian Scully.

Companion website: www.wiley.com/go/malamos/clinical_guide

Table 2 The most common causes of blue and black lesions.

Pigmentation

- **Related to melanin** (brown, black lesions)
  - *Increased melanin production only*
    - Related to race
      - Racial pigmentosaw
    - Related to hormone alterations
      - Chloasma
      - Addison disease
      - Ectopic ACTH production
      - Nelson syndrome
      - Acanthosis nigricans
      - Laugier-Hunziker syndrome
      - Leopard syndrome
      - Spotty pigmentation, myxoma, endocrine overactivity syndrome
      - Von Recklinghausen's disease
      - Albright syndrome
    - Related to consumption of
      - Drugs
      - Foods
    - Related to exposure in sun
      - Freckles
      - Solar lentigines
    - Related to smoking habits
      - Betel nut chewing
      - Smoker's melanosis
    - Related to inflammation
      - LP metachrosis
      - BMMP metachrosis
      - EM metachrosis
    - Related to various factors
      - Ephelides (simple)
      - Ephelides in Peutz-Jegher syndrome
  - Increased number of melanocytes
      - Lentigines simplex
      - Nevi
      - Melanoma
- **Related to hemosiderin** (blue, red lesions)
      - Angiomas
      - Kaposi's sarcoma
      - Epithelioid angiomatosis
      - Ecchymosis
      - Hemochromatosis/hemosiderosis
      - Beta thalassemia
- **Related to foreign material** (gray, black lesions)
      - Argyria
      - Heavy metal poisoning (lead, bismuth, arsenic)
      - Permanganate or silver poisoning
      - Tattoos (amalgam, lead pencils, ink, dyes, carbon)

Case 2.1

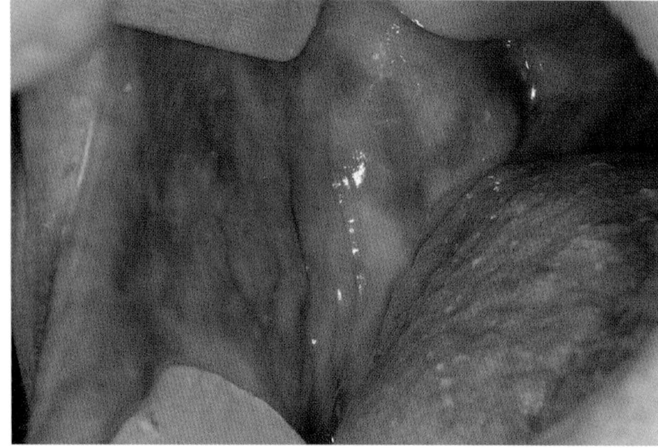

Figure 2.1

CO: A 65-year-old woman was referred by her dentist for evaluation of a black discoloration of her buccal mucosae and palate.

HPC: The discoloration was firstly noticed by her dentist during a routine examination for denture replacement one week ago.

PMH: She was a slim woman with dark skin and with no serious medical problems apart from low blood pressure and chronic allergic asthma which were controlled with a special salty diet and systematic steroids respectively. She also suffered from iron deficiency anemia at child bearing age, and had been on iron tablets only on the days of menstruation. Smoking had been stopped from the age of forty.

OE: The intra-oral examination revealed dark black–bluish discolorations on her buccal mucosae, soft palate and lips (Figure 2.1). This discoloration was diffuse, superficial, and prominent at areas of chronic friction such as at the occlusal line. Similar discolorations were seen on the skin of hands and feet. Fatigue, nausea, or even episodes of fainting during very tiring activities were occasionally reported.

Q1 Which is the possible diagnosis?

A Racial pigmentation
B Hemosiderosis
C Addison's disease
D Melasma
E Melanoma

Answers:

A No

B No

C Addison's disease is the cause of the dark pigmentation of her skin and oral mucosa (especially on buccal mucosae) which was attributed to the increased stimulatory action of adrenocorticotropic hormone (ACTH) in the melanocytes, changing the color of melanin pigment to black or dark. This disease is characterized with adrenal insufficiency (secondary) due to the chronic use of steroids for the patient's asthma, and with stimulation and overproduction of pituitary hormones like ACTH. Low blood pressure, weight loss, muscle and joint pain, nausea, diarrhea and fainting during exercise and increased pigmentation are among the commonest manifestations of this disease.

Comments: Dark pigmented lesions are common and distinguished in diffuse and discrete -localized lesions. Diffuse pigmentation is common in dark skin patients (see racial pigmentation).in pregnancy (melasma) or in diseases per ce (Addison) or induced by drugs (hemosiderosis) Localized lesions are common and some of them like melanoma jeopardize patient's life Their diagnosis is based on clinical characteristics like onset, location, type of discoloration location and progress. Racial pigmentation is usually noticed at an earlier age and not associated with general symptomatology. Hemosiderosis causes a similar discoloration but is not the cause as the patient did not have a history of blood dyscracias or overtaking of iron tablets, and her pigmentation remained unchanged. Melasma is also found in pregnant women, but restricted mainly on facial skin while melanoma is associated with satellite pigmented lesions and has a more aggressive clinical course.

Q2 Addison's disease is characterized by:

A Excess secretion of cortisol

B Increased secretion of ACTH

C Reduced secretion of aldosterone and cortisol

D Reduced production of thyroid-stimulating hormone (TSH)

E Increased secretion of prolactin

Answers:

A No

B No

C Reduced secretions of aldosterone and cortisol hormones are characteristic findings in Addison's disease, and caused either by disorders of the adrenal glands (primary) or inadequate secretion of ACTH from the pituitary gland (secondary).

D No

E Hyperprolactinemia is found in active phases of various autoimmune diseases such as systemic lupus erythematosus (SLE), rheumatoid arthritis, celiac disease, diabetes type 1 as well as Addison's disease.

Comments: An increased TSH, with or without low levels of thyroxine, occurs in patients with primary or secondary Addison's disease while increased cortisol and reduced ACTH levels are found in Cushing syndrome.

Q3 Addison's disease is commonly part of syndromes such as:

A Crouzon syndrome

B McCune-Albright syndrome

C Griscelli syndrome

D Peutz-Jeghers syndrome

E Autoimmune polyendocrine syndrome

Answers:

A No

B No

C No

D No

E Autoimmune polyendocrine syndrome (PAS II) is characterized by a drop in production of several essential hormones, commonly found in patients with Addison's disease; hypo or hyperthyroidism, hypogonadism, and diabetes mellitus type I.

Comments: Skin or oral mucosa discolorations are characteristically seen in various syndromes apart from Addison's disease. Skin hyperpigmentation is also seen in Cushing syndrome and in other syndromes combined with acanthosis nigricans and early craniosynostosis (Crouzon syndrome) and with polyostotic fibrous dysplasia, café au lait skin pigmentations (McCune Albright syndrome). Skin hypopigmentation together with silver gray hair discoloration alone, or combined with brain or autoimmune dysfunctions are characteristics of Griscelli syndrome.

Case 2.2

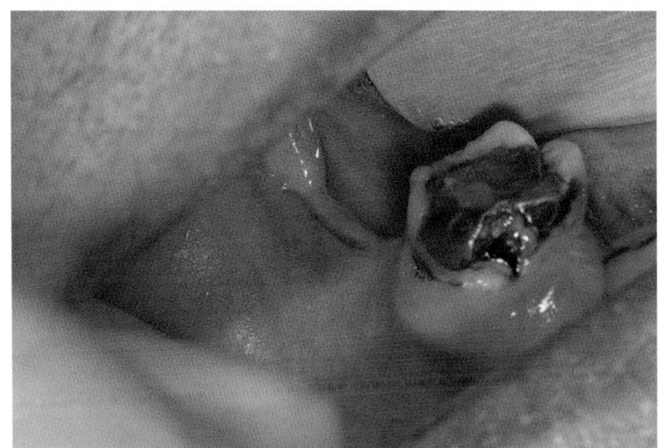

Figure 2.2a

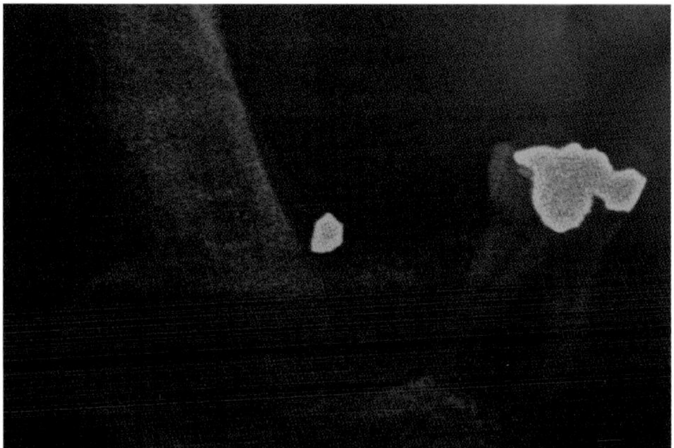

Figure 2.2b

CO: A 58-year-old woman was referred for evaluation of an asymptomatic black spot on the lower alveolar mucosa opposite the right second molar.

HPC: This black lesion was first noticed by her dentist two days ago when the woman visited him to relieve her severe throbbing pain which had arisen from her broken second molar.

HPC: Her medical history was clear from any serious diseases apart from allergic rhinitis which was treated with anti-histamine tablets. Her recent dental history revealed an extraction of her lower right third molar that had been heavily restored with amalgam.

OE: An isolated, flat black-gray lesion was seen on the alveolar mucosa covering her previously extracted lower right wisdom tooth. The lesion was asymptomatic, soft in palpation with irregular margins (max dimension of 1.6 cm) and not associated with similar skin and other mucosae lesions or general symptomatology and lymphadenopathy (local or systemic) (Figure 2.2a).The tooth next to the lesion also had an old broken filling with caries underneath causing severe pain. An intra-oral radiograph revealed a radiopaque material with the healing socket of the extracted molar (Figure 2.2b).

Q1 What is the possible diagnosis?

- **A** Amalgam tattoo
- **B** Melanoma
- **C** Cosmetic tattoo
- **D** Metal poisoning
- **E** Pigmented nevus

Answers:

- **A** Amalgam tattoo is the answer. Amalgam tattoo is the most common exogenous material implanted in the soft tissues of alveolar mucosae, buccal mucosae, gingivae, floor of the mouth, palate, or tongue. It appears as a solitary or multiple, flat black to gray or even blue discrete asymptomatic discoloration, thus causing the patient concern and often being misdiagnosed as melanoma.
- **B** No
- **C** No
- **D** No
- **E** No

Comments: Localized pigment lesions are common and induced by accumulations of melanine producing cells (macules) benign neoplasmatic cells (nevi) or malignant cell s(melanoma) or even external dyes used for cosmetic tatoos Pigmented nevus has a similar appearance as amalgam tattoo, but has a longer duration with no history of trauma or teeth with heavy amalgam restorations, or even having undergone surgery (apicectomy/extractions). Melanomas have more aggressive clinical appearance, satellite lesions in the skin or oral mucosa, and lymphadenopathy and early distant metastases. Cosmetic tattoos are usually done in visible parts of mouth and skin while poisoning with metals appears as an extensive discoloration of the gingivae and other parts of the human body associated with various toxicity symptoms.

Q2 The diagnosis of this lesion is based mainly on:

- **A** History
- **B** Clinical characteristics
- **C** Radiographic findings
- **D** Biopsy results
- **E** Oral photography

Answers:

- **A** History of previous extraction or renewing of old amalgam fillings by high speed drills or rotary instruments confirms the clinical suspicion of deposition of amalgam metallic particles into adjacent gingivae or other parts of the oral mucosa.

B The clinical examination together with the previous dental records of old amalgam fillings are useful in the diagnosis of the majority of amalgam tattoos.

C Intra-oral X-rays reveal radiopaque material only if it is adequate in size.

D Biopsy is the most accurate diagnostic test for amalgam tattoo, as it shows silver impregnation of the reticular fibers of small vessels and nerves that are usually surrounded by chronic inflammatory cells, forming reactive granulomas.

E No

Comments: A series of photos taken at intervals are very helpful to record changes of other pigmented lesions regarding their size, color, and morphology, while the amalgam photos are rather useless, as this stain does not show any alterations over time.

Q3 Which other oral conditions are related to amalgam fillings apart from amalgam tattoo?

A Aphthous stomatitis
B Lichenoid reactions
C Metallic taste
D Bullous disorders
E Teeth discoloration

Answers:

A No

B Lichenoid reactions are commonly seen in areas close to amalgam fillings at the result of an allergic reaction of the oral mucosato various metalic components of amalgam.

C Metallic taste is often reported among patients with very new amalgam fillings or with phobias.

D No

E Intrinsic teeth discoloration is common and formed from the deposition of zinc, silver, tin, copper granules and other metallic components within the dental tissues during an amalgam filling preparation (simple or reverse).

Comments: The roughness of an amalgam filling rather the filling per ce is implicated in the development of adjacent traumatic aphthous like ulcerations while bullous disorders are caused by a reaction of circulating auto-antibodies against various components of the oral mucosa and not against amalgam components.

Case 2.3

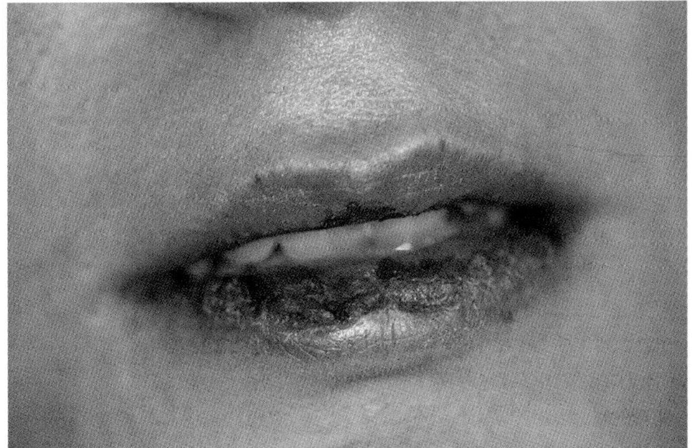

Figure 2.3

CO: A 24-year-old woman presented with painful black-dark brown scabs on both her lips.

HPC: The lip lesions were present for five days following an episode of painful ulcerations on her lips and mouth. The lesions were associated with sore throat, cervical lymphadenopathy, conjunctivitis, and areas of skin erythema. The ulcerations appeared one week after an upper respiratory infection, but similar episodes of skin and mouth lesions had been reported twice last year and resolved within three weeks without treatment.

PMH: Her medical history was unremarkable and no skin diseases, allergies, or drug use were recorded.

OE: The oral examination revealed black hemorrhagic scales covering the vermillion border of the upper, but mainly lower lip (Figure 2.3); these were easily removed leaving erythematous, bleeding areas underneath. Many superficial painful ulcers at the dorsum of the tongue, palate, and buccal mucosae were also seen and associated with bad breath and sialorrhea. The extra-oral examination revealed mild cervical lymphadenitis, conjunctivitis, and erythematous patches on both her hands and legs combined with myalgia, fatigue but no fever.

Q1 What is the possible cause of her lip scabs?

A Exfoliative cheilitis
B Allergic cheilitis
C Erythema multiforme
D Drug-induced cheilitis
E Primary herpetic stomatitis

Answers:

- **A** No
- **B** No
- **C** Erythema multiforme (EM) is an acute recurrent disease that affects the skin, mouth, and other mucosae of young patients and is triggered by certain infections or drugs. This disease may present with a variety and severity of lesions, and has a tendency to be resolved through the years. The oral lesions that involve the mouth appear with a variety of ulcerations and erythema, while the lips are covered with hemorrhagic exudates as seen in this patient "Target" lesions are characteristically seen on the skin.
- **D** No
- **E** No

Comments: The lesions on the vermillion border of lips differ among EM, cheilitis (exfoliative; allergic; drug-induced) or primary herpetic gingivostomatitis. Hemorrhagic, necrotic sloughs covering multiple painful ulcerations with minimal symptomatology were found in erythema multiforme, while small hyperkeratotic yellow scales which are easily removed by scrubbing the lips against the anterior teeth in young nervous women were seen in exfoliative cheilitis. In allergic cheilitis, the lips are swollen and erythematous with cracks, scales, and small ulcerations whenever they come in contact with allergens. Drug-induced cheilitis shares clinical characteristics with allergic cheilitis and appears one to two weeks after drug uptake, while it is resolved soon after its withdrawal. In primary herpetic stomatitis the lip lesions are always accompanied with fever and general symptomatology.

Q2 Which of the infections below mostly precedes the onset of erythema multiforme?

- **A** Staphylococcal infection
- **B** Herpetic infection
- **C** Hemolytic streptococcal infection
- **D** Toxoplasmosis
- **E** Coccidioidomycosis

Answers:

- **A** No
- **B** Erythema multiforme is precipitated mostly by a previous Herpes virus infection in the majority (>70%) of cases. Both HSV 1 and 2, Epstein-Barr, varicella zoster and cytomegalovirus DNA fragments trigger autoreactive T cells which via an inflammatory cascade release an interferon gamma that plays a crucial role in the development of EM lesions.
- **C** No
- **D** No
- **E** No

Comments: Bacterial, viral, fungal, or even parasitic infections have been involved in the pathogenesis of erythema multiforme. Bacterial infections such as diphtheria, streptococcal, legionellosis, leprosy, tuberculosis, or syphilis have been considered as triggering erythema multiforme. Infections from adenovirus, Coxsackie B5, enteroviruses, influenza, Herpes simplex virus (HSV), measles and mumps viruses or rare fungi such as *Histoplasma*, *Coccidioides immitis* and parasites such as *Toxoplasma gondii* and various species of *Trichomonas* often precede EM.

Q3 Which blood tests are abnormal in EM patients?

- **A** White blood account
- **B** Erythrocyte sedimentation rate (ESR)
- **C** Blood urea and creatinine
- **D** Electrolytes
- **E** Liver enzyme levels

Answers:

- **A** White blood count usually reveals moderate leukocytosis with atypical lymphocytes and lymphopenia but occasionally eosinophilia. Neutropenia is an indicator of bad prognosis.
- **B** ESR is an indicator of inflammation and can be elevated.
- **C** Blood urea and creatinine abnormalities are indicators of renal involvement and seen in severe cases with EM.
- **D** Electrolyte values are abnormal in severe cases of EM where fluid uptake could be extremely difficult, as it is hard for the patients to drink because of their mouth ulcerations.
- **E** No

Comments: None of these tests is pathognomonic for the disease and may be abnormal in severe cases. Specifically, the liver enzymes such as aspartate transaminase (AST), alanine transferase (ALT), alkaline phosphatase, and bilirubin are within the normal range in the majority but show an increased tendency in patients with EM due to acute hepatitis or due to antiviral treatment for HIV infection.

Case 2.4

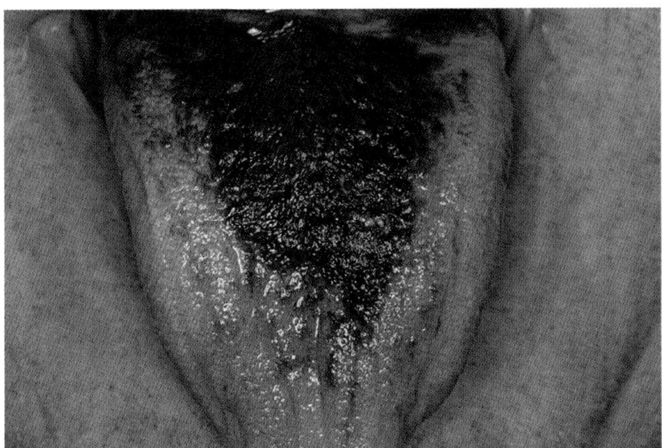

Figure 2.4

CO: A 72-year-old man presented complaining of a black coating on the dorsum of his tongue.

HPC: His black tongue appeared after one week of wide spectrum antibiotic uptake for an upper respiratory infection. This black discoloration appeared suddenly and became daily more dense during treatment. It was associated with mild xerostomia caused by his mouth breathing, and with metallic taste.

PMH: He was suffering from chronic sinusitis, mild hypertension and prostate hypertrophy that were controlled with antibiotics, irbesartan, and tamsulosin tablets respectively. He was an ex-smoker (stopped smoking eightyears ago) and non-drinker, but used strong mouthwashes on a daily basis.

OE: On examination, black hairy projections on the middle and posterior third of the dorsum of his tongue were seen, but the tip and lateral margins were clear (Figure 2.4). No other lesions were found within his mouth apart from cervical lymphadenopathy which was attributed to his previous upper respiratory infection. The black discoloration was not completely removed by scrubbing with a spatula.

Q1 Which is the possible diagnosis?

- **A** Hairy black tongue
- **B** Hairy oral leukoplakia
- **C** Tongue staining from colored foods
- **D** Racial pigmentation of tongue
- **E** Metal poisoning

Answers:

- **A** Black hairy tongue or lingua villosa nigra is a rare benign tongue condition characterized by elongation of filiform papillae where chromogenic bacteria grow. Poor oral hygiene, black stains from smoking, alcohol, or foods, hyposalivation and antibiotic intake capable to grow for anaerobic chromohenic bacteria or even excessive use of chlorhexidine mouth washes daily are among the possible causes for this condition.
- **B** No
- **C** No
- **D** No
- **E** No

Comments: Other conditions such as hairy leukoplakia, racial discoloration or that caused by colored foods or metal intake are easily excluded from the black hairy tongue case due to their differences in clinical characteristics such as the color and location, presence of similar or no lesions in the mouth, persistence with scrubbing as well as the patient's history of drug intake or habits. Therefore, in hairy leukoplakia, the lesions are white and usually located on the lateral margins of the tongue, while in racial pigmentation the lesions are located all over the mouth. The dark discoloration caused by colored foods is easily removed with scrubbing, while it remains fixed in metal poisoning and associated with general toxicity symptoms.

Q2 In which other tissues or organs, apart from the tongue, can chromogenic bacteria cause discoloration?

- **A** Bones
- **B** Teeth
- **C** Sclera
- **D** Skin
- **E** Heart

Answers:

- **A** No
- **B** Chromogenic bacteria in the mouth are responsible for the dark black linear stain that is seen on the cervical part of all teeth (deciduous and permanent) following the contour of gingivae. This stain comes from the deposition of insoluble ferric salts that are produced from the interaction of hydrogen sulfide released from chromogenic bacteria with iron, which is found in the saliva or gingival exudate.
- **C** No
- **D** No
- **E** No

Comments: Discoloration of bones and soft tissues of the skin, heart, and sclera of the eyes are caused by a number of local and systemic causes including trauma, metabolic diseases, tumors (de novo or metastatic) and metals or drugs such as minocycline deposition.

Q3 Which of the bacteria below is the most predominant in dark teeth stains?

- **A** *Porphyromonas gingivalis*
- **B** *Prevotella melaninogenica*
- **C** *Actinomyces*
- **D** *Fusobacterium nucleatum*
- **E** *Mycobacterium lepromatosis*

Answers:

- **A** No
- **B** No
- **C** *Actinomyces* species are predominant in saliva of patients with black stains on their teeth.
- **D** No
- **E** No

Comments: Other bacteria like *Porphyromonas gingivalis* and *Fusobacterium nucleatum* are implicated in various periodontal diseases while *Prevotella melaninogenica* and *Mycobacterium lepromatosis* cause anaerobic infections of the upper respiratory tract and leprosy respectively.

Case 2.5

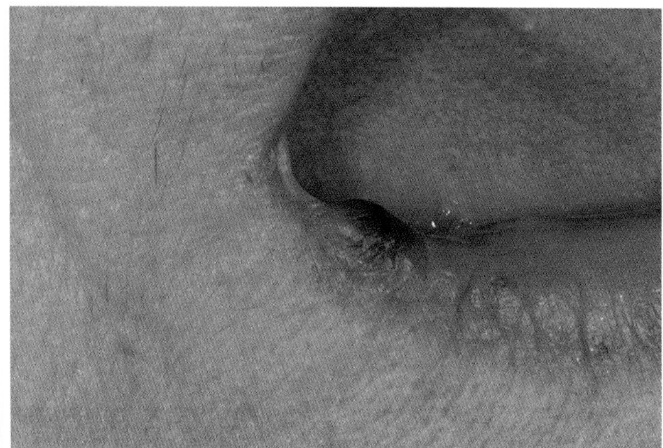

Figure 2.5

CO: A 58-year-old woman presented with a dark black to blue painless swelling in the vermillion border of her lower lip, close to the right commissure.

HPC: The lesion had been present for almost 25 years, and remained unchanged. A lip trauma caused a transient increase in the size of this swelling four years ago, but day by day it returned to its previous size.

PMH: Her medical history was free of any serious diseases, except for varicose veins on her legs which were dealt with by ligation and stripping surgery two years ago. She was a non-smoker or drinker and spent her free time gardening. She had no other similar lesions in her mouth or other parts of her body.

OE: The examination revealed a black swelling on the lower lip, approximately 5 mm in diameter, with a smooth surface but firm in palpation (Figure 2.5) which was not associated with other similar lesions within her mouth, skin, or other mucosae. Cervical lymphadenopathy was not detected. Biopsy confirmed that the lesion was vascular with amorphous calcifications at places.

Q1 What is the diagnosis?

- **A** Hemangioma
- **B** Melanoma
- **C** Phlebolith
- **D** Mucocele
- **E** Kaposi's sarcoma

Answers:

- **A** No
- **B** No
- **C** Phlebolith is the correct answer. This isolated lesion is relatively rare in the mouth of older people and is characterized by a relatively hard swelling, dark black or blue in color and associated with local vascular malformations and blood stasis causing dystrophic calcifications that are responsible for ts hard consistency.
- **D** No
- **E** No

Comments: The long but harmless course of this lesion easily allows the exclusion of aggressive neoplasms such as melanoma or Kaposi's sarcoma from the diagnosis. Hemangioma has also a similarly long course with the lesion, but appears in childhood with a tendency of being resolved over time. Mucocele sometimes has a similar color and location but is soft and fluctuant and is associated with previous trauma, but this was not reported from this lady.

Q2 Which is the most common dystrophic calcification, apart from phleboliths, in the head and neck region?

A Myositis ossificans
B Calcified epidermal cysts
C Calcified lymph nodes
D Calcified acne
E Osteitis deformans

Answers:

A No
B No
C Calcified lymph nodes are numerous small masses of calcification within the lymph nodes of the head and neck region due to chronic inflammation, infection, or neoplasia.
D No
E No

Comments:
The other diseases causes dystrophic calcifications in the head and neck region but their calcifications are rare and accompanied with lesions in jaws and other bones (osteitis deformans); the facial muscles (myositis ossificans), in the healing acne vulgaris lesions (calcinosis cutis) and within epidermal cysts.

Q3 Which is or/are the difference/s between a small phlebolith and salivary gland stone?

A Location
B Symptomatology
C Age of appearance
D Composition
E Radiological features

Answers:

A The calculus in the phlebolith is located within a vein while the sialolith is located within salivary gland or its duct respectively.
B Small phleboliths do not cause severe symptoms apart from esthetic problems, while sialoliths are associated with salivary gland enlargement, topical inflammation and pain.
C Phleboliths are "vein stones" and are presented in younger patients with vascular malformations, but sialoliths appear in older patients.
D Phleboliths are calcified thrombus of calcium carbonate and phosphorus within a dilated vessel, while sialoliths consist of a mixture of hydroxyapatite and carbonate-apatite, centrally, being surrounded by an organic component of glycoproteins, mucopolysaccharides, lipids and cell dendrites.
E Radiographically, phleboliths are presented as oval or round radiopacities with a radiolucent center while sialoliths are elongated following a ductal shape.

Case 2.6

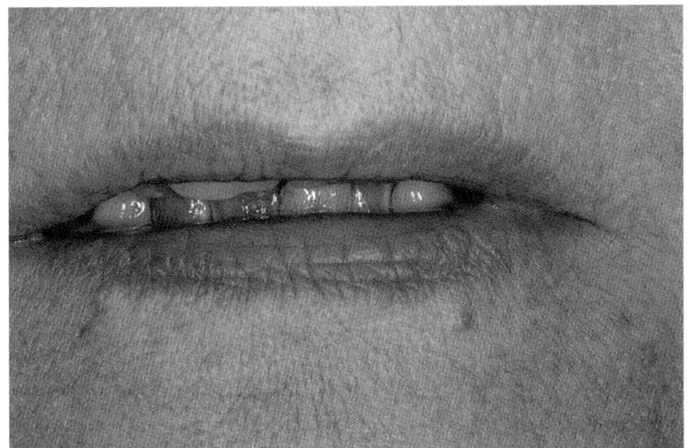

Figure 2.6

CO: A 67-year-old woman was referred for evaluation of a bluish discoloration of her lips.

HPC: Her lips had a blue hue which was first noticed by her dentist during her routine dental examination one week ago.

PMH: She suffered from mild diabetes, chronic asthma and congestive heart failure and was under a special diet and treated with systemic steroids and salbutamol inhaler (in crisis) and furosemide and metoprol tablets. She was an ex-smoker but never a drinker and had no history of facial trauma recently.

OE: The physical examination revealed an overweight lady with bluish discoloration of both her lips (Figure 2.6). Her lips were smooth, moist with no evidence of desquamation or atrophy but with a diffuse bluish discoloration that remained unchanged under pressure. No other similar lesions were found intra-orally. The patient also complained about shortness of breath and tiredness, while her face was pale and her legs were swollen.

Q1 What is the cause of her lip discoloration?

A Hemangioma
B Heart failure induced
C Blue nevus
D Hematoma
E Melanoma

Answers:

A No
B Congestive heart failure is the cause of the bluish color of her lips (cyanosis), skin and other mucosae and appears when the level of deoxygenated hemoglobin level is above of 5 g/dl. Cyanosis is more obvious in an acute crisis of asthma.
C No
D No
E No

Comments: In heart failure, the cyanosis is mixed (central and peripheral) and differs clinically from similar lesions such as hemangiomas, blue nevus, melanoma, or even hematomas. The stable blue color on the patient's lips regardless of its duration or absence of bleaching changes seen with local pressure exclude hematoma, hemangiomas, and blue nevus respectively. The fact, that her blue discoloration was diffuse, without overgrowths or satellite lesions or color variations equally found on both lips, rules out melanoma from diagnosis.

Q2 Cyanosis is more obvious in patients with:

A Dark complexion
B Vitamin C deficiencies
C Anemia
D Post-inflammatory pigmentation
E Bullous disorders

Answers:

A No
B Vitamin C deficiency causes scurvy, a condition that leads to abnormally pale skin and therefore the cyanosis is more obvious.
C Anemia is characterized by cyanosis when the oxygen saturation falls below hemoglobin levels. Cyanosis appears when the oxygen saturation in patients without anemia drops to <80–85 per cent and even lower than 60 per cent in patients with severe anemia (Hb < 6 g/dl).
D No
E No

Comments: The blue color is the result of deoxyhemoglobin's optical properties and especially its porphyrin rings; therefore it is more difficult to be seen in patients with dark skin due to racial or post-inflammatory pigmentation.

Q3 The differences between peripheral and central cyanosis are based on:

A Location of cyanosis
B Degree of cyanosis
C Temperature of affected parts
D Response to oxygen
E Duration of cyanosis

Answers:

A In central cyanosis the discoloration is generalized and affects the skin, oral and other mucosae while the peripheral cyanosis is localized only on the skin.
B No
C The limb temperature is unaffected in central, but is lower in peripheral cyanosis.
D The application of pure oxygen improves the central but not peripheral cyanosis.
E No

Comments: The duration of cyanosis reflects on the severity rather than the type of cyanosis. Cyanosis of a few seconds seems benign, while a prolonged or unresolved cyanosis may raise concerns of serious complications such as seen in heart, lungs, or brain.

Case 2.7

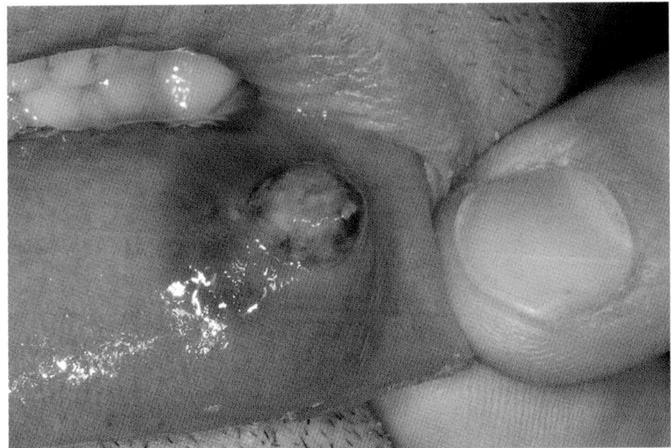

Figure 2.7

CO: A healthy young man of 18 years of age presented to the Emergency Dental Clinic for a bluish swelling on his lower lip.

HPC: The lesion appeared, one week ago, following a facial injury during a basketball game as a small, asymptomatic soft lump. The lesion has become bigger over the last three days when the patient bit accidentally his lip during eating again.

PMH: He has no serious medical problems apart from an atopic dermatitis, since the age of six, which was treated with topical glucocorticoid cream. Being a basketball player, his regular blood check-up did not reveal any bleeding conditions, while his habits do not include smoking or drinking.

OE: A large soft swelling of the inner surface of the lower lip. The swelling was painless and fluctuant with bluish color and with a size of 2 cm maximum in diameter and a superficial ulcer on top (Figure 2.7). It was associated with swollen minor salivary glands and topical ecchymosis due to previous trauma. No bruises or ecchymoses in other parts of his mouth and skin were found.

Q1 What is his most likely diagnosis?

- **A** Hemangioma
- **B** Mucocele
- **C** Hematoma
- **D** Fibroma (traumatic)
- **E** Lip abscess

Answers:

- **A** No
- **B** Mucocele is a common soft, cystic-like swelling seen on both lips but mainly in the lower caused by an extravagation of saliva into the submucosa due to the damage of minor salivary glands after a local injury. A repeated trauma increases mucocele size and changes its color from translucent to bluish, due to the accumulation of blood within the saliva and hematoma formation at the base of lesion as is exactly seen in this patient.
- **C** No
- **D** No
- **E** No

Comments: In contrast to the mucocele, hemangioma appears very early in the patient's lifewhile the hematoma is a blue discoloration which faints over the time; Fibroma is a soft but not fluctuated lesion; while abscess is a fluctuated, inflamed swelling containing pus and therefore its color ranges from red to yellow but rarely blue.

Q2 Which is/are the histological difference(s) between a mucous extravasation and retention mucocele?

- **A** Inflammation (type/density)
- **B** Epithelial lining
- **C** Associated closely with salivary acini
- **D** Location within submucosa
- **E** Presence of foam macrophages

Answers:

- **A** No
- **B** Epithelium lines the lumen of the mucous retention but not the extravasation cyst whose lining is from granulation tissue.
- **C** No
- **D** No
- **E** Macrophages with large foam or vacuolated cytoplasm are abundant within the mucous and the surrounded lumen of granulation tissue in mucous extravasation rather than retention cysts.

Comments: Both cysts are located superficially or deeply within the underlying connective tissue of the oral mucosa, where a mixed chronic inflammation and a few scattered ducts are seen.

Q3 Which of the cysts, found in the oral mucosa, do not have epithelial lining?
- **A** Ranula
- **B** Stafne cyst
- **C** Dermoid cyst
- **D** Aneurysmal cysts
- **E** Mucous extravasation cyst

Answers:
- **A** No
- **B** No
- **C** No
- **D** No
- **E** Mucous extravasation cyst is the answer.

Comments: Ranula and dermoid cysts, additionally to mucous extravasation cysts, are also found within the oral cavity but lined with stratified squamous epithelium. On the other hand, the Stafne cyst and aneurysmatic cyst are real pseudocysts that are not located within the oral mucosa but are found in the lower jaw, close to the apex of molars and at the angle of the mandible respectively.

Case 2.8

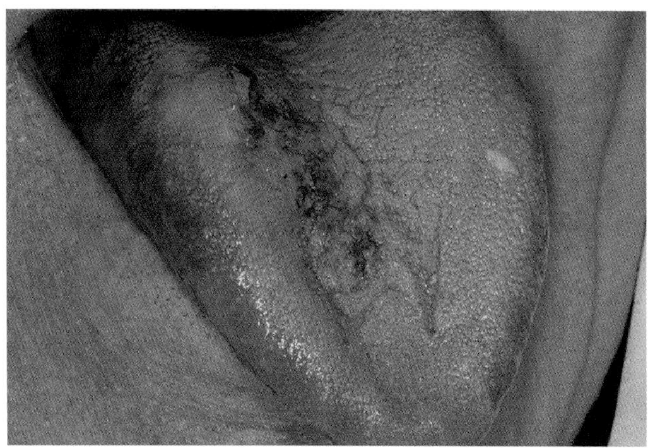

Figure 2.8

CO: A 52-year-old woman was admitted with one week history of bluish discoloration of her tongue.

HPC: Half of her tongue was swollen, sensitive on touching with a bluish discoloration which appeared after an episode of collapse one week ago.

PMC: She had no serious medical problems apart from low blood pressure which sometimes caused her dizziness and instability. She suffered from iron deficiency anemia, in the past, which was resolved as the patient entered the menopause. No other blood diseases or bleeding dyscrasias were reported. She is a non-smoker or drinker and has never chewed her lips or tongue.

OE: The oral examination revealed a diffuse swelling on the right part of her tongue that was associated with a small healing ulcer, yellow coat of debris and necrotic papillae. The swelling is painful on palpation and has a bluish discoloration extended to the lateral margin of her tongue (Figure 2.8). No other similar lesions, petechiae or ecchymoses were seen within the oral mucosa or other mucosae and skin nor evidence of bleeding in internal organs like liver, kidney or even brain .

Q1 What is the main cause of this blue discoloration?
- **A** Enlarged tongue vessels
- **B** Hemangioma
- **C** Hemosiderosis
- **D** Traumatic hematoma
- **E** Lymphangioma

Answers:
- **A** No
- **B** No
- **C** No
- **D** After a collapse, tongue biting commonly happens and can cause swelling and hematoma formation locally. The hematoma was formed by seeping and

accumulation of blood within the tongue submucosa from broken capillaries due to trauma causing a bluish discoloration of this area.

E No

Comments: Superficial vascular tongue lesions like hemangiomas and lymphangiomas or enlarged vessels cause often a bluish discoloration but are excluded as these malformations of the lymphatic system (lymphangiomas) or blood vessels (hemaniomas) are usually presented at a very early age (birth or infancy) and are unrelated to any local trauma. Hemosiderosis should also be ruled out from the diagnosis as the patient's medical history is negative for severe anemias or diseases requiring blood transfusion or drugs rich in iron, and this condition appears in many parts of the body apart from the mouth.

Q2 The necessity for urgent treatment of hematoma is mainly dependent on:

A Location
B Color
C Syptomatology
D Size
E Patient's age

Answers:

A Hematomas may occur anywhere in the body, but skull hematomas are the most dangerous and require immediate treatment, as they can increase intracranial pressure and seriously impair various brain functions.

B No

C Symptomatology of hematoma (swelling or pain) is sometimes very alarming and patients must seek immediate surgical (drainage) or clotting treatment (altering or stopping the responsible medicines).

D Large hematomas have a higher risk of altering basic functions of the tissues involved such as the brain and other vital organs, and require immediate treatment.

E No

Comments: Hematomas appear initially as dark blue or black lesions whose color is dependent on the amount of accumulated blood or its location's depth and duration, but is not associated with prognosis. Hematomas that are resolved within one to two weeks despite the patient's age, change their color from dark blue to yellow, and do not pose a risk to the patient's life.

Q3 Which investigations are required for the diagnosis of a traumatic-induced skull hematoma?

A Neurological tests
B Cerebrospinal fluid analysis
C Skull CT/MRI
D Clotting blood tests
E Respiratory tests

Answers:

A Neurological tests should be undertaken to examine the degree of consciousness, ataxia, or nystagmus as well as the sensory or motor deficits which might have been provoked by a subdural hematoma.

B Analysis of the cerebrospinal fluid in patients with traumatic intracranial hematoma reveals an increased level of glucose, lactate, and lactate dehydrogenase (LDH) as well as a predominance of monocytes or polymorphonuclear cells at the cellular level.

C CT or MRI of the skull shows the location and severity of skull hematoma and its response to treatment.

D No

E No

Comments: Clotting tests are useful for the detection of hemostasis dysfunctions rather than trauma-induced intracranial hemorrhage, while the respiratory tests are only required when the hematoma is severe and might affect the respiratory centers in the pons and medulla oblongata in the brainstem.

Case 2.9

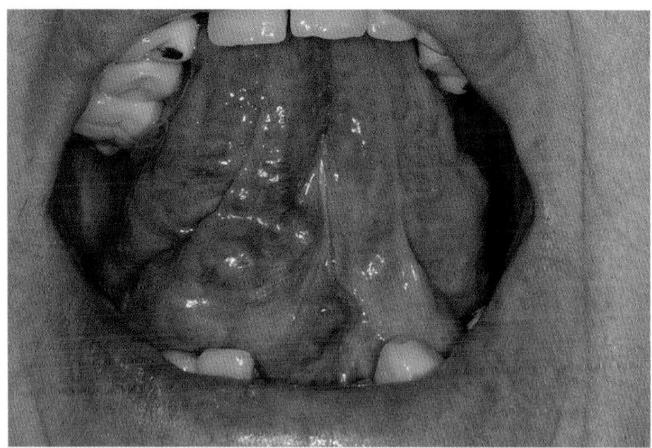

Figure 2.9

CO: A 67-year-old woman presented with bluish swellings on the ventral surface of her tongue.

HPC: The lesions were discovered accidentally by the patient a few years ago and have remained the same since then.

PMH: Hypertension was treated with captopril (angiotensin converting enzyme [ACE]-analog) drugs, hyperlipidemia (mild) controlled with atorvastatin and sleeping apnea which responded well to the use of a continuous positive pressure airway ventilator during sleeping. No local trauma was reported and only vascular surgery for enlarged veins of both her legs three years ago was reported.

OE: Two large corrugated blue lesions on the ventral surface of the tongue extending from the floor of the mouth to the tip of tongue. The lesions are located symmetrically to the lingual frenum, but the right lesion showed an enlargement close to the floor of the mouth (Figure 2.9). By applying a mild pressure, their color and width was reduced, but returned when the pressure was released. These lesions are asymptomatic, but cause mild discomfort with eating or speaking. No other similar lesions were found within the mouth or other mucosae in this patient or among her close relatives.

Q1 What is the diagnosis?

- **A** Hemangioma
- **B** Eruption cysts
- **C** Kaposi sarcoma
- **D** Hemorrhagic ranula
- **E** Lingual varicosities

Answers:

- **A** No
- **B** No
- **C** No
- **D** No
- **E** Enlarged lingual varicosities are abnormal, dilated lingual veins, highly visible in older patients (> 60 years old) and are sometimes associated with thrombophlebitis of the legs as seen in this lady.

Comments: The lack of trauma at the ventral surface of the tongue excludes hemorrhagic ranula from diagnosis. Hemangiomas can bleach or reduce their size with pressure, but in contrast to the lady's lesion, they have a tendency to shrink over time. Sarcoma Kaposi is a vascular neoplasia that is mainly seen in patients with immunodeficiencies, while eruption cysts are bluish lesions which are found in the alveolar mucosa and associated with the crowns of unerupted teeth.

Q2 What is/are the difference(s) between varicoses and spider veins?

- **A** Location
- **B** Color
- **C** Size
- **D** Symptomatology
- **E** Predilection (age or sex)

Answers:

- **A** Spider veins are seen only on the skin of the face or associated with varicose veins on the legs, while varicoses are seen on the skin of the legs, but also on other parts of body.
- **B** No
- **C** Spider veins are smaller in size than varicose veins
- **D** No
- **E** No

Comments: Both veins have a tendency to appear in middle-aged women and cause patients cosmetic concern due to their skin distribution and/or dark red or bluish discoloration, as well as their symptomatology of burning sensation, pain, or even ulcer formation.

Q3 Which is the treatment for asymptomatic lingual varicosities?

- **A** Use beta blockers
- **B** Laser application
- **C** Band ligation
- **D** Embolization
- **E** None required

Answers:

- **A** No
- **B** No
- **C** No
- **D** No
- **E** Asymptomatic lingual varicoses do not require any treatment apart from reassurance for patients with a fear of cancer.

Comments: Laser application is useful for the elimination of facial spider veins and not of tongue varicoses. The systematic use of beta blockers reduces the risk of venous hemorrhage in patients with portal hypertension due to cirrhosis, while embolization and band ligation are widely used to cope with an acute hemorrhage that arises from large esopharyngeal and gastric rather than lingual veins.

Case 2.10

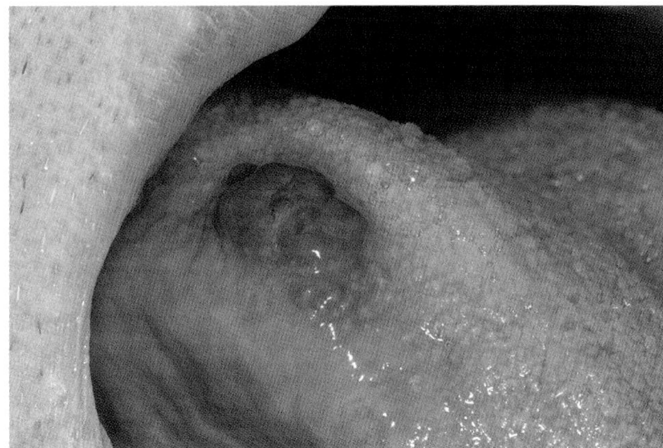

Figure 2.10

CO: A 62-year-old man presented to the Oral Medicine Clinic with an enlarged bluish-red lesion on his tongue.

HPC: The lesion had been present since the age of two, and showed a tendency to expand during adolescence, but had remained unchanged in size and color since then.

PMH: Asbestosis was his main serious problem. This is chronic respiratory failure due to chronic exposure to asbestos at work, and was treated with bronchodilator inhalers; oxygen supply and wide spectrum antibiotics in crisis. He had no history of other serious diseases, apart from two minor operations, one for removal of his appendix and the other for hemorrhoids.

OE: Oral examination revealed a rubbery, spongy bluish mass located at the dorsum of the tongue adjacent to the right lower molars (Figure 2.10). According to the patient, this lesion is asymptomatic, but unstable as it changes its color and size with pressure and consumption of hot foods or drinks respectively. No other similar lesions within his mouth or on the facial skin or cervical lymphadenopathy were recorded.

Q1 What is the possible diagnosis?

- **A** Cyanosis
- **B** Hemangioma
- **C** Melanoma
- **D** Lingual arteritis
- **E** Kaposi's sarcoma

Answers:

- **A** No
- **B** Hemangioma is a benign vascular lesion characterized by an abnormal proliferation of blood vessels that appears at birth or during the patient's early life with a tendency to subside over time. This lesion is formed by blood vessels and its color ranges from dark red to blue. Local pressure moves blood from the lesion and makes it brighter in color and smaller in size.
- **C** No
- **D** No
- **E** No

Comments: Kaposi's sarcoma and melanoma are malignant tumors but their clinical characteristics (i.e. presence of similar local or distant and satellite lesions associated with lympho-adenopathy and a lethal course) do not fit with patient's lesion characteristics. Oral cyanosis is a common sign of chronic respiratory failure as was diagnosed in this patient, but cyanosis is not the cause as this is a diffuse and flat rather than localized swelling. Lingual arteritis is a very painful inflammation of the lingual artery, short in duration and causes severe tongue necrosis, and is therefore easily excluded from the diagnosis.

Q2 Which are the common histological characteristics of capillary and cavernous hemangiomas?

- **A** Increased proliferation of endothelial cells
- **B** Calcified thrombus formation (phlebolith)
- **C** Fibrous septa
- **D** Dense accumulation of inflammatory cells within the submucosa
- **E** Cholesterol crystals

Answers:

- **A** Endothelial cell hyperplasia with or without lumen formation is characteristic of hemangiomas, especially at their proliferative phase. The endothelial cells are dense and form clusters or small vascular channels prominent at the proliferative phase (capillary hemangiomas) or they form large cystic dilated vessels with thin walls (cavernous type).
- **B** No
- **C** Fibrous septa separate the neoplastic vascular lumens and are more numerous and dense at the involuting phase of the hemangiomas.
- **D** No
- **E** No

Comments: Cholesterol crystals are associated with chronic vascular inflammation, as well as being commonly seen in atheromatous plaques and in the inflamed cystic wall of dental cysts, but not in hemangiomas. Inflammation of the fibrous hemangioma's stroma is rare and mainly consists of chronic inflammatory cells, mast cells and a few macrophages. Phleboliths are formed from clots within the lumen of cavernous hemangiomas only.

Q3 Which of the syndromes below is/or are associated with cavernous hemangiomas?

- **A** Sturge-Weber syndrome
- **B** Maffucci syndrome
- **C** Blue rubber bleb nevus
- **D** PHACE syndrome
- **E** Klinefelter syndrome

Answers:

- **A** No
- **B** Maffucci syndrome is associated with multiple enchondromas, mainly on the bones of hands and feet as well as hemangiomas.
- **C** Blue rubber bleb nevus syndrome is characterized by multiple hemangiomas (cavernous in majority) in the skin and visceral organs.
- **D** PHACE syndrome is a cutaneous syndrome characterized by multiple congenital abnormalities of posterior fossa, hemangiomas, and other vascular abnormalities, cardiac, and eye defects, sternal clefts and supraumbilical raphe syndrome.
- **E** No

Comments: Klinefelter syndrome is characterized by a number of oral abnormalities apart from hemangiomas and occurs exclusively in males, while Sturge-Weber syndrome is characterized by capillary lesions of leptomininges and facial skin (nevus flammeus) along the distribution of ophthalmic and maxillary divisions of the trigeminal nerve.

3

Brown Lesions

Brown lesions are commonly seen in the oral mucosa and characterized by accumulations of endogenous or exogenous pigments in the superficial subepithelial connective tissue. These lesions appear as punctuate (macular) or diffuse and have a variety of clinical courses and prognosis (Figure 3.0a and b). Some of them are innocent lesions like racial, physiological mucosal pigmentation or those induced by drugs, diseases like Addison's or syndromes like Peutz-Jeghers, and others are dangerous like complex nevi or melanomas.

Table 3 shows the most common oral brown pigmented lesions.

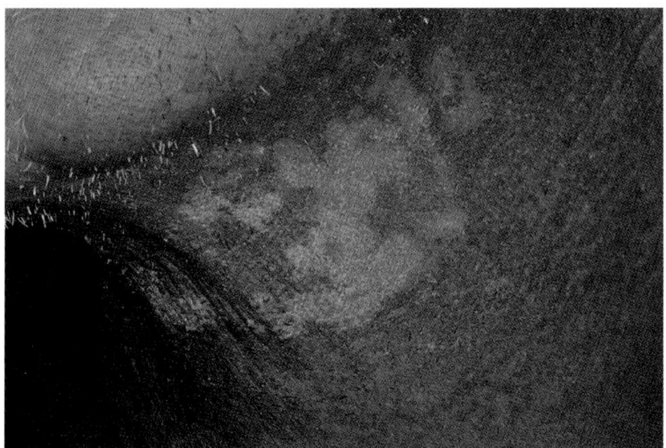

Figure 3.0a Brown discoloration of neck skin after radiation.

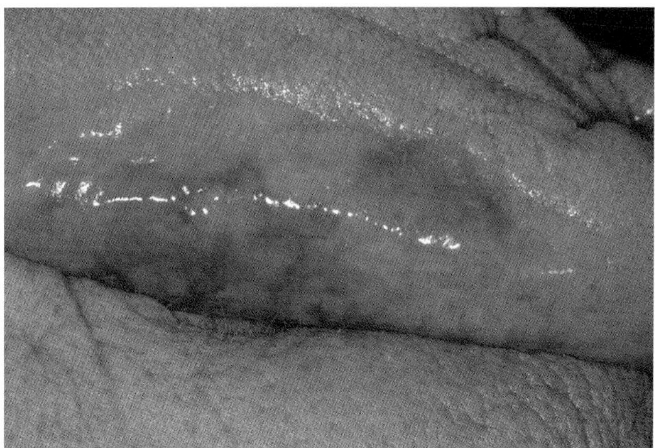

Figure 3.0b Hydroxyurea-induced oral brown pigmentation.

Clinical Guide to Oral Diseases, First Edition. Dimitris Malamos and Crispian Scully.

Companion website: www.wiley.com/go/malamos/clinical_guide

Table 3 The most common oral brown lesions.

In brown oral lesions the pigmentation (exogenous or endogenous) is superficial, while in black or blue lesions is deep into the submucosa

Endogenous pigmentation

- *Related to melanin*
  - Increased melanin production only
    - Related to: race
      - Racial pigmentosa
    - Hormone alterations
      - Chloasma
      - Addison's disease
      - Ectopic ACTH production
      - Nelson syndrome
      - Acanthosis nigricans
      - Laugier-Hunziker syndrome
      - Leopard syndrome
      - Spotty pigmentation, myxoma, endocrine overactivity syndrome
      - Von Recklinghausen's disease
      - Albright syndrome
    - Use of
      - Drugs
        - Oral contraceptives
        - Cytostatics
        - Antimicrobials
        - Antiarrythmics
- Foods
- Sun exposure
  - Freckles
  - Solar lentigines
- Smoking
  - Betel nut chewing
  - Smoker's melanosis
- Inflammation
  - LP melachrosis
  - BMMP melachrosis
  - EM melachrosis
- Infections
  - HIV
- Syndromes
  - Peutz-Jegher syndrome
  - Abnormal distribution of melanin
    - Tumors
      - Basal cell carcinomas
      - Melanoacanthoma
  - *Increased number of melanocytes*
    - Lentigines simplex
    - Nevi
    - Melanoma

Exogenous pigmentation

- Foreign materials
  - Tattoos
    - Amalgam
    - Graphite
    - Tribal
    - Tar
- Medications
  - Local
    - Potassium permanganate

Case 3.1

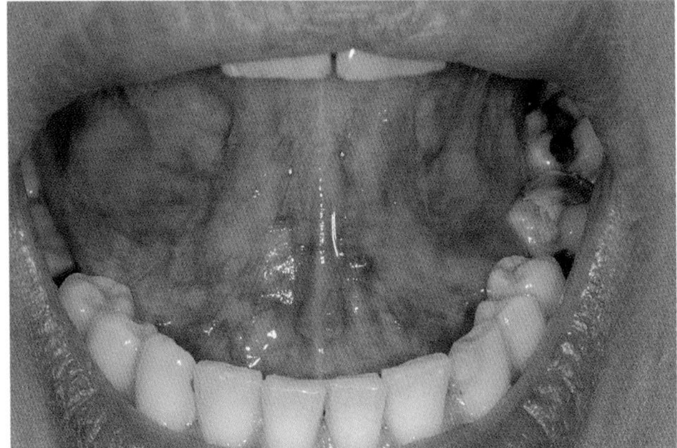

Figure 3.1

CO: A 43-year-old woman was evaluated for multiple brown lesions scattered in her mouth.

HPC: The brown lesions were first noticed by her dentist 10 years ago, but had remained unchanged since then. The lesions were asymptomatic and did not cause any patient concern until two years ago when she lost her sister from lung cancer and started her menopause.

PMH: She suffered from carpal tunnel syndrome on her right hand, exacerbated due to her job as a secretary and allergic keratitis on both eyes relieved with steroid eye drops (in crisis). She used no other medications or other known allergies. She was a chronic smoker of 8–10 cigarettes daily, and an occasional drinker.

OE: A middle-aged lady with dark complexion, with no other lesions on her mouth apart from a few pigmented brown lesions on her gingivae, buccal mucosae, floor of the mouth (Figure 3.1) and lips. The discoloration was more obvious on the gums and floor of the mouth. No other lesions were found on her skin or other mucosae.

Blood pressure and hormone tests were within the normal range.

Q1 What is the cause of the discoloration?

- **A** Addison's disease
- **B** Racial pigmentation
- **C** Drug-induced discoloration
- **D** Heavy metal poisoning
- **E** Melasma

Answers:

- **A** No
- **B** Racial pigmentation is a common condition among darker skinned individuals, and is presented as multifocal brown to black discoloration of gingivae (mainly) but also the tongue (dorsum and inferior) (Figure 3.1), floor of the mouth and soft palate. This discoloration is the result of increased production of melanin pigment by normal melanocytes.
- **C** No
- **D** No
- **E** No

Comments: Brown pigmentation is the result of increased melanin production and deposition in the melanocytes of the basal layers of the epithelium. Apart from racial pigmentation other conditions may be the cause such as Addison's disease, melasma, heavy metals, or drug effects. Drugs induced or metal poisoning pigmentation was easily discounted as the patient did not take any causative drugs nor was she exposed to chemicals in her hob or at home.. In melasma, the pigmentation is limited to facial skin and never involves the oral mucosa, and it mainly appears in young women during pregnancy. Normal blood pressure and Na, K, Ca, and cortisol levels as well as a normal Synacthen test excludes Addison's disease from the diagnosis

Q2 Which are the histological characteristics of racial pigmentation?

- **A** Increased production of melanin from an adequate number of melanocytes
- **B** Increased number of melanocytes at the basal layer
- **C** Presence of melanophages within the superficial lamina propria
- **D** Atrophic epithelium
- **E** Reduced number of melanocytes

Answers:

- **A** Racial pigmentation is connected with the increased production of melanin from melanocytes at the basal layer which is transported to adjoining keratinocytes through membrane-bound organelles known as melanocytes.
- **B** No
- **C** Melanophages are macrophages within the upper corium containing melanin.
- **D** No
- **E** No

Comments: The brown discoloration is the result of increased melanin production in normal or increased number of melanocytes. The brightness or not of this discoloration depends on the epithelial thickness' atrophic epithelium presents melanin pigment closer to the examiners' eyes,

Q3 In which other parts of the human body apart from the mouth is melanin commonly found?

- **A** Heart
- **B** Skin and its appendages (hairs/nails)
- **C** Brain
- **D** Joint cartilage
- **E** Eyes

Answers:

- **A** Heart valves, aortic sinuses and coronary vessels are often found with increased melanin pigmentation induced by antibiotics such as minocycline.
- **B** Increased skin pigmentation is often seen among patients with dark complexion and nails (melanonychia) or in patients exposed to solar radiation (solar dermatitis, lentigines, freckles), or in chronic inflammation (lichen planus), and hormone changes (melasma). Hair pigmentation is the result of sequential interaction between follicular melanocytes, matrix keratinocytes and dermal papillae fibroblasts. Hair color is also based on the ratio between eumelanin and pheomelanin. The higher the level of eumelanin, the darker the hair.
- **C** Brain pigmentation is seen in catecholaminergic cells of the substantia nigra of the brain and is caused by the accumulation of neuromelanin (one of the three components of melanin), the role of which remains obscure.
- **D** No
- **E** Eye color is the result of iris pigmentation, as dark brown eyes have a higher quantity of melanin than blue eyes.

Comments: Cartilage pigmentation is rarely seen and is associated with the accumulation of homogentisic acid rather than melanin in the connective tissues of nails, cartilage and bones.

Case 3.2

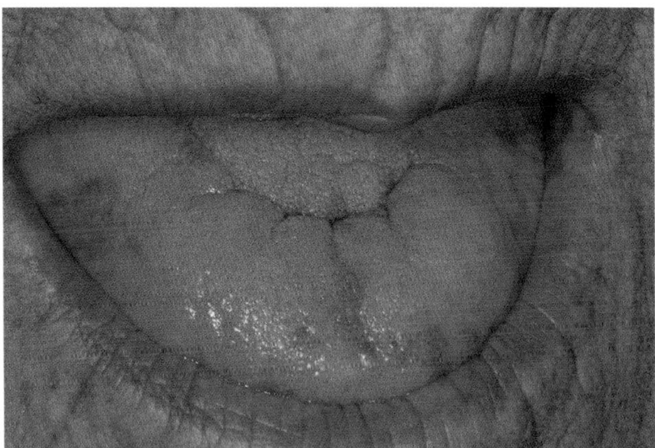

Figure 3.2a

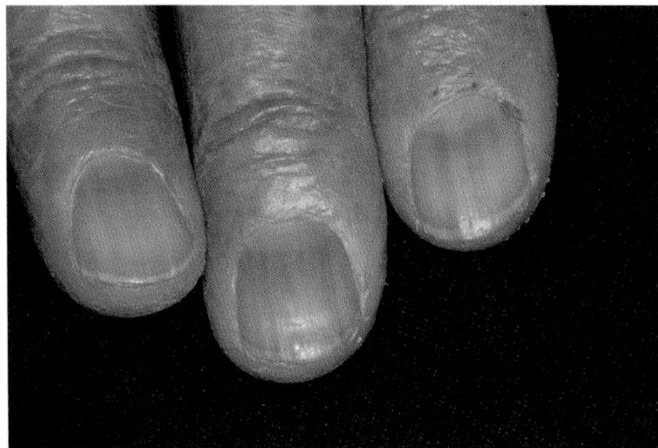

Figure 3.2b

CO: A 72-year-old woman was referred for evaluation of multiple brown lesions in her mouth.

PMH: She suffered from polycythemia vera which was diagnosed 15 years ago. It was controlled with hydroxyurea tablets. A small hormone-sensitive carcinoma in situ of her right breast was removed; letrozole tablets are now her maintenance treatment. She has never been hypotensive or allergic to various drugs or foods, nor a smoker or drinker.

HPC: The brown lesions in her mouth were accidentally found during a clinical examination by her physician two weeks ago.

OE: During the examination, multiple brown lesions scattered on the dorsum and lateral margins of the tongue (Figure 3.2a), buccal mucosae and soft palate and were linked with skin pigmentation and brown discoloration of the nail hands and feet (melanonychia) (Figure 3.2b). No other abnormalities either on the skin or other organs were reported, and her blood tests, including various hormone tests, were in a normal range.

Q1 What is the cause of her oral and skin pigmentation?

- **A** Addison's disease
- **B** Melanoma, widespread
- **C** Chemical poisoning
- **D** Drug-induced pigmentation
- **E** Cushing's disease

Answers:

- **A** No
- **B** No
- **C** No
- **D** The use of hydroxyurea and not letrozole has been associated with the increased pigmentation in this patient. Hydroxyurea is routinely used as an anti-neoplastic agent for the treatment of various myeloproliferative disorders such as leukemias, thrombopenias, polycythemia, and sometimes in psoriasis. Hydroxyurea can cause increased melanin production thus showing dark brown pigmentation of skin, sclera, nails of hands and feet and oral mucosa within a few months of treatment.
- **E** No

Comments: The normal blood pressure together with the normal hormone levels and the clinical characteristics and slow pigmentation progress exclude Cushing's, Addison's diseases and melanoma from the diagnosis.

Q2 What other drugs can cause hyper-pigmentation?

- **A** Anti-malarials
- **B** NSAIDs
- **C** Antibiotics
- **D** Cytotoxic drugs
- **E** Anti-emetics

Answers:

- **A** Anti-malarials such as chloroquine or hydroxychloroquine, having been used for months, can cause blue or gray pigmentation on face, neck, legs, and nails.
- **B** NSAIDs are used for pain or inflammation relief and sometimes cause a fixed drug reaction which initially appears in the form of erythematous

lesions on the face, lower extremities or genitalia, leaving, eventually, a brown discoloration.
- **C** Antibiotics and especially tetracyclines cause brown discoloration of nails, sclera, skin, and bones.
- **D** Cytotoxic drugs cause a brown discoloration as a transverse or longitudinal band of the nail bed and other mucosae which gradually fades with drug withdrawal.
- **E** No

Comments; Anti-emetic drugs are widely used against nausea and vomiting in motion sickness, gastroenteritis and during chemotherapy, and are mostly related to dry mouth, constipation, fatigue, and drowsiness rather than skin discoloration.

Q3 Which drug mechanism induces pigmentation?
- **A** Activation of melanocytes for melanin production
- **B** Inhibition of melanophage action
- **C** Deposition of drug into the tissues
- **D** Extravagation and disintegration of red blood cells from the small vessels in the lamina propria
- **E** Vasodilatation due to drug-induced inflammation

Answers:
- **A** Various drugs increase the production of melanin from active melanocytes within the basal layer.
- **B** No
- **C** Deposition of the causative drug or its complex with melanin can cause discoloration of the tissues.
- **D** No
- **E** No

Comments: Certain drugs could trigger local inflammation causing vasodilation and in some places hemorrhage, and breakdown of hemoglobulin of the red blood cells, with final production of hemosiderin. This is an iron storage complex whose excessive accumulation into various tissues, known as hemosiderosis, causes secondary black to brown discoloration. The presence and the number rather than the action of melanophages seems to play a role in inflammatory pigmented skin lesions.

Case 3.3

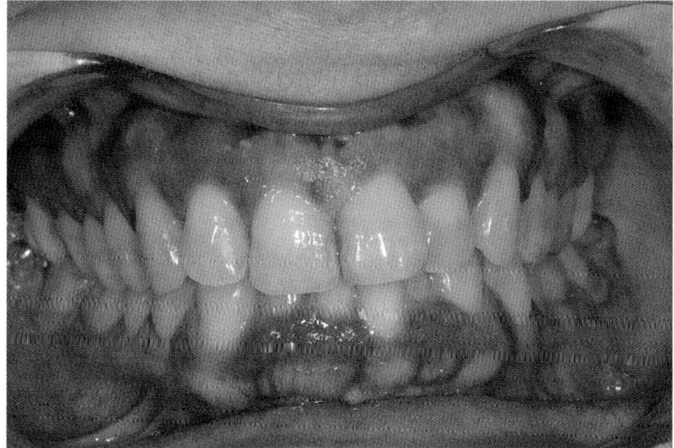

Figure 3.3

CO: A 42-year-old Caucasian men presented with dark brown discoloration of his gingivae.

HPC: The gingival discoloration had been observed in the patient over the last 10 years, but became more intense within the last 2 years when the patient started smoking cigars.

PMH: This patient suffered from a mild hypertension and hyper-cholesterolemia, both being controlled with the help of a special diet. He was allergic to pollen and suffers from hayfever; when severe, anti-histamines are used. He is a workaholic and started smoking cigarettes from the age of 14. However, over the last two years the patient switched to cigars (>15/day).

OE: Physical examination revealed a tall, thin, dark complexioned man with no serious skin problems apart from a yellow stain on his right hand and especially on the nails of the middle and index fingers. His intra-oral examination showed multiple brown patchy discolorations of the upper and lower gingivae extended to the inter-dental papillae and the attached gingivae and buccal sulcus (Figure 3.3). This discoloration was darker in the anterior lower gingivae than in the buccal mucosae and dorsum of the tongue and lower lip, where the patient lights up his cigar.

Q1 What is/or are the possible cause(s) of gingival pigmentation?
- **A** Metal poisoning
- **B** Smoker's melanosis
- **C** Drug-induced melanosis
- **D** Gingival melanoma
- **E** Racial pigmentation

Answers:

- **A** No
- **B** Smoker's melanosis is confirmed by the dark gingival pigmentation especially on his anterior lower gingivae with a benign course and reinforced by yellow staining from nicotine on the middle and index finger nails, where his cigars were hold.
- **C** No
- **D** No
- **E** Having in mind the patient's race (Caucasian) and his dark complexion, the gingival pigmentation could be attributed to racial pigmentation in addition to smoker's melanosis.

Comments: The characteristics of the patient's gingival pigmentation regarding the color (brown rather than blue or black), distribution (all gingivae and not ion-free or mesio-dental gingivae), type (band and not zone) in combination with the lack of recent exposure to toxic chemicals, exclude metal poisoning from the diagnosis. The homogeneity and not the gradation of brown discoloration, along with its morphology (plaque and not growth) or its progress (slow and not rapid) and lack of symptomatology and lympho-adenopathy rule out oral melanoma from the diagnosis.

Q2 Which of the oral lesions below is/or are not related to smoking?

- **A** Leukoplakia
- **B** Nicotinic stomatitis
- **C** Hairy leukoplakia
- **D** Acute ulcerative gingivitis
- **E** Oral squamous cells carcinoma

Answers:

- **A** No
- **B** No
- **C** Hairy leukoplakia in contrast to hairy tongue lesion is not related to smoking. Hairy leukoplakia appears as a white corrugated lesion on the lateral margins of the tongue and is strongly related to Epstein-Barr virus (EBV) infection in immunocompromised patients, which is partially responding to anti-viral therapy.
- **D** No
- **E** No

Comments: Smoking can be involved in the pathogenesis of various oral lesions in several ways. The heat produced with smoking causes mouth dehydration, leading to difficulties in removal of dead epithelial cells (washing), retardation of the normal rate of desquamation on the dorsal surface of tongue, producing a hair-like appearance which is susceptible to colonization of chromogenic bacteria as seen in a hairy-coated tongue. The carcinogenic chemicals that are released with smoking damage the DNA, and delay the healing process, causing the accumulation of abnormal cells, with cancer development. Smoking provokes xerostomia, together with nicotine which induces gingival vasoconstriction. This as well as the impaired host immunity, enhances the pathogenic action of various bacteria in gingival diseases, especially in acute ulcerative gingivitis/stomatitis. The nicotine causes vasoconstriction of the palatal blood vessels and at the same time, the irritation of the mucosa from heat and various toxic irritants cause hypertrophy of the mucosa and inflammation of the ducts of minor salivary glands, as has been observed in nicotinic stomatitis.

Q3 Which of the tobacco chemicals below is/or are NOT related to cancer development?

- **A** Nicotine
- **B** Polycyclic aromatic hydrocarbons (PAHs)
- **C** Essence oils
- **D** Herbs
- **E** Nitrosamines

Answers:

- **A** No
- **B** No
- **C** Essence oils embedded on rolling papers or blends have been used in some tobacco products in small quantities, having a minimum risk of cancer development.
- **D** Various products from thyme, rosemary, and chamomile, intermingled with tobacco blends and essence oils increase the flavor and make cigars more attractive.
- **E** No

Comments: The most important carcinogens in tobacco products are nicotine, nitrosamines, and PAHs which affect cell growth and apoptosis, expression of oncogenes, neovascularization, and treatment response.

Case 3.4

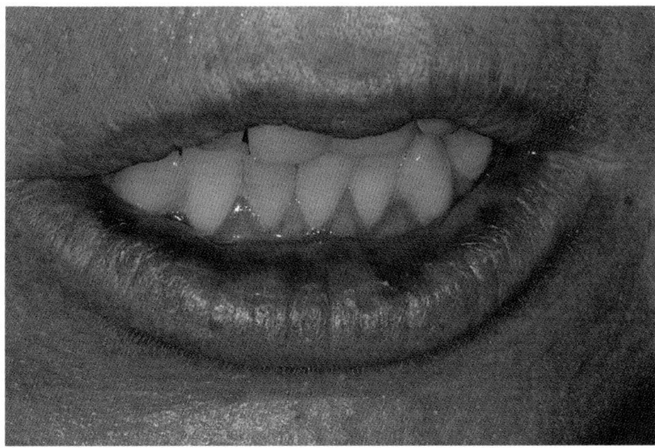

Figure 3.4

CO: A 23-year-old woman is referred by her physician to be evaluated for the brown patchy discoloration of her lips.

HPC: The lesions were first noticed by her mother at the age of 10, increasing in number and intensity during puberty and fading over the last three years.

MH: She suffered only from an iron deficiency anemia and bowel problems (constipation) which were initially attributed to the use of iron supplement tablets during the days of her heavy menstrual cycle, but recently, to the two small benign polyps in her small intestine. It has to be underlined that her father had a history of a colorectal carcinoma. Recent blood tests (hematological/biochemical) were within a normal range, as was her blood pressure. She was an occasional smoker and drinker, as she enjoyed mountain climbing in her free time.

OE: A thin, woman with brown lesions on the vermilion borders of her lips (lower lip mainly) (Figure 3.4), lower gingivae and buccal mucosae and on the skin around her right eye. The lesions were flat, superficial, brown discolorations with no evidence of induration or bleeding on palpation, and not associated with local lymphadenopathy or other mucosal lesions.

Q1 What is the possible cause?

A Solar melanosis
B Hemosiderosis
C Cushing syndrome
D Peutz-Jeghers syndrome
E Laugier-Hunziker syndrome

Answers:

A No
B No
C No
D Peutz-Jeghers syndrome (PJS) is the cause and characterized by numerous brown pigmented lesions on the skin, mouth, and other mucosae together with hamartomatous polyps in the gastrointestinal tract. It is an autosomal dominant genetic disease with an increased risk of developing cancer in a number of organs as found in her father with similar oral pigmentation.
E No

Comments: The pigmented skin lesions could be attributed to chronic skin exposure to solar radiation during her mountain climbing, but the presence of intra-oral lesions together with the presence of polyps exclude solar melanosis and Laugier-Hunziker syndrome from the diagnosis. The abnormal laboratory tests and characteristic clinical features found in Cushing syndrome and hemosiderosis includes these conditions in the diagnosis.

Q2 Which is the major complication of Peutz-Jeghers syndrome?

A Melanoma
B Blindness
C Carcinoma
D Bowel obstruction
E Osteoporosis

Answers:

A No
B No
C Increased risk of gastrointestinal carcinomas and other extra-intestinal malignancies occur in patients with Peutz-Jeghers syndrome even at an early age.
D No
E No

Comments: The pigmented oral and skin lesions in PJS are characterized by increased melanin production, which derives from an increased number of normal melanocytes, which do not show architectural or cytologic atypia or the great number of mitoses as seen in melanoma. In patients with PJS, bowel obstruction is common and arises from the polyps, while osteoporosis induced from pituitary adenomas is rare, yet neither of them jeopardize patient's life. Blindness is not characteristic clinical finding of PJS.

Q3 Which of the laboratory tests below may be done in patients with PJS on a regular basis?

A Endoscopy/colonoscopy
B U/S of the abdomen

- **C** Stool analysis
- **D** Mammography
- **E** Blood tests for anemia

Answers:

- **A** Endoscopy and colonoscopy are useful investigations for detecting intestinal polyps.
- **B** No
- **C** Stool analysis and particularly fecal occult blood tests can be used to diagnose gastrointestinal bleeding from an ulcerated polyp or colorectal or stomach cancer, while other tests such as colonoscopy, double control barium enema or stool DNA tests, seem to be more useful.
- **D** No
- **E** Anemia, especially due to iron deficiency, is a common finding among PJS patients due to chronic intestinal bleeding from polyps.

Comments: Mammography is an irrelevant test and used for detection of breast anomalies, especially in women, while the abdominal U/S is useful for anomalies of the structures of the upper abdomen in both sexes.

Case 3.5

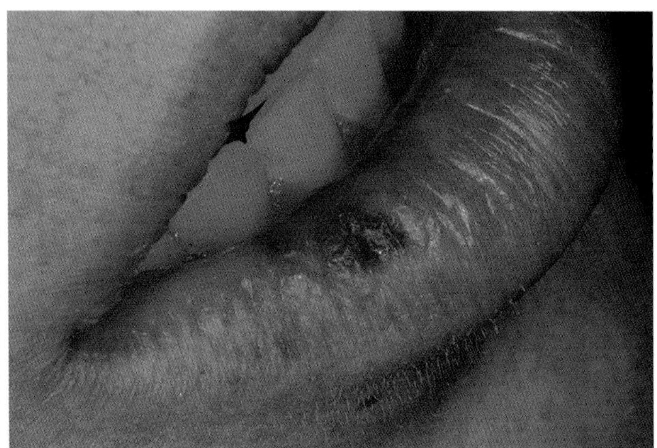

Figure 3.5

CO: A 25-year-old woman was evaluated on a brown lesion on her lower lip.

HPC: The lesion was first noticed during her dental visits for a root canal treatment five months ago and since then, remains asymptomatic, although having a slight tendency of worsening during the last summer vacation.

PMH: A healthy young woman with no serious medical or dental problems who likeed to spend most of her free time in sea sports. She was not allergic to any foods or drugs and is averse to unhealthy habits such as smoking and drinking.

OE: The oral examination revealed a brown, well demarcated, superficial, discoloration on the vermillion border of the lower lip (Figure 3.5). The lesion was asymptomatic, soft in palpation, unchanged in pressure, without color variation or other similar, satellite-like lesions on the lips and oral mucosa. The lower lip did not show any dryness, desquamation, or atrophy associated with bleeding. A few pigmented lesions on the skin of her nose and cheeks (freckles) were seen, which became darker in summers.

Q1 What is the possible diagnosis?

- **A** Melanotic macula
- **B** Fixed drug reaction
- **C** Melanoma
- **D** Actinic cheilitis
- **E** Hemangioma

Answers:

- **A** Melanotic macule or lentigolabialis is an asymptomatic brown lesion on the vermilion border of lower lip (mainly), tongue, buccal mucosae and gingivae (Figure 3.5).The lesion is well demarcated and uniformly pigmented with no proneness of malignant transformation.
- **B** No
- **C** No
- **D** No
- **E** No

Comments: The clinical characteristics (absence of satellite lesions or local lymphadenopathy as well as color variation with or without pressure) rules out labial melanoma and hemangioma from the diagnosis, respectively. The patient's preoccupation with sea sports, resulted in enhanced melanin production in summer, but this did not cause any dryness, desquamation, or lip atrophy as seen in actinic cheilitis. Fixed drug reaction requires drug uptake, but this is easily ruled out as the patient was not under any medication.

Q2 Which histological feature is/are pathognomonic of a melanocytic macule?

- **A** Increased size of melanocytes
- **B** Increased number of melanocytes
- **C** Elastosis
- **D** Hemosiderin deposition among epithelial layers
- **E** Atrophic mucosa

Answers:

- **A** No
- **B** Melanocytic macula is characterized by increased melanin production due to the increased number of melanocytes within the dermal–epidermal junction.
- **C** No
- **D** No
- **E** No

Comments: Chronic exposure of the labial mucosa to the sun can cause a great number of alterations ranging from innocent lesions as a result of increased melanin production (melanocytic macules) to those of intermediate risk due to any possible alteration in the epithelium atrophy and underlying submucosa (elastosis as seen in actinic cheilitis), or more severe effects threatening the patient's life (carcinomas) or melanomas. Haemosiderin deposition is irrelevant to solar radiation and strictly related to excess iron deposition within the body tissues.

Q3 What is the difference between café au lait lesions and melanotic macules?

- **A** Association with genetic disorders
- **B** Color
- **C** Presence of giant cell melanocytes in histological sections
- **D** Onset
- **E** Risk of malignant transformation

Answers:

- **A** Numerous café au lait lesions are associated with genetic disorders (i.e. neurofibromatosis 1) while melanotic macules are not.
- **B** No
- **C** Both lesions are characterized by increased melanin production but only café au lait lesions show giant cell melanocytes in microscopic examination.
- **D** Café au lait lesions are related to genetic disorders and appear from birth or childhood while melanotic macules can make their appearance at any age.
- **E** No

Comments: Both pigmented lesions clinically appear as brown to black discolorations with no tendency of malignancy.

Case 3.6

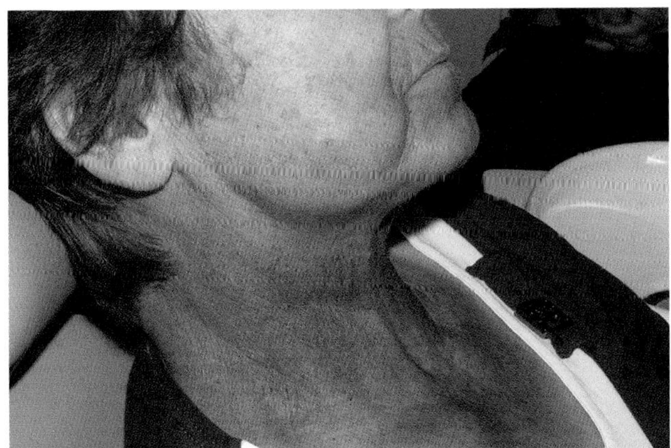

Figure 3.6

CO: A 68-year-old woman presented with a diffuse skin discoloration on her neck.

HPC: This discoloration appeared two weeks ago, coming after an erythema on the sun-exposed skin of her neck and was associated with dryness and mild pruritus.

PMH: This lady suffered from a mild rheumatoid arthritis which had being controlled with sulfasalazine and ibuprofen tablets. However, the latter seemed to cause her mild hypertension and therefore, it had been recently replaced with paracetamol. Her medical records revealed a meningioma which was removed five years ago along with a squamous cell carcinoma on her tongue, and ipsilateral lymph nodes, which were also removed two months ago. Additionally, the patient had undergone a course of chemo- and radiotherapy which had just been completed on the examination day. She has no other serious skin, hormone, or allergy problems and was an ex-smoker but not a drinker.

OE: Clinical examination revealed a diffuse brown discoloration on her neck extending from the area below the mandible to the suprasternal notch. The pigmentation is darker in the middle of the neck, near the surgical incision, but fades away at the periphery (Figure 3.6); it is currently associated with mild pruritus caused by her skin dryness.

Q1 What is the possible cause of her neck pigmentation?

- **A** Melasma
- **B** Drug-induced pigmentation
- **C** Solar pigmentation
- **D** Addison's disease
- **E** Radiation-induced pigmentation

Answers:

- **A** No
- **B** No
- **C** No
- **D** No
- **E** The radiotherapy for head and neck cancers creates severe side effects, among them an hyper pigmentation as it seems to activate rather than to destroy melanocytes as obviously seen in this woman's facial and neck skin. This pigmentation begins as a dispersed erythema which finally, within the next one or two weeks, changes to a brown pigmentation that persists for up to four weeks after the end of the therapy.

Comments: The skin pigmentation, caused by solar rays, is not only restricted to the area of irradiation, but affects all parts of the body which are exposed to sun. Addison's disease pigmentation is seen as isolated or diffused pigmentation in the whole body, including the mouth, in contrast to melasma which is mainly restricted to the face. Hyper-pigmentation is a phototoxic effect of various drugs, including sulfasalazine, but this was not the case here as the pigmentation only appeared during radiotherapy.

Q2 Which of the skin alterations below is/are not side effects of radiotherapy?

- **A** Edema
- **B** Desquamation
- **C** Ulceration
- **D** Rosacea
- **E** Skin tags

Answers:

- **A** No
- **B** No
- **C** No
- **D** Rosacea is a chronic skin disease, unrelated to irradiation and characterized by facial erythema, papules, pustules and swellings and dilation of superficial blood vessels.
- **E** Mucosal tags are benign growths on the skin of the neck, chest, underneath the breasts and surrounding groin. These lesions have been connected with a number of conditions such as Crohn's disease, polycystic ovary syndrome, acromegaly, and diabetes mellitus type 2, but not with radiation.

Comments: Among the side effects of radiation, erythema and edema are common and usually appear after the first two weeks of treatment, while ulcerations and atrophy are observed at the end of radiotherapy.

Q3 Which of the chemotherapeutic agents below cause increased facial pigmentation?

- **A** 5-fluorouracil
- **B** Cyclophosphamide
- **C** Dasatinib (tyrosine kinase inhibitor)
- **D** Melphalan
- **E** Bleomycin

Answers:

- **A** 5-Fluorouracil is widely used against carcinomas of the skin, oral mucosa, esophagus, stomach, pancreas, breast, and cervix by blocking the action of thymidylate synthase and DNA synthesis and stimulates the production of melanin.
- **B** Cyclophosphamide is used as a chemotherapeutic agent for lymphoma multiple myelomas, ovarian and breast carcinomas, sarcomas as well as neuroblastomas, as an alkylating agent which blocks DNA and RNA synthesis but increases pigmentation.
- **C** No
- **D** Melphalan induces alkylation of the DNA nucleotide guanine, thus causing alteration and inhibition of DNA and RNA synthesis in various body tumors such as multiple myelomas, malignant melanomas and ovarian cancers but associated with a number of side effects including melanosis.
- **E** Bleomycin is used for treatment of oral, lung, and genital carcinomas and gliomas by intercalating into DNA and reacting with ferrous ions, therefore producing free radicals capable of inducing DNA fragmentation and accumulation of neoplasmatic cells in the G2 phase of the cell cycle. Skin hyperpigmenation is rare.

Comments: Dasatinib is a tyrosine kinase inhibitor and is used for the treatment of chronic myelogenous leukemia and acute lymphoblastic leukemia with Philadelphia positive chromosome, by constraining lymphocyte-oriented kinase (LOK) activity. As a tyrosine kinase inhibitor, it is able to cause hypopigmentation, especially in black patients who are treated with this drug for leukemia, over a long period.

Case 3.7

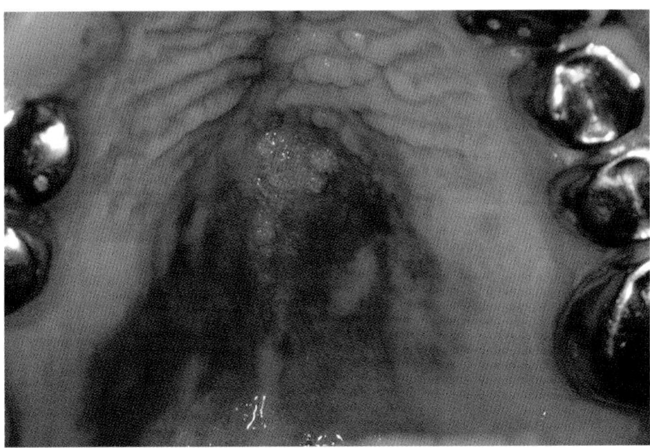

Figure 3.7

CO: A 64-year-old deaf man presented for assessment of a brown lesion on his palate.

HPC: The lesion was asymptomatic and accidentally discovered many years ago during a dental check-up; it has become slightly bigger and more nodular over the last three months.

PMH: He had got a complete hearing loss due to his premature birth and a history of a healing gastric ulcer, which had being controlled with diet. He was not taken any medicine apart from anti-acids for stomach pain when needed. His recent clinical and laboratory investigations did not reveal any other serious medical problems. He was an ex-smoker, but with no history of alcohol use. None of his close relatives had similar oral lesions.

OE: A thin Caucasian male with grade III skin pigmentation, according to the Fitzpatrick scale, presented a diffuse brown discoloration spread out in the middle of his hard palate (Figure 3.7). This pigmentation depicts a color variation as it is lighter at the apex and darker at the center where the mucosa is more nodular. Neither other pigmented lesions in his mouth, other mucosae and skin, nor local lymphadenopathy were detected.

Q1 What is the possible diagnosis of his palatal pigmentation?

- **A** Melanoma
- **B** Fixed drug reaction
- **C** Deep hemangioma
- **D** Nevus
- **E** Hemosiderosis

Answers:

- **A** No
- **B** No
- **C** No
- **D** Melanocytic oral nevus is the answer. It presents as benign isolated, single, or multiple asymptomatic lesions caused by the accumulation of nevus cells within the basal layer, underling the corium or deep in the sub-mucosa. It appears as flat or slightly raised nodular lesions on the lips, buccal mucosae, palate tongue or gingivae. The color ranges from pale to dark brown, gray, black, or blue and is mainly based on the location of nevi cells and the lesion's duration.
- **E** No

Comments: Looking at the patient's history, the absence of any systemic diseases or drug uptake responsible for the deposition of iron (hemosiderosis), or other pigments such as melanin (drug induced pigmentation), enables the clinicians to exclude hemosiderosis or drug-induced pigmentation from the diagnosis. Also, the long duration of the lesion accompanied with no serious complications combined with the clinical characteristics (absence of bleeding or local lymphadenopathy at palpation) excluded melanoma from the first clinical diagnosis, making biopsy the only tool for this to be confirmed.

Q2 Which is the commonest oral melanocytic nevus?

- **A** Blue nevus
- **B** Intramucosal nevus
- **C** Junctional nevus
- **D** Compound nevus
- **E** Spitz nevus

Answers:

- **A** No
- **B** Intramucosal nevi are the most common nevi in the oral cavity (>65%, of all) and are presented as small (<1 cm), brown, dome-shaped lesions anywhere in the mouth. This type of nevus is characterized by the accumulation of nevi cells within the lower spinous and basal layers, with no atypia or tendency for melanoma transformation.
- **C** No
- **D** No
- **E** No

Comments: Oral nevi are benign tumors which are mostly noticed in patients over the age of 30 (acquired) and very rarely as a patient's characteristic from birth (congenital), while they are associated with a number of genetic disorders. Intramucosal is the commonest type, followed by the blue (16–35%), compound (6–16.5%) and junctional (3–6%).

Q3 What are the differences between melanocytes and nevi cells?

The differences are in:

A Morphology
B Location
C Origin
D Organization
E Functions

Answers:

A Nevi cells are small, round, dark pigmented cells while the melanocytes are irregular with large dendritic processes and larger cytoplasm full of granules. Dendritic processes are also found in some blue nevi.
B Melanocytes are located among basal cells of the epithelium, while the nevi cells are additionally found in the upper and lower parts of the submucosa.
C No
D Melanocytes are single cells among basal cells, while nevi cells are organized in clusters of up to 30–40 cells.
E Melanocytes produce melanin for sun protection, while the role of the nevi remains unknown.

Comments: Both cells seem to originate from neural crest cells. Melanocytes initially migrate to the epidermis and settle at the basal layer and in the hair follicles as melanoblasts, which finally mature into melanocytes. Nevi cells originate from melanocytes at the dermo-epidermal junction and sometimes proliferate and migrate into the sub-mucosa or from dermal pluripotent congenital precursors

Case 3.8

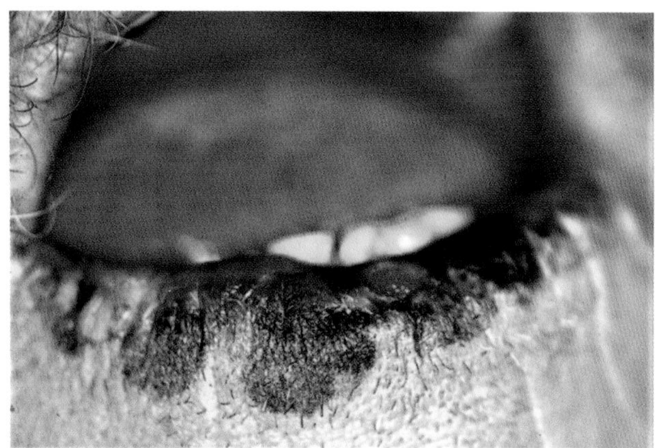

Figure 3.8

CO: A 70-year-old man presents with an extensive brown lesion covering most of his lower lip.

HPC: The lesion had existed for almost one year and started as a small pigmented plaque which had gradually increased in size, and finally covered the whole of his lower lip over the last three months (Figure 3.8).

PMH: His medical history revealed a prostate cancer, removed with radical prostatectomy eight years ago, and a mild heart attack treated with coronary artery bypass, antiplatelets, cholesterol agents, and angiotensin converting enzyme (ACE) inhibitor tablets. He was a chronic smoker (>40 cigarettes/day) as well as a drinker (up to 5 glasses of wine/meal) and he used to go for fishing before his heart attack three years ago. His family history was negative.

OE: The examination revealed a large superficial lesion of a very dark brown discoloration, covering all the length of his lower lip vermillion border and submerging into his adjacent chin with bulbous brighter leaf-like lesions. This lesion showed a small ulcer of 0.8 cm in maximum diameter centrally and three (small) satellite pigmented lesions at the inner labial mucosa, both being associated with two submental and one left submandibular palpable. lymph nodes. No other pigmented lesions were found on his skin or oral and other mucosae.

Q1 What is the possible diagnosis?

A Solar lentigo
B Actinic prurigo
C Lip cyanosis
D Smoking melanosis
E Lentigo maligna melanoma

Answers:

A No
B No

C No
D No
E Lentigo maligna melanoma is the cause. Lentigo maligna melanoma affects old patients especially at the peak of their 7th or 8th decade of life, who have had chronic exposure to ultraviolet radiation. It appears as a very extensive pigmented lesion on the sun-exposed skin of face or lips with irregular borders, large diameter (>4 mm), heterogeneous coloration and follows a pigmented lesion (lentigo maligna). The present patient was 70 years old, a heavy smoker and drinker, and had spent most of his time fishing; so he was totally exposed to sun radiation. He had a lip discoloration ranging from dark to light brown color and a former pigmented lesion from which the present lesion originates.

Comments: Chronic exposure to sun is responsible, apart from lentigo maligna melanoma, for other lesions like solar lentigo and actinic prurigo. Solar lentigo is a small (<1 cm) innocent pigmented lesion while solar prurigo affects certain groups of patients from North America and Asia, and is presented as numerous lip and skin lesions with a small risk of malignant transformation. Cyanosis and smoking melanosis are easily excluded from the diagnosis as the first one affects the vermillion border of both lips and its color is dark blue, which is closely related to the level of deoxyhemoglobin in the blood, while smoking melanosis is mostly observed in the anterior gingivae and inner surface of the lower lip.

Q2 Which of the tools below is/are not that useful for clinicians' diagnosis of solar lentigo melanoma?
A Biopsy
B Dermoscopy
C Photography
D PET scan
E CT/MRI

Answers:
A No
B No
C Photography is useful for the mapping of moles, rather than pigmented lesions with supraclavicular lymph node metastases (SLM) diagnosis. By comparing a series of photos taken at different intervening periods, clinicians try to recognize any changes in morphology, structure, and color of suspicious moles, as well as to detect any early melanoma.
D No
E No

Comments: Dermoscopy is a useful tool for distinguishing suspicious melanoma lesions from inflammatory dermatoses by using a high quality magnified lens and a strong lighting system. Biopsy is mandatory to confirm the clinical diagnosis of melanoma, while CT or MRI detect possible metastases (local/systemic). PET scan shows the presence of active disease in the whole body.

Q3 Which is the best treatment for lentigo maligna melanoma?
A Cryotherapy
B Radiotherapy
C Laser CO_2 therapy
D Imiquimod cream application
E Surgery

Answers:
A No
B No
C No
D No
E Surgery is the best treatment possible, as the wide removal of tumor with clear margins of 9 mm has the smallest recurrence rate (<10%).

Comments: All the other techniques are less invasive, but show a high rate of recurrence. This could be attributed either to failure of laser CO_2 to reach the whole lesion (in depth or size) or to treatment delay of secondary misdiagnosed depigmented lesions after imiquimod application.

Case 3.9

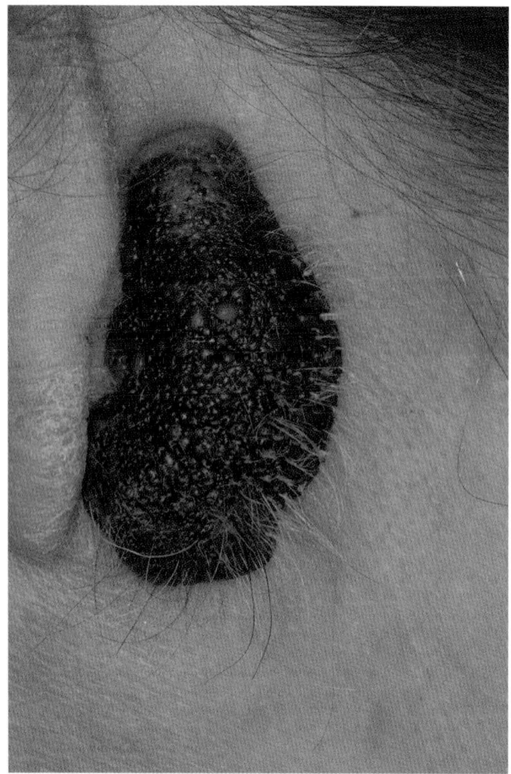

Figure 3.9

CO: A 56-year-old woman was presented for a routine medical–dental check-up and during her examination a dark brown lesion behind her right ear lobe was found.

HPC: The lesion had been present since childhood, but increased in size and color during puberty and had remained unchanged since then.

PMH: This middle-aged post-menopausal woman had a history of mild hypertension, dislipidemia, and depression which were treated with an ACE inhibitor, fluvastatin plus diet and psychological counseling respectively. She had a basal cell carcinoma on the skin of her nose that was removed in surgery two years ago. She used to smoke two to five cigarettes on a daily basis and had no history of alcohol use. None of her close relatives had similar brown lesions.

OE: Clinical examination revealed a dark brown oval lesion on the skin behind her right ear lobe with a larger dimension of 3.5 cm. The lesion was well-defined, soft with a nodular surface, unique color and contained few hairs (Figure 3.9). No other similar lesions were found apart from a few small moles on her back.

Q1 What is the diagnosis?

- **A** Pigmented basal cell carcinoma
- **B** Melanocanthoma
- **C** Congenital melanotic nevus
- **D** Melanoma
- **E** Neurocutaneous melanosis

Answers:

- **A** No
- **B** No
- **C** Congenital melanotic nevus is the cause and is characterized by a well-defined, dark pigment lesion on the skin of the face with a nodular appearance, containing hairs. Congenital nevus is characterized by its large size (>3.5 cm in diameter) and early onset (from birth). Acquired melanotic nevi are usually numerous, of small size (<1 cm) and develop later in puberty or adolescence.
- **D** No
- **E** No

Comments: Although the lesion is congenital, the absence of other melanocytic tumors in the leptomeninges of the central nervous system (CNS) excludes neurocutaneous melanosis from the differential diagnosis. The lack of induration or bleeding at palpation as well asymmetry and color variation together with the satellite new lesion formation ruled out melanoma from diagnosis. Another benign pigmented lesion that mainly affects female skin, especially the face, is melanoacanthoma; it differs in that it affects older women with dark skin (>30 years of age) and is characterized histologically by proliferation of epithelial and nevus cells.

Q2 What are the differences between congenital and acquired nevi apart from the year of onset?

- **A** Size
- **B** Skin distribution
- **C** Color
- **D** Risk for melanoma transformation
- **E** Location of nevi cells

Answers:

- **A** The acquired nevi are smaller than the congenital ones. Congenital nevi can be small (<2 cm); intermediate (>2 cm but <20 cm) or giant covering a whole part of the body such as the face, back, or legs.

B No
C No
D No
E The congenital nevi cells are usually found deeper into the dermis, within neurovascular bundles.

Comments: Both types of nevi have been observed in the skin and oral mucosa as benign pigmented lesions with color ranging from brown to dark black. Both are asymptomatic and do not show any indication of melanoma following the asymmetry, border, color, diameter, evolving (ABCDE) rule. Only the giant congenital nevus has an increased risk of developing melanoma and that is why it should be closely monitored.

Q3 Which other treatment options are available apart from surgical excision for congenital melanocytic nevi?
A Phototherapy
B Corticosteroid creams
C Chemical peeling
D Hyperbaric oxygen
E Dermabrasion

Answers:
A No
B No
C Chemical peeling with trichloracetic acid or phenol solutions lighten the color of nevus but cause local skin irritation.
D No
E Dermabrasion involves the partial removal of a large congenital nevus causing its color lighting, although it can be scarring.

Comments: Phototherapy involves the exposure of skin to ultraviolet light. On a regular basis, this is used for the treatment of psoriasis, and not for nevus disappearance. This therapy may stimulate nevi cells and produce melanin. Hyperbaric oxygen is used to treat wrinkles induced by ultraviolet radiation, and steroids are used for the eczema around the nevus, but not for the nevus.

Case 3.10

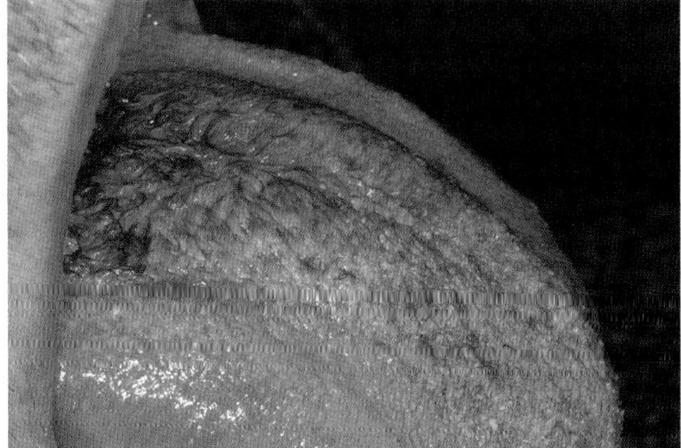

Figure 3.10a

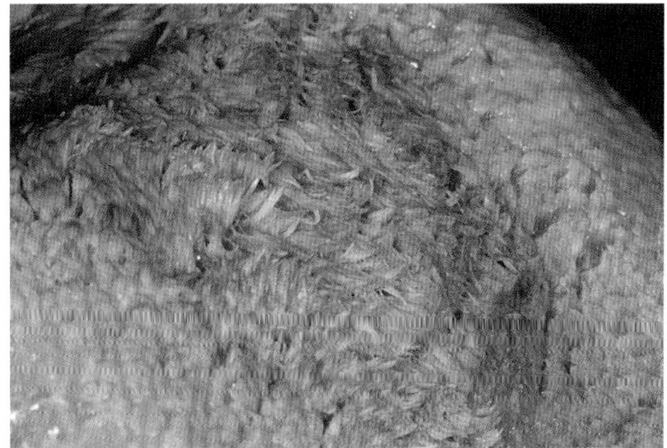

Figure 3.10b

CO: A 22-year-old student was evaluated for a brown discoloration of his tongue.

HPC: The tongue became brown after a course of antibiotics for pericoronitis on his lower left wisdom tooth two weeks ago.

PMH: His medical history is clear from any serious diseases except for a few episodes of aphthous stomatitis, two to three times a year. He is not on any medicines apart from antibiotics and chlorhexidine mouthwash recently. He is a chronic smoker of 10 to 15 cigars per day and chews mint flavor chewing gum on a regular basis.

OE: The oral examination revealed a brown discoloration on his dorsum of his tongue (Figure 3.10a) associated with hypertrophy of filiform papillae (Figure 3.10b).This discoloration covered the middle of the area, but was more prominent on the posterior part of the tongue and was related to mild halitosis. This discoloration was partially wiped off by scrubbing his tongue with a wooden spatula, and it had no other connection with similar lesions on the oral and other mucosae.

Q1 What is the cause?
- **A** Pseudomembranous candidiasis
- **B** Brown hairy tongue
- **C** Hairy leukoplakia
- **D** Mint-induced stomatitis
- **E** Smoking melanosis

Answers:
- **A** No
- **B** No
- **C** Brown hairy tongue is a variation of hairy tongue and is presented with an abnormal keratin coating of the elongated filiform papillae on the dorsum of the tongue. It is commonly found among young anxious patients with poor oral hygiene, who smoke, take antibiotics – metronidazole in particular – or use strong mouthwashes on a regular basis, as in the case of this young man.
- **D** No
- **E** No

Comments: The lesions in pseudomembranous candidiasis are white creamy lesions that are spread all over the oral mucosa apart from the tongue, and can be easily removed with a spatula, leaving only an erythema underneath. Hairy leukoplakia lesions appear as white fixed lesions on the lateral margins and not on the dorsum of tongue in immuno-compromised patients, while the mint induced stomatitis lesions are not only restricted to the area of tongue (lateral margins) but can be also be seen in other parts that are exposed to mint flavor. Cigar smoking may contribute to the brown discoloration through the accumulation of nicotine stains within filiform papillae in hairy tongue, but also by stimulating the gingival melanocytes to produce melanin, therefore causing a gingival melanosis.

Q2 The diagnosis of this lesion is based mainly on:
- **A** Intra-oral examination
- **B** History
- **C** Culture
- **D** Biopsy
- **E** Allergic tests

Answers:
- **A** Intra-oral examination shows the brown covering of the dorsum of tongue.
- **B** History of drug/smoking or drinking habits allows clinicians to identify the possible risk factors of hairy tongue.
- **C** No
- **D** No
- **E** No

Comments: Although cultures and biopsies show the presence of various chromogenic bacteria and *Candida* species within the elongated filiform papillae in hairy tongue lesions, these techniques are not widely used for diagnosis as they are expensive, time consuming and their results do not seem to alter the clinical course of this disease.

Q3 What symptom is/or are commonly associated with brown hairy tongue?
- **A** Pruritus
- **B** Metallic taste
- **C** Belching
- **D** Fatigue
- **E** Nausea

Answers:
- **A** No
- **B** Metallic taste is a common complaint of patients with hairy tongue as it is induced by the alteration of gustatory papillae (proliferation or delayed apoptosis) as a result of the excessive smoking, drinking, or use of strong mouthwashes.
- **C** No
- **D** No
- **E** No

Comments: The excessive tongue coating sometimes causes a local irritation on the palate that provokes nausea, belching, or even pruritus, especially in anxious patients.

4

Malodor

Malodor, also known as halitosis, is unpleasant bad breath that causes severe patient concern and a negative effect on the patient's life. Halitosis is caused by the release of various volatile gases, either during food breakdown from various bacteria that are normal inhabitants in the patient's mouth, or during expiration of odorous substances which are moved via circulation from the periphery. Halitosis can easily be detected by other people (real) or not (fake). The majority of causes of real halitosis come from disorders inside the mouth (>85%) and the remaining are from nose, sinuses, throat, lungs, stomach, pancreas, and liver. Fake halitosis (halitophobia) is common in patients with severe anxiety, depression, or obsessive compulsive disorder. The basic step in halitosis treatment is the recognition and treatment of its underlying cause (Figure 4.0a and b).

The more common causes of halitosis are listed in Table 4.

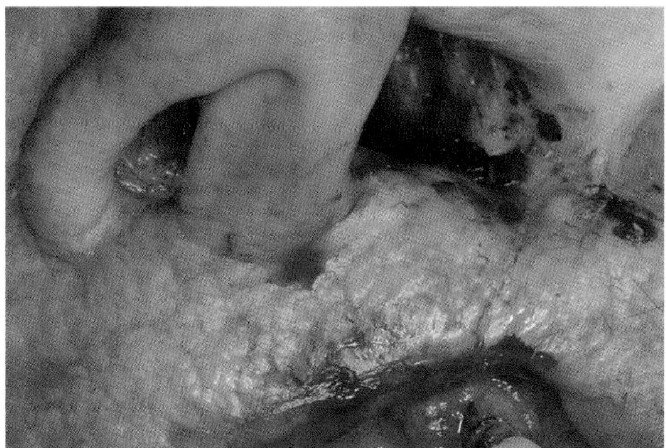

Figure 4.0a Halitosis from a patient with advanced oro-nasal carcinoma.

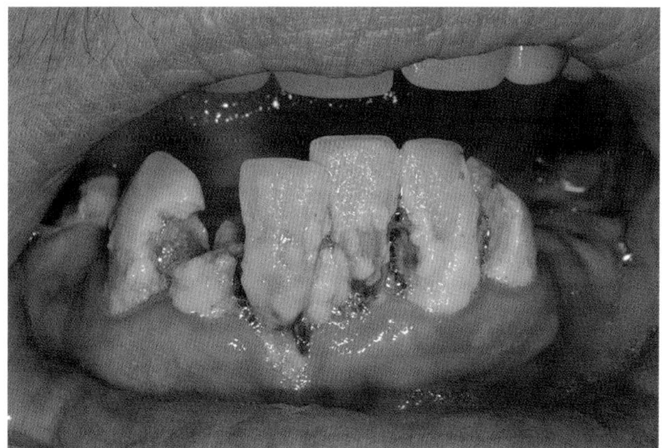

Figure 4.0b Halitosis from a patient with a neglected mouth.

Clinical Guide to Oral Diseases, First Edition. Dimitris Malamos and Crispian Scully.

Companion website: www.wiley.com/go/malamos/clinical_guide

Table 4 Common and important conditions associated with malodor

Malodor
• Physical causes
○ Food or fluid ingredients
▪ Onions/garlic
▪ Foodstuffs/additives
▪ Spice
▪ Alcohol
○ Food or fluid lack
▪ Starvation or dehydration
○ Habits
▪ Smoking
▪ Heavy drinking
• Local causes
○ Related with the mouth
▪ Caries
▪ Acute ulcerative gingivitis
▪ Pericoronitis
▪ Chronic periodontitis
▪ Chronic dental abscess
▪ Osteo
- necrosis
- myelitis
▪ Medicated osteonecrosis (due to bisphosphonates, denosumab, bevacizumab)
▪ Dry socket
▪ Noma
▪ Oroantral fistula
▪ Sinusitis
▪ Ulcerations, i.e. pemphigus vulgaris (PV)
▪ Sialdenitis
▪ Neoplasms
○ Related with pharynx/esophagus
▪ Tonsillitis
▪ Esophangeal infection
- reflux
- pouch
▪ Neoplasms
• Systemic causes
Diseases from
○ liver
▪ Hepatic failure
○ Kidney
▪ Renal failure
○ Lungs
▪ Infections
▪ Bronchiectasis
▪ Neoplasms
○ Gut
▪ Gastric regurgitation
○ CNS
▪ Temporal lobe epilepsy
▪ Temporal lobe tumors
▪ Delusions
○ Metabolism
▪ Trimethylaminuria
- Drugs
○ Associated with xerostomia
▪ Antihistamines
▪ Diuretics
▪ Narcotics
▪ Antidepressants
▪ Decongestants
▪ Antihypertensive
▪ Antipsychotics

Case 4.1

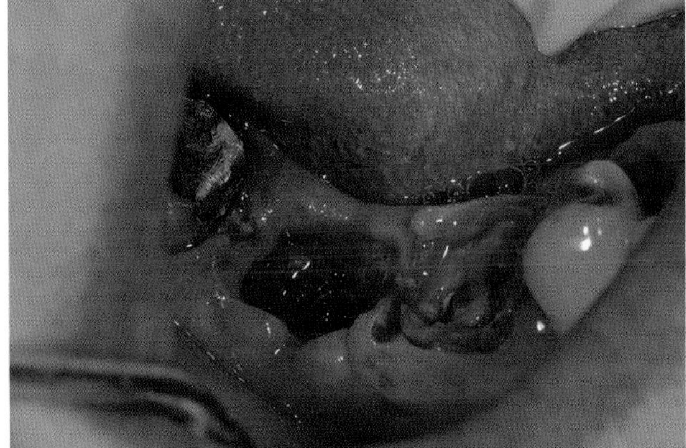

Figure 4.1

CO: A 43-year-old woman presented with halitosis and severe pain in the area of a recent extraction.

HPC: The pain started immediately after a difficult extraction of a severely decayed second lower molar, becoming even more intense over the following three days and radiating toward the ipsilateral upper molars and ear. One day later, a bad rotten smell coming from her mouth was noted and remained unchanged at her last dental examination.

PMH: Her medical history did not reveal any serious diseases or drug uptake, and her dental history recorded only occasional visits to her GDP for dental pain relief. Smoking (>25 cigarettes daily) was reported.

OE: Oral mucosa did not show any oral lesions apart from erythematous and tender gingivae around the socket of the extracted molar. The socket was empty of clot and showed a partially exposed alveolar bone which was covered with debris and saliva (Figure 4.1). Pain was coming from the socket and was exacerbated with probing. No evidence of a dental abscess, facial swelling or cervical lympho-adenopathy was noticed, except that a bad, rotten smell was arising from the socket. Her mouth and dentition was neglected and many decayed teeth and roots due to her poor oral hygiene were recorded.

Q1 What is the cause of her bad breath?

- **A** Tooth avulsion
- **B** Intra-alveolar carcinoma
- **C** Dry socket
- **D** Metastatic tumors
- **E** Osteonecrosis induced by drugs

Answers:

- **A** No
- **B** No
- **C** Dry socket or alveolar osteitis is the cause and is the most common complication after a tooth extraction. It is characterized by the absence of blood clot within the socket due to its incomplete formation, disintegration, or removal. The empty socket can be easily infected and inflammatory products could activate pain, taste, and smell receptors thus causing pain, dysgeusia, and halitosis.
- **D** No
- **E** No

Comments: The lack of severe trauma on either mouth or head excludes tooth avulsion, while the severe symptomatology despite its short duration rules out intra-alveolar carcinomas and metastatic tumors from diagnosis. Osteochemonecrosis is not the cause, as the lady was not under any medications such as biphosphonates which could be responsible for bony necrosis.

Q2 Which is/or are the main predisposing factors for this condition?

- **A** Preexisting infection
- **B** Anemia
- **C** Poor oral hygiene
- **D** Smoking
- **E** Vitamin deficiency

Answers:

- **A** Preexisting inflammation of the teeth or gingivae cause inflammation and disintegration of the blood clot.
- **B** No
- **C** Poor oral hygiene allows pathogenic germs to inoculate and grow into the socket of a recently extracted tooth, causing inflammation and lysis of the clot as well as necrosis of adjacent alveolar bone.
- **D** The sucking action of cigarette smoking dislodges the clot from the socket while at the same time, the smoking chemical, i.e. nicotine, causes local vasoconstriction thus delaying the healing.
- **E** No

Comments: Severe anemia, especially due to iron or vitamin deficiency, causes low oxygen compilation in the tissues, and indirectly may halt or delay wound healing stages increasing the risk of local infection and secondarily the disintegration of the clot.

Q3 Which is/or are the complication(s) of an untreated dry socket?

- **A** None
- **B** Osteomyelitis
- **C** Low quality of life
- **D** Increased risk of malignant transformation
- **E** Paresis of the trigeminal nerve

Answers:

- **A** No
- **B** Osteomyelitis is an infection (acute or chronic) of the bone marrow of the mandible or maxilla, induced by various bacteria or fungi, that occurs after a local trauma or difficult extractions, and rarely from dry sockets.
- **C** Dry socket is characterized by an intense pain which often interferes with the patient's work or social activities in the community, thus reducing his quality of life.
- **D** No
- **E** No

Comments: Chronic local irritations and not dry socket inflammation are believed to participate in the development of some oral carcinomas. In dry socket the inflammation is acute and does not have enough time to provoke changes in the affected tissues capable for malignant transformation. Dry socket can rarely cause the spread of pathogenic bacteria into the surrounding tissues at such degree that the induced inflammation can cause pressure and dysfunction of the trigeminal nerve.

Case 4.2

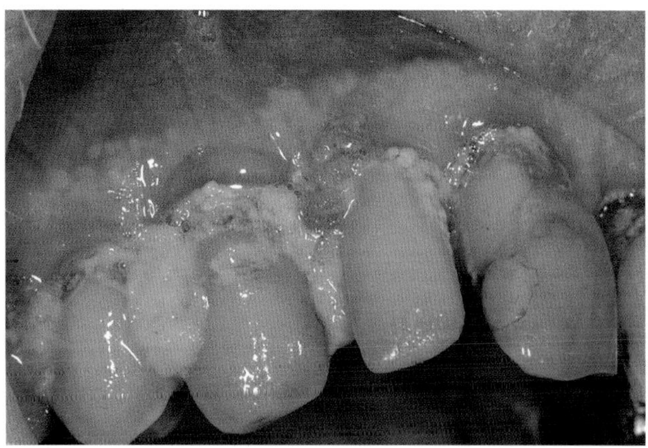

Figure 4.2

CO: A 68-year-old man was referred for evaluation of his dental status and his rotten breath before the beginning of zoledronic acid treatment for his lung cancer spine metastases.

HPC: His bad breath was first noticed by his clinician one month ago when the patient visited him for back pain. His halitosis was constant, worse at mornings and night, and unrelated to his meals.

PMH: His medical history revealed hypertension and respiratory problems such as chronic bronchitis and a small cell carcinoma in the left lung diagnosed two years ago which was surgically removed (lobectomy), unsuccessfully, as recent metastasis into the spine had been shown. His smoking or drinking habits had stopped since the diagnosis of his cancer.

OE: Examination revealed a cachectic man with periodontitis with gingival pockets depth from 4 to 8 mm depth forming thus a suitable place for accumulation of excessive plaque and food debris on his remaining decayed teeth (Figure 4.2). No other oral lesions were detected. His breath was bad, rotten and repulsive. Severe pain and difficulties in posture were reported and according to his oncologist were related to his spine metastasis.

Q1 What is the origin of the bad breath?
- **A** Smoking
- **B** Poor oral hygiene
- **C** Spine metastasis
- **D** Antihypertensive drugs
- **E** Periodontitis

Answers:
- **A** No
- **B** Anaerobic bacteria are easily found in mature dental plaque, capable of disintegrating food debris and releasing a plethora of volatile molecules which are responsible for the patient's malodor.
- **C** No
- **D** No
- **E** No

Comments: Smoking can cause halitosis in some patients but is not the cause here, as this habit was stopped two years ago. Spine metastasis is associated with pain and moving difficulties and spinal cord decompression, but never with halitosis. Periodontitis and some antihypertensive drugs have been related to chronic halitosis, but cannot be the cause as his bad breath was recent and detected one month ago.

Q2 Which of the volatile gases is mainly responsible for the patient's halitosis?
- **A** Alcohol
- **B** Fatty acids
- **C** Amines
- **D** Sulfur compounds
- **E** Nicotine

Answers:
- **A** No
- **B** Volatile gases of fatty acids like butyric, valeric, and propionic acids are the result of anaerobic degradation of carbohydrates, which gives rise to oral malodor.
- **C** No
- **D** Sulfur compounds such as methyl mercaptan, hydrogen sulfide and methyl sulfide are responsible for his halitosis.
- **E** No

Comments: As the patient had stopped smoking or drinking for many months, his halitosis was not caused by the volatile gases released from alcohol metabolism and tobacco or its smoke-related amines.

Q3 Which of the volatile substrates has/or have sulfur components that are involved with halitosis?
- **A** Cysteine
- **B** Methionine
- **C** Isoleukine
- **D** Histidine
- **E** Valine

Answers:

A Cysteine is a non-essential sulfur containing amino acid that is found in foods with high protein content like meat and eggs. Cystine and cysteine are metabolized under the presence of sulfhydrase positive bacteria, and release H_2S, a very high volatile gas.

B Methionine and cysteine are the two sulfur containing amino acids that play an important role in halitosis (cysteine > methionine).

C No

D No

E No

Comments: All the other amino acids do not have sulfur components and do not participate in sulfur production during the degradation of food debris with bacteria.

Case 4.3

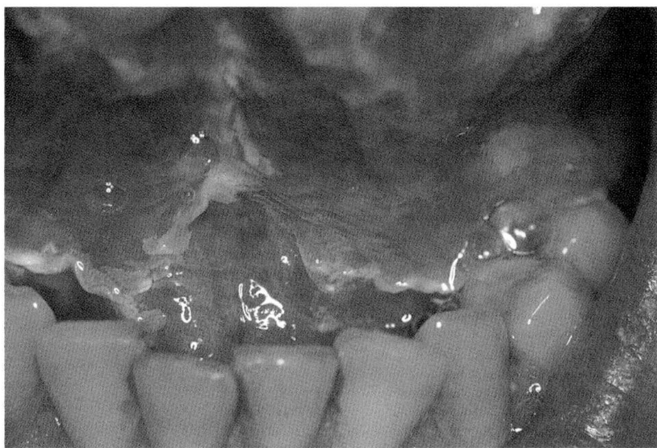

Figure 4.3

CO: A 38-year-old woman was referred for white oral lesions and severe halitosis of one month's duration.

HPC: The white lesions were first found by her dentist following a detailed examination before receiving a kidney transplant. Her bad breath was first noticed by her husband over a year ago, and had become more obvious over the last five months when her kidney deteriorated.

PMH: An unhealthy married woman, suffering from chronic renal failure due to recurrent episodes of pyelonephritis and hypertension, anemia, and hypercalcemia; all these conditions were partially controlled with hemodialysis and medication.

OE: A thin lady with yellow to brown skin with an edema on her face and legs, showed a number of scattered white, undetached, oral lesions on the floor of her mouth, lateral margins of tongue and buccal mucosae (Figure 4.3). A bad smell was easily detected and had a characteristic fish-like odor.

Q1 Which disease(s) below is/are associated with this fish odor?

A Uncontrolled diabetes mellitus

B Intestinal obstruction

C Kidney insufficiency

D Phenylketonurea

E Alcoholic ketoacidosis

Answers:

A No

B No

C Kidney insufficiency is the cause. Its failure is associated with high blood and saliva urea and nitrogen concentration. Degradation of these components release a number of volatile gases causing the characteristic uremic fish-like odor which was reinforced by the xerostomia, a common finding in patients with kidney failure.

D No

E No

Comments: A great number of diseases are associated with bad breath, but the type of halitosis could be an indicator of certain diseases. A fruity odor is detected among patients with diabetes I or II and in alcoholic ketoacidosis; mouse odor in phenylketonurea and fish or fecal odor are commonly accompanied with kidney diseases or intestinal obstruction respectively.

Q2 Which other factors apart from urea can participate in fishy breath among patients with chronic kidney diseases (CKDs)?

A Reduced flow rate

B Type of dialysis treatment

C Duration (acute vs. chronic)

D Poor oral hygiene status

E Electrolyte imbalance

Answers:

A Reduced salivary flow rate (stimulated and unstimulated) is often found in CKDs. This hyposalivation allows the accumulation of sulfur producing

bacteria within the mouth that are capable of producing urea, the basic component of fish odor.
- **B** No
- **C** No
- **D** Poor oral hygiene allows the accumulation of a number of bacteria, alters the pH of the biofilm matrix and causes tooth decay and gingival disease. All of these factors play an indirect role in halitosis production.
- **E** No

Comments: Halitosis is related to the severity and not to the duration or type of dialysis (peritoneal vs. hemodialysis). Electrolyte imbalance is a common finding but does not seem to play a role in halitosis.

Q3 Which is/or are the main component(s) of fish malodor?
- **A** Ketones
- **B** Cholines
- **C** Methylamines
- **D** Acetone
- **E** Carbon dioxide

Answers:
- **A** No
- **B** No
- **C** Methylamines (mono, di, or tri) are considered as the major components of uremic toxins which are poorly removed with dialysis and play an important role in the production of fish odor.
- **D** No
- **E** No

Comments: Acetone and other ketones are products of fatty metabolism in patients with uncontrolled diabetes where the metabolism of glucose is impaired due to low insulin synthesis. Carbon dioxide is the major gas component of exhaled air and altered in various conditions or diseases but has never been linked with fish odor.

Case 4.4

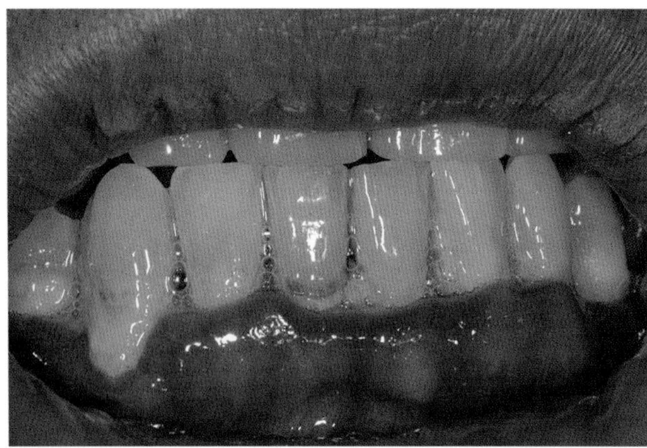

Figure 4.4

CO: A 23-year-old man presented with painful gums and bad breath.

HPC: His gums had been sore over the last ten days and associated with sialorrhea, metallic taste and bad breath.

PMH: This man had no serious medical problems, but his diet was inadequate and poor in proteins and fresh vegetables/fruits. He had lost his job last year and since then started to smoke more than 30 cigarettes daily.

OE: Erythematous gingivae with necrotic interdental papillae covered with whitish slough (Figure 4.4). The gingivae were sore on probing and associated with sialorrhea, metallic taste and bad fecal breath. No other lesions were found in his mouth and other mucosae apart from a mild cervical (sub-mental/maxillary) lymphadenitis.

Q1 What is the cause of his bad breath?
- **A** Smoking
- **B** Chronic gingivitis
- **C** Acute necrotizing gingivitis
- **D** Malnutrition
- **E** Plasma cell gingivitis

Answers:
- **A** No
- **B** No
- **C** Acute necrotizing gingivitis is the cause of this condition, and is characterized by painful gums and inter-dental papillae necrosis, both being associated with metallic taste and halitosis.
- **D** No
- **E** No

Comments: Oral malodor in young patients can be chronic or acute and seems to be related to local causes rather than systemic diseases. Among the local causes, oral infections and particularly of gingivae (gingivitis) and throat (pharyngitis); neglected mouth due to poor OH or bad habits like smoking , drinking and excessive diet are included. Some but not all the types of gingivitis have been associated with halitosis. Plasma cell gingivitis is characterized by accumulation of mature plasma cells in the free and attached gingivae, but is not associated with interdental necrosis or halitosis. Chronic gingivitis and smoking are often associated with chronic and not with acute halitosis as seen in this man;

therefore are easily excluded. Malnutrition causes degradation of fat and release of ketones which are responsible for halitosis as long as the malnutrition lasts. His poor diet was recorded since the day of his job loss and is therefore is not a recent cause of halitosis.

Q2 Which other conditions are associated with this gingival condition?

- **A** Diabetes, mild
- **B** Drug (heroin) addiction
- **C** HIV-AIDS +ve
- **D** Vitamin deficiency
- **E** Respiratory diseases

Answers:

- **A** No
- **B** Patients addicted to heroin and other drugs have neglected oral hygiene, which is the main predisposition factor for the development of acute necrotizing gingivitis (ANG).
- **C** Immunodeficiencies caused by HIV viruses are often associated with a number of oral conditions including ANG, especially when the number of circulated CD4 lymphocyte count is lower than 200 cells/μL in their bloods.
- **D** Deficiency of various vitamins, especially B12 and C due to malnutrition seems to play an important role in ANG and other periodontal diseases by affecting DNA synthesis, cellular maturation and immunity.
- **E** No

Comments: Although smoking is a causative factor for both respiratory and periodontal diseases including ANG, ANG tends to appear among younger patients with poor oral hygiene or uncontrolled severe diabetes mellitus or with psychological stress and immune-suppression. Chronic respiratory diseases affect older patients, are progressive and can jeopardize the patient's life but not provoke the development of this type of gingivitis.

Q3 The microbiota pathogens of ANUG are:

- **A** *Treponema* spp.
- **B** *Fusobacterium* spp.
- **C** *Selenomonas* spp.
- **D** *Streptococcus viridans*
- **E** *Lactobacillus acidophilus*

Answers:

- **A** *Treponema* species are a group of spiral-shaped bacteria that play a role in the pathogenesis of several diseases including syphilis (*Trep. pallidum*); periodontal and pulp diseases (*Trep. denticole* and *Trep. lecithinolyticum*).
- **B** Fusobacteria are anaerobic Gram −ve, non-spurring, rod-shaped bacilli, inhabitants of the oropharynx which cause several human diseases such as ANG and other periodontal diseases, skin atypical ulcerations and thrombophlebitis (Lemierre syndrome).
- **C** Selenomonas are anaerobic, Gram −ve, curved or crescent-shaped rods that are isolated mainly from human oral cavity and play a crucial role in ANUG and other periodontal diseases.
- **D** No
- **E** No

Comments: *Streptococcus viridans* belong to a large group of Gram +ve bacteria that are isolated within the oral cavity and are mainly related to caries and not to periodontal diseases. *Lactobacillus acidophilus* is also a Gram +ve bacterium, but is part of the vaginal microbiota and does not play a role in the pathogenesis of ANUG.

Case 4.5

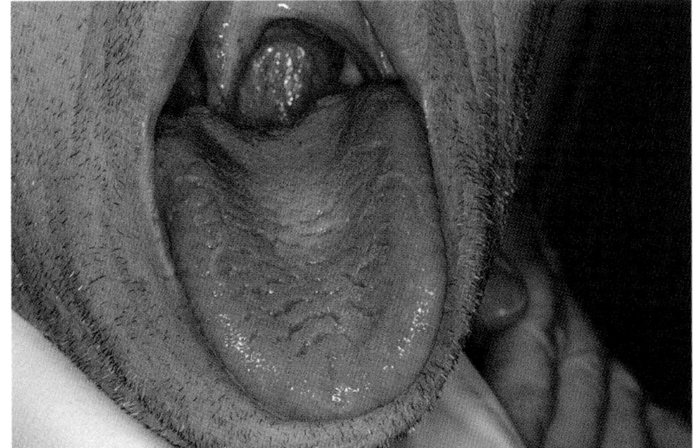

Figure 4.5

CO: A 46-year-old man presented complaining of bad smell and breath over the last one and a half years.

HPC: According to the patient, his bad breath was first noticed during the period of his divorce, and became more severe during the last six months. His halitosis was constant during the day, easily noticed by him but not by his close relatives. At the same time, body odor problems were reported. Both complaints gave him serious concerns about meeting with other people at his job.

PMH: He had no serious medical problems apart from being carcinophobic, as he lost his best friend from a lung carcinoma five years ago. He was not under any medicine uptake and never a smoker or drinker.

OE: Physical examination revealed a healthy middle-aged man with no obvious respiratory or gastroenterology problems. His mouth was in a good condition, with a complete dentition having a few fillings but no caries, healthy gingivae and absence of serious oral diseases (Figure 4.5). Breathing his exhaled air from his mouth by closing his nose did not reveal bad breath. Smelling common odors did not reveal any disturbances.

Q1 What was the cause of the patient's halitosis?

- **A** Early morning halitosis
- **B** Halitophobia
- **C** Smoking
- **D** Drug-induced
- **E** Inadequate oral hygiene

Answers:

- **A** No
- **B** The fear of having bad breath (halitophobia) was the cause, despite that no one else could notice it. This halitosis is present all day, slightly improved during tooth-brushing or eating chewing-gum, causing the patient to brush his teeth and chewing-gum many times during the day.
- **C** No
- **D** No
- **E** No

Comments: All the other causes of bad breath are easily detected by the people close to the patient, but this did not happen in this case. The early morning halitosis appears in healthy patients only in early mornings, but disappears with teeth brushing or eating breakfast. The absence of smoking or drug use together with the patient's good oral hygiene confirms the fear of non-existing halitosis.

Q2 What other symptoms accompanied this breath disturbance?

- **A** Metallic taste
- **B** Burning sensation
- **C** Sense of xerostomia
- **D** Stomatodynia
- **E** Pruritus

Answers:

- **A** Taste alteration like metallic taste is a common symptom in patients with severe anxiety, and especially in those with halitophobia.
- **B** Burning sensation is part of the burning mouth syndrome and often appears together with the delusion of bad breath.
- **C** The sense but not the presence of dry mouth is a common finding in patients under severe stress, depression, and halitophobia.
- **D** Stomatodynia is a clinical complaint of patients with severe depression and anxiety and sometimes comes together with halitophobia.
- **E** Pruritus is a chronic itching of the skin of face and body that is caused by a number of factors among which anxiety plays an important role and is sometimes accompanied with halitophobia.

Q3 Which other conditions have been linked with this condition?

- **A** Hypochondria
- **B** Brain tumor
- **C** Obsessive compulsive syndrome
- **D** Olfactory reference syndrome
- **E** Parkinson's disease

Answers:

- **A** Hypochondria is a somatic symptom disorder characterized by a persistent fear of having an undiagnosed disease which sometimes could cause bad breath.
- **B** No
- **C** This disorder is characterized by chronic, uncontrollable thoughts (i.e. worry about bad breath or fear of germs) and continuously repeated behaviors.
- **D** Olfactory reference syndrome is a psychiatric condition which involves a false belief of an existing body odor that is offensive to other individuals.
- **E** No

Comments: Both Parkinson's disease and brain tumors cause existing and not hallucinated bad breath, as it is easily detected by other people as a result of xerostomia, poor oral hygiene and main treatment side effects (drugs or surgery).

Case 4.6

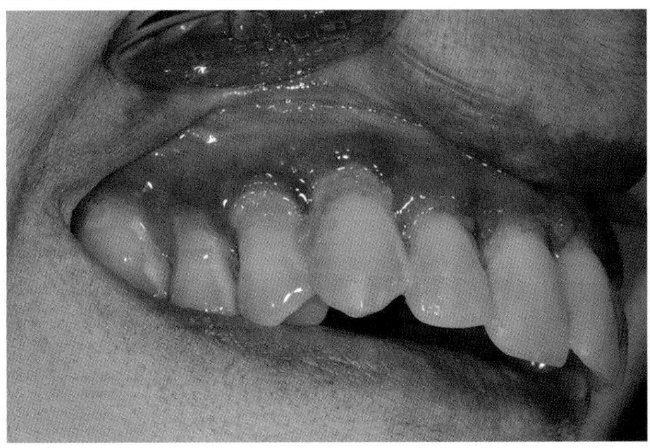

Figure 4.6

CO: A 67-year-old woman was presented with multiple bullae on her mouth which could easily break and leave painful ulcerations and bad breath as well.

HPC: The oral lesions appeared one year ago, as flaccid small bullae on the floor of the mouth and buccal mucosae which were easily broken with mastication, thus leaving scattered painful ulcerations. These lesions were accompanied by bad breath.

PMH: Chronic lymphocytic leukemia was diagnosed two months ago and partially responded to two courses of a combined chemotherapy with fludarabine, cyclophosphamide, and rituximab together with plasmapheresis.

OE: Multiple superficial erosions and not intact bullae were found on her palate, floor of the mouth and buccal mucosae. Her gingivae were erythematous, swollen, and bled with probing (Figure 4.6). Nikolsky sign was positive as a small bulla which appeared with gingival rubbing, but is easily broken with slight pressure. Her oral hygiene was poor, causing periodontal problems and caries in her remaining teeth. Gingival biopsy revealed acantholysis at the lower epithelial layers with intra-epithelial bulla formation and positive immune-fluorescence (direct and indirect). The bad breath like rotten fruit was obvious and remained unchanged over the days.

Q1 Which is the main cause of her bad breath?
- **A** Pemphigus vegetans
- **B** Paraneoplastic pemphigus
- **C** Benign mucous membrane pemphigoid
- **D** Caries
- **E** Periodontitis

Answers:
- **A** No
- **B** Paraneoplastic pemphigus was the cause of halitosis. This bad breath was attributed to excessive volatile gas production from numerous pathogenic bacteria which grew within the inflamed oral ulcerations in this woman with a positive history of hematological malignancy.
- **C** No
- **D** No
- **E** No

Comments: The halitosis from pemphigus vulgaris, pemphigoid, or paraneoplastic lesions is indistinguishable and the diagnosis of the responsible bullous disorder should be based on the patient's clinical and histological characteristics, immunological profile and association or not with serious diseases. The bad breath was also reinforced by the patient's chronic periodontitis, caries, and inadequate tooth brushing.

Q2 Which of the neoplasms below is mostly related with this bullous condition?
- **A** Carcinomas
- **B** Non-Hodgkin lymphoma (NHL)
- **C** Thymoma
- **D** Sarcomas
- **E** Melanomas

Answers:
- **A** No
- **B** NHL is the most frequent hematologic neoplasm that is associated with paraneoplastic pemphigus.
- **C** No
- **D** No
- **E** No

Comments All these tumors usually preexist the oral lesions in paraneoplastic pemphigus, with a declining association starting with NHL, followed by a chronic lymphocytic leukemia, carcinomas, sarcomas, and least likely, melanomas.

Q3 Which auto-antibodies (abs) are characteristics of a paraneoplastic pemphigus?
- **A** Desmoglein 1 abs
- **B** Desmoglein 3 abs
- **C** Anti-smooth muscles abs

D Anti-neutrophil cytoplasmic abs
E Plakins (envo; peri; desmo) abs

Answers:
A No
B Desmoglein 3 rather than 1 Abs have been implicated with the pathogenesis of paraneoplastic pemphigus.
C No
D No
E Envoplakins (210 kDa); periplakins (190 kDa) and desmoplakins (250 kDa) play a crucial role in combination with cellular immunity in the pathogenesis of paraneoplastic pemphigus.

Comments: Auto abs against desmoglein 1 are detected in pemphigus foliaceus but rarely in paraneoplastic. Anti-smooth muscle and anti-neutrophils cytoplasmic abs are not found in paraneoplastic pemphigus, but are pathognomonic of autoimmune liver disease and necrotizing vessel vasculitides.

Case 4.7

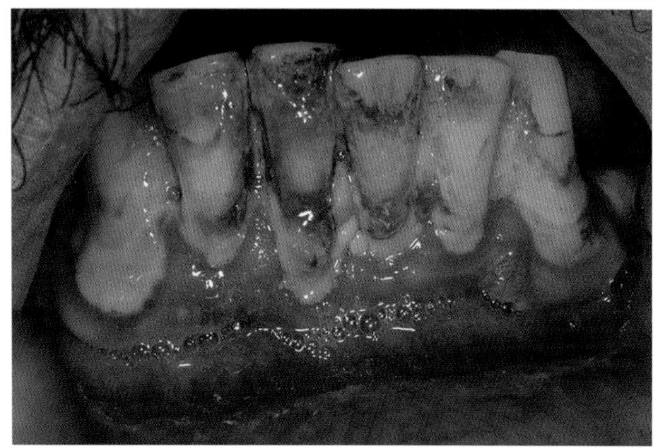

Figure 4.7

CO: A 37-year-old man presented for an evaluation of his repellent odor.

HPC: His breath had a strong acetone like odor and was first perceived two months ago by his therapist who tried to help him to stop his drinking habit.

PMH: His medical history did not reveal any serious diseases or drug abuse apart from alcoholism that was diagnosed five years ago, and treated with counseling and use disulfiram (Antabuse) drug over the last two months.

OE: The oral examination revealed a neglected dentition with missing teeth, decays, and external stains as well as mature plaque and food debris on most of his remaining teeth whose gingivae were inflamed (Figure 4.7). A strong acetone-like odor was easily noticed and remained unchanged during his examination.

Q1 Which is the main cause of his halitosis?
A Alcohol overuse
B Poor oral hygiene
C Caries
D Gingival disease
E Drug-induced

Answers:
A No
B No
C No
D No
E Dusilfiram-induced halitosis is the answer. This drug is used to stop alcoholism by inhibiting acetaldehyde dehydrogenase and inducing a hangover effect after alcohol consumption. The metabolism of this drug enhances the acetone concentration in the blood which is finally transferred to the pulmonary alveoli and excreted into exhaled air, thus producing the characteristic odor.

Comments: Halitosis induced by periodontitis has a chronic, constant fruity odor in contrast with the acetone-like odor induced by dusilfiram, while the halitosis from poor oral hygiene, caries, and alcohol use are temporary and can disappear with brushing, restorations, and withdrawal of alcohol.

Q2 Which other drugs are responsible for unpleasant odor when are metabolized?
A Penicillamine
B Valsartan
C Paraldehyde
D Tetracyclines
E Dimethyl sulfoxide

Answers:
A Penicillamine is the drug of choice for rheumatoid arthritis which releases malodor components, rich in hydrogen sulfide, during its degradation. These components are responsible for rotten egg-like halitosis.
B No
C Paraldehyde is used intravenously in epileptic crisis and is related to pungent odor.
D No

E Dimethyl sulfoxide or DMSO is an anti-inflammatory and antioxidant drug with good results in interstitial cystitis. This drug is metabolized into dimethyl sulfide which is a stable malodor component in the blood and released into exhaled air, causing a garlic odor.

Comments: Tetracyclines are widely used antibiotics for various bacterial infections including acne, and sometimes cause a metallic taste. Valsartan is an angiotensin II blocker that is used for hypertension, causing a dry mouth but not bad breath.

Q3 Which drug components are related to garlic-like odor?

- **A** Methyl mercaptan
- **B** Hydrogen sulfate
- **C** Ammonia
- **D** Allyl mercaptan
- **E** Allyl methyl sulfide

Answers:

- **A** No
- **B** No
- **C** No
- **D** Allyl mercaptan is a small molecule in the blood, which in adequate concentration in the alveolar air, can cause a garlic odor.
- **E** Allyl methyl sulfide is an organosulfur compound with the chemical formula CH_2-$CHCH_2SCH_3$, which releases garlic odor when it is metabolized.

Comments: Drugs containing hydrogen sulfate, methyl mercaptan or ammonia when released in the exhaled air give a characteristic odor of rotten fruit, pungent, and a pleasant odor respectively.

Case 4.8

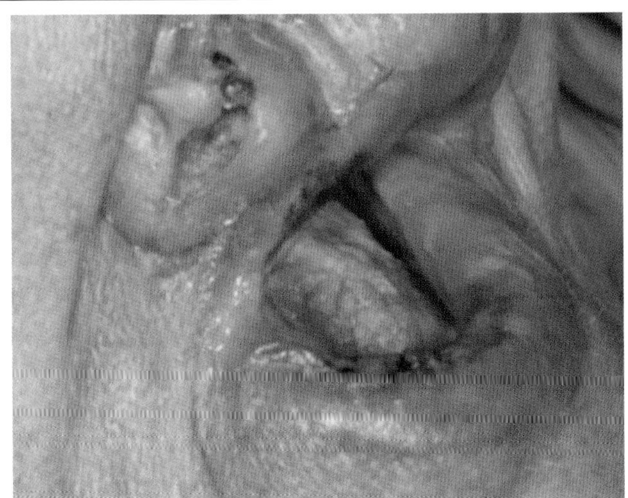

Figure 4.8

CO: An 81-year-old man presented with severe pain in his mouth, and bad breath after a course of chemo-radiotherapy for carcinoma of his palate–anterior gingivae.

HPC: The pain started after the surgical removal of a carcinoma from his palate six months ago and worsened from the end of the third week of chemo-radiotherapy. Together with his pain, bad breath like rotten fruit was detected, remaining unchanged during the course of his treatment.

PMH: He was an old man with cachexia due to his recent treatment for an extensive oral carcinoma, while his hypertension and respiratory failure was controlled with drugs and ceasing smoking.

OE: His examination revealed a large indurate ulcer with raised margins on the skin above the right corner of his mouth (Figure 4.8). The ulcer was deep and extended to the adjacent alveolar mucosa and hard palate, and infiltrated facial skin close to his right nostril. Some superficial ulcerations covered most of his oral mucosa (mucositis grade III) together with xerostomia, halitosis, and difficulties in consuming food and drinks.

Q1 Which is/are the possible cause/s of the patient's halitosis?

- **A** Resistant carcinoma
- **B** Mucositis
- **C** Xerostomia
- **D** Malnutrition
- **E** Mouth breathing

Answers:

- **A** His extensive oral cancer and local necrosis–sepsis allow a number of anaerobic bacteria to grow and produce strong volatile gases which are easily detected by the patient and his close relatives.

B Mucositis causes difficulties in brushing his remaining teeth, and allows the accretion of halitosis-induced pathogenic bacteria.

C Xerostomia occurs with halitosis in various ways. Oral dryness assists the growth of various pathogenic halitosis bacteria, by reducing the mechanical washing–cleaning action of saliva or eliminating various antimicrobial components (enzymes, immunoglobulins). Xerostomia was seen and induced by the damage of the salivary glands (minor and major) with radiotherapy and boosted with the reduced fluid consumption due to patient's mucositis-induced dysphagia.

D The malnutrition of this patient, due to his eating and swallowing problems from mucositis, causes his liver to break down the lipids and proteins for energy and release of ketones into the blood. When these substances reach the lungs, they are exhaled into the air, producing breath smelling of rotten fruit.

E No

Comments: Mouth breathing causes a temporary oral dryness and halitosis that easily go with fluid and food consumption and teeth brushing.

Q2 What are the other causes of cachexia apart from oral cancer?

A Acquired immunodeficiency syndrome
B Diabetes mellitus
C Anorexia nervosa
D Kwashiorkor
E Hyperthyroidism

Answers:

A Patients with full-blown AIDS are often characterized by loss of weight, muscle atrophy, fatigue, weakness, and loss of appetite (typical characteristics of cachexia).

B No

C No

D No

E No

Comments: Diseases such as uncontrolled diabetes mellitus and hyperthyroidism are characterized by weight loss due to increased metabolism of fat and muscles. Anorexia nervosa is a typical example of marasmus; a condition characterized by energy deficiency due to severe malnutrition, while in Kwashiorkor, the malnutrition involves only protein intake.

Q3 Which pathogens are isolated in oral mucositis lesions?

A *Candida* spp.
B *Pseudomonas aeruginosa*
C *Herpes simplex*
D *Mycobacterium ulcerans*
E *Treponema pallidum*

Answers:

A Radio-chemotherapy disrupts the epithelial barrier and alters the host immunity allowing the entrance and growth of *Candida* species such as *albicans*, *glabrata*, *krusei*, and *tropicalis* in mucositis lesions.

A *Pseudomonas aeruginosa* and *Escherichia coli* are among the Gram-negative bacteria which grow in increased numbers in oral mucositis lesions.

B Alterations in a patient's immunity allow the growth of fungi and viruses like *Candida* and *Herpes* species in oral mucositis.

C No

D No

Comments: Mycobacterium ulcerans is a slowly growing mycobacterium infecting the skin and subcutaneous tissues but not oral mucosa causing non-ulcerated nodules/plaques and ulcerated lesions. *Treponema pallidum* is responsible for ulcerations in syphilis and not in mucositis.

Case 4.9

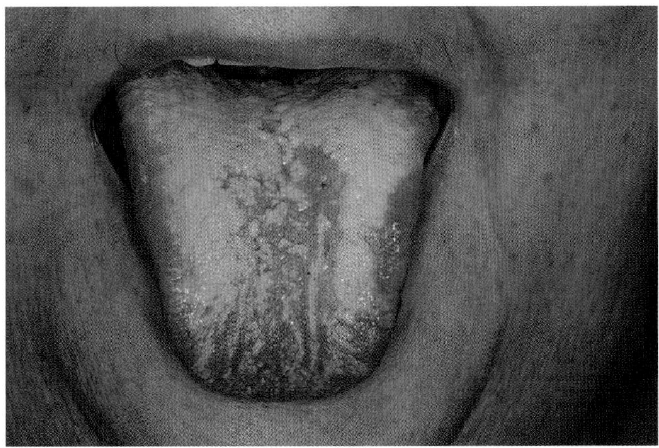

Figure 4.9

CO: A 62-year-old woman was presented for evaluation of her bad breath.

HPC: Her bad breath was first noticed by her husband four days ago, and was more intense in the mornings and slightly improved during eating or brushing her teeth. Her halitosis appeared at the same time with a febrile viral infection of her mouth and throat.

GMH: Diabetes and mild hypertension were her main medical problems and were under control with drugs and daily exercise. Smoking was stopped after an episode of pneumonia last year.

OE: A whitish yellow asymptomatic thick coating was found, on the dorsum of her tongue, which was partially removed with scraping (Figure 4.9) and associated with sore throat, stuffy nose, mild fever (<38 C) and cervical lymphadenitis. Her oral hygiene was inadequate and the patient wore partial ill-fitted dentures. Malodor was noted during examination.

Q1 Which is the main origin of her bad breath?

- **A** Furry or coated tongue
- **B** Stuffy nose
- **C** Mouth breathing
- **D** Fever-induced dehydration
- **E** Bad prostheses

Answers:

- **A** Bad breath was caused mainly by degradation of food debris and necrotic epithelial cells from various anaerobic bacteria that located on the dorsum of the tongue (white coat), found in large quantities in upper respiratory viral infections.
- **B** No
- **C** No
- **D** No
- **E** No

Comments: The oral dehydration facilitates the growth of a number of bacteria, including those responsible for bad breath. However, in this patient, the dehydration was not severe, as the mouth breathing and fever were neither intense nor high. Her poor OH and bad prosthesis caused constant malador, which was not restricted to the period of her febrile illness.

Q2 Which other diseases have similar clinical features with this condition?

- **A** Acute pseudomembranous candidiasis
- **B** Black hairy tongue
- **C** Hairy leukoplakia
- **D** Lichen planus
- **E** Geographic tongue

Answers:

- **A** Acute pseudomembranous candidiasis, or thrush, also develops white lesions on the dorsum of the tongue which are easily scraped off, but cause a tingling or burning sensation and leaving erythematous areas underneath.
- **B** No
- **C** No
- **D** No
- **E** No

Comments: Other white lesions on the dorsum of the tongue are persistent as in lichen planus and hairy leukoplakia, or transient as in geographic tongue. However all the above lesions are not associated with halitosis and have different symptomatology and clinical features. The black hairy tongue lesion differs in the color and the length of the filiform papillae, as the patient's tongue coat is whitish and not black, while the length of the filiform papillae is normal.

Q3 Which other conditions are associated with similar furry tongue lesions?

- **A** Scarlet fever
- **B** Cold
- **C** Sjogren syndrome
- **D** Chronic pneumonia
- **E** Hyperplastic candidiasis

Answers:

- **A** Scarlet fever is an acute infection from *Streptococcus* A bacterium and characterized by white coating on the tongue, gradually changing into a strawberry-like appearance due to the inflammation of taste papillae and associated with sore throat, fever, swollen glands as well as a generalized sandpaper skin rash.
- **B** Cold is an acute viral infection of the upper respiratory system that is characterized by sore throat, runny nose, white furry tongue and accompanied with cough, fever, muscle aches and general fatigue as well.
- **C** No
- **D** No
- **E** No

Comments: Sjogren syndrome, chronic pneumonia, and hyperplastic candidiasis are often associated with furry tongue but with different etiology clinical picture or and duration.

Case 4.10

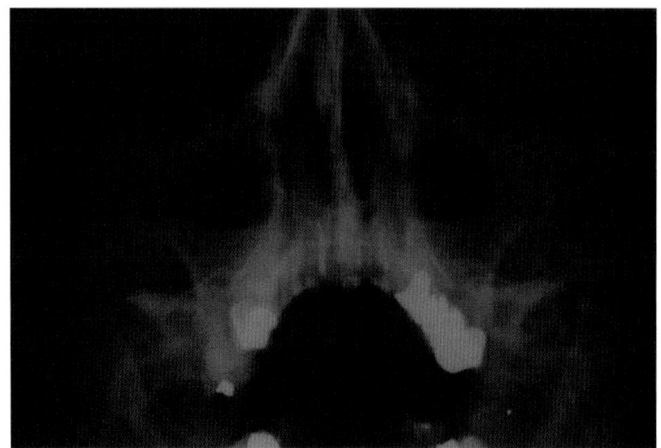

Figure 4.10

CO: A 58-year-old woman presented for an evaluation of some pain from her upper teeth and bad breath.

HPC: The pain was located at the upper molars area and characterized as a constant, dull ache without exacerbations from various cold or hot stimuli. It appeared gradually after a severe cold infection three weeks ago and became associated with a partial loss of smell and taste, as well as bad breath. This was more obvious in the mornings, slightly improved with teeth and mouth cleaning, but remained unchanged with eating.

PMH: She was an overweight lady with no serious medical problems apart from a few episodes of hay fever in spring which were controlled with antihistamine sprays. She was not under any drugs and only a few paracetamol tablets were taken for a flu infection three weeks ago. She had never been a smoker, drinker, or consumer of spicy foods.

OE: The oral examination revealed oral mucosa and dentition in good condition. Despite her heavy restorations (crowns and fillings) her teeth responded well to pulp vitality tests. A slight tenderness around her molars together with stuffy nose, nasal drip secretions and slight cervical lymphadenopathy were seen. A rotten-like bad breath was detected during the examination. Laboratory investigations revealed hematological and biochemical tests within normal values but sinus X-rays revealed opacification of the lower third part of both maxillary sinuses (Figure 4.10). The nasal septum and the rest of the visualized sinuses and teeth were normal. A similar episode of pain was reported one year ago and gone with wide broad antibiotics.

Q1 What is the cause of her bad breath?

- **A** Cystic fibrosis
- **B** Fungal sinusitis
- **C** Foreign bodies in maxillary sinuses
- **D** Sinus malignancies
- **E** Chronic sinusitis

Answers:

- **A** No
- **B** No
- **C** No
- **D** No
- **E** Chronic sinusitis is the cause. Chronic sinusitis is characterized by a chronic infection of the sinuses causing an increased production of mucus with bad odor, which drains down the back of the throat. There, the odor of the infected mucus is intermingled with the exhaled air and causes malodor.

Comments: Halitosis is also detected in deep fungal infections (mainly from *Aspergillus* or *Mucor* species) and various sinus malignancies, but these affect a certain group of patients (with immunodeficiencies or with uncontrolled diabetes) and is associated with severe bony and soft tissue destruction. These features are not seen in this patient. Cystic fibrosis is often the cause of antrum infection, but in contrast to this case, is associated with other endo-bronchial infections, pancreatic insufficiency and intestinal malabsorption. Foreign body in the antrum is usually seen only in one antrum and is often associated with head trauma during surgical or patients' manipulations.

Q2 Which is the major complication of an untreated chronic sinusitis for patient's life?

- **A** Infections of surrounding bone or soft tissues
- **B** Vision problems
- **C** Loss of smell and/or taste
- **D** Meningitis
- **E** Increased risk of sinus malignancy

Answers:

- **A** No
- **B** No
- **C** No
- **D** Meningitis is very rare, but is the most dangerous complication and caused by the extension of the antral infection to the fluid that surrounds the brain.
- **E** No

Comments: Uncontrolled infection of the maxillary antrum spreads to the adjacent soft tissues or to the bone causing cellulitis or osteomyelitis respectively. In some cases, infections of the olfactory and optic nerve cause partial or total smell or even vision problems. However, none of the above complications jeopardize the patient's life.

Q3 Which other cause(s) apart from chronic sinusitis is/are not associated with post-nasal discharge?

- **A** Allergic rhinitis
- **B** Acute sinusitis
- **C** Cold or flu infection
- **D** Gastroesophageal reflux disease (GERD)
- **E** Medications

Answers:

- **A** No
- **B** No
- **C** No
- **D** Gastroesophageal reflux is characterized by acid fluid reflux from the stomach to the throat, leaving the patient with a sense of a lump or post-nasal sour secretion.
- **E** No

Comments: Allergic rhinitis, acute sinusitis and flu are characterized by increased production of mucus from the glands of the nose or antra, giving the sense of accumulation of fluid in the throat. Rarely, drugs such as anti-hypertensives and birth control drugs cause an increased thin clear secretion dropping from the back of nose.

5

Muscle Deficits (Trismus/Paralysis)

Muscular deficits are common and occur at all ages and cause weakness, pain or even paralysis of the body muscles to such a degree that it may affect the patient's quality of life. Muscular deficits may be congenital and appear at an early age, as is seen in muscular dystrophies, or at a later age, when it is known as acquired. The acquired conditions may be due to increased muscular contraction or overuse due to local trauma, infiltration of muscles with inflammatory or neoplasmatic cells, as well as new fibrous tissue. Over-contraction of the masticatory muscles leads to reduced mouth opening (trismus or lockjaw) and temporal or permanent weakness of the head muscles, especially those controlling facial expression or tongue movements, leading to facial palsy or hypoglossal paralysis (Figure 5.0a and b).

Table 5 shows the most common and important causes of muscle dysfunction.

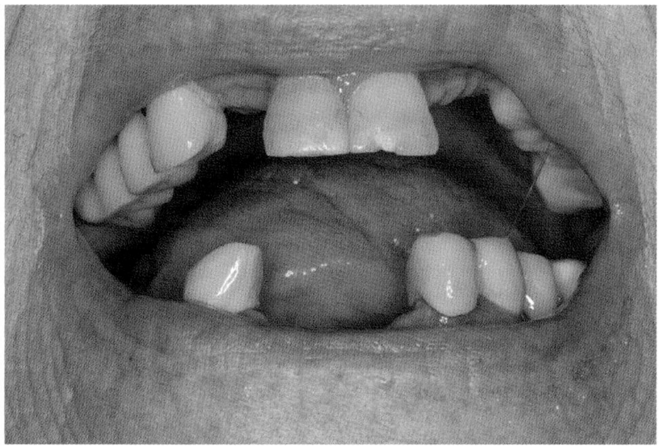

Figure 5.0a Trismus.

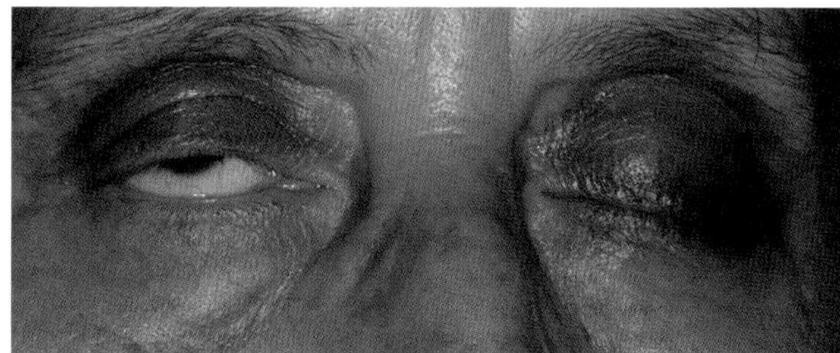

Figure 5.0b Facial palsy.

Clinical Guide to Oral Diseases, First Edition. Dimitris Malamos and Crispian Scully.

Companion website: www.wiley.com/go/malamos/clinical_guide

Table 5 Common and important conditions related to muscle dysfunctions.

Motor defects

- Caused by lesions in the brain above or below motor nerve nucleus
  - Vascular
    - Stroke
    - Ischemia
    - Kawasaki disease
  - Neoplasia
    - Cerebral tumor
  - Injuries
    - Cerebral palsy
- Peripheral nerves
  - Related to the nerve
    - Facial palsy due to nerve injuries
    - Bell's palsy
    - Moebius syndrome
    - Diabetes
    - Connective tissue diseases
    - Reiter's syndrome
    - Viral infections
      - Herpes
      - Retroviruses
      - Guillain-Barré syndrome

Table 5 (Continued)

  - Related to the adjacent tissues of the nerve
    - Bacteria; infections
      - Otitis media
      - Botulism
      - Leprosy
      - Lyme disease
    - Middle ear diseases
      - Cholesteatoma
      - Malignancy
      - Mastoiditis
    - Parotid diseases
      - Trauma
      - Tumors
    - Granulomatous diseases
      - Crohn's disease
      - Orofacial granulomatosa
      - Melkersson-Rosenthal syndrome
      - Sarcoidosis (Heerfordt syndrome)
- Muscles
    - Myopathies
    - Trismus
    - Paralysis

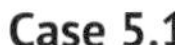

Case 5.1

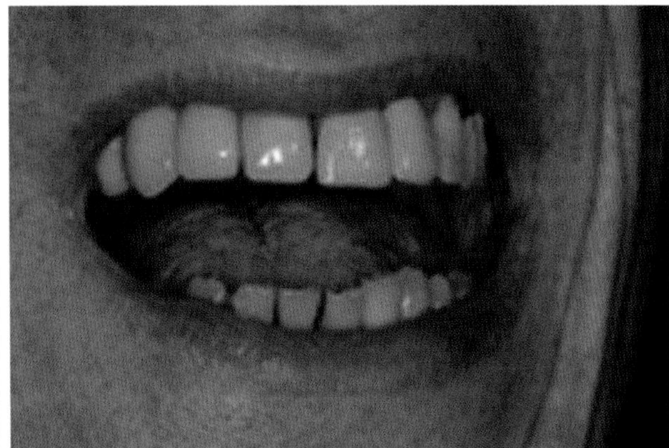

Figure 5.1

CO: A 42-year-old man presented with trismus over the last five days.

HPC: The problem started the day after an episode of severe pain and swelling of his lower second right decayed molar. It appeared as a painful reduction of mouth opening (trismus) which gradually reached a maximum opening of 18 mm.

PMH: His medical history revealed no serious medical problems such as connective tissue diseases, allergies, drug use or surgery apart from a tonsillectomy at the age of 10 as well as an appendectomy at the age of 25. His dental history revealed numerous caries due to high sugar consumption, which were fully restored with large fillings. Local trauma had not been recently reported.

OE: A diminished mouth opening of 18 mm was measured between the central upper and lower incisors (Figure 5.1), recorded and associated with pain from a periodontal abscess on the second severely decayed second lower right molar and in the ipsilateral temporomandibular joint (TMJ), The swelling was diffuse and extended into the floor of the mouth, towards the lingual tonsils causing difficulties during the full mouth examination while the pain was constant, increased and exacerbated with hot stimulus and mouth opening. The right sub-mandibular lymph nodes were enlarged and sensitive in palpation.

Q1 What is the cause of trismus?
- **A** Odontogenic infection
- **B** TMJ disorder
- **C** Local trauma
- **D** Tetanus
- **E** Rheumatoid arthritis

Answers:
- **A** Odontogenic infection is the cause. Trismus is the result of a bacterial infection that spreads from the necrotic pulp, periodontal and pericoronal tissues into the masticatory space. It therefore requires immediate therapy, otherwise the infection will spread and may cause cervical cellulitis or mediastinitis.
- **B** No
- **C** No
- **D** No
- **E** No

Comments: The trismus differs in clinical characteristics of various conditions like TMJ dysfunction, rheumatoid arthritis, tetanus disorders and local trauma. Firstly, in TMJ disorders, the trismus is associated with pain and with no signs of inflammation on the soft tissues around the suspected tooth, while in arthritis, the inflammation is found in a number of joints except for the TMJ, and is associated with morning stiffness. Tetanus or post-traumatic trismus is not the cause as the spasm is found in a number of muscles apart from masseter or not associated with history of either dental and facial trauma or recent surgery.

Q2 What is/are the characteristic(s) associated with a trismus?
- **A** Smiling difficulties
- **B** Pain
- **C** Fever
- **D** Chewing or swallowing problems
- **E** Cramping jaws

Answers:
- **A** No
- **B** Pain is present and always elicited with jaw movements to a wider mouth opening.
- **C** No
- **D** The chewing or swallowing process is difficult due to the constriction of the masticatory muscles.
- **E** Jaw cramping is commonly seen temporarily or permanently and can affect several activities of daily living.

Comments: Fever comes usually together with trismus in infections (odontogenic or not). The masticatory muscle's constriction participates in trismus while the muscles of the facial expression play a secondary role, as seen in facial palsy.

Q3 Which of the facial space infections do not play a role in trismus?
- **A** Perimandibular spaces
- **B** Masticatory spaces
- **C** Mental spaces
- **D** Submasseteric spaces
- **E** Fascia lata

Answers:
- **A** No
- **B** No
- **C** No
- **D** No
- **E** Fascia lata is the deep fascia of the thigh, and its role is to encircle muscles of the thigh in order to be bound together tightly.

Comments: The perimandibular (submandibular/lingual or mental) together with masticatory spaces (submasseteric, pterygomandibular and temporal) play an important role in the transmission of an odontogenic infection into the head, thus causing trismus.

Case 5.2

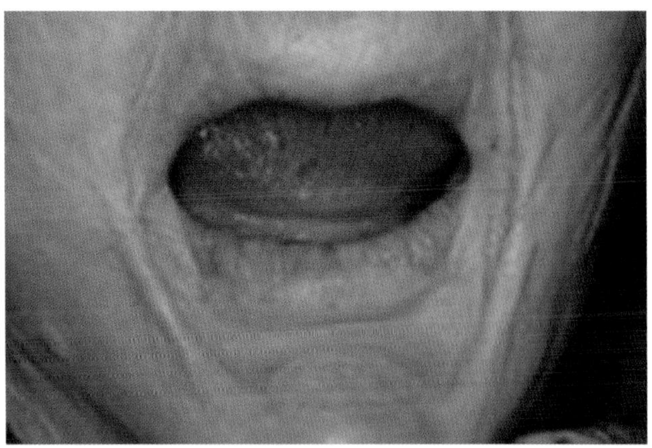

Figure 5.2

CO: A 72-year-old lady presented with difficulties with her dentures due to a limited mouth opening.

HPC: The problem became obvious when the patient lost her last remaining lower molars and had to replace her partial ones with a new full denture. The new denture did not fit properly due to her thin alveolar mucosa and restricted mouth opening.

PMH: Mild hypertension and spine osteoarthritis were controlled with exercise, special diet and drug uptake (valsartan and NSAIDs). A case of extensive facial skin burn was reported from an accident with boiling water during childhood.

OE: The examination revealed a lady with a mask-like face due to burn scarring. Her oral mucosa was normal apart from an atrophic lower alveolar mucosa, which was partially ulcerated due to a badly fitted denture. The facial skin was anelastic, causing her to have a distorted facial expression. While any local infection was not evident, a limited, slightly painful, mouth opening of 16 mm (Figure 5.2) was recorded early in the morning but reached the 20 mm during the day with jaw movements and speaking.

Q1 What is the cause of her trismus?
- **A** Burn scarring
- **B** Osteoarthritis
- **C** Post-traumatic ulcerations
- **D** Local infections
- **E** Drug-induced

Answers:
- **A** Burns cause the replacement of the elastic with inelastic fibrous tissues, with a direct effect on tightness of the facial skin and dysfunction of masticatory muscles, resulting in the limitation of mouth opening (trismus).
- **B** No
- **C** No
- **D** No
- **E** No

Comments: Traumatic ulcerations of the soft oral tissues such as in the alveolar mucosa did not cause any severe local infections which could spread into the facial spaces, and thus were not involved with trismus development. Osteoarthritis in the spine and not in the TMJ was reported and the drugs (NSAIDs and valsartan) used did not cause muscle contraction or trismus.

Q2 Which are the available treatments for a facial scar to reduce trismus?
- **A** Scar massage
- **B** Exercise therapy
- **C** Skin moisturizing applicants
- **D** Systemic antibiotics
- **E** Systemic steroids

Answers:
- **A** Scar massage helps the remodeling process by breaking the strong bonds between the fibers and moving the interstitial fluid. It involves cross-friction and myofascial release massage that can apply gentle pressure. The skin and the underlying tissues around scar may also be rubbed with vitamin E or baby oil, or in some cases with stainless instruments in various directions.
- **B** Gentle stretching and flexibility exercises help to remodel the scar tissues.
- **C** Skin moisturizing agents may be creams, ointments, unguents, pastes and oils that contain ingredients such as water, oils, herbal extracts and glycerol. These ingredients are capable of moisturizing and remodeling the scarred tissue by using various rehabilitation techniques.
- **D** No
- **E** No

Comments: Systemic use of steroids and various antibiotics do not prevent or improve scars. Instead, the intra-lesional injection of steroids or antibiotics like bleomycin within the keloid scars can only soften them by decreasing inflammation, increasing breakdown and reducing collagen.

Q3 Which type(s) of facial scarring is/are found in the patient?
- **A** Keloids
- **B** Widespread hypertrophic scarring
- **C** Widespread stretching
- **D** Contractures
- **E** Mature scarring

Answers:
- **A** No
- **B** No
- **C** No
- **D** Contractures are the scars induced by skin burns that are not fully mature, and usually disabling or dysfunctional, as those seen in this lady.
- **E** Mature scars are also seen on the patient's face and characterized by light colored and flat scars around the mouth corners.

Comments: Keloids (linear and hypertrophic), widespread hypertrophic and stretching are characterized by hyperplastic, pruritic scars that are more often seen after a surgery rather than after burns.

Case 5.3

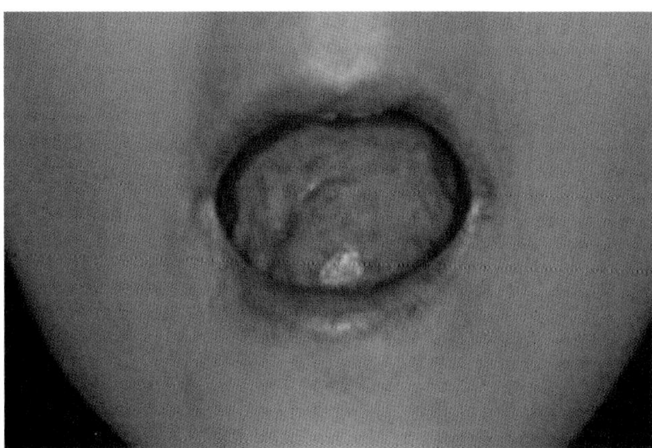

Figure 5.3

CO: A 20-year-old woman was referred for an evaluation of a pain on her upper left wisdom tooth and reduced mouth opening.

HPC: A pain from her upper left decayed wisdom tooth started six days ago and was relieved by putting a cotton enriched with eugenol while trismus appeared two days before her dental examination.

PMH: She suffered from Fanconi anemia since the age of 10, and squamous cell carcinoma of her tongue two years ago. The tumor was surgically removed twice; the first surgery was done two years ago while the second one 14 months later after a relapse. She had never been a smoker or drinker, but used to grind her teeth at night.

OE: A young woman with short stature and hyperpigmented skin showed a reduced mouth opening of 16 mm (Figure 5.3). The oral examination found chronic gingivitis and numerous caries as well as xerostomia together with lingual atrophy of a partially glossectomized tongue. Her upper left wisdom tooth was decayed and vitality tests confirmed the clinical suspicion of having acute pulpitis. No evidence of previous trauma or new tumor recurrence was found.

Q1 What is the cause of her trismus?
- **A** Periodontal infection
- **B** Fanconi anemia
- **C** Oral carcinoma surgery
- **D** TMJ disorder
- **E** Local anesthesia

Answers:
- **A** No
- **B** Fanconi anemia (FA) may play a role as patients with this genetic condition are characterized with microcephaly and microstomia.
- **C** The surgery for the removal of her tongue carcinoma caused some limitation of movements and fibrosis of adjacent tissues leading to the reduced mouth opening.
- **D** No
- **E** No

Comments: The dental infection was not enough to spread into the masticatory muscles and spaces, but it was restricted within the pulp and therefore did not cause trismus. On the other hand, the local anesthesia for the removal of caries from the wisdom teeth was not related with trismus as the trismus was preceded. Other symptoms from a TMJ disorder were not recorded, so this is easily excluded.

Q2 Which is/are the complication/s of trismus to this patient?
- **A** Difficulty of re-examination
- **B** Aspiration difficulties
- **C** Communication problems
- **D** Susceptibility to opportunistic infections
- **E** Increased hemorrhagic tendency

Answers:

- **A** The limited opening makes oral examination difficult, especially in the areas at the back of her tongue and pharynx.
- **B** The surgical removal of her cancer caused reduced tongue control, while trismus caused some chewing and eating difficulties with increased risk of entrance of fluids or pieces of food into the airway (aspiration) provoking thus an aspiration pneumonia.
- **C** Her microstomia and trismus decreased the size of the resonating oral cavity and diminished the vocal quality, resulting in problems in speaking.
- **D** No
- **E** No

Comments: Fanconi anemia but not trismus, is characterized by a progressive bone marrow failure leading to aplastic anemia that is responsible for hemorrhagic lesions like petechiae and ecchymoses, as well as opportunistic infections.

Q3 What are the other manifestations of Fanconi anemia apart from trismus?

- **A** Oral hyperpigmentation
- **B** Dental anomalies
- **C** Desquamative gingivitis
- **D** Oral ulcerations
- **E** Angina bullosa hemorrhagica

Answers:

- **A** Increased pigmentation on the skin (extra-orally) and gingivae and buccal mucosae (intra-orally) are common and also seen in this patient seen.
- **B** Dental anomalies such as microdontia, taurodism, enamel hypoplasia, tooth discoloration, and agenesia have been sporadically reported in patients with FA.
- **C** No
- **D** Atypical and recurrent oral ulcerations are seen in patients with pancytopenia due to FA.
- **E** No

Comments: Although FA anemia affects gingivae causing gingivitis/periodontitis but never desquamative gingivitis. In FA petechiae and ecchymoses are common but not hemorrhagic bullae in the oral mucosa skin and other mucosae.

Case 5.4

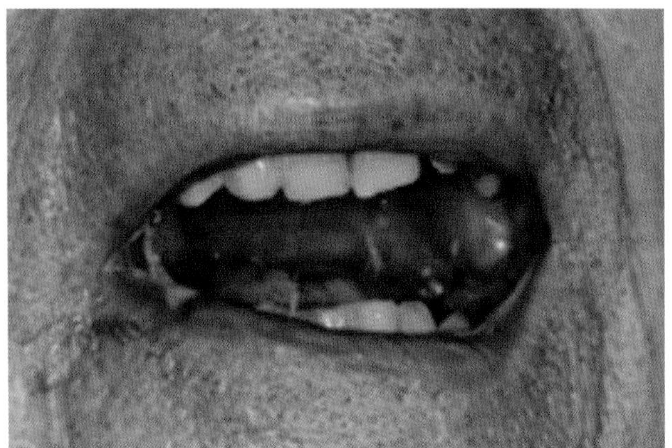

Figure 5.4

CO: A 69-year-old man presented for his weekly check-up during radio-chemotherapy for a carcinoma of his oropharynx, when a reduced mouth opening was detected.

HPC. His mouth opening was 22 mm at the beginning and dropped to 17 mm in width during the fourth week of treatment of his tumor. His trismus was painful and associated with the inflammation of the oral mucosa (mucositis) grade III and very thick, sticky saliva.

PMH: His medical history revealed many episodes of gastritis that were treated with omeprazole and special diet, as well as chronic bronchitis which was treated with O_2, antibiotics and bronchodilators in crisis. An oropharyngeal squamous cell carcinoma (Sca) was diagnosed three months ago in the area behind his right tonsils and was surgically removed, and followed by a supplementary course of 35 sessions of radiotherapy and 5 sessions of cisplatin chemotherapy. He was a heavy smoker (>2 packets of cigarettes) and drinker (>5 glasses of heavy spirit) per day for more than 40 years.

OE: A reduced mouth opening at 17 mm was measured and associated with multiple painful superficial oral ulcerations, especially at the side of his mouth where the radiotherapy was more intense (Figure 5.4). The skin of his neck was erythematous and very dry with signs of desquamation.

Q1 Which is/are the main causes of his trismus?
- **A** Local infiltration from oral cancer
- **B** Radiotherapy side-effects
- **C** Xerostomia
- **D** Surgical intervention
- **E** Mucositis

Answers:
- **A** Oral cancer can infiltrate the masticatory muscles and tissues around the TMJ, causing limitations of jaw movements and trismus.
- **B** Radiotherapy causes the destruction of cancer and adjacent tissues and fibrosis to such a degree that it affects mouth opening. The degree of fibrosis is closely related with the number and dose of radiotherapy sessions.
- **C** No
- **D** The removal of the tumor through surgery and reconstruction of tissues with flaps causes scar formation and limitation of mouth opening.
- **E** The oral pain in mucositis may be so severe that the patient would be afraid to move his mouth, thus deteriorates his mouth opening.

Comments: Xerostomia makes eating or swallowing difficult and aggravates symptoms of mucositis, but does not affect directly trismus. Trismus may be secondarily affected by the degree of mucositis and a secondary infection.

Q2 What are the predisposing factors for trismus development in head and neck carcinoma patients?
- **A** Previous irradiation
- **B** Location of tumor
- **C** Total irradiation dosage
- **D** Patient's age
- **E** Stage of tumor

Answers:
- **A** Previous irradiation increases fibrosis and is one of the causes of trismus in recurrent oral carcinoma patients as the effect of radiation is cumulative.
- **B** Trismus occurs more often in patients who are treated for carcinomas on the base of the tongue, oropharynx, mandible or maxillae and parotid glands, as the field of irradiation covers the masseter, lateral pterygoid and TMJ.
- **C** The increased dose of irradiation above 60 Gr causes trismus as the production of collagen is more rapid and extensive.
- **D** No
- **E** A carcinoma with stage 3 or 4 has a worse prognosis than those with stage 1 or 2, and therefore its treatment is more radical and extensive, causing severe destruction of tissues adjacent to the tumor, more collagen production and consequently more fibrosis leading to trismus.

Comments: The age of patients does not seem to directly affect the presence or not of trismus, but tumors in young patients seem to be more aggressive and their treatment is more intense, causing severe complications including trismus.

Q3 Which is/or are other complications of irradiation of the jaws of patients with head and neck tumors?
- **A** Reduction of jaw movements
- **B** Osteoradionecrosis
- **C** Bone hypovascularity
- **D** Osteopenia
- **E** Fracture

Answers:
- **A** The movements of jaws after irradiation may be impaired due to collagen overproduction and fibrosis of masseter and median pterygoid muscles.
- **B** Osteoradionecrosis is the most important complication affecting both jaws, and causes severe bony necrosis, even many years after radiotherapy.
- **C** Hypovascularity is a common finding due to the destruction of bony vascular tissue from radiation and is one of the factors to participate in osteoradionecrosis formation.
- **D** Osteopenia is temporal and characteristically seen in irradiated bones due to the destruction of osteocytes.
- **E** Excessive osteopenia leads to an increased risk of bone fracture in those areas that are under excessive pressure such as mandibles, and other bones with the highest ratio of trabecular to cortical structure.

Case 5.5

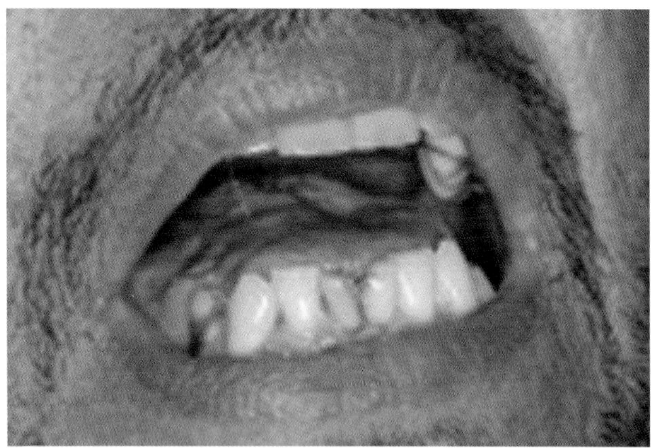

Figure 5.5

CO: A 42-year-old man was referred for an evaluation of his painful limited mouth opening that appeared one day after a fight.

HPC: His mouth was almost locked during the time of examination with the maximum opening to be 12 mm and accompanied with severe pain at the right TMJ and adjacent ear. The pain was sharp, deep and provoked by various mandible movements; it appeared after a blow to his chin during a fight last night.

PMH: His previous medical history was unremarkable despite his unhealthy diet of canteen food and a high consumption of sweets, heavy smoking (>2 packets of cigarettes) and spirits (up to 4 drinks a day).

OE: The physical examination revealed a patient experiencing severe pain with bruises on his chin and edema below his eyes and right TMJ, along with limited jaw movements and reduced mouth opening (Figure 5.5). The oral examination revealed a superficial cut at the right lateral margins of his tongue from the broken cusps of the lower first premolar and caries in the remaining teeth due to his poor oral hygiene. X-rays did not reveal any skull bone fractures, especially in his jaws.

Q1 Which is the cause of trismus?
- **A** Head injury
- **B** Periodontal abscess
- **C** Tetanus
- **D** Fracture of the mandible
- **E** TMJ disorder

Answers:
- **A** Head injury is the cause. The blow caused trauma of the TMJ components, jaws and masticatory muscles, leading to edema and hematoma formation that inhibits jaws movement and restricts the width of mouth opening
- **B** No
- **C** No
- **D** No
- **E** No

Comments: The lack of toothache and periodontal swelling as well as the negative X-rays excludes the possibility of a periodontal abscess or fractures from the diagnosis. The pain characteristics and the short duration of symptoms in TMJ and lack of other muscles involvement therefore ruled out tetanus.

Q2 Which other facial lesions could be detected immediately after a head injury?
- **A** Periorbital ecchymoses
- **B** Facial edema
- **C** Facial lacerations
- **D** Facial apathy
- **E** Hyperpigmentation

Answers:
- **A** Periorbital ecchymoses occur as the hematoma produced by facial injury is accumulated within the periorbital tissues.
- **B** Facial edema is common and is induced by the leakage of fluid from ruptured vessels from the punch.
- **C** Facial blow often cuts the skin and causes superficial lacerations or deep skin defects.
- **D** Crushing the facial nerve throughout its root can sometimes cause sensory deficits which is well-known as facial palsy. This condition can be temporal or permanent and is characterized by inability to control the facial muscles on the affected side and the face looks without any expression (apathy).
- **E** No

Comments: Hyperpigmentation is not an early effect of head injury, but may be presented later as a result of chronic irritation like trauma, chronic infection or foreign body deposition through skin lacerations.

Q3 Which is the major complication of head injuries additionally to trismus?
- **A** Diplopia
- **B** Esthetic disfiguration

C Sensory nerve damage
D Sialorrhea
E Cerebrospinal fluid rhinorrhea

Answers:

A No
B No
C No
D No
E Cerebrospinal fluid leakage, via broken ethmoid bone in fractures Le Fort type II and III, is very dangerous with a risk of spread of a bacterial infection to the brain causing severe meningitis. Therefore, a broad spectrum antibiotic therapy together with an early fixation of the responsible fracture is mandatory.

Comments: Diplopia is persistent and caused by the damage of suspensory ligaments or trapping of the extraocular muscles in the orbital or malar fractures and recovers as soon as the fracture is repaired. Esthetic disfiguration due to facial injuries or jaw fractures can be easily restored with plastic and jaw immobilization therapies, while sialorrhea is caused by difficulties in swallowing rather than increased saliva secretion. Sensory deficits due to crushing of the trigeminal and facial nerves are often reported, but these deficits (transient or permanent) do not jeopardize the patient's life.

Case 5.6

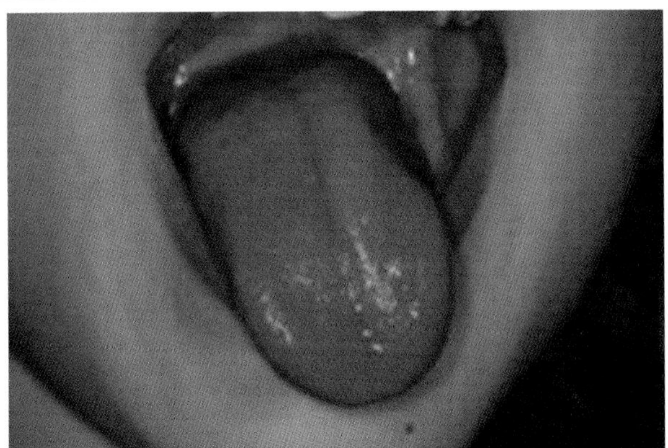

Figure 5.6

CO: A 4½-year-old boy was referred for an evaluation of paralysis of his tongue over the last 10 days.

HPC: The paralysis of the left side of his tongue was first noticed by his mother when the patient showed some speaking difficulties in pronouncing certain letters. However, his paralysis disappeared gradually within the next 15 days.

PMH: His medical history was unremarkable apart from an episode of a Coxsackie viral infection of his throat five months ago, while his family history was unspecific. No history of head trauma or drug uptake was recorded except for a vaccination against measles rubella, mumps and chicken pox which was given 10 days before the onset of his paralysis.

OE: A young boy with tongue paralysis with left side deviation upon protrusion (Figure 5.6). His tongue showed some side weakness and fasciculation on the left side that was also accompanied with dysarthria. His neurological examination, at the same time, was normal as all cranial nerves apart from the hypoglossal worked properly and their upper motor nerve function was not specific. MRI and virology examinations were normal as well.

Q1 Which is the possible cause of his tongue paralysis?

A Idiopathic
B Tumor
C Vaccination-induced
D Local trauma
E Infections

Answers:

A No
B No
C The quadruplicate vaccination may be the cause as this drug was given right before the patient's tongue paralysis. As additional proof, tongue and leg weakness or paralysis have also been reported with other vaccines such as polio, chicken pox and hepatitis B. This vaccine is used in children in order to prevent measles, mumps, German measles and chicken pox, by introducing a small amount, but weakened version, of the above viruses into the child's body.
D No
E No

Comments: Based on the previous patient's history together with his negative MRI and virology tests, it is easy for local trauma, tumor or viral infection to be excluded as a possible cause of his tongue paralysis. The case of an idiopathic paralysis could be considered as a possible cause when there was no evidence of other causes.

Q2 Which of the test/s below is/are useful in the diagnosis of this condition?
- **A** Virology tests
- **B** Plain X-rays of the skull
- **C** MRI skull/brain
- **D** Glucose blood tests
- **E** Cranial nerve function tests

Answers:
- **A** Virology tests are useful to detect a present or recent viral infection that affects the route of cranial nerves from the periphery to the CNS.
- **B** Skull X-rays are useful to detect any possible fracture that compresses the cranial nerves and induces paralysis.
- **C** The MRI is very useful to detect tumors or signs of multiple sclerosis as possible causes of tongue paralysis.
- **D** No
- **E** The neurological examination of cranial nerves helps clinicians to define which nerves are involved in this paralysis.

Comments: Glucose blood tests are useful to diagnose diabetes and its neuropathies, but not hypoglossal nerve paralysis.

Q3 Which is/are the contraindications of this vaccination?
- **A** Older patients
- **B** Allergies to vaccine ingredients
- **C** Active tuberculosis infection
- **D** Pregnant women
- **E** Patients in immunosuppression treatment

Answers:
- **A** Adults and older patients may have already antibodies for mumps, measles or chicken pox and therefore their immunization is useless.
- **B** Allergies to vaccine ingredients cause hives, edema, flu symptoms, redness and swelling at the injection site.
- **C** The vaccination can worsen any preexisting infection such as tuberculosis.
- **D** Immunizing pregnant women with live, attenuated viruses and bacteria is a risk (theoretical?) for the fetus and clinicians should take under consideration the risks and benefits of such vaccination as well.
- **E** A patient who is a under pharmaceutical immunosuppression has the risk of reduced ability of his immune system to fight the infection.

Case 5.7

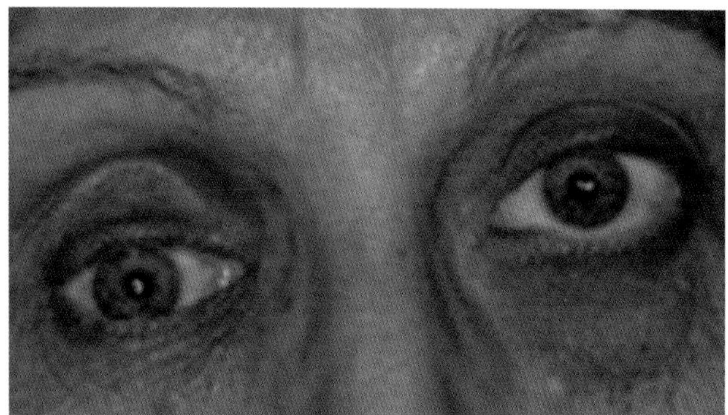

Figure 5.7

CO: A 58-year-old woman was referred for an evaluation of a unilateral blepharoptosis that was detected during her routine dental examination right before the construction of an upper full denture.

HPC: Her eyelid ptosis was discovered accidentally and did not cause any vision problems or other symptomatology.

PMH: Her medical history was clear apart from serious encephalitis which was diagnosed four months ago, after an episode of varicella zoster infection along the ophthalmic branch of the right trigeminal nerve. This infection was treated with a long course of antiviral drugs and steroids. No other serious neuromuscular diseases, drug uptake, recent head injury or smoking and drinking habits were recorded.

OE: The examination revealed a partial ptosis of her right upper eyelid (2mm) together with some irregularities of pupil but with no effect on her vision (Figure 5.7).

Facial muscles did not show any clinical signs of paralysis while the expression and mastication movements were stable. No other lesions were found intra- or extra-orally.

Q1 What is the cause of blepharoptosis in this patient?

- **A** Head injury
- **B** Old age
- **C** Eye tumor
- **D** Myasthenia gravis
- **E** Complications from encephalitis

Answers:

- **A** No
- **B** No
- **C** No
- **D** No
- **E** Her eyelid ptosis was a complication of encephalitis induced by her previous herpetic infection Encephalitis is a serious brain inflammation caused by a number of viruses (mainly herpes), bacteria (syphilis), fungi (*Cryptococcus*) or even parasites (toxoplasma) in patients with a weakened immune system. It is a rare complication that requires patient hospitalization and appears with fever, malaise, headaches, ptosis of the eyelids, diplopia, neck stiffness, tremor and other motor dysfunctions.

Comments: Blepharoptosis is also a clinical finding on old patients, those with head injury, eye tumors or myasthenia gravis. However, in this case, these can be easily excluded as the patient was not very old and with no history of recent head injury. For the above disorders the ptosis should be in both eyelids due to a weakness of the levator palpabrae and tarsalis, and other symptoms such as vision and myoskeletal problems would be recorded.

Q2 Which is the most preferable treatment for this patient?

- **A** Treatment of the main cause
- **B** Plastic surgery
- **C** Physiotherapy
- **D** None
- **E** Antibiotics

Answers:

- **A** Treating encephalitis with steroids to reduce edema in the brain and anti-virals reduces the compression of superior division of oculomotor nerve.
- **B** No
- **C** Physiotherapy such as eyelid exercises or topical massage strengthens the affected elevator muscles and improves eyelid drooping.
- **D** No
- **E** No

Comments: Plastic surgery of the elevator muscles of the eye and antibiotic treatment are not useful for this woman as her ptosis is only mild (2 mm), short in duration and not associated with bacterial encephalitis.

Q3 Which of the tests below is/or are mandatory in the diagnosis of this condition?

- **A** Brain MRI
- **B** Cerebrospinal fluid analysis
- **C** Encephalography
- **D** Vision test
- **E** Electromyography

Answers:

- **A** Brain MRI distinguishes a brain inflammation from other causes of ptosis such as tumors, abscesses or other malformation lesions.
- **B** Cerebrospinal fluid analysis determines the presence of inflammation or not and especially the polymerase chain reaction (PCR) analysis may show the presence of viral or bacterial DNA as possible etiological factors.
- **C** No
- **D** No
- **E** No

Comments: Vision tests help to detect the presence or absence of diplopia or other vision problems, while electro-encephalography and electromyography monitor the brain changes and the extent of muscles dysfunction, respectively.

Case 5.8

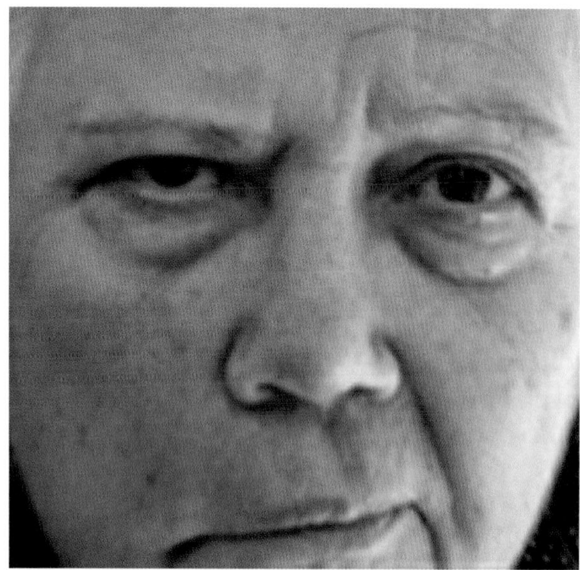

Figure 5.8

CO: A 72-year-old woman was referred by her dentist for an evaluation of her difficulties on smiling.

HPC: Her problem started one week ago with a small transient numbness of the right part of her face which gradually became permanent and associated with a paralysis of all the ipsilateral muscles of her face. She recalled a right inner ear infection three weeks ago which was treated with a broad course of antibiotics.

PMH: Her medical history revealed hypertension which had been controlled with diuretics and angiotensin converting enzyme (ACE) inhibitor, and hypercholesterolemia, controlled with statins. Allergies or other serious myoskeletal problems or habits such as smoking or drinking were not reported.

OE: The physical examination revealed a lady with a lack of symmetry on her face, absence of wrinkles on the right part of her forehead, smoothness of her right nasolabial fold, together with drop in the of corner of her mouth, causing her difficulties in speaking, whistling or laughing (Figure 5.8). Intra-orally, no indications of oral and dental infections were found.

Q1 Which is the cause of paralysis of her facial muscles?

A Stroke
B Brain tumor
C Bell's palsy
D Head trauma
E Multiple sclerosis

Answers:

A No
B No
C Bell's palsy is the most common cause of an acute paralysis of the facial nerves and it can be either idiopathic, or it appears after an infection (viral or bacterial) in the area. It is presented with a loss or weakness of the ipsilateral facial muscles along with facial asymmetry and loss of facial expression and wrinkling. The mouth corner drops and is associated with problems in drinking, eating or whistling as seen in this lady.
D No
E No

Comments: Stroke and brain tumors cause not only facial paralysis, but also provoke weakness of leg muscles, excessive tearing, reduced salivation and dysgeusia and sometimes hyperacusis. The absence of other systematic symptoms and a negative history of recent trauma excludes the case of head injury or multiple sclerosis from the diagnosis.

Q2 Which of the characteristic(s) below is/are favorable prognostic factor/s for an acute facial nerve paralysis?

A Complete nerve paralysis
B Rapid progression
C History of recurrence
D Early treatment
E Presence of other motor or sensory deficits

Answers:

A No
B No
C No
D Early beginning of the treatment (<7 days from the day of onset) of the facial muscle paralysis is a favorable prognostic factor. A series of early uptake of steroids and antivirals helps to eliminate the inflammation of the facial nerve and enables quick nerve recovery.
E No

Comments: The presence of other sensory or motor deficits like hearing loss, and recurrence of severe or complete paralysis induced in a very short period after diagnosis are considered among the unfavorable prognostic factors.

Q3 Which of the characteristics below differentiate/s the upper from the lower motor neuron paralysis?
- **A** Location of the facial paralysis in relation to the cause
- **B** The duration of paralysis
- **C** The response or not to antibiotics
- **D** Abnormal corneal reflexes
- **E** Forehead winkles

Answers:
- **A** The paralysis of the facial muscles ipsilateral to the cause are seen in lower motor nerve lesions.
- **B** No
- **C** No
- **D** Abnormal corneal reflex is only seen in lower motor nerve paralysis.
- **E** Forehead wrinkles are found in the upper but disappear in the lower motor neuron paralysis.

Comments: The facial palsy can be partial or complete, ipsilateral or bilateral, congenital or acquired, mild or severe, regardless of the duration of the palsy. The treatment of choice is a combination of steroids and antivirals and not antibiotics.

Case 5.9

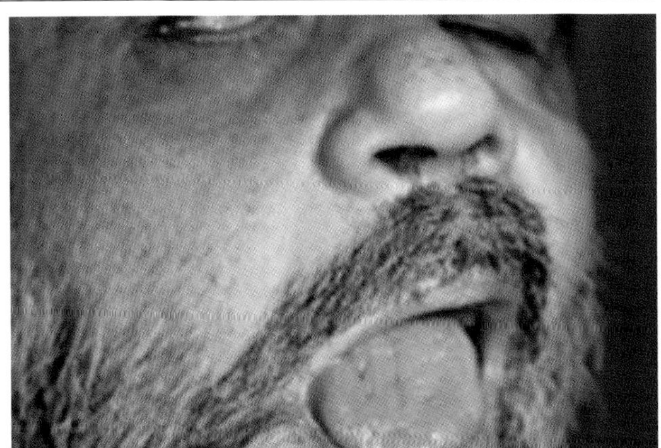

Figure 5.9

CO: A 56-year-old man presented with pain in his right ear, and facial muscle and tongue paralysis.

HPC: The pain in his ear was dull, constant and associated with hearing problems over the last two months. Paralysis of the muscles on half of his face as well as the ipsilateral right part of his tongue had appeared gradually over the last month, but no other muscle weakness of his arms or legs were recorded.

PMH: His medical history revealed an aggressive oropharyngeal carcinoma 10 months ago that was initially treated with chemo- and radiotherapy but relapsed, and resulted in metastases to the posterior part of his pharynx and the inner part of his ear.

OE: The extra-oral examination revealed a paralysis of the right part of his face, drop of the corner of the mouth and incomplete eyelid closure (Bell's phenomenon) together with tongue movement to his right side on protrusion (Figure 5.9). Moreover, a partial loss of hearing and a dull constant pain inside his right ear, as well as a number of episodes of headaches but with no weakness of his legs and arms or balance problems were recorded.

Q1 What is the cause of facial and lingual paralysis?
- **A** Guillain-Barré syndrome
- **B** Ischemic stroke
- **C** Multiple sclerosis
- **D** Radio-chemotherapy-induced neuritis
- **E** Metastatic carcinoma

Answers:
- **A** No
- **B** No
- **C** No
- **D** No
- **E** Metastatic oropharyngeal carcinoma may infiltrate or compress the facial and hypoglossal nerve or their anostomosis and can gradually cause paralysis of facial and tongue muscles.

Comments: The generalized muscle paralysis together with different symptomatology, the acute onset (ischemic stroke) and the gradual progress (Guillain-Barré syndrome and multiple sclerosis) along with the presence of tingling, numbness, or burning sensation rather than a muscle paralysis (radiation-induced neuritis) rule out these diseases from the diagnosis.

Q2 Which of the tongue muscles below is/are not innervated with hypoglossal nerve?
- **A** Styloglossus
- **B** Palatoglossus
- **C** Hyoglossus
- **D** Superior longitudinal
- **E** Genioglossus

Answers:

- **A** No
- **B** Palatoglossus muscle is an intrinsic muscle and arises from palatinal aponeurosis and enters into the posterior part of tongue which is elevated via activation of vagus (X) cranial nerve.
- **C** No
- **D** No
- **E** No

Comments: All the other intrinsic muscles and all the extrinsic muscles are innervated from the hypoglossal nerve.

Q3 Which is/or are the effect/s of a low dose of radiation on the tongue?

- **A** Muscle atrophy
- **B** Muscle fibrosis
- **C** Reduced speed of contraction
- **D** Increased apoptosis of taste buds
- **E** Loss of microvilli of taste buds

Answers:

- **A** No
- **B** No
- **C** The speed of contraction may be reduced and is dependent on the patient's age.
- **D** Taste cells degenerate within six to seven days after radiation while taste alterations are seen earlier.
- **E** Taste bud microvilli are damaged with radiation, thus leading to a reduced reception of taste stimulants.

Comments: Muscle atrophy or increased fibrosis are not found in patients treated with low amounts of radiation for short periods.

Case 5.10

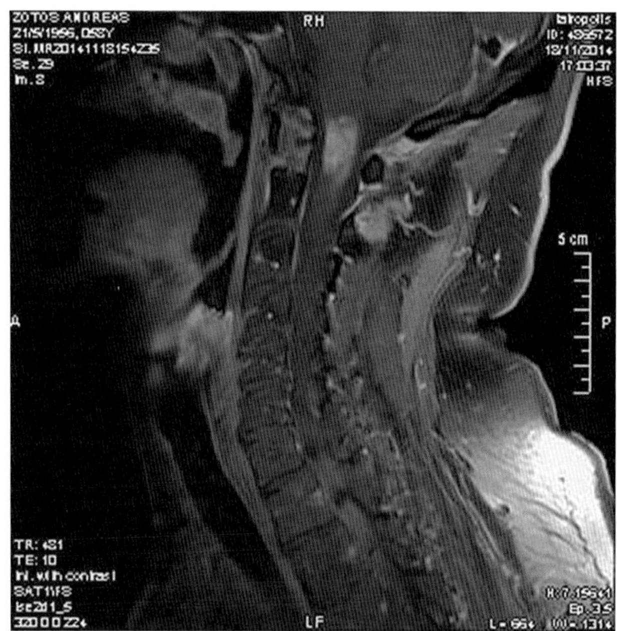

Figure 5.10

CO: A 58-year-old man presented for a regular oral examination five months after the end of a course of chemo-radiotherapy for recurrent squamous cell carcinoma (Sca; spindle type) on his tongue and neck. He complained about a progressive weakness of his lower extremities over the last three weeks.

HPC: His weakness appeared four months ago initially as a difficulty in moving of his right foot, sensory deficit and mild hyperreflexia of his lower limbs and extensor palmar reflex, as well as a loss of proprioception in his legs.

PMH: His medical history revealed a small SCA on his right lateral margin of his tongue which was surgically removed and successfully treated with radium implantation 20 years ago. Another more aggressive SCA was also detected two years ago in the same place with as the previous one, and was treated with surgical excision and a course of radio-chemotherapy. However, it resulted in metastasis into the lymph nodes of his neck, and two other courses of cisplatin chemotherapy and selected CyberKnife radiation was undertaken and ended five months ago, just before his leg problems appeared.

OE: The examination revealed no evidence of tumor or any other sign of infection intra-orally or on the skin. His skin was dry, hyperpigmented and atrophic, due to his previous radiotherapies. The patient often suffered with headaches and progressive weakness of both his legs which showed positive electromyography. On the other hand, a PET scan did not identify any active or residual tumor, while the MRI of the brain did not reveal any other lesions capable of inducing body paralysis. MRI of his neck revealed a mild spinal cord swelling where an area of intensity at the level of the atlas was detected (Figure 5.10).

Q1 What is the cause of his leg paralysis?

- **A** Oral cancer metastasis
- **B** Trauma of the spine
- **C** Myelopathy induced by radiotherapy
- **D** Multiple sclerosis
- **E** Congenital vascular spine lesion

Answers:

- **A** No
- **B** No
- **C** Radiation-induced myelopathy is the cause. This is a rare complication (transient or permanent) of radiotherapy for carcinomas of the head and neck. It is characterized by a slowly progressing ascending sensory motor disturbance due to a myelin breakdown caused by a breakdown of oligodendrocytes. This disturbance appears as a tingling or burning sensation, leg or hand paralysis, and in severe cases bowel or bladder dysfunction few months after radiotherapy.
- **D** No
- **E** No

Comments: The negative PET scan or MRI of his neck easily excludes oral carcinoma metastasis and other spinal malignancies or vascular congenital lesions from the diagnosis. Trauma from a recent head or spine accident had not been reported, while the symptomatology and brain MRI of multiple sclerosis differs and therefore these conditions are ruled out.

Q2 Which is/are the requirement/s of a radiation-induced myelopathy development?

- **A** Radiotherapy dose
- **B** Radiation region related with a spinal lesion
- **C** Latent period
- **D** Vertebral anomalies
- **E** Spinal trauma prerequisite

Answers:

- **A** Excessive radiotherapy causes damage of the spine marrow whose severity is dependent on the dose and the number of radiotherapy sessions.
- **B** The irradiation field must be slightly above the demyelinated spinal cord.
- **C** Myelopathy must appear a few months or years after radiotherapy.
- **D** No
- **E** No

Comments: Radiation-induced myelopathy does not require previous spinal trauma, although trauma can be a possible cause of myelopathy. Vertebral anomalies may cause pressure, spinal cord edema, and be unrelated to radiation myelopathy.

Q3 What is/are the best treatment/s of radiation-induced myelopathy?

- **A** Hyperbaric oxygen
- **B** Muscle relaxant drugs
- **C** Antibiotics
- **D** Steroids
- **E** Physiotherapy

Answers:

- **A** Hyperbaric oxygen alone or in combination with other treatments is effective in the recovery of some but not all patients with myelopathy.
- **B** No
- **C** No
- **D** Steroids are very useful for reducing spinal cord edema and for giving a quick but short improvement for muscle weakness.
- **E** Physiotherapy helps patients with myelopathy to relieve their pain, improve their muscle function, or reverse neurological defects.

Comments: Antibiotics may be useful in spinal bacterial infection, but not in radiation-induced myelopathy, while muscle relaxant drugs may worsen leg paralysis as they reduce the nerve transmission from the spinal cord to skeletal muscles.

6

Orofacial Pain

Orofacial pain is the pain that affects mouth, jaws, or face. Orofacial pain is a symptom and not a disease, with a great number of causes implicated in its pathogenesis such as local causes, neoplasms, neurological, vascular, muscular, or even psychiatric problems. Orofacial pain can be primary or secondary in presentation.

Oral pain affects the mouth (oral mucosa, teeth, and underlying jaws) and is the commonest cause for patients to seek medical help. Dental and periodontal infections, oral ulcerations, tumors or jaw lesions and temporomandibular joint (TMJ) dysfunctions or even neuralgias require a comprehensive medical evaluation for the best treatment path forward. Delayed diagnosis and inappropriate treatment can lead to patients with prolonged pain suffering with serious implications in their life (Figure 6.0).

The most important causes of orofacial pain are listed in Table 6.

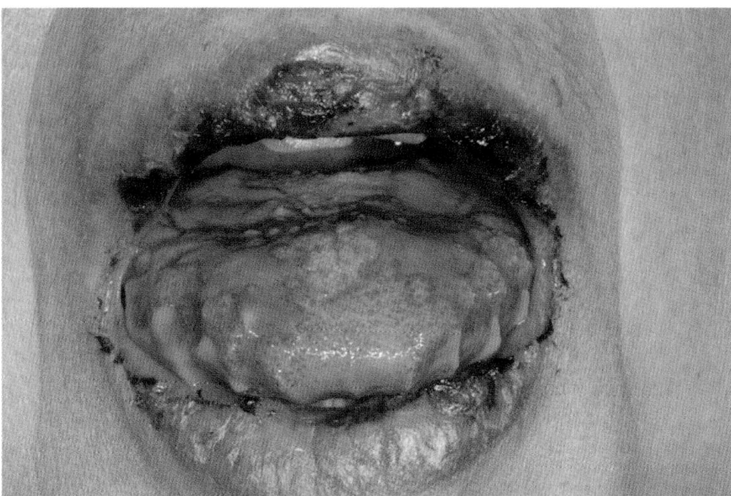

Figure 6.0 Pain from the ulcerated oral mucosa of a patient with graft-versus-host disease (GVHD).

Clinical Guide to Oral Diseases, First Edition. Dimitris Malamos and Crispian Scully.

Companion website: www.wiley.com/go/malamos/clinical_guide

Table 6 Common and important conditions in orofacial pain.

- Real pain
  - **Local**
    - Related to teeth
      - Eruption
        - Teething
        - Impaction
      - Structure loss
        - Abfraction
        - Attrition
        - Erosion
        - Caries
        - Cracking
        - Hypersensitivity to cold
        - Pulpitis (acute, chronic)
        - Dental abscess
    - Related to periodontium
      - Inflammation
        - Pericoronitis
        - Periodontal abscess
        - Acute ulcerative gingivitis
    - Related to oral mucosa with the following subdivisions
      - Traumatic ulcerations
        - Mechanical
        - Thermal
        - Chemical
        - Electrical burns
      - aphthous stomatitis
        - simple (minor; major; herpeiform) associated with syndromes (Bechet; PFAPA)
      - neoplasmatic
        - squamous cell carcinoma
      - local infections
        - bacterial

Table 6 (Continued)

        - fungal
        - viral
  - **Systemic causes**
    - related to skin
      - bullous diseases
      - erosive lichen planus
    - related to blood
      - anaemia
    - related to gut
      - Cronh's disease
  - **Referral from**
    - Adjacent tissues
      - Antrum
        - Sinusitis
      - Salivary glands
        - Sialadenitis
      - Joints/muscles
        - TMJ syndrome
    - Distant organs
      - Heart
        - Angina pectoris
        - Acute myocardial infarct
      - Blood vessels
        - Migraine
        - Cluster headaches
        - Temporal arteritis
      - Nerves
        - Herpes zoster neuralgia
        - Trigeminal neuralgia
        - Multiple sclerosis
- Psychogenic (fake) pain from
  - Depression
  - Anxiety

Case 6.1

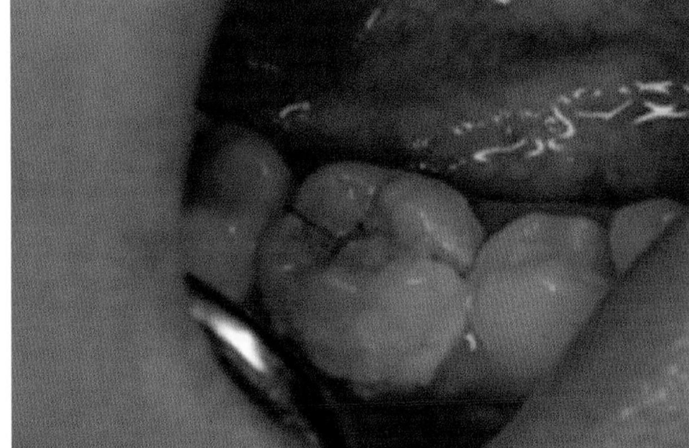

Figure 6.1

CO: An 11-year-old boy was presented with pain from his lower posterior teeth.

HPC: The pain was acute, sharp on biting and exacerbated with thermal changes. It appeared for the first time after eating a hard candy.

PMH: His medical record was clear from any serious diseases, allergies or drug use while the chewing of hard candies, since the age of 6, has been a habit that caused him a number of dental problems.

OE: The oral examination revealed an incomplete fracture in the lower right deciduous second molar across the middle line from the enamel and through the dentin to the pulp (Figure 6.1). Vitality tests revealed an increased response to cold stimulus (acute pulpitis). Gingival infection or other oral lesions were not found.

Q1 What is the cause of pain?

A Cracked tooth syndrome

B Sinusitis

C Trigeminal neuralgia
D Atypical stomatodynia
E Acute periodontal disease

Answers:
A Cracked tooth syndrome is the cause. It is characterized by an incomplete fracture of the dentin in the vital mandibular and maxillary posterior teeth of patients with grinding or clenching, or biting hard food habits.
B No
C No
D No
E No

Comments: The patient's pain characteristics such as location, sensitivity to cold stimulus, and frequency of attacks can easily exclude pain from diseases such as sinusitis where the pain is constant, dull and arisen from the antra; trigeminal neuralgia where the pain is sharp and has a trigger zone, but is not usually found at such a young age; or atypical facial pain (AFP) where the pain is diffuse and not coming from a certain area such as the broken molar. The lack of gingival involvement rules out the possibility of an acute periodontal disease from the diagnosis.

Q2 Which of the tests below are less useful in the diagnosis of this condition?
A Visual inspection
B Percussion test
C Intraoral radiographs
D Dye test
E Periodontal probing

Answers:
A No
B No
C Intraoral radiographs have some limitations as the fracture line tends to have a mesiodistal direction parallel to the plane of film, and it is therefore very difficult to be detected.
D No
E No

Comments: The visual inspection alone or together with specific dyes allows the detection of the fracture line while the percussion test and the periodontal probing reveal the pulp reaction and the extension of the fracture beyond the tooth to the periodontal ligament, respectively.

Q3 What is/are the differences between a broken cusp and this condition?
A Location
B Movement
C Discoloration
D Symptomatology
E Dentition (deciduous or permanent)

Answers:
A No
B The movement of broken parts of a cracked tooth is not detected, while a slight pressure can easily detach the broken cusp.
C Changes in tooth color are not seen in teeth superficially fractured, and in teeth with attrition or broken cusps, but are seen in deeply cracked teeth with pulp necrosis.
D No
E No

Comments: Teeth with cracks or broken cusps are both found in the mandible rather than the maxilla and mainly in the posterior rather than anterior teeth which do not show any severe symptomatology.

Case 6.2

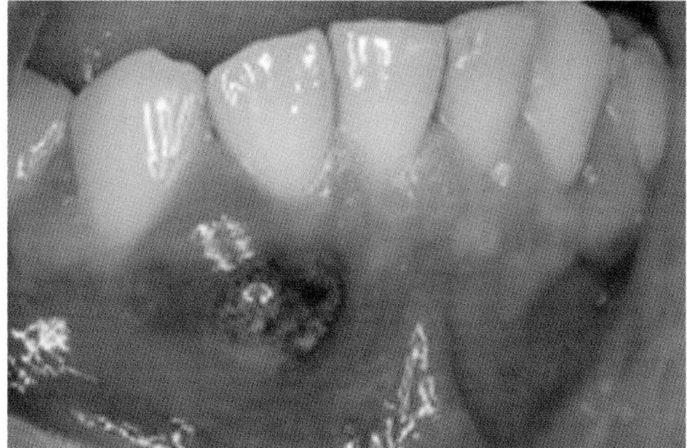

Figure 6.2

CO: A 38-year-old woman was presented with a soft swelling of the anterior gingivae between lower right lateral incisor and canine associated with deep throbbing pain.

HPC: The pain preceded two days earlier from the onset of this soft, fluctuant gingival swelling.

PMH: Her medical history was clear apart from a juvenile diabetes that was controlled with the daily use of insulin, while her dental history revealed some chronic gingival problems despite her adequate oral hygiene. She was a chronic smoker of less than six cigarettes per day, but a drinker only on occasions.

OE: A black lady with a soft swelling on the anterior lower gingivae, distally to the vital right lateral incisor. The lesion was fluctuant, consisting of pus and covered with thin, slightly inflamed hyperpigmented oral mucosa (Figure 6.2) and associated with deep throbbing pain which was worse on biting or on palpation. Two similar lesions had also been recorded at the same place in the past, but were resolved with antibiotics. Cervical lymphadenopathy or general symptomatology was absent. A number of intra-oral radiographs revealed a vertical alveolar bone loss with periodontal pocket formation.

Q1 What is the cause of pain?

- **A** Periapical abscess
- **B** Periodontal abscess
- **C** Pericoronitis
- **D** Lateral periodontal cyst
- **E** Gingival abscess

Answers:

- **A** No
- **B** Periodontal abscess is the cause and characterized by the accumulation of pus within tissues adjacent to the periodontal pocket, that may lead to the destruction of the periodontal ligament and alveolar bone. The accumulation of pus induces a deep throbbing pain that is prominent with biting and thermal changes, but not with pulpal necrosis.
- **C** No
- **D** No
- **E** No

Comments: The presence of vital fully erupted teeth adjacent to the lesion easily excludes a periapical or pericoronal abscess, while the radiographic finding of bone loss (vertical or horizontal) locally and not forming well-defined radiolucent lesions or being extended to large parts of the jaw and other bones, can rule out gingival abscess, lateral periodontal cysts and eosinophilic granuloma from the diagnosis.

Q2 What are the first steps of treatment for this condition?

- **A** Eliminate pain
- **B** Drainage of abscess
- **C** Endodontic treatment
- **D** Periodontal surgery
- **E** Extraction of related teeth

Answers:

- **A** The elimination of pain was the initial step by giving NSAIDs alone, or together with antibiotics for a short time.
- **B** Drainage of pus via the pocket or external incision relieves the pressure and the pain, thus allowing the antibiotics to act properly.
- **C** No,
- **D** No
- **E** No

Comments: Endodontic treatment is useless as no pulpal necrosis is present, while a periodontal surgery or extraction of the related teeth must be done after having controlled the gingival infection first.

Q3 Which are the major complications if this condition remains untreated?

- **A** Tooth loss
- **B** Dissemination of infection
- **C** Trigger trigeminal neuralgia
- **D** Induce sickle cell crisis
- **E** Deregulate diabetes

Answers:

- **A** No
- **B** Dissemination of the infection could cause extensive cellulitis or necrotizing fasciitis; conditions which require special care and a long antibiotic treatment.
- **C** No
- **D** Periodontal abscess, in patients with sickle cell anemia, has been recorded as causing severe body pain, difficulties in breathing, headaches or dizziness or even jaundice (sickle cell crisis).
- **E** No

Comments: Trigeminal neuralgia is provoked by a topical compression or abnormalities of peripheral nerve endings of the trigeminal nerves at the trigger zone, and not by the products of an acute gingival inflammation. The level of inflammatory cytokines is low as the inflammation is restricted and therefore is not capable of altering insulin action, especially in diabetic patients.

Case 6.3

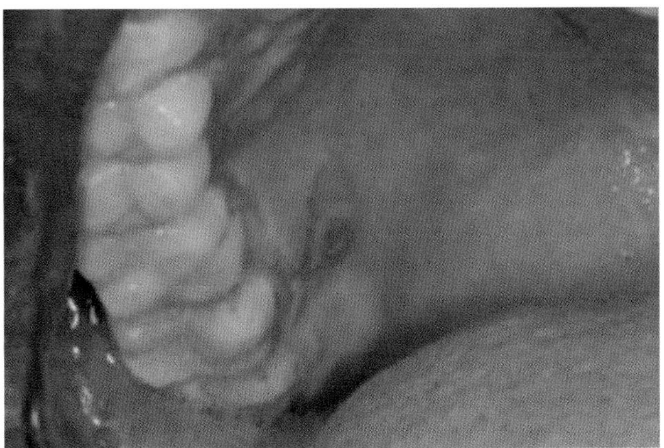

Figure 6.3

CO: A 48-year-old man was presented for an evaluation of his pain in his palate.

HPC: The pain was initially sharp, throbbing and deep, but gradually decreased and finally disappeared leaving a diffuse swelling with a sinus tract at the palatal mucosa between the 1st and 2nd molar.

PMH: His medical history was clear apart from gut problems (gastro-esophageal reflux and chronic gastritis) which were controlled with proton pump inhibitors, anti-acids and a suitable diet.

OE: The oral examination revealed a diffuse palatal swelling with a sinus releasing pus and blood, with pressure in the area of the 1st and 2nd upper right molars (Figure 6.3). Both teeth had an intact composite filling at the occlusal surface, and did not show periapical lesions with intra-oral radiographs. while the first molar did not respond to vitality tests. No other similar oral lesions or cervical lymphadenopathy was detected.

Q1 What is the cause of pain?

- **A** Acute necrotizing sialometaplasia
- **B** Osteonecrosis due to biphosphonate drugs
- **C** Periapical infection due to pulp necrosis
- **D** Palatal antral fistula
- **E** Actinomycosis

Answers:

- **A** No
- **B** No
- **C** Composite restorations are often highly toxic to pulp causing irreversible pulpitis and necrosis that leads to periapical infection. This infection was initially responsible for the acute and severe pain that developed later as the inflammation moved from the pulp to the periapical alveolar bone, and finally stopped when it was drained via sinus to the palatal mucosa. The negative pulp test was an indication of the 1st molar pulp necrosis.
- **D** No
- **E** No

Comments: Palatal sinuses are commonly seen in other inflammatory jaw conditions such as osteonecrosis due to the chronic use of biphosphonate drugs, or due to infection from *Actinomyces* species, but are easily excluded as the patient did not take any drugs inducing osteonecrosis, and did not show clinical and radiographic features of actinomycosis. Oro-antral fistula sometimes resembles a hypertrophic sinus, but requires an open oro-antral communication due to a recent extraction, while the acute necrotizing sialometaplasia appears as a necrotic palatal lesion after a local trauma or local anesthetic injection. However, neither extractions or local trauma were recorded in this patient.

Q2 Which is/or are the major complication(s) of this condition capable of jeopardizing his patient's life?

- **A** Endocarditis
- **B** Trismus
- **C** Ludwig's angina
- **D** Cellulitis
- **E** Cavernous sinus thrombosis

Answers:

- **A** No
- **B** No
- **C** No
- **D** No
- **E** Cavernous sinus thrombosis is the result of expansion of an odontogenic infection to the middle face where the local edema causes the blood to stagnate and clot. As a result, the new clots often escape into the blood circulation and form infective emboli, which are extremely dangerous for the affected tissues or organs.

Comments: The spread of a periapical infection into surrounding fasciae causes a severe infection that is known as cellulitis, while in the masticatory muscles does trismus. Bacteria, via the circulation, can reach the heart and damage its valves leading to heart failure. All the above complications are under drug control, allowing the patients to live longer. Ludwig's angina is a serious complication of a dental abscess and characterized by a large neck swelling due to the extension of an odontogenic infection into the sublingual/submandibular and submental space. This case may cause severe breathing problems and a potential lethal airway obstruction and is associated with necrosis of lower bud not the upper teeth.

Q3 Which are the factors that determine the spread of a periapical infection into the fascial spaces of the head and neck?

- **A** Patient's age
- **B** Location of tooth apex
- **C** Thickening of underlying bone
- **D** Patient's oral hygiene status
- **E** Previous medication

Answers:

- **A** No
- **B** The location of the suspected tooth apex in relation to its overlying buccal and lingual cortical plates, close to the lingual and submandibular space, play the most important role in the spread of the infection.
- **C** The thickness of an overlying bone is also another factor, as the spread of the infection is easier when the bone which covers the root is thin.
- **D** No
- **E** No

Comments: The older age of patients or their previous medications are factors that could initially define the patient's health status, and secondarily, their defense against pathogenic bacteria which are predominant in patients with poor oral hygiene.

Case 6.4

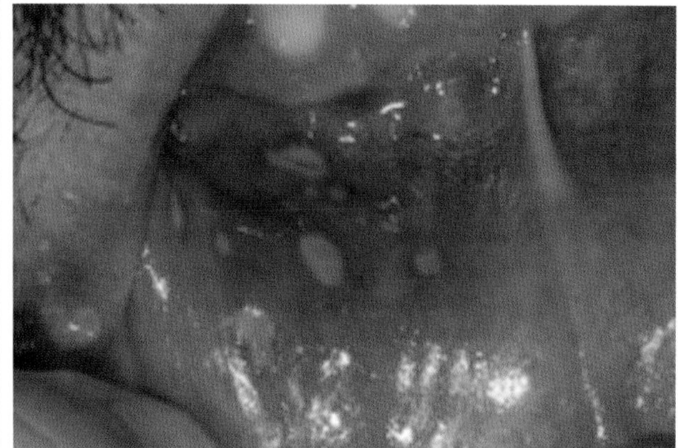

Figure 6.4

CO: A 23-year-old man was referred for examination of several painful ulcers spread all over his mouth, particularly on the inner surface of the lower lip.

HPC: His ulcers appeared initially as small, painful, pinhead like red spots or ulcerations one week ago, and gradually became bigger and became covered with whitish pseudomembranes.

PMH: His medical history was unremarkable apart from a few episodes of pain and diarrhea due to irritable bowel syndrome, recently diagnosed, and controlled with special diet. Allergies, anemia, drug use, or smoking and drinking habits were not recorded.

OE: Multiple painful ulcerations of various sizes, covered with yellow pseudomembranes and surrounded by erythematous halo in places were found scattered in the mouth, but organized in clusters on the inner surface of the lower lip (Figure 6.4). The lesions are extremely painful with the consumption of acidic, salty or spicy foods, leaving a burning sensation and causing increased sialorrhea and halitosis. No other lesions were found on the skin, genitals or other mucosae, while fever, general malaise or cervical lymphadenitis was not detected.

Q1 What is the cause of pain?

A Herpangina
B Hand, mouth, and foot disease
C Aphthous stomatitis
D Drug-induced stomatitis
E Primary herpetic stomatitis

Answers:

A No
B No
C Aphthous stomatitis is the cause. This condition is characterized by one or more painful discrete ulcerations of various sizes on erythematous oral mucosa. There are four types; minor, major or herpetiform aphthae and aphthous-like lesions in association with various systemic disorders. Herpetiform type are the aphthae found in this patient based on their number (>10 in. clusters), location and symptomatology. The irritable bowel syndrome seems to play a role in the aetiology of aphthae for this patient.
D No
E No

Comments: The absence of similar lesions in other mucosae and skin, general symptomatology like fever, malaise and lymphadenopathy, excludes diseases like the hand, mouth and foot disease as well as primary herpetic stomatitis from the diagnosis. Drug-induced stomatitis is easily ruled out as the patient was not under any medication. As the patient did not have palatal lesions and had no symptomatology of a viral infection or history of similar lesions among his close relatives and friends herpangina is easily excluded.

Q2 Which other diseases have almost identical oral lesions with the patient's condition?

A Cyclic neutropenia
B Anemia (iron or B12)
C Leukemia
D HIV infection
E Sweet syndrome

Answers:

A No
B Anemia due to iron, folate or B12 deficiency is often associated with atrophic glossitis and recurrent painful aphthous ulcerations. Atrophic oral mucosa is more vulnerable to trauma and to the penetration of various bacteria and viral agents. These are important factors have been implicated in the pathogenesis of aphthae and therefore clinicians should consider hematinic deficiencies as crucial etiological factors among middle-aged or elderly patients.
C No
D No
E No

Comments: Although diseases like cyclic neutropenia HIV or leukemiae (acute or chronic) are often presented with aphthous-like lesions, are entirely different from recurrent aphthous stomatitis (RAS). Cyclic neutropenia lesions show a periodicity of around three weeks while in RAS it varies. HIV infection also presents with oral ulcerations some of which resemble aphthae and last longer, but some others are irregular and cause necrosis of underlying tissues. Leukemia often presents with shallow painful ulcers, but differs as their ulcers lack the erythematous halo and are associated with systemic lymphadenopathy and symptomatology while in Sweet syndrome, high fever precedes the oral ulcers and skin lesions.

Q3 Which of the therapeutic agents below should be used firstly to reduce the intensity and duration of his pain?

A Laser
B Cryotherapy
C Cauterization
D Systemic steroids
E Topical anesthetic/antiseptics

Answers:

A No
B No
C No
D No
E Topical anesthetics, anti-inflammatory and antiseptic agents provide satisfactory and rapid symptomatic pain relief with the anti inflammatory agent diclofenac 3% in 2,5 hyaluronic acid gel being the best.

Comments: The destruction of peripheral nerve endings (necrosis) at the base of an ulcer with cryotherapy, cauterization or even recently with CO_2 and Nd YAG laser, gives immediate pain relief, but these techniques should be used only by experts and in special clinics. Systemic steroids should be used at the secondary stage when all the other topical agents have failed.

Case 6.5

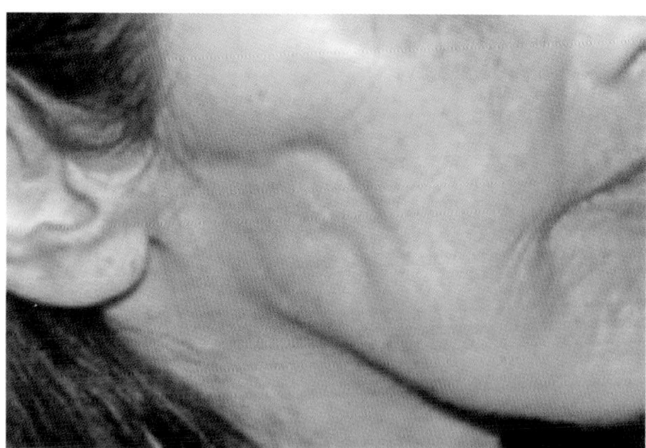

Figure 6.5

CO: A 45-year-old woman was referred for an evaluation of her one-year long facial pain.

HPC: The pain started firstly after a long visit to her dentist for the removal of a decayed lower right second molar. It lasted for two to three weeks, and reappeared six months later when she started to use nicotine chewing-gum regularly.

PMH: She was diagnosed with systemic sclerosis since the age of 40, and took methotrexate, methylprednisolone, together with omeprazole and nifedipine. No history of trauma or facial infection was recorded apart from a periapical infection which ended with the extraction of the responsible molar tooth. She had no parafunctional habits such as grinding or clenching her teeth, apart from using nicotine chewing-gum at regular base recently.

OE: She was a thin lady with a mask-like face, with smooth and tight facial skin without lines or wrinkles. An area of atrophy on the right part of her face, induced by a topical application of steroid cream, was found while the palpation of the masticatory muscles showed bilateral stiffness and dull pain which was reflected to her isilateral ear and upper teeth (Figure 6.5). Despite her good OH her dentition was heavily restored with fillings and crowns. Her mouth opening was limited to 21 mm and her mandible deviated to the left side when opened. No other lesions were recorded except for a mild xerostomia. Orthopantogram (OPG)-X rays did not reveal any inflammation or infection in both jaws.

Q1 What is the cause of pain?

- **A** Eagle syndrome
- **B** Otitis
- **C** Parotitis
- **D** Temporomandibular joint disorder
- **E** Mandibular osteomyelitis

Answers:

- **A** No
- **B** No
- **C** No
- **D** Temporomandibular joint disorder is the cause, and characterized by pain and dysfunction of masticatory muscles and temporomandibular joint. The pain is dull, poorly localized and reflected to the adjacent ear, face, back of the head and molar teeth, while it can be intermittent or permanent and worsen with eating or on waking. The pain began with the traumatic extraction of a lower molar bur worsened by using nicotine chew-gums at daily base to stop smoking.
- **E** No

Comments: The lack of parotid swelling or erythematous sensitive ears on palpation associated with fever, lymphadenitis, and general fatigue, easily excludes parotitis and otitis (external or medial) from the diagnosis. Elongation of the styloid processes and alveolar bone necrosis were not recorded in the patient's radiographs and as a result, Eagle syndrome and osteomyelitis are withdrawn from the diagnosis.

Q2 Which is/are the cardinal sign(s) of this condition?

- **A** Dull pain on muscles of mastication
- **B** Limited mandible movement
- **C** TMJ noises
- **D** Headache
- **E** Referred pain to ears and teeth

Answers:

- **A** Pain is a constant finding and may be presented as a dull intermittent or constant tenderness of the masticatory muscles and face around the joint, while it may worsen on waking up, eating, yawing, and speaking.
- **B** Impairment of mandibular movements are characteristic and presented as jaw locking, stiffness or deviation toward left or right.
- **C** The abrupt condyle movement against the articulator disc produces characteristic noises (clicking, crepitus) on mouth opening or closing movements.
- **D** No
- **E** No

Comments: Referred pain in the temple, behind the eyes, back of head or even around the ears and teeth is common, but not seen in every patient with this condition.

Q3 Which of the conditions below are related to this disorder?

A Irritable bowel syndrome
B Migraine
C Interstitial cystitis
D Fibromyalgia
E Atypical odontalgia

Answers:

A Irritable bowel syndrome has been associated with TMJ disorders and this correlation is more prominent in women under stress rather than men.
B An association between TMJ disorder and migraine has been established via the malfunction of the trigeminal nerve and is more obvious in chronic but not episodic migraines.
C Interstitial cystitis is common in patients with TMJ disorder.
D Fibromyalgia and TMJ disorder are also characterized by chronic muscle pain and share many epidemiological, clinical findings and symptoms.
E No

Comments: Atypical odontalgia and TMJ disorders share some characteristics, but differ in pain duration or location and jaw function as well.

Case 6.6

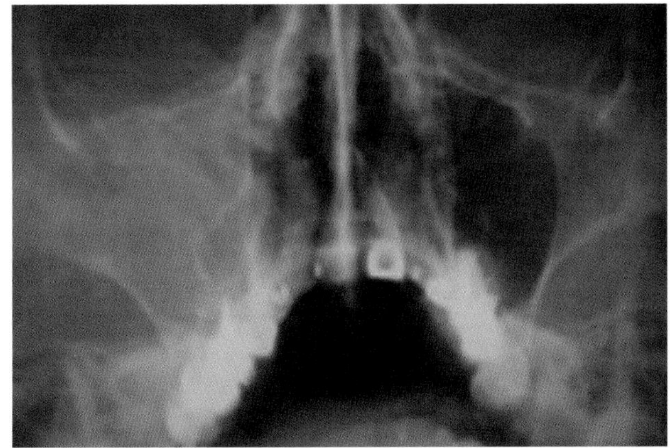

Figure 6.6

CO: A 48-year-old man presented for an evaluation of the pain in his upper right molars over the last week.

HPC: The pain was dull, constant and was affecting the upper right molars and their overlying maxilla and face. The pain did not show any alterations in cold or hot stimuli or exacerbate during food consumption, but it worsened with the downward motion of his head or its lifting up and laying down.

PMH: His medical history was remarkable apart from a few episodes of allergic rhinitis and hyperlipidemia that were controlled with antihistamines, diet and statins as well. His dental records revealed regular visits to his GDP in order to keep his heavily restored dentition intact.

OE: A healthy middle-aged man with a complete dentition whose teeth were vital and responded well to hot and cold stimuli. The pulp test did not confirm any pulp necrosis while his mouth did not show any oral lesions capable of eliciting pain. Moreover, halitosis was recorded and was not coming from his mouth but from his runny and congested nose. However, the palpation on the facial skin of the suspected molars area released pain. Intraoral radiographs did not reveal any periapical infections. A thick mucus coming from both his nostrils (mainly from the right) intermingled with pus and blood was detected and a right antrum was congested as seen in (paranasal radiograph).

Q1 Which of the conditions below is responsible for the pain?

A Antral foreign body
B Acute sinusitis
C Antral polyp
D Antral malignancy
E Molar periapical abscess

Answers:

A No
B Acute sinusitis is the cause. It is an acute inflammation of the tissues lining one or two antra and characterized by a dull facial pain, stuffy, and runny nose, loss of smell and in severe cases is associated with fever, fatigue bad breath, and dental pain.
C No

D No
E No

Comments: The short period of his pain and lack of serious symptomatology excludes malignancy from the diagnosis. The irregular-defined radiopaque lesion and a negative history of trauma or an accidental entrance of material into the antrum can easily exclude antral polyp and foreign body from the diagnosis. Periapical infection requires pulp necrosis, which was not found in none of the upper molars and therefore it could be easily discounted.

Q2 Which of the pain characteristics is/are indicator(s) of sinusitis rather than pulpitis?
A Type of pain
B Duration
C Response to mild painkillers
D Worse when patient is lying down
E Worse with head movements

Answers:
A No
B No
C No
D No
E Head movements such as moving up or down, exacerbate the pain from antral inflammation, while the pain in pulpitis remains unchanged.

Comments: The pain from pulpitis and sinusitis has similar characteristics such as the type, location and response to painkillers, and both become more intense by lying down.

Q3 Which of recommendations below is/are not useful for the treatment of acute viral sinusitis?
A Resting
B Surgery
C Decongestants
D Antibiotics
E Painkillers

Answers:
A No
B Surgery can be used for severe forms of chronic sinusitis, but always taking into consideration the possible complications.
C No
D Antibiotics should be useful only in bacterial and rarely in neglected viral sinusitis, in order to avoid serious complications such as secondary bacterial infections spreading into the jaws, eyes or brain.
E No

Comments: As the acute viral sinusitis lasts for 4–10 days, the best way to be treated is to advise the patient to take some rest, take enough liquids and fruits rich in vitamin C. In case the symptoms remain stable after four days, then the uptake of decongestants and painkillers should be suggested.

Case 6.7

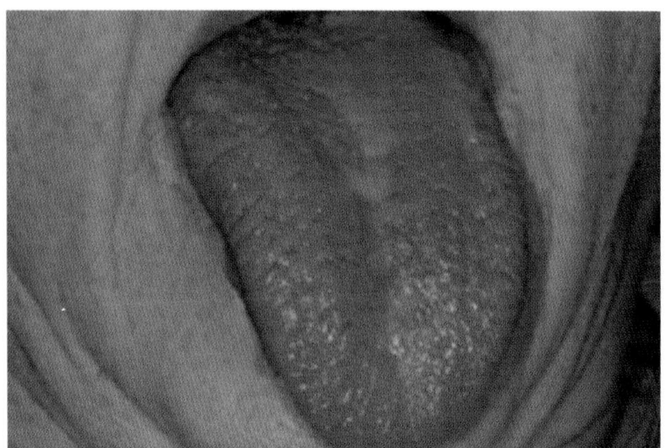

Figure 6.7

CO: A 62-year-old woman presented with pain and a burning sensation of her tongue.

HPC: This painful burning sensation started two years ago and since then remained constant during the day and worsened from midday to night with sleeping interference.

PMH: Her medical history revealed a mild hypertension and hypercholesterolemia that were controlled with amlodipine and statins respectively. Carcinophobia was diagnosed two years ago since her niece's death from breast carcinoma, but the patient refused any medication for her depression. She was an ex-smoker since the beginning of the mouth symptoms, but liked to consume spicy hot drinks and food during her meals.

OE: She is a post-menopausal woman with an extreme burning sensation of her tongue (mainly on the tip), inner surface of her lower lip and palate in clinically normal oral mucosa. Her tongue was mild fissured with no clinical evidence of atrophy or local irritation. This burning sensation was associated with a metallic-like taste and mouth dryness although the saliva flow rate was normal. Complete blood count (CBC) and biochemical blood investigations were not indicative for anemia or hormone disorders.

Q1 What is the cause of the pain-burning sensation?

- **A** Burning mouth syndrome
- **B** Multiple sclerosis
- **C** B12 or iron deficiency
- **D** Sjogren syndrome
- **E** Submucous fibrosis

Answers:

- **A** Burning mouth syndrome (BMS) is the cause and is characterized by an extreme burning sensation or pain, particularly on the tip of the tongue. It appears every day for more than two months without any clinical evidence of causative lesions and is seen predominantly at the afternoon or nights among pre- or post-menopause women, as well as patients with neuropsychiatric disorders.
- **B** No
- **C** No
- **D** No
- **E** No

Comments: The absence of atrophic glossitis helps clinicians to withdraw iron or B12 deficiencies from the diagnosis. The presence of burning sensation without white lesions or xerostomia rule out Submucous fibrosis and Sjogren syndrome. Multiple sclerosis sometimes appears with burning sensationin mouth or extremities but is always accompanied with peripheral and central neuropathies which were not seen in this lady. The absence of oral lesions such as atrophic glossitis, white lesions and xerostomia, peripheral or central neuropathies together with negative blood results easily rule out iron or B12 deficiencies, submucous fibrosis or even Sjogren syndrome and multiple sclerosis from the diagnosis respectively.

Q2 Which is/are the cardinal sign/s of burning mouth syndrome?

- **A** Burning sensation or pain
- **B** Headache
- **C** Metallic or bitter taste
- **D** Halitosis
- **E** Sialorrhea

Answers:

- **A** The chronic intermittent or constant burning sensation all over the mouth and particularly on the tongue is always reported and may last a few months or more.
- **B** No
- **C** Taste alterations such as metallic or bitter taste are common patients complains.
- **D** No
- **E** No

Comments: Headaches such as migraine or cluster/tension type are only seen in patients with BMS having neuropsychiatric disorders, while a sense of dryness and not a sense of excessive saliva or halitosis is reported in the majority of BMS patients.

Q3 Which is/are the differences between BMS and other neuropathic conditions in the mouth?

- **A** Type of complain
- **B** Onset of pain
- **C** Location of pain
- **D** Reaction with eating
- **E** Taste alterations

Answers:

- **A** In BMS patients the main complaint is pain together with a burning or tingling sensation, while in neuropathic conditions it is mostly pain.
- **B** In BMS the pain is spontaneous or idiopathic, while in neuropathic it is always associated with dental treatments.
- **C** In BMS, the pain is usually bilateral while in neuropathic conditions it is always unilateral.
- **D** Eating procedures improve symptoms in BMS, but make them worse in neuropathic conditions.
- **E** No

Comments: Taste is often altered in both conditions; reduced taste or metallic and bitter taste in BMS, and a mixed decrease or increase of sense of taste in neuropathic conditions are often reported.

Case 6.8

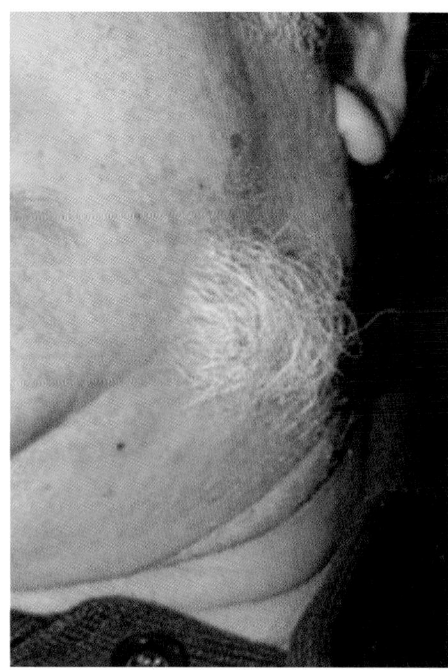

Figure 6.8

CO: A 67-year-old man asked for medical help for a severe pain in his mouth and left cheek over the last three years.

HPC: His pain was extremely severe and presented as a cluster of sharp, stabbing or throbbing aches lasting only a few seconds and affecting the lower left part of his face and adjacent teeth. It appeared initially with two to three episodes a week three years ago, but worsened and became a daily phenomenon over the last five months. The pain did not respond to cold or hot stimulus and could not be relieved with mild painkillers.

PMH: Hypertension and chronic bronchitis as well as an episode of herpes zoster on the waist that happened two months ago were the only serious medical problems recorded. He used to smoke one or two cigars occasionally, and his diet was poor in vegetables and fruit.

OE: The physical examination did not reveal any local cause of pain inside his mouth and facial skin, but when touching the facial skin around the molar area, a severe shooting pain was provoked and lasted a few seconds. According to the patient, this was the area that usually triggers the onset of pain and therefore it remained unshaved and unclean (Figure 6.8).

Q1 What is the cause of pain?

- **A** Pulpitis
- **B** Post-herpetic neuralgia
- **C** Scurvy
- **D** Trigeminal neuralgia
- **E** Multiple sclerosis

Answers:

- **A** No
- **B** No
- **C** No
- **D** Trigeminal neuralgia is the cause and characterized by a number of episodes of sharp stabbing, electric shock-like pain affecting usually one branch of the trigeminal nerve. It does not respond well to painkillers, but instead, is provoked by speaking or touching a certain area that is known as the trigger zone.
- **E** No

Comments: Neuropathic pain from multiple sclerosis or post-herpetic neuralgia is similar to the patient's pain, but could be easily ruled out as the location of pain was on his face and not on the waist, while other symptoms from the central nerve system are missing. Neuropathies are also seen in scurvy patients but easily excluded by the absence of hemorrhagic lesions like petechiae or ecchymosis in the mouth and skin of this patient.

Q2 Which are the diagnostic criteria for this condition?

- **A** Type of pain
- **B** Location of pain
- **C** Frequency of pain
- **D** Association with trigger zones
- **E** Response to painkillers

Answers:

- **A** In this neuralgia, the pain can be either a sharp, stabbing and throbbing pain in clusters (type I) or a constant dull burning sensation (type II).
- **B** The pain follows the distribution of one or two branches of the trigeminal nerve, usually on one side, and that is where its name comes from.
- **C** No
- **D** This neuropathic pain is always provoked by an irritation of the trigger zones which are certain areas either in the face or in the mouth that can be irritated by washing and touching or by teeth brushing and eating, respectively.
- **E** No

Comments: The pain at the early stage of trigeminal neuralgia is sharp, throbbing, lasting a few seconds and is spontaneously resolved. Nevertheless, as time goes on it may become more intense, and have minimal or no response at all to mild painkillers.

Q3 Which of the characteristics below differentiate the pain of this condition from atypical facial pain (AFP)?
- **A** Prevalence
- **B** Location
- **C** Duration
- **D** Provoking factors
- **E** Associated symptoms

Answers:
- **A** Trigeminal neuralgia is rare, while AFP is a common condition.
- **B** In the first condition, the pain is located along a branch of trigeminal nerve, while in AFP it could involve the whole face, neck etc.
- **C** The pain lasts a few hours or days in AFP, while it is a matter of only a few seconds in trigeminal neuralgia.
- **D** Light touching, shaving, brushing the teeth or hair, eating or speaking could trigger pain in trigeminal neuralgia, while stress is the trigger in AFP.
- **E** Secondary anosmia or taste alterations are often reported in AFP, but neither of them are reported in trigeminal neuralgia.

Case 6.9

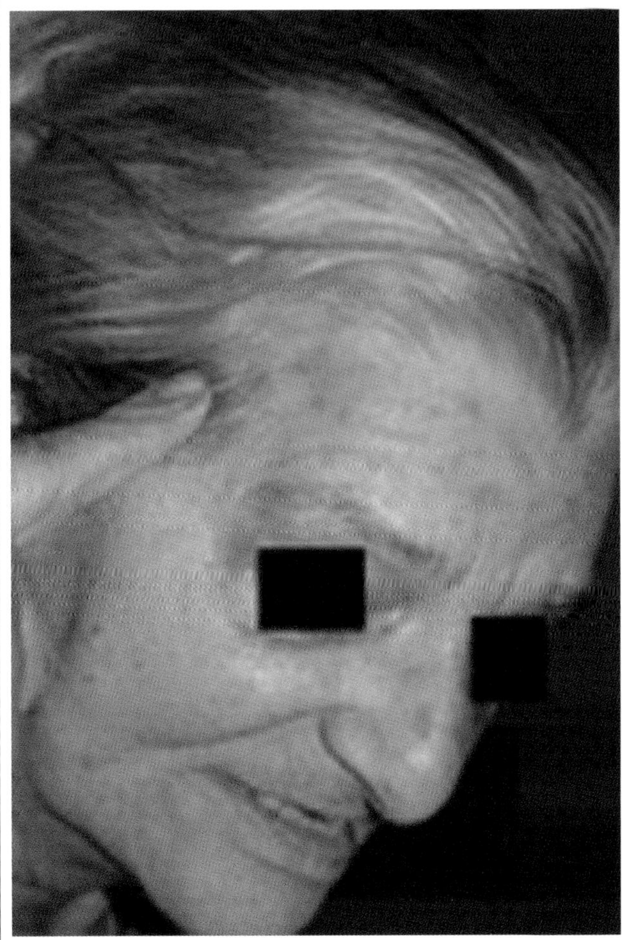

Figure 6.9

CO: A 72-year-old lady presented with severe headache located on her right temple over the last week.

HPC: The pain was an acute, continuous, throbbing type and was located on her right temple which is very sensitive to touch, as when hair combing. The pain was reflected towards her eye that show diplopia and spontaneous flashing lights, being associated with jaw claudications and polymyalgia.

PMH: Her medical record was clear apart from a few episodes of orthostatic hypotension due to hyperthyroidism which was controlled with methimazole, fluid, and salty food consumption. She was a chronic smoker of five cigarettes per day.

OE: A very thin lady with severe pain on her right temple which is partially resolved with rubbing of the area, but worsens with various head movements (Figure 6.9). Her pain was constant and associated with eye problems and generalized myalgia. No other local or systemic causes of pain were found intra or extra-orally. Her face was normal for her age with a few wrinkles on her temple which became deeper as the pain continued. Her blood results with normal range apart from ESR and CRP that were high.

Q1 What is the cause of pain?
- **A** Migraine
- **B** Temporomandibular dysfunction disorder
- **C** Herpes zoster
- **D** Wegener's granulomatosis (granulomatosis with polyangiitis)
- **E** Temporal arteritis

Answers:

- **A** No
- **B** No
- **C** No
- **D** No
- **E** Temporal arteritis is the cause. This condition is characterized by an acute throbbing, continuous pain that is located on the temporal and occipital area, predominantly affecting elderly female patients. It is strongly associated with vision problems (transient or permanent); jaw claudications, fatigue and rarely with fever and elevated erythrocyte sedimentation ratio (ESR). The scalp and especially the area where the superficial temporal artery lies is very sensitive in palpation and shows signs of ischemia due to the stenosis of the vessel.

Comments: Clinical characteristics and symptomatology allow clinicians to differ this condition from migraine, Wegener grannulomatosis, herpes zoster and TMJ dysfunction. In migraine, prodromal aura precedes migraines, while in Wegener grannulomatosis, loss of weight fever and lung and kidney involvement are common. Locally, the lack of vesicular rash along the 2 nd or 3 rd branch of trigeminal nerve excludes herpes zoster while dysregulation of TMJ is accompanied with pain in the area but without raised ESR or C-RP.

Q2 Which are the characteristics of this condition?

- **A** Youtng age
- **B** Localized pain
- **C** Reduced pulsation of temporal artery
- **D** Negative histological findings
- **E** Elevated erythrocyte sedimentation ratio (ESR)

Answers:

- **A** No
- **B** The pain is located along the route of a temporal artery in temple.
- **C** On palpation, the temporal artery is swollen and tender with a reduced pulse which is unrelated to atherosclerosis of the cervical arteries.
- **D** No
- **E** The ESR is elevated >50mm/h and is an indicator of temporal vasculitis.

Comments: Temporal arteritis is a vascular inflammation of the temporal artery which affects patients older than 50 years, and is characterized by an accumulation of inflammatory cells within the thick arterial wall (inner intima; media and inner adventitia), mostly of multinuclear giant cells.

Q3 Which is/or are the complication(s) of an untreated temporal arteritis?

- **A** Hearing loss
- **B** Blindness
- **C** Skin necrosis
- **D** Dementia
- **E** Difficulties with hair combing

Answers:

- **A** Sensorineural hearing loss can be a preceding or concurrent finding of a temporal arteritis.
- **B** Temporal or permanent loss of vision and other eye problems are related to the central retinal arterial occlusion due to the narrowing of the lumen from the inflammatory cells – giant cells within the underlying intima.
- **C** Skin necrosis can be a rare complication and is attributed to the ischemia induced by the narrowing of the lumen of the responsible vessel.
- **D** Dementia is a rare complication and must always be considered as a possible cause in older patients with any sudden onset of mental retardation.
- **E** Hair combing can be very difficult especially in ladies with long hair, as the skin of the scalp and especially its temporal part is extremely sensitive on touching.

Case 6.10

CO: A 32-year-old man presented with severe pain on the back of his tongue and his throat over the last three months.

HPC: The pain started at the same time as the beginning of mucositis induced by chemo-radiotherapy for a non-surgical carcinoma on the base of his tongue and right palatinopharyngeal folds. Two months after the end of his treatment, the mucositis was almost completely gone, but the pain in his throat remained and was reflected towards his upper and lower molars as well as the temporomandibular joint. The pain was deep and constant, lasting for hours, with daily variations in severity. It was more intense in the early mornings, with the first attempts at swallowing, and late at night when lying down for sleep. Days without pain were not recorded.

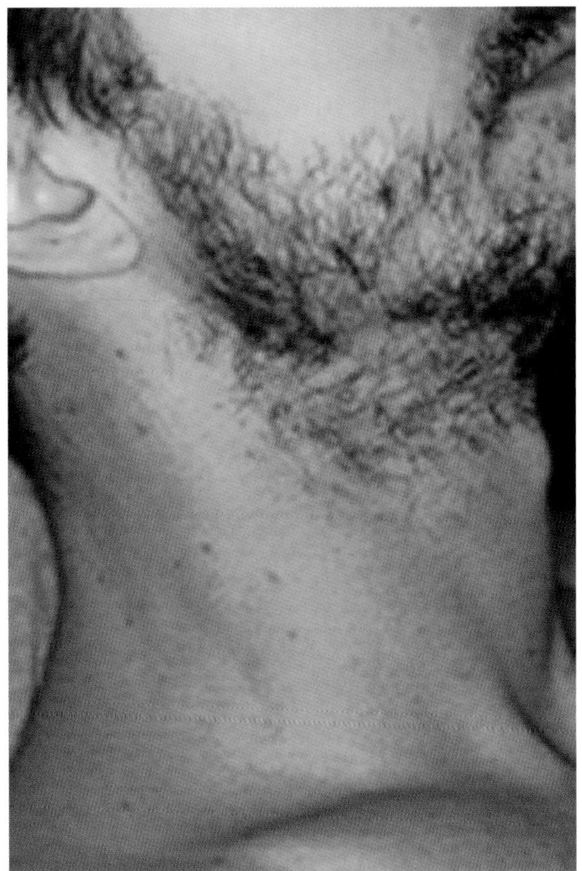

Figure 6.10

PMH: His medical history was unremarkable apart from a recently diagnosed oropharyngeal carcinoma which was possibly related to his previous human papillomavirus (HPV) infection and treated with cisplatin chemotherapy (seven sessions once a week) and 30 sessions of radiotherapy. This resulted in an oropharyngeal mucositis grade III, which was symptomatically treated (hydration, rinses with chamomile, moisturizing gels). He was a passive smoker but never a drinker.

OE: The examination did not show any clinical evidence of a remaining tumor inside his mouth or other causes of local pain such as mucositis or infections. Xerostomia and dysgeusia were stable. Additionally, some pressure on the area of his neck behind the right submandibular gland triggered a deep and severe pain that reflected towards the adjacent upper and lower molars and ipsilateral ear. A similar pain was induced when the patient choked on water. No other lesions were detected on his neck apart from a diffuse skin erythema and dryness due to his previous radiotherapy (Figure 6.10). Endoscopy and MRI did not reveal any suspicious lesions inside his oropharynx.

Q1 What is the cause of pain?

- **A** Angina pain
- **B** Glossopharyngeal neuralgia
- **C** Mucositis
- **D** Odynophagia
- **E** Tumor (previous or new)

Answers:

- **A** No
- **B** No
- **C** No
- **D** Odynophagia is the cause and characterized by sharp, stabbing pain during swallowing in a number of conditions. Some of them are transient such as a cold, flu infection or injury, and some other chronic conditions such as like heartburn or gastroesophageal reflux disease (GERD), immune deficiency such as HIV, acquired immunodeficiency syndrome (AIDS) and radiotherapy or even esophageal carcinomas.
- **E** No

Comments: The patient's pain characteristics such as its long duration (hours) rules out glossopharyngeal neuralgia from the diagnosis, despite the fact that the pain is also sharp there and triggered by swallowing. Angina can also cause pain in the neck and teeth, but this pain can be triggered by exercise or activities and not by swallowing, lasts a few minutes and may disappeared with rest. The absence of ulcerations or suspicious lesions inside his mouth and throat excludes mucositis or tumor (new or old) from the diagnosis.

Q2 What is the main difference between odynophagia and dysphagia?

- **A** Symptomatology
- **B** Location
- **C** Pathogenesis
- **D** Spontaneous resolution
- **E** Risk patients

Answers:

- **A** Odynophagia is the condition in which pain is elicited with swallowing, while dysphagia is a clinical term given for various difficulties in swallowing regardless of the induced pain.
- **B** No
- **C** No
- **D** No
- **E** No

Comments: Both conditions share common etiological factors such as *Candida* or *Herpes* infections, topical inflammation such as esophagitis and pharyngeal abscesses, immunodeficiencies induced by HIV infection, chemo/radiotherapy, and tumors in patients regardless of their age or sex.

Q3 Which of the laboratory investigations below is/are mandatory for the diagnosis of this condition?

- **A** Endoscopy
- **B** Biopsy
- **C** MRI
- **D** Blood tests
- **E** Cultures

Answers:

- **A** Endoscopy is the most important tool that helps us to detect digestive lesions such as constrictions, tumors, ulcerations, or infections.
- **B** Biopsy is sometimes useful to confirm or not any suspicious pharyngeal lesions.
- **C** MRI. It allows the identification of changes in lesions, previously seen with the endoscopic method, that were related to the pain induction.
- **D** No
- **E** No

Comments: Blood and culture tests are used for the exclusion of various immunodeficiencies or bacterial and fungal infections that may participate in the pathogenesis of odynophagia.

7

Red Lesions

Red lesions are large group of diseases with various etiology; some of them are traumatic, infective, reactive, premalignant or malignant or even congenital or idiopathic. Their red color could be attributed to the proximity of local blood vessels to a thin oral mucosa, dilation or increased in number of existing vessels, or blood extravasations into oral mucosa (See Figure 7.0).

Table 7 lists the common causes of oral red lesions.

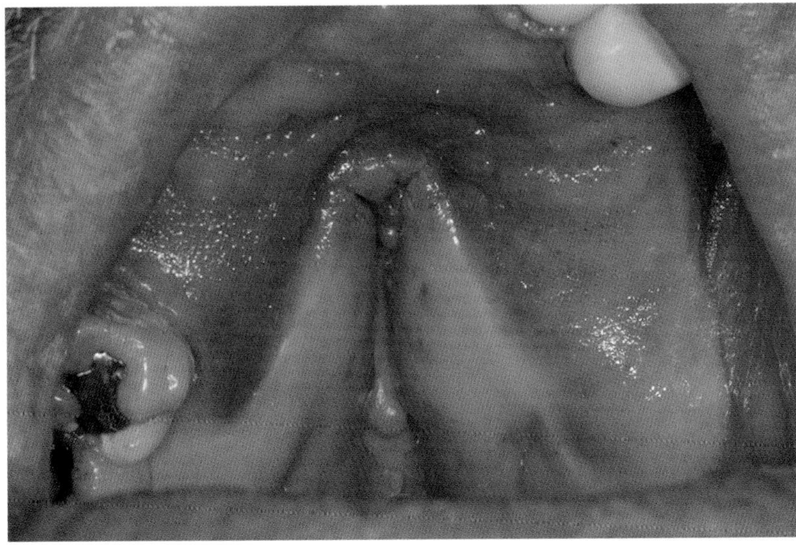

Figure 7.0 Erythematous candidiasis in the palate: induced by constant wear of a partial denture.

Clinical Guide to Oral Diseases, First Edition. Dimitris Malamos and Crispian Scully.

Companion website: www.wiley.com/go/malamos/clinical_guide

Table 7 The common causes of oral red lesions.

- Localized
    - Atrophy of mucosa
    - Trauma
    - Burns
    - Geographic stomatitis
  - Vascular changes
    - Increased vascularity
      - Angiomas (purple)
      - Chronic renal failure
      - Telangiectasias
      - Vasculitis
      - Wegener's granulomatosis
      - Henoch-Schonlein purpura
      - Polyarteritis nodosa
    - Increased fragility
      - Senile purpura
    - Increased permeability
      - Ehlers-Danlos syndrome
  - Inflammation
    - Burns
    - Denture-induced stomatitis
    - Psoriasis
    - Plasma cell gingivitis
    - Lichen planus
    - Lichenoid reaction
    - Lupus erythematosus
    - Median rhomboid glossitis
    - Desquamative gingivitis
    - Fixed drug eruption
  - Infections
    - HIV
    - Measles
    - Rubella
    - Infection mononucleosis
    - Syphilis

Table 7 (Continued)

    - Candidiasis
  - Neoplasia
    - Cancer
    - Erythroplakia
    - Mucoepithelial dysplasia
    - Kaposi sarcoma
  - Bleeding
    - Amyloidosis
- Diffused
  - Atrophy of mucosa
    - Avitaminosis (B12)
  - Vascular changes
    - Increased vascularity
      - Hyperglobulinemia purpura
    - Increased fragility
      - Scurvy
      - Marfan syndrome
    - Increased permeability
      - Ehlers-Danlos syndrome
      - Drug allergies
  - Inflammation
    - Erythema nodosum in Crohn's disease
    - Sarcoidosis
  - Infections
    - Cellulitis
    - Erythematous candidiasis
  - Neoplasia
    - Wallenstrom macroglobulinemia
    - Leukemia
    - Malignant histiocytosis
    - Multiple myeloma
  - Bleeding
    - Polycythemia
    - Thrombopenia

Case 7.1

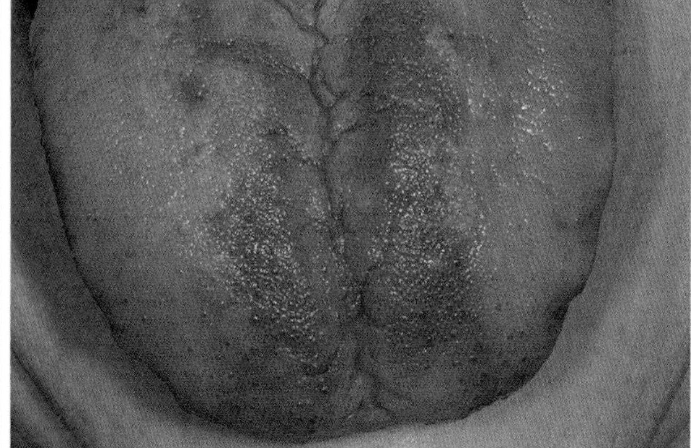

Figure 7.1

CO: A 32-year-old woman presented for an evaluation of a number of red lesions inside her mouth.

HPC: The lesions appeared gradually two months ago when the patient gave birth to her child, but became more serious over last two weeks.

PMH: The patient had a clear medical history apart from a history of an iron deficiency anemia which was more obvious during her pregnancy and controlled with regular iron tablets. She did not report allergies or other serious diseases apart from a periapical infection from her lower right first molar that was relieved with a wide spectrum of antibiotics last week. She was a vegetarian, non-smoker or drinker and none of her close relatives had similar red lesions.

OE: Diffuse erythematous lesions on the dorsum of the tongue (Figure 7.1), buccal mucosae, inner surface of both lips and soft palate. The oral lesions were associated in places with atrophic but not ulcerated oral mucosa. A burning sensation rather than itching or pain was reported which was being exacerbated with spicy foods and remained stable all day. No other oral, skin, or other mucosae lesions were seen.

Q1 What is the diagnosis?

- **A** Erythematous candidiasis
- **B** Erythroplakia
- **C** Allergic reaction to foods
- **D** Deficiency of vitamin B12
- **E** Burning mouth syndrome

Answers:

- **A** No
- **B** No
- **C** No
- **D** A deficiency of vitamin B12 appears with erythematous oral mucosa, pale skin, fragile nails and is associated sometimes with neurological and heart problems such as tingling sensation in the hands and feet, paresthesia, neuropathic pain, numbness, and poor reflexes, tachycardia and altered blood pressure. The oral mucosa presents focal or diffuse erythematous red areas causing a constant burning sensation.
- **E** No

Comments: Burning sensation is also found in burning mouth syndrome, candidiasis or food allergies, but differs, In burning mouth syndrome the mucosa is normal and not red, in candidiasis induced by antibiotics the mucosa is white covered with pseudomembranes or erythematous and in allergies is accompanied with facial swelling and an itching sensation. Erythroplakia appears as a red lesion, but differs as it is single rather than multiple and has a raised velvety surface with long duration and is usually seen in smokers and heavy drinkers.

Q2 Which is the less frequent cause of B12 deficiency?

- **A** Asthma
- **B** Gastrectomy
- **C** Pregnancy
- **D** Myeloma
- **E** Folate deficiency

Answers:

- **A** Asthma is the less frequent cause of B12 deficiency. This vitamin deficiency is seen only in a minority of patients with asthma especially in women aged 50–59 years old who have a gastroesophageal disease.
- **B** No
- **C** No
- **D** No
- **E** No

Comments: Pernicious anemia is a classic example of B12 deficiency and characterized by the reduced absorption of B12 in the ileum and small intestine due to the lack of (i) intrinsic factor; (ii) after gastric surgery for tumors; (iii) malabsorption in alcoholic patients or by increased demand in pregnancy or/and poor diet. It often comes with folate deficiency causing abnormal large red cells production and heart and neurological problems.

Q3 Which of the laboratory findings is/or are NOT characteristic of B12 deficiency?

- **A** Presence of drepanocytes in blood smears
- **B** Reduced level of serum folic acid
- **C** Low number of parietal cells in stomach biopsies
- **D** Increased level of homocysteine and methylmalonic acid in the blood
- **E** Increased intrinsic factor in stomach juices

Answers:

- **A** The detection of drepanocytes (sickled-shaped cells) is characteristic of sickle cell and not B12 deficiency anemia.
- **B** No
- **C** No
- **D** No
- **E** The intrinsic factor is produced by the parietal cells and helps the absorption of vitamin B12, whose deficiency has been credited to reduced number of the parietal cells.

Comments: The Schilling test was initially used for the detection of B12 deficiency, but has been recently replaced by simpler tests such as the measurement of serum protein levels of homocysteine or methylmalonic acid and intrinsic factor These proteins are secreted by the parietal cells that were found in reduced numbers with biopsies of the fundus and body of the stomach.

Case 7.2

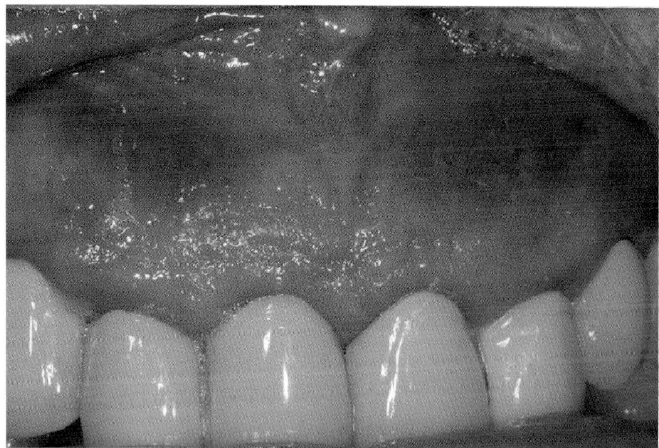

Figure 7.2

CO: A 56-year-old woman presented with complaints about a burning and itching sensation of her mouth.

HPC: The burning sensation started two to three months from the beginning of treatment for multiple sclerosis with Interferon beta 1a.

PMH: Multiple sclerosis was diagnosed 25 years ago and remained asymptomatic apart from a few episodes of atypical pain along the third branch of right trigeminal nerve and a lichenoid rash on both her legs. She started to take interferon once a week for the last year and recently venlafaxine hydroxide 75 mg daily. Blood or other serious diseases were not recorded. Smoking and drinking were limited on social occasions only.

OE: The oral examination revealed two areas of diffuse erythema with superficial small ulcerations in the anterior upper alveolar mucosa, causing her mild itching but no pain (Figure 7.2).

No other oral lesions apart from a lichenoid reaction to both her legs were seen.

Q1 What is the cause of these oral lesions?

- **A** Erythroplakia
- **B** Plasma cell gingivitis
- **C** Drug reaction
- **D** Traumatic erythema
- **E** Multiple sclerosis

Answers:

- **A** No
- **B** No
- **C** Drug reaction could be the cause. This is a hypersensitivity reaction to interferon rather than to venlafaxine and is characterized by oval erythematous patches on the oral mucosa which appeared a few months later after the interferon started, accompanied with itching sensation in the mouth and skin.
- **D** No
- **E** No

Comments: Erythematous gingival lesions are common and are the results of local trauma (traumatic erythema) or cosmetic or food allergies(plasma cell gingivitis) or even neoplasies (erythroplakia)However these lesions differs from interferone induced erythema as there is not a history of trauma, allergies and the lesions are multiple with shiny red surface and slow progress Multiple sclerosis appears with atypical neuropathic pain from the trigeminal nerve but never with red lesions.

Q2 Which of the investigations below can be used for the diagnosis of multiple sclerosis?

- **A** Cerebrospinal fluid analysis
- **B** Urine analysis
- **C** MRI of brain
- **D** Chest X-rays
- **E** Blood tests

Answers:

- **A** Cerebrospinal fluid analysis will show chronic inflammation mediators such as prostaglandins, chemokines, myelin, neurofilament proteins, and the presence of oligoclonal bands of IgG in electrophoresis.
- **B** No
- **C** MRI shows disseminated demyelinated areas in the brain which look like small hypo- or hyperintense lesions that are surrounded by edema (acute) or atrophy (chronic phase).
- **D** No
- **E** No

Comments: Chest X-rays, blood tests and urine analysis cannot be done to confirm multiple sclerosis, but to rule out other diseases such as Lyme disease, syphilis, HIV/AIDS and other genetic disorders that affect the nerves.

Q3 Which phenomenon is a characteristic finding of multiple sclerosis?

- **A** Raynaud's phenomenon
- **B** On–off phenomenon
- **C** Iceberg phenomenon
- **D** Uhthoff's phenomenon
- **E** Counter-steal phenomenon

Answers:

- **A** No
- **B** No
- **C** No
- **D** Uththoff's phenomenon is characterized by a worsening of neurological symptoms in multiple sclerosis patients in the cases when their body is exposed to very hot conditions (weather, exercise, fever, sauna).
- **E** No

Comments: The other phenomena characterize different other diseases irrelevant to multiple sclerosis. Specifically Raynaud's phenomenon shows as a vasospasm of the fingers and toes of patients with connective tissue disorders when they are exposed to cold temperature. The on–off phenomenon is seen in patients with Parkinson's disease and is referred to as the switch between mobility and immobility in levodopa treated patients, while the iceberg phenomenon is not a characteristic of solely one disease, but a spectrum of diseases (clinical, preclinical, subclinical, and undiagnosed) in a community. The counter-steal phenomenon occurs during hyperventilation in patients with cerebrovascular diseases due to focal loss of autoregulation to CO_2.

Case 7.3

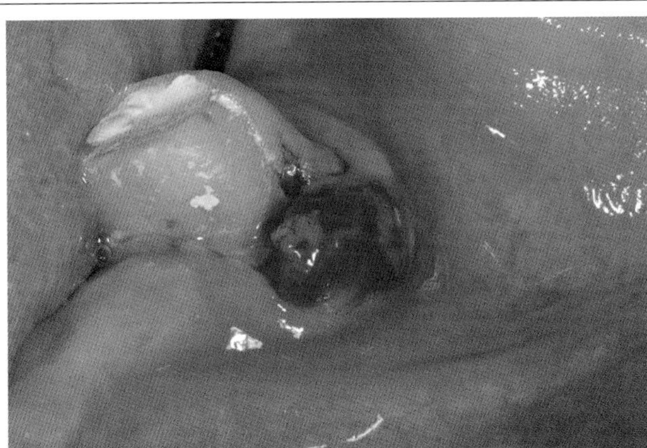

Figure 7.3

CO: A 64-year-old woman was referred for examination of a red swelling in the gingivae of her second lower molar.

HPC: The lesion was noticed two weeks ago by her dentist who removed her old broken bridge on the gingivae along the bifurcation of her previously capped molar.

PMH: She suffered from mild diabetes and hypertension which were both controlled by diet. No other serious medical problems, allergies or surgeries were recorded apart from a basal cell carcinoma that was removed on the skin of her forehead three years ago.

OE: A red, soft and fragile mass had arisen from the facial gingivae of the second left lower molar (Figure 7.3). The lesion was asymptomatic and easily bled with touching while the adjacent molar did not respond to various pulp tests. The patient is partially edentulous and her oral hygiene was not very good. No other lesions were recorded in her mouth or other mucosae.

Q1 What is the possible diagnosis?

- **A** Gingival carcinoma
- **B** Giant cell epulis
- **C** Parulis
- **D** Traumatic fibroma
- **E** Hemangioma

Answers:

- **A** No
- **B** No
- **C** Parulis is a red, fragile, soft nodule on the facial or lingual gingival surface of a non-vital tooth or one with a deep periodontal pocket, and it can easily bleed with pressure, leaving a sinus opening to drain the periapical infection into the mouth.
- **D** No
- **E** No

Comments: The very soft consistency of the lesion excludes gingival carcinomas from the diagnosis. Giant cell and traumatic fibroma lesions are seen close to vital teeth and their histological picture includes giant cell cells and fibrous cells (mature mixed with immature) rather than granulation tissue as seen in this patient if biopsy was taken.

Q2 Which is/or are the LESS diagnostic test/s for parulis?
- **A** Biopsy
- **B** Pulp testing
- **C** Periodontal probing
- **D** Periapical X-rays
- **E** Culture

Answers:
- **A** Biopsy is rarely used to exclude any gingival neoplasias (carcinomas; sarcomas) and recommended only to patients with carcinophobia or previous cancer history.
- **B** No
- **C** No
- **D** No
- **E** Culture is not useful for diagnosis as a great number of germs have been isolated in parulis, among them are *Bacteroides*, *Treponema denticola*, *Eubacterium*, *Fusobacterium*, *Peptostreptococcus*, *Actinomyces*, and *Enterococcus faecalis*.

Comments: The dentist should diagnose the cause of parulis and in the case of a pulp necrosis or periapical infection with pulp testing and x-rays or periodontal abscess with probing, to do a root canal treatment of the suspected tooth or deep scaling respectively. In the case of treatment failure, the suspected tooth should be extracted.

Q3 Which other oral diseases are accompanied with granulomatous fistulae lesions?
- **A** Dens in dente
- **B** Osteomyelitis
- **C** Peri-implantitis
- **D** Fluorosis
- **E** Scleroderma

Answers:
- **A** Dens in dente. These teeth are characterized by the invagination of enamel and dentine into the dental papillae and remnants of food that are easily lodged in the abnormal tooth surface. These cause caries which rapidly grow, causing pulp necrosis and periapical infections.
- **B** Chronic osteomyelitis of the jaws is characterized by an intense periosteum inflammation and bony destruction as well as a sequestration with numerous intra- and extra-oral granuloma fistulas.
- **C** Peri-implantitis is the common cause of an implant loss and is characterized by an inflammation around the implant causing bony loss, forming in this way soft hemorrhagic lesions similar to parulis.
- **D** No
- **E** No

Comments: Other diseases affect the teeth structure and color like fluorosis or the periodontal ligament of gingivae in sclerodema but are rarely responsible for periapical or periodontal abscesses with or without grannulation fistula.

Case 7.4

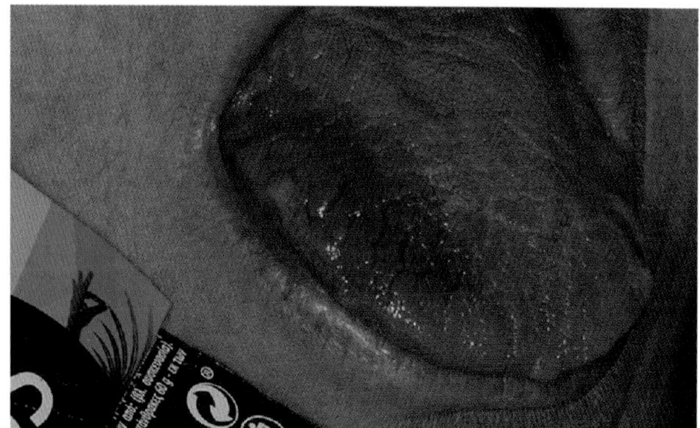

Figure 7.4

CO: A 58-year-old woman presented with a red area on the dorsum of her tongue.

HPC: The lesion appeared three days ago and was associated with a tingling and burning sensation. Similar lesions were seen close to her buccal mucosae adjacent to her molars.

PMH: She suffered from mild diabetes and had been on venlafaxine hydrochloride tablets over the last eight years for her depression, and anti-histamine drugs when needed only for her hay fever. She is allergic to pollen and oysters. She is a chronic smoker, but she has recently tried to quit smoking by using cinnamon or menthol chewing gums, which she used to keep in her right buccal sulcus for many hours in the day.

OE: The oral examination revealed a red well-defined area on the right side of the dorsum of the tongue, which was extended from the tip to the follate papillae areas. This lesion showed a lack of filiform papillae and was sensitive to touch, but did not bleed, was non-indurate, or associated with cervical lymphadenopathy (Figure 7.4).

No other lesions were seen apart from a mild erythema and a few superficial erosions at the buccal mucosa close to the tongue lesion.

Q1 What is the diagnosis?

- **A** Erythroplakia
- **B** Erythematous candidiasis
- **C** Plasma cell glossitis
- **D** Cinnamon-induced contact stomatitis
- **E** Geographic tongue

Answers:

- **A** No
- **B** No
- **C** No
- **D** Cinnamon-induced stomatitis is the cause. The daily and constant use of cinnamon or menthol products can cause allergic stomatitis which might be manifested either as an erythematous lesion associated with small vesicles and erosions (acute phase) as is seen in this lady, or as hyperplastic white plaques (chronic phase). The holding of cinnamon flavored gum in the buccal sulcus causes a restricted irritation of the buccal mucosa and lateral margins of tongue, Similar lesions are more extensive and diffuse in the gums and oral mucosa appear when toothpaste or mouth washes with cinammon or mint flavor are over used.
- **E** No

Comments: The cinnamon induced lesions differentiate from other similar tongue lesions such as geographic tongue, erythematous Candidosis, erythroplakia and plasma cell glossitis. In cinnamon glossitis , the lesion is usually in contact with the irritant (chew gum) while in geographic tongue , erythmatous Candidosis, plasma cell glossitis and erythroplakia is irrelevant . In plasma cell glossitis similar lesions are found in other mucosae while in erythematous Candidosis the tongue lesion is so closely related with palatal lesion giving the impression of kissing each other. In geographic tongue the margins are white and hyperplastic and changeable with time. In cinnamon stomatitis the margins are red and ill defined. Erythroplakia has a velvety appearance and a long aggressive course while in cinnamon stomatis the lesion is soft and last as long the irritant used.

Q2 Which of the dental materials below rarely cause contact allergic stomatitis?

- **A** Mercury in amalgams
- **B** Acrylic monomer for denture construction
- **C** Palladium in fixed prosthesis
- **D** Ethylene amine activator in impression material
- **E** Latex in gloves or rubber dams

Answers:

- **A** No
- **B** No
- **C** Palladium rarely causes contact stomatitis and is dependent on the water solubility of the palladium components, especially its nickel. It is usually seen close to the palladium based alloys.
- **D** No
- **E** No

Comments: Contact stomatitis is a delayed hypersensitivity reaction (type IV) of oral mucosa against previously exposed dental material via a cascade of cellular immunity steps. Mercury is highly toxic in large quantities and not in those found in amalgam fillings. Latex allergies are common among patients with hay fever or their work in the rubber industry. Acrylic resin and impression material activators cause an allergic reaction closely related with areas of contact with the oral mucosa.

Q3 Which of the lesions below is/or are NOT oral delayed hypersensitivity reaction/s type IV)?

- **A** Plasma cell stomatitis
- **B** Pemphigus
- **C** Angioedema
- **D** Granulomatous disorders
- **E** Lichenoid reactions

Answers:

- **A** No
- **B** Pemphigus is a hypersensitivity reaction of type II in which desmoglein 1 and 3 abs formed and attract the epithelial desmosomes, causing the loss of their integrity-epithelial separation and intra-epithelial bullae formation.
- **C** Angioedema is an anaphylactic hypersensitivity reaction type I.
- **D** No
- **E** No

Comments: Hypersensitivity reactions are a series of reactions that are produced by a normal immune system and categorized by four types. Type I is responsible for asthma, atopy or anaphylaxis; type II for autoimmune diseases; type III for immune-complex deposition diseases; type IV for contact dermatitis, multiple sclerosis and celiac diseases. Plasma cell gingivitis and lichenoid reaction to amalgam and chronic granulomatous conditions are hypersensitivity reactions type IV.

Case 7.5

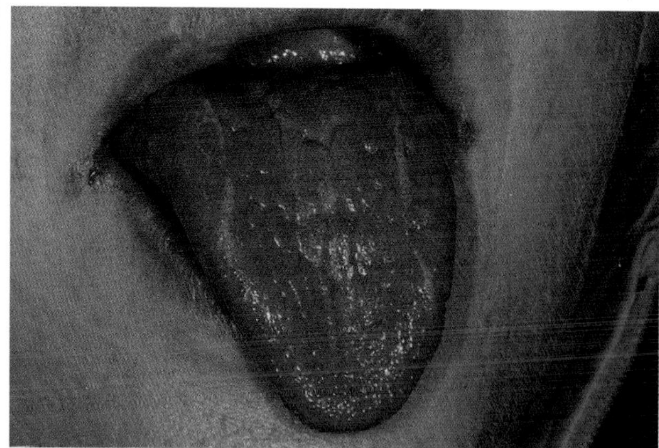

Figure 7.5

CO: A 26-year old man presented with a burning sensation of his red tongue.

HPC: The burning sensation appeared one week after an upper respiratory infection and associated with an erythematous burning tongue, and inflammation of the angles of his mouth.

PMH: He was a heroin addict who was recently diagnosed positive for HIV virus, because of his frequent respiratory, mouth, or genital fungal infections. He had not taken any medicines for his HIV infection at that time apart from a course of wide spectrum antibiotics for his recent upper respiratory infection.

OE: The oral examination revealed an erythematous, sensitive tongue, which easily bled with touching (Figure 7.5). No other lesions were seen apart from an inflammation and crusting of the angles of his mouth. Cervical lymphadenopathy was detected and was possibly related to his previous upper respiratory infection. No other skin lesions or general symptomatology was recorded.

Q1 What is the diagnosis of his red tongue?

- **A** Pernicious anemia
- **B** Allergic stomatitis
- **C** Sideropenic anemia
- **D** Erythematous candidiasis
- **E** Median rhomboid glossitis

Answers:

- **A** No
- **B** No
- **C** No
- **D** Erythematous candidiasis is the cause. This fungal infection usually affects patients with immunodeficiencies due to HIV infection, immunosuppressive drugs, and rarely antibiotics. It is characterized by diffuse erythematous patches on the whole dorsum of the tongue, palate and commissures (angular cheilitis) and is also accompanied by a burning sensation.
- **E** No

Comments: In erythematous candidiasis, the lesions are covered over the whole of the dorsum of the tongue, in contrast with the median rhomboid glossitis where they are restricted only to the middle. Diffuse erythema is also seen in sideropenic and pernicious anemia, as well as in allergic stomatitis. Angular cheilitis is common in iron deficiency anemias in which the tongue is pale, smooth and shiny due to the loss of filiform and fungiform papillae, and accompanied with a pallor of the skin and oral mucosa and koilonychias, but these findings were not found in this patient. Diffuse erythema is also seen in allergic stomatitis, but the lesions are scattered and sometimes associated with oral ulcerations and skin pruritus.

Q2 Which of the parameters below is/or are NOT associated with oral candidiasis?

- **A** Hypersalivation
- **B** Reduced occlusal height
- **C** Immunodeficiencies
- **D** Glucagonoma
- **E** Smoking

Answers:

- **A** Hypersalivation is characterized by excessive production and secretion of saliva in the mouth. The increased saliva cleans the mouth from debris, bacteria and fungi, thus making an unfriendly environment for fungi to grow.
- **B** No
- **C** No
- **D** No
- **E** No

Comments: *Candida albicans* is the most common fungus which is responsible for infection in the angles of the mouth (angular cheilitis) in patients with a reduced occlusal vertical dimension or anemia, infections in the tongue and the rest of mouth (candidiasis) in patients with immunodeficiencies (i.e. HIV); or systemic diseases affecting sugar metabolism (diabetes, glucagonoma); or xerostomia. Drugs (cytotoxic, steroids; antibiotics) together with harmful habits such as smoking alter the oral microflora leading to the oral mucosa being vulnerable to fungal infection.

Q3 Apart from *albicans*, which other *Candida* species have been isolated exclusively in HIV +ve patients?

A *Candida tropicalis*
B *Candida krusei*
C *Candida glabrata*
D *Candida parapsilosis*
E *Candida dubliniensis*

Answers:

A No
B No
C No
D No
E *Candida dubliniensis* is an opportunistic yeast which is isolated in few incompetent patients (<3%) but is mainly found in HIV +ve patients and responds well to voriconazole, itraconazole and amphotericin and sometimes to fluconazole.

Comments: All the other *Candida* species are isolated in acute and chronic fungal infections regardless the patient's HIV status.

Case 7.6

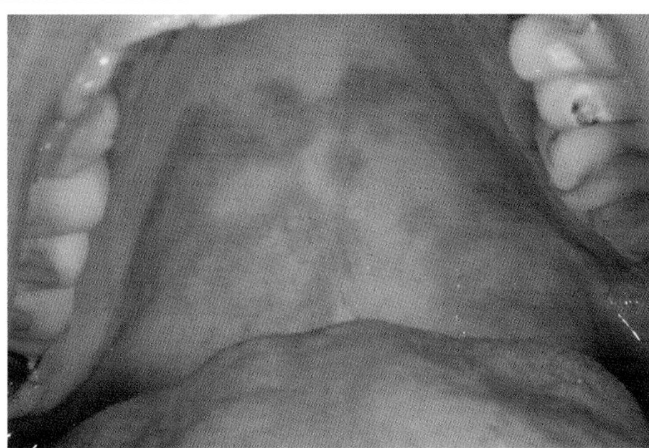

Figure 7.6

CO: A 39-year-old woman presented for an evaluation of red lesions on her palate.

HPC: The red lesions were first noticed by the patient two months ago after an episode of vomiting. The lesions have come and gone since then, leaving no scars and associated with a mild burning sensation.

PMH: The patient had no serious medical problems apart from chronic gastritis and the presence of *Helicobacter pylori* found with endoscopy. Allergies to various cosmetics or foods were not reported, while laboratory investigations did not confirm the presence of any blood dyscrasias, connective tissue disorders or recent infections.

OE: Oral examination revealed multiple superficial red lesions on her soft palate which form a network of red patches intermingled with zones of normal mucosa (Figure 7.6). The lesions lasted one to two weeks and reappeared very soon, forming different shaped lesions and being associated with a mild burning sensation. No other oral, skin and other mucosae lesions or cervical lymphadenopathy were found, apart from a few depapillated areas on the dorsum of her tongue forming ring-like erythematous lesions with white margins.

Q1 What is the cause of her palatal lesions?

A Syphilis (plaques)
B Reiter syndrome
C Geographic stomatitis
D Polycythemia vera
E Psoriasis

Answers:

A No
B No
C Geographic stomatitis is the cause. This is a benign condition characterized by multiple circinate erythematous patches on the palate, but mainly seen on the dorsum and lateral margin of the tongue which last from a few days to one or two weeks causing mild symptomatology.
D No
E No

Comments: Other diseases such as polycythemia vera, syphilis, Reiter syndrome and psoriasis could present with similar mucosa lesions, but were easily excluded, as having additional clinical and laboratory findings. Polycythemia vera is characterized by abnormal platelets in number or function; syphilis by *Treponema* Abs in the serum and systemic lymphadenitis; Reiter syndrome associated with inflammatory arthritis, conjunctivitis, and cervicitis; while psoriasis with numerous itchy, scaling red skin plaques, arthritis, and nail involvement.

Q2 Which histological features are NOT characteristic of geographic stomatitis?

A Parakeratosis
B Acanthosis
C Accumulation of polymorph white cells within the epithelium
D Civatte bodies
E Sub-mucosa fibrosis

Answers:

A No

B No

C No

D Civatte bodies are characteristic histological findings in a great number of diseases such as lichen planus; discoid lupus erythematosus; sarcoidosis; erythema multiformis; and bullous pemphigoid, but is never seen in geographic tongue lesions. These bodies appear as homogeneous eosinophilic masses of keratin, intermediate filaments covered with immunoglobulins, mainly IgM at the junction of the epithelium with the corium and are the result of basal cell apoptosis.

E Sub-mucous fibrosis is commonly seen in patients who are exposed to extreme weather conditions (sun); chronic anemia (iron) or areca nut (chewing instead of smoking) and characterized by an juxta epithelial inflammation leading to increased fibroblastic activity, delayed collagen breakdown and replacement of elastin with fibrin fibers.

Comments: The histological findings in geographic stomatitis include parakeratosis; hyperplasia of the spindle cell layer, accumulation of polymorphs in the epithelium forming Munro microabscesses, but with no *Candida albicans* hyphae colonization. Dilatation of superficial vessels and perivascular inflammation with chronic inflammatory cells are also seen.

Q3 Which of the conditions below is/or are characterized by the formation of neutrophils-microabscesses within the epithelium?

A Psoriasis

B Dermatitis hepertiformis

C Geographic tongue

D Mycosis fungoides

E Candidiasis

Answers:

A Psoriasis is characterized by the accumulation of polymorphs within the stratum corneum (Munro-microabscess).

B No

C Geographic tongue has similar histological microabscesses as psoriasis.

D No

E In acute oral candidiasis, the upper layers of the epithelium are penetrated by *Candida* hyphae and polymorphs; the last accumulate and form microabscesses.

Comments: Microabscess is a focal accumulation of inflammatory cells within or below the epithelium. The microabscesses seen within the epithelium are from neutrophils (psoriasis and geographic tongue), lymphocytes (lymphoma type of mycoses fungoides), and eosinophils (eosinophilic esophangitis). In pemphigus and dermatitis herpetiformis the microabscesses are located within the upper corium.

Case 7.7

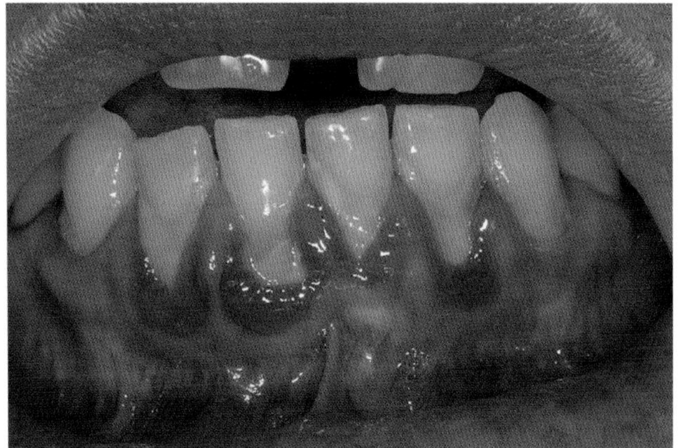

Figure 7.7

CO: A 52-year-old woman presented with halitosis and spontaneous bleeding from her gums.

HPC: Her halitosis was first noticed by her husband over the last six months, first in the mornings, but gradually during the whole day, while the bleeding from her gums was initially seen with tooth-brushing but recently appeared automatically, without any local irritation.

PMH: She was an overweight post-menopausal lady with no serious medical problems apart from a familiar hypercholesterolemia and mild diabetes that were controlled with statins and diet. She did not have a history of skin or venereal diseases or allergies, but was a chronic smoker of >30 cigarettes, and used chewing gum with strong flavor on a daily basis to improve her halitosis.

OE: The oral examination revealed swollen erythematous gingivae characterized by an enlargement of interdental papillae and gingival recession at some places closely related to calculus accumulations. The anterior gingivae (free and attached) of the lower incisors were red and bled easily with probing (Figure 7.7). No other lesions were detected intra- or extra-orally. Bad breath was noticed when the patient was asked to breathe out. Recent blood tests did not reveal any blood dyscrasias but OPG revealed severe alveolar bone loss mainly on upper and lower molars area.

Q1 What is the possible diagnosis?

- **A** Acute necrotizing gingivitis
- **B** Herpetic gingivostomatitis
- **C** Linear gingival erythema
- **D** Chronic periodontitis
- **E** Plasma cell gingivitis

Answers:

- **A** No
- **B** No
- **C** No
- **D** Chronic periodontitis is the cause. This condition is characterized by a chronic inflammation of the gingivae (free and attached), seen in patients with poor oral hygiene and associated with gingival enlargement or recession, bleeding during tooth brushing, alveolar bone loss and pocket formation (pocket depth>3 mm) as well as loose teeth.
- **E** No

Comments: The inflamed gingivae close to the plaque and calculus, may become flabby and purple or deep red, as was seen in this patient with chronic periodontitis. The long duration of her gingival lesions and the lack of necrosis of inter-dental papillae or the absence of superficial vesicles or erosions in the gums and other parts of oral mucosa excluded acute ulcerative periodontitis and primary herpetic gingivostomatitis from the diagnosis. The absence of general symptomatology did not indicate the presence of any severe infections such as HIV that cause a linear gingival erythema regardless of plaque or calculus. The absence of other similar lesions in the tongue and other parts of the oral or genital mucosa, and lack of known allergies ruled out plasma cell gingivitis from the diagnosis.

Q2 Which is/are NOT characteristic finding/s in chronic periodontitis?

- **A** Gingival inflammation mainly from of neutrophils and eosinophils
- **B** Destruction of periodontal ligament
- **C** Resorption of the alveolar bone
- **D** Pocket formation
- **E** Migration of epithelial attachment to the root apex

Answers:

- **A** In chronic periodontitis, the gingival inflammation is characterized by a dense accumulation of chronic inflammatory cells such as lymphocytes, plasma cells and macrophages. Eosinophils are rarely seen, while neutrophils are present only when a periodontal abscess appears.
- **B** No
- **C** No
- **D** No
- **E** No

Comments: Alveolar bone loss is the hallmark of periodontitis and is mediated by the host immune and inflammatory response to various pathogenic germs causing destruction of the periodontal ligament, migration of gingival epithelium towards the tooth apex and pocket formation.

Q3 Which of the germs below play an important role in the pathogenesis of chronic periodontitis?

- **A** *Actinomyces israelii*
- **B** *Porphyromonas gingivalis*
- **C** *Treponema pallidum*
- **D** *Escherichia coli*
- **E** *Helicobacter pylori*

Answers:

- **A** No
- **B** *Porphyromonas gingivalis* is a Gram –ve anaerobic bacterium that is a normal oral inhabitant which plays an important role in the pathogenesis of chronic periodontitis. It does this by producing factors such as enzymes, collagenases, and lypopolysaccharides that are responsible for alveolar bone loss.
- **C** No
- **D** No
- **E** No

Comments: All the above germs have been isolated in normal and inflamed gingivae, but seem to play an important role in other pathological conditions such as actinomycoses (*Actinomyces israelii*), syphilis (*Treponema pallidum*), infections of the urinary and digestive system (*Escherichia coli*) and gastritis or peptic ulcer (*Helicobacter pyloris*).

Case 7.8

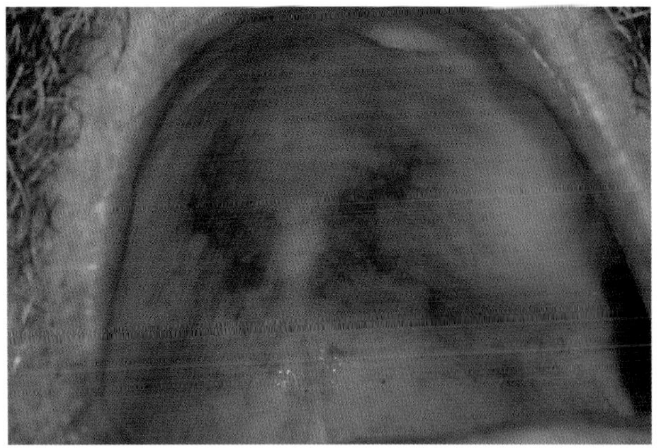

Figure 7.8

CO: A 62-year-old man presented with two red patches on his palate.

HPC: The red patches were first noticed by the patient when he tried to remove his new upper denture one week ago. According to his dentist, these lesions were not seen three weeks ago when impressions were taken for the construction of a new denture.

PMH: His medical history revealed mild hypertension which was controlled by an ACE Inhibitor and history of a heart operation for mitral valve replacement five years ago. Since then he had taken clopidogrel bisulfate, an anti-platelet drug, on a daily basis. Blood dyscrasias or other serious diseases or allergies were not recorded. He was an ex-smoker and drinker, but used to eat very hot foods.

OE: Two red non-elevated, painless hemorrhagic (ecchymose-like) lesions on both sides of his hard palate, symmetrically along the middle palatal raphae (Figure 7.8). The lesions did not bleach with pressure and were gone after the removal of his upper denture for one week. No other similar lesions inside his mouth or other mucosae or lymphadenopathy (local or systemic) were found, and his blood results were within the normal range.

Q1 What is the possible diagnosis?

- **A** Infectious mononucleosis
- **B** Antiplatelet drug side-effect
- **C** Thrombocytopenic purpura
- **D** Traumatic ecchymoses
- **E** Kaposi sarcoma

Answers:

- **A** No
- **B** No
- **C** No
- **D** Trauma is the cause of these ecchymoses and could be caused either by his dentist during the procedure of taking impressions for a new upper denture construction, or by overpressure from the new denture
- **E** No

Comments: The normal blood test results together with the lack of other similar hemorrhagic lesions inside his mouth, skin and other mucosae, in combination with the absence of general symptomatology and lymphadenopathy, can easily lead to the exclusion of thrombocytopenic purpura, anti-platelet drug reaction, or infectious mononucleosis from the diagnosis, respectively. Kaposi sarcoma lesions are usually seen in palate but their clinical course is unrelated to denture use.

Q2 Which of the diseases below do not cause regularly ecchymoses in the mouth?

- **A** Osler-Weber-Rendu syndrome
- **B** Liver cirrhosis
- **C** Acute leukemia
- **D** Amyloidosis
- **E** Gardner-Diamond syndrome

Answers:

- **A** No
- **B** No
- **C** No
- **D** No
- **E** Gardner-Diamond syndrome, or painful bruising syndrome, is seen in young to middle-aged women with personality disorders and is characterized by pruritus, followed by painful ecchymosis especially on the legs, trunk and face but rarely on the oral mucosa.

Comments: Oral ecchymoses appear as large (>1 cm) areas of sub-mucosal bleeding due to number of factors such as blood vessel fragility (amyloidosis); dilatation (Osler-Weber-Rendu syndrome) or an increased bleeding tendency caused by impaired absorption of Vitamin K (liver cirrhosis), waste products (kidney failure) or abnormal white cells in the circulation (leukemia).

Q3 Which of the syndromes below do not include ecchymoses among their clinical characteristics?

- **A** Blue rubber bleb nevus syndrome
- **B** Ehlers-Danlos syndrome
- **C** Stevens-Johnson syndrome
- **D** Antiphospholipid syndrome
- **E** McCune-Albright syndrome

Answers:

- **A** No
- **B** No
- **C** Stevens-Johnson syndrome is a serious disease involving the skin with the characteristic target-like lesions and mucous membranes of the mouth, eyes, genitals, gastrointestinal and upper respiratory tract with scattered atypical ulcerations but not cchymoses.
- **D** No
- **E** McCune-Albright syndrome is characterized by polyostotic fibrous dysplasia and precocious puberty, as well as café au lait pigmentation, but not ecchymoses.

Comments: The vascular type of Ehlers-Danlos syndrome is characterized by rupture of some blood vessels, leading to a great number of complications ranging from local simple ecchymoses to involvement of large and significant vessels like the aorta. The blue rubber bleb syndrome is a series of multifocal venous malformations of the skin, oral mucosa and gastrointestinal tract, developing severe anemia, nose epistaxis and skin as well as mouth ecchymoses. Venous thromboses, necrotic vasculitis and ecchymoses are often the first sign of antiphospholipid syndrome.

Case 7.9

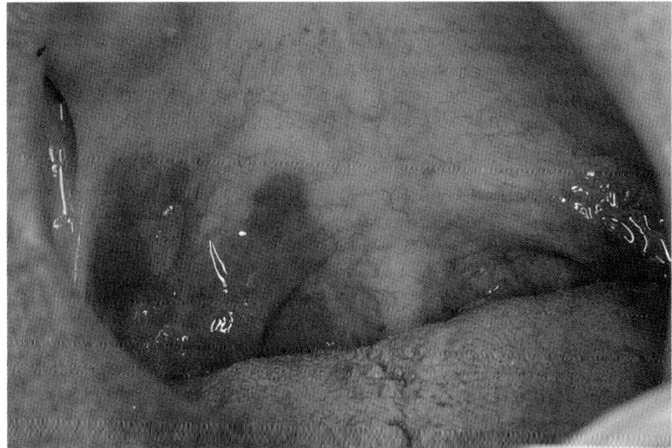

Figure 7.9

CO: A 72-year-old man presented with a red plaque on his soft palate.

HPC: The lesion was discovered accidentally by the patient four days ago during a self-examination for his sore throat.

PMH: This man had no serious medical problems apart from prostate hypertrophy, which had responded well to finasteride and a mild anemia controlled with a supplementary uptake of vitamin B12. He had no other blood, skin diseases, or known allergies. He liked to eat and drink hot foods and tea although a thermal burn had not been recorded in his mouth recently. He was a heavy smoker (>40 cigarettes/day) and drinker (>5 alcoholic drinks/day) for many years.

OE: A bright red plaque extending from the beginning of the right side of soft palate towards the ipsilateral pillars area (Figure 7.9). The lesion is painless, flat with irregular margins, with no clinical evidence of induration or bleeding tendency. No other similar lesions within his mouth, other mucosae or cervical lymphadenopathy were found.

Q1 What is the possible diagnosis?

- **A** Erythroplakia
- **B** Plasma cell stomatitis
- **C** Vitamin B12 deficiency
- **D** Mucositis
- **E** Syphilis (second stage)

Answers:

A Erythroplakia or erythroplasia is the diagnosis. It is a clinical term to describe any red lesion that cannot be characterized clinically or pathologically to any recognizable known condition/or disease. It is commonly seen among middle-aged or older men, heavy smokers, and found in the soft palate, dorsum of the tongue and buccal mucosa. The lesion, histologically, shows in the majority, a severe dysplasia; carcinoma in situ or even invasive carcinoma.

B No

C No

D No

E No

Comments: Red lesions have also been found on the palate of patients with other conditions such as plasma cell stomatitis, B12 deficiencies, syphilis or even early mucositis, but their clinical characteristics together with the history exclude them from the diagnosis. In mucositis, the redness is rather diffused and follows a course of radiotherapy, while in syphilis the lesions are multiple and associated with lymphadenopathy. Multiple lesions have been reported in plasma cell stomatitis and vitamin B12 deficiency, but these diseases are characterized by a history of allergies and abnormal serum B12 concentration respectively.

Q2 Which is the first step that a dentist should do in a patient with a similar red lesion?

A To give an antifungal treatment

B To replace patient's amalgam fillings

C None (follow-up, only)

D To prescribe antibiotics

E Biopsy

Answers:

A No

B No

C No

D No

E Biopsy is mandatory to identify whether the red lesion has a dysplasia or in situ or invasive carcinoma. The majority of these lesions (>40%) are already carcinomas in situ or invasive at the time of biopsy.

Comments: Having the histological diagnosis, patients should be referred for complete removal of this red lesion. In the case of dysplasia, the excision must be done with laser or scalpels, while in the case of carcinoma the removal must be more aggressive and should be extended at least 1 cm from the lesion margins. Treatment with antifungals or antibiotics are useless, while the replacement of amalgam fillings can only improve any lichenoid reaction but not erythroplakia.

Q3 Which of the diseases below is/or are NOT premalignant?

A Bowen's disease

B Paget's disease of the breast

C Psoriasis

D Oral erythroplakia

E Bowenoid papulosis

Answers:

A No

B No

C Psoriasis is characterized by red itchy scaly patches that are located on the skin of the back of the forearms, shins, and cover the whole body, including the nails, and rarely the oral mucosa. Psoriasis has not a high risk for malignancy although its chronic inflammation has been accused for some malignancies.

D No

E No

Comments: Premalignant diseases are the diseases in which there is a high risk of a carcinoma development. These are Bowen's disease and Bowenoid papulosis in the skin, Paget's disease in the breasts and erythroplasia of Queyrat in the penis, prepuce or vulva, while oral leukoplakia has a lower risk than erythroplakia (30% vs. 90%) for developing oral carcinomas.

Case 7.10

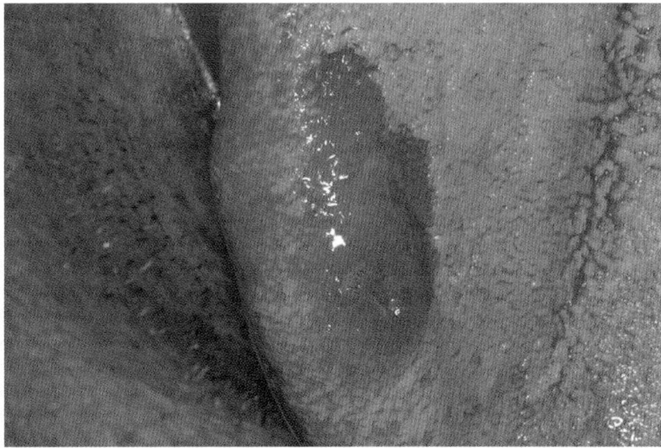

Figure 7.10

CO: A 21-year-old man presented with a painful area on the right side of his tongue.

HPC: The lesion started accidentally as a small traumatic ulcer due to tongue biting five days ago, but got worse over the last two days when the patient applied crashed raw garlic in order to accelerate the ulcer's healing.

PMH: He was an athletic, non-smoking young man with no serious medical problems apart from a few episodes of aphthae over the last eight years. Allergies or drugs use were not recorded.

OE: A red well-defined superficial ulceration in an erythematous base, found on the right lateral margin of his tongue opposite his first lower molar (Figure 7.10). The lesion was sensitive in touching and caused a burning sensation, but was not associated with other similar lesions in the mouth, skin or cervical lymphadenopathy in this patient or his close relatives.

Q1 What is the possible cause?

- **A** Aphtha
- **B** Chemical burn
- **C** Geographic tongue
- **D** Chancre
- **E** Fixed drug reaction

Answers:

- **A** No
- **B** A chemical burn was the possible cause, and was produced by the direct contact of various garlic products to the oral mucosa such as mono, di and trisulfides, whose final metabolites can cause acantholis *in vitro*, but also formation of small vesicles *in vivo* which are finally broken, leaving superficial ulcerations on an erythematous demarcated base, as it was seen in this patient.
- **C** No
- **D** No
- **E** No

Comments: It is very easy for the clinicians to exclude fixed drug reaction and geographic tongue from the diagnosis as the patient was not under any medication at that time and his lesion is single transient causes slight discomfort respectively. Although pain is a common symptom of an aphtha, this lesion should not be included in the diagnosis as aphthae are usually more than one, recurrent ulcerations surrounded by a well-defined erythematous halo. Chancre was not included as it is a painless ulcer associated with cervical lymphadenopathy, and such findings were not seen in this patient.

Q2 The severity of a chemical burn is NOT related to the:

- **A** Concentration of the chemical
- **B** Color of the chemical
- **C** Frequency of exposure
- **D** pH of the chemical
- **E** Form of applied chemical

Answers:

- **A** No
- **B** The color of the chemical is not related to its toxicity and severity of the burn but is dependent on the excitation of electrons during absorption of energy.
- **C** No
- **D** No
- **E** No

Comments: The direct contact of acids or base (alkali) with mucosa can cause necrosis the severity of which depends on their pH, form (solid, liquid, gases) and concentration, the duration and frequency of application as well as the type of tissues affected.

Q3 Which of the terms below is/or are NOT restricted with tissue necrosis?

- **A** Coagulation
- **B** Liquefaction
- **C** Gangrene
- **D** Apoptosis
- **E** Saponification

Answers:

- **A** No
- **B** No
- **C** No
- **D** Apoptosis, is a normal process which is sometimes accelerated or not with external factors (toxins; infections; burns) and acts as a defense mechanism during the healing process.
- **E** No

Comments: Necrosis is a type of injury with the premature death of cells in living tissues as a final result. Acids cause chemical burns via a coaqulative necrosis, forming eschars, while alkalis cause liquefaction with viscous liquid mass production. Gangrene is a form of a coagulative necrosis and appears in tissues with inadequate blood supply, while saponification is seen in fatty necrosis where triglyceride esters of cell membranes via enzymes produce glycerol and fatty acids.

8

Saliva Disturbances (Xerostomia/Sialorrhea)

Saliva is the fluid which is secreted by major and minor salivary glands in the mouth and plays an important role in various functions such eating and swallowing procedures, taste, food digestion and protection against caries and various oral infections (Figure 8.0a and b).

The most important conditions related to salivary disturbances are listed in Tables 8.1 and 8.2.

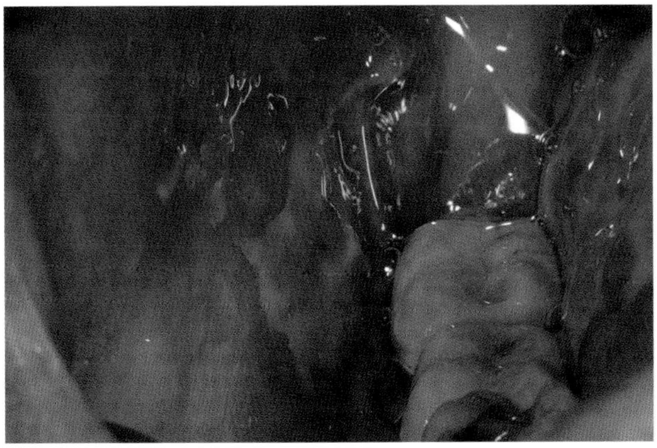

Figure 8.0a Increased saliva in a patient with graft versus host disease (GvHD).

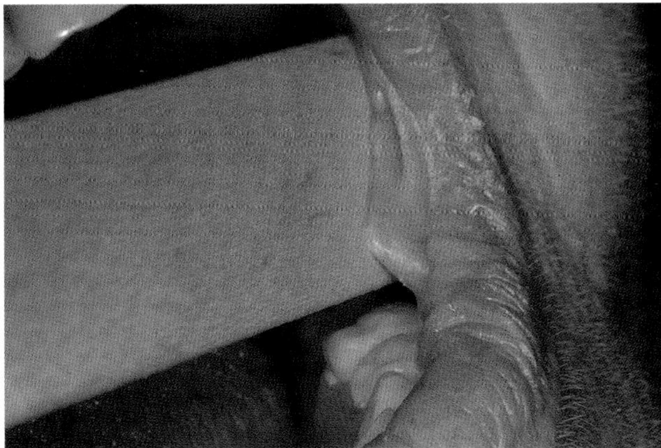

Figure 8.0b Xerostomia.

Table 8.1 Drooling and sialorrhea: Common and important conditions.

- Local
    - Painful oral ulcerations
    - Foreign bodies in the mouth
- Systemic:
    - Related to normal conditions
        - Pregnancy
    - Related to head diseases
        - Esophangitis
        - Viral labyrinthitis
        - Surgery or obstruction (lingual, esophageal or pharyngeal)
    - Related to the nerves
        - Alzheimer's disease
        - Facial palsy
        - Poor neuromuscular coordination
        - Other physical disability
    - Related to psychiatric diseases
        - Schizophrenia
    - Related to drugs
        - Anticholinesterases
        - Antipsychotics
    - Related to chemical contact
        - Copper sulfate
        - Heavy metals
        - Mercury
        - Strychnine
    - Related to toxins
        - Insect bites
        - Rabies

Clinical Guide to Oral Diseases, First Edition. Dimitris Malamos and Crispian Scully.

Companion website: www.wiley.com/go/malamos/clinical_guide

Table 8.2 Dryness: common and important conditions.

- Dehydration
  - Normal conditions
    - Mouth breathing
    - Low consumption of fluids
  - Pathological conditions
    - Excessive sweating
    - Vomiting
    - Fever
    - Diarrhea
    - Bleeding
    - Diuresis
    - Burns
- Side-effects of diseases:
  - Genetic
    - Cystic fibrosis
    - Salivary gland aplasia
  - Infections
    - HCV
    - HIV

Table 8.2 (Continued)

  - Autoimmune
    - Sjogren syndrome
    - Sarcoidosis
    - Amyloidosis
    - GvHD
  - Endocrine
    - Diabetes insipidus
    - Diabetes mellitus
  - Nerves
    - Cholinergic dysautonomia
  - Psychiatric
    - Anxiety
    - Depression
    - Bulimia nervosa
- Side-effects of medical interference
  - Drugs
    - With anti-cholinergic or sympathomimetic effects
  - Medical treatment
    - Irradiation
    - Chemotherapy

Case 8.1

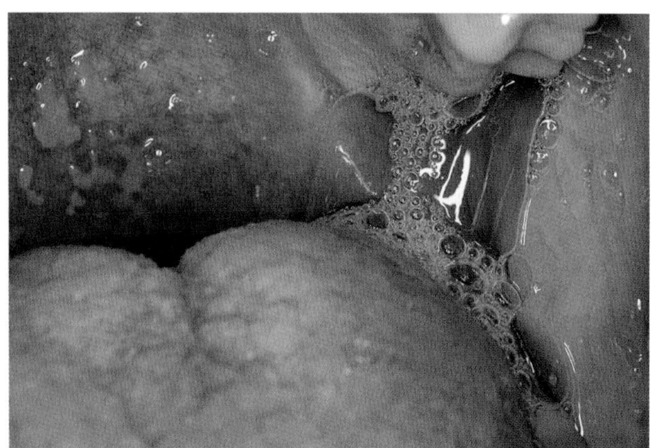

Figure 8.1

CO: A 48-year-old man was referred by his oncologist for an evaluation of his sore throat and increased salivation.

HPC: His throat was sore and his mouth showed increased saliva concentration over the last week after the 1st chemotherapy session for a carcinoma on his rhino-pharynx.

PMH: His medical history revealed an extensive rhino-pharyngeal carcinoma which was initially treated with strong chemotherapy for a quick size reduction, which was followed later by a combination of chemo-radiotherapy. An allergic rhinitis and a mild hypertension were reported and controlled with anti-histamine drugs and diet, respectively. He was an ex-smoker of eight cigarettes per day, but never a drinker.

OE: The oral examination revealed numerous painful superficial ulcerations that were scattered on his soft palate and the back of his throat and covered with yellowish pseudomembranes (Figure 8.1). A mild leukoedema on both buccal mucosae and dorsum of the tongue were seen, while an elongation of filiform papillae was found in several places. Excessive saliva was accumulated at the back of his mouth and throat.

Q1 What is the main cause of his excess saliva?

A Chemotherapy-induced early mucositis
B Carcinoma of the rhinopharynx
C Allergy
D Smoking cessation
E Antihistamine drug side-effects

Answers:

A Very strong chemotherapy can cause early side-effects in the patient's mouth and throat as well, such as a diffuse erythema and multiple ulcerations. These ulcerations are painful and can cause throat soreness, which makes swallowing very difficult, so that the patient prefers to keep his saliva in his mouth, giving the false impression of excessive saliva production.

B No

C No

D No

E No

Comments: Mouth breathing due to nose block from tumors or allergies induces xerostomia which exacerbated with smoking. The large carcinoma of his rhinopharynx blocks his nose breathing, and causes the patient to breathe through his mouth causing xerostomia rather than hypersalivation. Similarly, his allergic rhinitis is a seasonal disease which is characterized by a runny/stuffy nose, therefore causing mouth breathing and secondly a temporal oral dryness that is aggravated with antihistamine drugs. Heavy smoking increases oral dryness and only the quitting of it may restore saliva.

Q2 Drooling is characterized by:

A Normal salivary secretion and handling

B Normal salivary secretion and disturbed handling

C Increased saliva secretion and disturbed handling

D Reduced saliva secretion and normal handling

E Increased saliva secretion and normal handling

Answers:

A No

B Neuromuscular diseases, drugs and poisonous chemicals disturb the masticatory muscle function, thus causing difficulties in swallowing and finally increased saliva accumulation in the mouth. Excess saliva coming out of the corner of the mouth appears as drooling or ptyalism.

C Drooling is characterized by excess saliva in the mouth beyond the lip margins and caused mainly by increased saliva production in conjunction with insufficient saliva handling.

D No

E Increased saliva production and secretion over the lip margins appears as drooling, even in patients with normal swallowing function.

Q3 Which of the cranial nerves are responsible for saliva secretion via their parasympathetic fibers?

A Facial nerve

B Glossopharyngeal nerve

C Olfactory nerve

D Vestibulocochlear nerve

E Vagus nerve

Answers:

A The parasympathetic efferent fibers of the facial nerve, release acetylcholine via the submandibular ganglion, which acts on muscarine M_3 receptors of submandibular and sublingual glands, and the minor salivary glands of the mouth, pharynx and nasopharynx to produce low protein serous saliva.

B Parasympathetic fibers of the small petrosal nerve that come from the tympanic plexus of the glossopharyngeal nerve, arise into the otic ganglion. There, the postganglionic fibers are converged into the parotid gland and secrete a high amount of watery saliva when activated.

C No

D No

E No

Comments: The only cranial nerves that transmit parasympathetic fibers are the oculomotor, facial, glossopharyngeal and vagus, although the oculomotor and vagus nerves do not affect the salivary glands secretion. The olfactory and vestibulocochlear nerves do not carry parasympathetic fibers.

Case 8.2

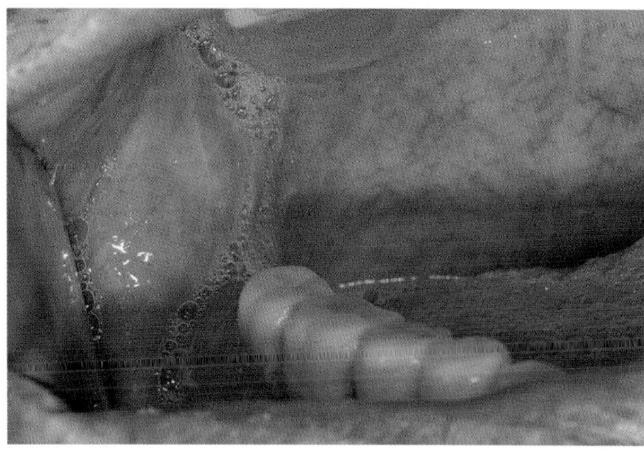

Figure 8.2

CO: A 68-year-old man complained about the increased saliva in his mouth over the last month.

HPC: His increased saliva was first noticed by the patient one month ago after wearing his first new dentures.

PMH: His medical history revealed allergic asthma and Parkinson's disease since his early 30s and late 50s respectively. Steroids were systematically used in asthma crisis and carbidopa for tremor control of his Parkinson's disease on a regular daily dose.

OE: The oral examination revealed an edentulous patient with full upper and lower dentures. The upper denture was overextended to the soft palate where the mucosa was previously treated with antifungals. The accumulated saliva at the retromolar area (Figure 8.2) was interfered with the patient's speech, therefore causing him concern.

Q1 Which is/or are the cause(s) of the increased saliva in the patient's mouth?

- **A** Fungal infection
- **B** Aging
- **C** Irritation of badly fitted complete dentures
- **D** Parkinson's disease
- **E** Allergic asthma

Answers:

- **A** No
- **B** No
- **C** The effect of hypersalivation after wearing complete dentures for the first time is a short-term problem, as the brain naturally recognizes them as a foreign material like food, stimulating the secretion of saliva to dissolve it. The fear of keeping new dentures in the patient's mouth may also accelerate salivation.
- **D** Drooling is a common finding in patients with Parkinson's disease and is the result of lingual bradykinesia, esophageal dysphagia or dysmobility and abnormal posture rather than increased salivary flow rate.
- **E** No

Comments: Aging has been accused as being the cause of deficits of various senses and functions, including salivation. Some diseases like allergic asthma or candidosis cause xerostomia but not sialorrhea.

Q2 Which other habits could be related to patient's sialorrhea?

- **A** Eating mushrooms
- **B** Keeping betel nut in the labial sulcus
- **C** Excessive consumption of cinnamon flavor chewing gum daily
- **D** Outdoor hobbies
- **E** Mouth piercing

Answers:

- **A** Toxins from poisonous mushrooms can cause a variety of symptoms; from the simplest ones such as sialorrhea, cramps, and diarrhea to more serious manifestations like a comatose state which if untreated, can jeopardize the patient's life.
- **B** Betel nut leaves are usually embedded with pilocarpine, a muscarinic analog which increases saliva secretion.
- **C** No
- **D** No
- **E** No

Comments: Chewing cinnamon flavored gum acts as a saliva secretion stimulant for a short period. However, the long and constant use of it may induce a local allergic reaction to cinnamon products which is known as cinnamon-induced stomatitis. This appears as a diffuse erythema or a combination of white and red lesions which are superficial erosions associated with a burning, tingling sensation rather than sialorrhea. Piercing acts as a foreign body and increases saliva for a short period only, while various outdoors sports lead to dehydration through increased sweating.

Q3 Which are the constituents of saliva?

- **A** Water
- **B** Electrolytes
- **C** Proteins
- **D** Enzymes
- **E** Nitrogenous products

Answers:

- **A** Water constitutes 95 per cent of saliva, which is used for the lubrication of the oral mucosa, softening of foods during mastication and swallowing procedures, transfer of various tasteful stimulants to the taste receptors and carrying antimicrobial as well as other chemical agents to various parts of the mouth.
- **B** Electrolytes such as calcium, phosphate, sodium, potassium and fluorine are used for the demineralization and remineralization of the teeth.
- **C** Proteins and mucins act to cleanse, aggregate and attach various oral microorganisms to the surface of the teeth (plaque formation and maturation).
- **D** Enzymes such as amylases and lipases are used as the first step in digestion of starch and fat containing foods.
- **E** Urea and ammonia (nitrogenous components) act to modulate pH and buffering capacity of saliva.

Case 8.3

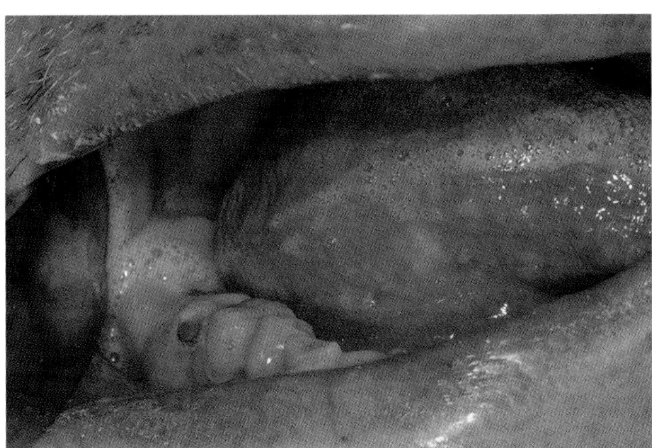

Figure 8.3

CO: A 42-year-old man was presented with an acute abdominal pain which was associated with increased salivation, nausea, vomiting, and diarrhea.

HPC: The patient complained about some abdominal pain a couple of days ago, which was transient and exacerbated with fatty foods, making the pain more constant over the last 12 hours.

PMH: His medical history did not reveal any serious diseases or drugs uptake. However, his diet was poor in fruits and vegetables, but rich in fatty foods together with a high alcohol consumption (>150 g/daily).

OE: The physical examination revealed an unwell middle-aged man with severe abdominal pain, nausea and fatigue, whose oral examination showed no oral lesions but a barely adequate hygiene with big fillings or crown restorations on the majority of his remaining teeth. An excessive salivation and alcohol-induced halitosis were present (Figure 8.3). Finally, among his blood investigations, only the biochemical blood tests revealed raised pancreatic and hepatic enzymes.

Q1 What is the cause of this sialorrhea?

- **A** Alcohol-induced pancreatitis
- **B** Malnutrition
- **C** Appendicitis
- **D** Peptic ulcer
- **E** Intestinal infections

Answers:

- **A** Alcohol-induced pancreatitis is a serious complication of alcohol overuse and confirmed by fatty stools and increased amylase and lipase in the blood. This complication may cause irreversible damage on the gland and predispose the development of diabetes or even carcinomas. It is presented with, swollen abdomen severe abdominal pain accompanied with nausea, vomiting, sialorrhea and occasionally fever.
- **B**
- **C** No
- **D** No
- **E** No
- **F** No

Comments: Appendicitis and other intestinal infections are always accompanied by a great number of white blood counts which were not found in this particular patient. The lack of anemia or bloody stools excludes malnutrition and peptic ulcer from the diagnosis.

Q2 Which are the other clinical indications of sialorrhea?

- **A** Perioral dermatitis
- **B** Commissure infections
- **C** Muscular fatigue
- **D** Contact cheilitis
- **E** Lip dryness

Answers:

A Perioral skin contact with saliva causes local irritation, erythema and scaling (perioral dermatitis).
B Local moisture due to saliva leaking allows the growth of pathogenic germs in the area. Bacteria such as *Staphylococcus aureus* and fungi like *Candida albicans* appear in the angles of the mouth and cause erythema, superficial ulcerations or deep groves that are covered with hemorrhagic crusts (angular cheilitis).
C The presence of increased saliva in the patient's mouth causes him swallow too many times per minute, and thus causes fatigue of the muscles related to this function.
D The dryness of the excess saliva from the lips with tissues removes the protective lip barrier, and causes the inflammation of the lips, known as contact cheilitis.
E No

Comments: Lip dryness is a manifestation of xerostomia and not of sialorrhea.

Q3 Which other drugs cause sialorrhea?
A Acetyl-cholinesterase inhibitors
B Parasympathomimetic drugs
C Anti-psychotic drugs
D Anti-vomiting drugs
E Anti-hypertensive drugs

Answers:

A Parasympathomimetic drugs, like pilocarpine, are widely used in patients with xerostomia especially those with Sjogren syndrome in order to increase salivation.
B The drugs for Alzheimer's disease treatment such as Donepezil, rivastigmine, and galantamine inhibit the action of acetylcholinesterase and increase the assemblage of acetylcholine which is the major muscarinic M_3 receptor stimulant for saliva production.
C Anti-psychotic drugs like clozapine may cause sialorrhea, due to their agonistic effect on the M_3 and M_4 glandular muscarine receptors as well as their antagonistic alpha-2 adrenergic receptors of the sympathetic nervous system.
D No
E No

Comments: Anti-emetic drugs such as scopolamine, in doses of 0.3-0.65 mg tds or qds, relieve nausea and vomiting, but then only increase salivation. Anti-hypertensive drugs like captopril and enalapril induce xerostomia.

Case 8.4

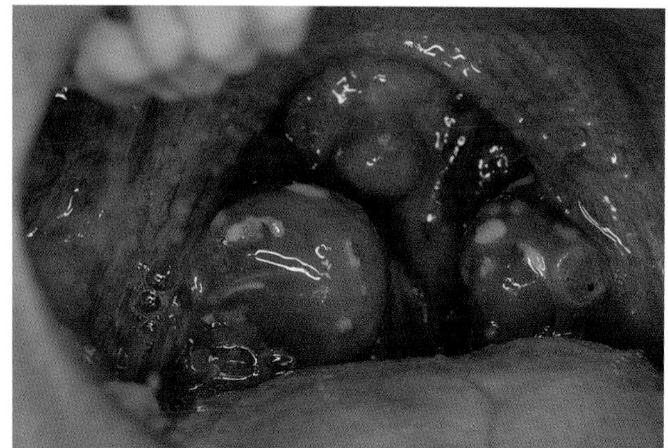

Figure 8.4

CO: An 18-year-old student presented with sore throat, fever and sialorrhea.

HPC: His symptoms started three days ago with fever, malaise and red swollen tonsils causing him difficulties in swallowing.

PMH: He was a young, first year university student, with no history of any serious diseases, allergies or drug use as well as no smoking or drinking habits.

OE: The examination revealed erythematous swollen tonsils with white exuded spots on the surface, associated with soreness, high fever, halitosis, sialorrhea and enlarged cervical nodes (Figure 8.4). Streptococcus was isolated from the cultures while heterophile antibodies for Epstein-Barr virus were not found. A broad-spectrum antibiotic was given, with a very short response.

Q1 Which is the cause of the sialorrhea?
- **A** Tonsillitis
- **B** Infective mononucleosis
- **C** Herpangina
- **D** Diphtheria
- **E** Acute pseudomembranous candidosis

Answers:
- **A** Tonsillitis is the cause. This is an acute infection of the tonsils which is induced by a variety of pathogens and associated with sore, inflamed tonsils together with the general symptomatology. The enlarged tonsils cover the largest part of the oropharyngeal entrance causing swallowing problems. For this reason, saliva remained in the patient's mouth and gave in this way, the false impression of increased saliva production (sialorrhea).
- **B** No
- **C** No
- **D** No
- **E** No

Comments: Enlarged tonsils are characteristic of bacterial infections like diphtheria viral infections like infective mononucleosis and herpanginaand fungal infevtions like pseudomembranous Candidosis. In the diagnosis infective mononucleosis was excluded as the patient did not show generalized lymphadenitis or other organ involvement (liver, spleen, skin) and his laboratory tests did not reveal marked monocytosis, EBV in cultures or positive mononucleosis test. Diphtheria was not the cause, as the inflammation exceeds the tonsils with characteristic formation of pseudomembranous and mucosal bleeding, while candidosis shows multiple whitish pseudomembranes on the tonsils and oropharynx, yet milder symptomatology. The absence of small vesicles and ulcerations in the soft palate and posterior oropharynx, apart from the tonsils, excludes herpangina.

Q2 Which is/or are the more serious complications of an untreated tonsillitis?
- **A** Scarlet fever
- **B** Peritonsillar abscess
- **C** Middle ear infection
- **D** Rheumatic fever
- **E** Glomerulonephritis

Answers:
- **A** No
- **B** No
- **C** No
- **D** Rheumatic fever is a serious complication of sore throat and especially of tonsillitis, caused by *Streptococcus* A, and characterized by an inflammation of the heart, joints, skin and brain, leading to aortitis and congestive heart disease as well as meningoencephalitis.
- **E** Streptococcal glomerulonephritis is a complication of streptococcal infection (impetigo, tonsillitis) which is characterized by the inflammation of glomeruli and small vessels of the kidney, leading to kidney failure.

Comments: Tonsillitis induced by bacteria (*Streptococcus* A) causes generalized inflammation of the skin (scarlet fever) as well as localized infection of the middle ear (otitis) or on the area between the tonsils and capsules (peritonsillar abscess). Their early diagnosis and antimicrobial treatment reduces the risk of any serious complications.

Q3 Which other viruses are responsible for acute tonsillitis?
- **A** Rhinoviruses
- **B** Adenoviruses
- **C** EBV
- **D** Rabies
- **E** Fifth herpes virus

Answers:
- **A** Rhinoviruses cause common infections in the throat, ear and sinuses and less commonly pneumonia and bronchiolitis.
- **B** Adenoviruses and especially their types 1, 2, 4, 5, and 16 cause febrile exudate tonsillitis.
- **C** No
- **D** No
- **E** No

Comments: Although EBV and HSV5 belong to the same family of viruses and cause sore throat, they are responsible for different diseases such as infective mononucleosis and fifth disease respectively. Rabies is a deadly virus affecting the central nerve system and not the tonsils.

Case 8.5

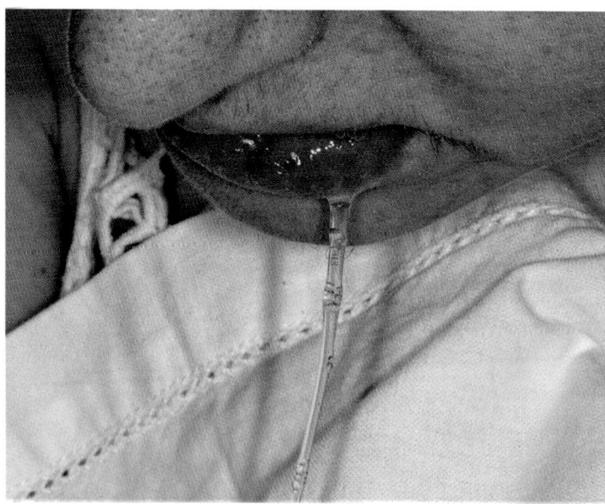

Figure 8.5

CO: A 36-year-old woman was referred by her mother for her uncontrolled saliva drooling.

HPC: Her drooling had become more obvious over the last eight years, when her medical problems became more serious.

PMH: She suffered from a serious motor nerve disorder known as amyotrophic lateral sclerosis. This condition appeared eight years ago and her treatment was only symptomatic. She had never smoked or drank.

OE: A women in a wheelchair with severe difficulties in controlling her body. Her mouth was constantly open and drooling of her saliva was obvious (Figure 8.5). No other intraoral lesions were found and her oral hygiene was adequate.

Q1 What is the cause of saliva drooling in this young woman?

- **A** Heavy metal poisoning
- **B** Pregnancy
- **C** Brain tumor
- **D** Amyotrophic lateral sclerosis
- **E** Pancreatitis

Answers:

- **A** No
- **B** No
- **C** No
- **D** Amyotrophic lateral sclerosis is the cause. This belongs to a rare group of neurological diseases affecting the neurons responsible for the control of voluntary muscle movement for walking, standing, talking, chewing, or even swallowing. The failure of the motor muscles to work properly seriously affects the patient's quality of life. Inadequate swallowing causes saliva accumulation and drooling.
- **E** No

Q2 What other neurological diseases apart from amyotrophic lateral sclerosis can cause drooling?

- **A** Myasthenia gravis
- **B** Facial palsy
- **C** Guillain-Barré syndrome
- **D** Trigeminal neuralgia
- **E** Parkinson's disease

Answers:

- **A** Myasthenia gravis is a neurovascular disease characterized by weakness of skeletal muscles including those of mastication and swallowing affecting the saliva.
- **B** Facial palsy is characterized by paralysis of all or some of the muscles of facial expression leading to incomplete lip closure, thus allowing saliva to drop out of patient's mouth.
- **C** Guillain-Barré syndrome is an acute inflammatory demyelinating polyradiculoneuropathy that starts from the lower limbs and progressively moves upwards. Its facial variant is characterized by hemicrania headaches, dysarthria, and sialorrhea.
- **D** No
- **E** Parkinson's disease is often accompanied with sialorrhea due to the dysfunction of muscles related with swallowing rather than being caused by the excess production of saliva.

Comments: Trigeminal neuralgia appears in the form of acute unilateral electric-shock-like episodes of pain which involve one or two branches of the trigeminal nerve. Sialorrhea is not a classic finding and most of the time is accompanied by euphoria and other precursory signs before the pain starts.

Q3 Neurological diseases are involved in drooling via:

- **A** Incomplete lip closure
- **B** Low suction pressure
- **C** Prolonged delay between suction and propulsion
- **D** Deficit of palatal reflex
- **E** Cricopharyngeal achalasia

Answers:

- **A** Paralysis of the facial muscles leads to incomplete lip-mouth closure, so that saliva or food escape from the patient's mouth.

B Incomplete or low suction is a common effect of muscle myopathies or neuropathies.

C The delay between suction and propulsion leads to the accumulation of an amount of saliva which drools out of patient's mouth.

D Absence of palatal reflex (total or partial) is a common finding in neuromuscular disorders and leads to the accumulation of saliva which comes out of patient's mouth due to an abnormal function of muscles that are related to mastication and swallowing.

E Cricopharyngeal achalasia is a rare clinical complication in which the upper esophageal sphincter does not open adequately during swallowing, leading to increased saliva accumulation within the patient's mouth due to the fear of drowning or coughing.

Case 8.6

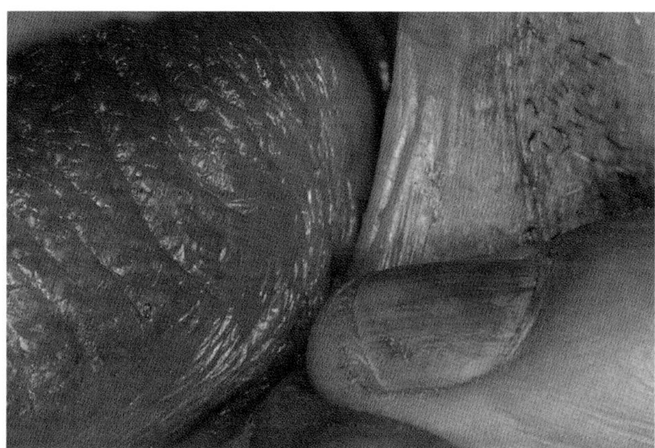

Figure 8.6

CO: A 52-year-old man presented complaining about his severe oral dryness.

HPC: His dryness appeared one year ago when he started to visit his cardiologist to control his hypertension.

PMH: His medical history revealed hypertension and familiar hyperlipidemia which were controlled with a combination of irbesartan and hydrochlorothiazide drugs as well as with diet and statins respectively. He was a chronic smoker (mainly of cigarettes, >2 packets per day) since the age of 18 and consumer of 5 cups of coffee daily.

OE: He is a thin, middle-aged man with severe xerostomia as was shown by the almost complete lack of saliva and the presence of a sticky lobulated tongue and atrophic buccal mucosae (Figure 8.6). His tongue was erythematous with many superficial grooves and fissures and was sensitive to touch, associated with erythematous angles of his mouth. No other lesions were found in his mouth or in the perioral skin, apart from a nicotine stain on his fingers and nails due to the holding of cigarettes.

Q1 What is/are the cause/(s) of his xerostomia?

A Smoking
B Antihypertensive drugs
C Diuretics
D Fungal infection
E Coffee overuse

Answers:

A Smoking can affect saliva secretion in two ways. On the one hand, chronic smoking causes xerostomia due to reduced secretion of saliva and its poor quality, while on the other hand, recent smoking causes irritation of the salivary glands and on the contrary increases secretion. Oxygen and nitrogen radicals as well as volatile aldehydes of tobacco may destroy various biomolecules in the saliva, and amylases may change the composition of saliva in smokers giving the impression of xerostomia.

B No

C Diuretics reduce saliva flow rate and composition significantly. This may explain the high incidence of fungal infection and other mucosal lesions or dental decays in patients taking those tablets.

D Reduced saliva may alter the oral microbiota and increase the risk of opportunistic infections such as candidiasis.

E Drinking coffee can also affect oral salivation in two ways. Having one or two cups per day helps in watering the balance of homeostasis, but overuse has controversial diuretic results, along with heart palpitations, breathing muscle switching or even dizziness.

Comments: The irbesartan rarely affects saliva secretion rate on its own, but it can cause bladder, chest and back pain, dark urine, chills, and cold sweating.

Q2 Which other oral lesion/(s) is/are related to smoking?

- **A** Oral carcinoma
- **B** Palatal leukokeratosis
- **C** Submucous fibrosis
- **D** Acute ulcerative gingivitis/periodontitis
- **E** Actinic cheilitis

Answers:

- **A** Tobacco is a well-known cause of oral cancer via its carcinogenic contents such as nitrosamines, polycyclic aromatic hydrocarbons and aromatic amines. All forms of tobacco play an important role in the development of oral cancer alone, or combined with other carcinogenic factors such as heavy alcohol use.
- **B** Palatal leukokeratosis or nicotine stomatitis, is a reaction of the oral mucosa and especially of the palate to the concentrated heat of smoke rather than that commonly found in nicotine in pipe and reverse cigarette smokers. It is characterized by white hyperkeratotic plaque which is presented in the form of lesions intermingled with red dots that represent the inflamed openings of minor salivary glands in palate.
- **C** No
- **D** Smoking is one of the predisposing factors in acute necrotizing gingivitis/periodontitis by affecting the vascular and cellular elements of gingival inflammation.
- **E** No

Comments: The chronic exposure to very spicy, hot foods and especially areca nut (the main component of betel quid) can cause submucous fibrosis while the chronic exposure of the lips to solar radiation (UVB mainly) may induce actinic cheilitis. Both conditions have a tendency to develop oral cancer (actinic>fibrosis) but their carcinogenesis is not associated with smoking.

Q3 Which factors affect the hyposalivation induced by smoking?

- **A** The patient's age
- **B** Number of cigarettes per day
- **C** Duration of smoking
- **D** Patient's sex
- **E** Patient's medications

Answers:

- **A** The older patients seem to show a decline in various body functions; among them is the reduced saliva production and secretion that is more obvious among smoker patients.
- **B** The frequent exposure to oral mucosa to heat released from smoking causes xerostomia especially in patients with neglected mouth, poor diet and increased alcohol but low water consumption.
- **C** The long duration of smoking seems to be related to a reduced salivary flow rate as seen in chronic smokers.
- **D** No
- **E** The tobacco seems to exacerbate oral dryness in patients induced by certain medication.

Comments: The gender does not have an impact on salivation in experimental models and patient studies

Case 8.7

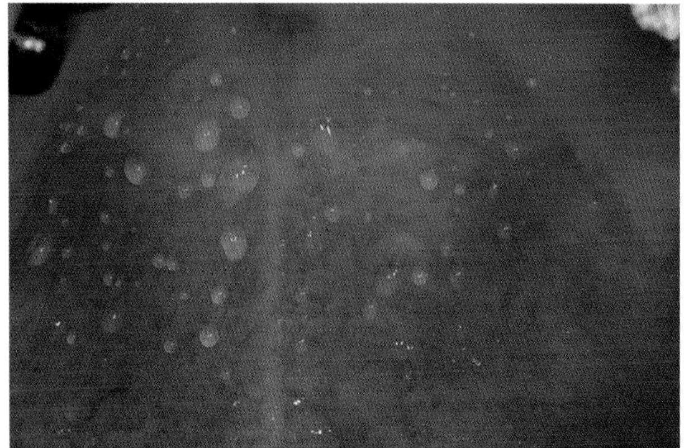

Figure 8.7

CO: A 32-year-old man presented with multiple vesicle-like lesions on his palate. This was found during his regular oral check-up after the end of a chemo-radiotherapy course for a non-surgical carcinoma on the base of his tongue.

HPC: The clear fluid of vesicle-like lesions on the palate was seen seven weeks after the end of six sessions of cisplatin chemotherapy in combination with 35 fractions of 7000 cGy radiation for a carcinoma in the space between the base of the tongue and epiglottis (vallecula).

PMH: His medical history was unremarkable apart from a carcinoma on the base of his tongue three months ago. He was also a human papilloma virus (HPV) positive patient and an ex-smoker from the day of his tumor diagnosis.

OE: Multiple asymptomatic vesicles-like lesions, scattered on the normal palatal mucosa and composed of a clear fluid, (Figure 8.7) were found and associated with superficial painful erosions on the posterior pharynx, xerostomia and metallic taste.

Q1 Which is the origin of these lesions?
- **A** Paraneoplastic pemphigus
- **B** Primary herpetic stomatitis
- **C** Impaired function of minor salivary glands
- **D** Erythema multiforme
- **E** Allergic denture stomatitis

Answers:
- **A** No
- **B** No
- **C** The fluid was an amount of thick saliva released from the openings of impaired minor salivary glands during the recovery phase after the radio-chemotherapy had been completed.
- **D** No
- **E** No

Comments: Despite the fact that vesicles – bullae with clear fluid, are characteristic of various oral conditions such as primary herpetic stomatitis, erythema multiforme, and paraneoplastic pemphigus, these conditions can be easily excluded as their bullae real are not only restricted to palate, and their underlying mucosa is erythematous and sensitive. The allergic denture stomatitis is closely related to the denture, but in this case the patient did not wear dentures.

Q2 Which body function(s) is/are less affected by inadequate saliva secretion?
- **A** Taste
- **B** Ingestion
- **C** Swallowing
- **D** Speech
- **E** Oral homeostasis

Answers:
- **A** No
- **B** No
- **C** No
- **D** Saliva lubricates the oral mucosa and facilitates the tongue's movements. Speech is affected by impaired tongue movements only in severe xerostomia cases.
- **E** No

Comments: Saliva and its enzymes such as amylases and lipases participate at the start of digestion of various foods containing starch and fats. Also, its mineral contents play an important role in oral homeostasis, through the neutralization of oral acids from food, drinks and drugs, thus preventing the development of caries. The high percentage of water content in saliva (>95%) enables food wetting during mastication, and accelerates swallowing. Saliva is used to dissolve and transport various tasteful stimulants to the taste receptors, playing a fundamental role in taste perception.

Q3 Which changes are seen in saliva content during irradiation for treatment of a head and neck tumor?
- **A** Alterations in electrolytes
- **B** Increased concentration of bicarbonates
- **C** Reduced concentration of immunoglobulins
- **D** Increased amylase concentration
- **E** Increased lactate dehydrogenase concentration

Answers:
- **A** The concentration of sodium, chloride, calcium, and magnesium is increased, while potassium is slightly affected.
- **B** No
- **C** No
- **D** Although the concentration of amylase has been greater during the chemo/radiotherapy, the salivary flow rate is reduced to such a degree that it may lead to immune deficits.
- **E** The increased lactate dehydrogenase concentration, during radiotherapy, seems to be associated with an increased tendency for tumor necrosis.

Comments: During radiotherapy, the concentration of bicarbonate in saliva is low, therefore leading to low pH and buffering capacity against the acids that are produced by dental plaque. On the contrary, the increased concentration of IgA, and IgM immunoglobulins has an antibacterial action which is eliminated with the reduced saliva secretion.

Case 8.8

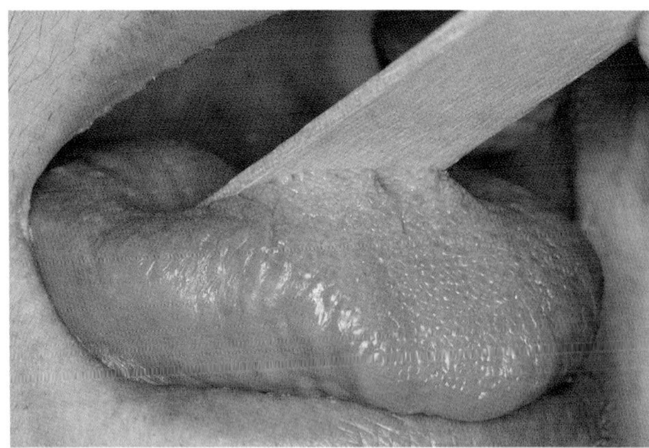

Figure 8.8

CO: A 67-year-old woman was evaluated for oral dryness.

HPC: Her dryness initially appeared on her lips, after spinal disc surgery that took place eight months ago, but became gradually extended to her whole mouth. This caused the patient eating as well as speaking problems.

PMH: Her medical history revealed severe depression and uncontrolled diabetes type II which were treated with duloxetine and metformin respectively. No other drugs – apart from NSAIDs for her back pain – or smoking and heavy drinking habits were recorded. Water or other fluid uptake was limited.

OE: The examination revealed an overweight lady with standing problems, who showed severe xerostomia. Her xerostomia was easily detected by the reduced amount of saliva and the presence of thick sticky saliva. The latter made it difficult for a wooden spatula to be detached from the dorsum of her tongue (Figure 8.8). No other lesions were found in the mouth, eyes or other mucosae.

Q1 Which is/or are the causes of her xerostomia?

- **A** Dehydration
- **B** Drug-induced
- **C** Uncontrolled diabetes
- **D** Old age
- **E** Spine surgery

Answers:

- **A** Dehydration may be induced by reduced water consumption, or loss of fluids due to fever, excessive sweating, diarrhea, or hemorrhage, and burns can cause xerostomia.
- **B** Antidepressant drugs act on muscarinic receptors and cause reduced salivary flow rate.
- **C** Uncontrolled diabetes II causes dry mouth in up to 62 per cent of patients, possibly due to polyuria and dehydration.
- **D** No
- **E** No

Comments: Older patients sometimes complain about their dry mouth due to an increased number of systemic disease side-effects rather than their actual age. Spinal surgery does not affect the routes of peripheral nerves related with salivation to the CNS. So, the surgery was not the actual cause.

Q2 Which are the main complications of xerostomia?

- **A** Halitosis
- **B** Decays
- **C** Gingival diseases
- **D** Dysphagia
- **E** Viral infections

Answers:

- **A** Halitosis is common and noticeable, especially in the mornings when xerostomia is intense and allows the growth of various anaerobic bacteria responsible for bad breath.
- **B** The reduced cleaning capacity of saliva encourages the growth of pathogenic carcinogenic bacteria.
- **C** The combination of reduced antimicrobial action of diminished saliva with the growth of pathogenic bacteria on the gingivae and teeth leads to periodontal infection.
- **D** The reduced saliva makes the swallowing of hard foods difficult.
- **E** No

Comments: The low saliva encourages the entrance and growth of various pathogenic germs like bacteria and fungi, but not of viruses in the oral mucosa. The viral infections are rather secondary, due to the immunodeficiency that is induced by the main disease which is responsible for the xerostomia.

Q3 Which blood tests could be regularly used for the diagnosis of hyposalivation?

- **A** Antinuclear antibodies (ANA) test
- **B** Glucose test
- **C** Cardiolipin antibodies test
- **D** SSA/SSB antibodies test
- **E** Parietal cell antibodies test

Answers:

A ANA test is an antinuclear antibody test which is widely used to diagnose various autoimmune diseases such as Sjogren, lupus, and rheumatoid arthritis which are strongly related to hyposalivation.

B The increased level of glucose in the blood is an indication of diabetes that is a condition strongly connected with hyposalivation.

C No

D Anti-SSA/SSB autoantibodies are useful for detecting Sjogren syndrome. This is an autoimmune disease, closely related to reduced saliva production/secretion.

E No

Comments: Cardiolipin antibodies are useful for the detection of a recent clot formation, the investigation of the cause of recurrent miscarriage, and the evaluation of antiphospholipid syndrome. Parietal cell antibodies distinguish pernicious from other anemias.

Case 8.9

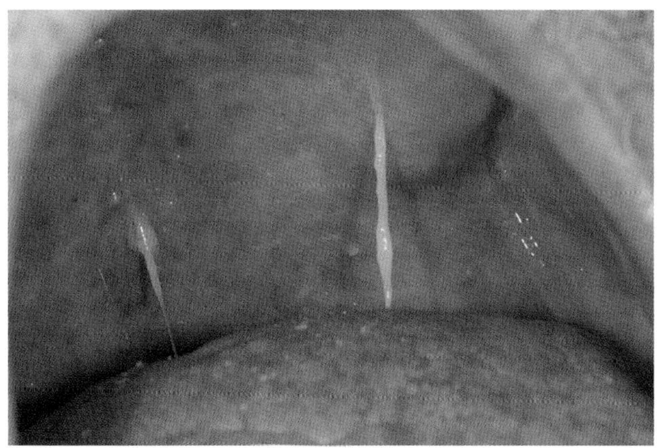

Figure 8.9

CO: A 69-year-old man complained about his dry mouth over the last year.

HPC: His dryness appeared at the same time as bladder incontinency problems, appeared causing him severe emotional stress and a negative impact on the quality of his life.

PMH: Hyperlipidemia, hypertension and prostate benign hypertrophy were his main medical problems, and were controlled with special diet and drugs such as atorvastatin, prazosin, and solifenacin, respectively. NSAIDs such as ibuprofen were occasionally taken during back pain crises, while a course of antibiotics such as azithromycin was taken three months ago for an atypical pneumonia. Smoking cessation was also recorded since the onset of pneumonia.

OE: An overweight, elderly edentulous man with severe mouth dryness and atrophic oral mucosa. His saliva was very thick and forming froth or strings in several places (Figure 8.9), thus making the use of dentures almost impossible. No skin or eye dryness were reported, while his major salivary glands were normal in size.

Q1 Which of the drugs below is/or are suspected for causing the patient's oral dryness?

A Anti-lipidemics (atorvastatin)
B Anti-hypertensive (prazosin)
C Dugs for bladder incontinence (solifenacin succinate)
D NSAIDs (ibuprofen)
E Antibiotic macrolides (azithromycin)

Answers:

A No

B No

C Solifenacin is a drug with antimuscarinic action that is used to treat contraction of overactive bladder and often causes xerostomia.

D No

E No

Comments: All the other drugs are irrelevant with saliva secretion.

Q2 Which is/are the objective sign(s) of xerostomia?

A Frothy, sticky saliva
B Atrophic oral mucosa
C Caries in the central incisors
D Swelling of the salivary glands
E Necrosis of inter-dental papillae

Answers:

A The saliva is limited, frothy and thick to such a degree that a spoon or spatula (metallic-wooden) sticks to the oral mucosa.

- **B** The oral mucosa is atrophic, while in severe cases of xerostomia, the tongue loses its filiform papillae and shows a shiny, smooth, lobulated, red surface.
- **C** Caries are seen even in resistant lower central incisors.
- **D** Swelling of the major salivary glands is a common finding in patients with severe xerostomia induced by Sjogren's disease, diabetes, HIV+ disease or alcoholism.
- **E** No

Comments: Necrosis of the inter-dental papillae is the landmark of necrotizing gingivitis. It is a special form of periodontal tissue infection related to the patient's poor oral hygiene and malnutrition rather than xerostomia.

Q3 Which of the ducts below are not anatomical structures of salivary glands?

- **A** Stensen ducts
- **B** Wharton ducts
- **C** Bartholin's ducts
- **D** Rivinus ducts
- **E** Bellini ducts

Answers:

- **A** No
- **B** No
- **C** No
- **D** No
- **E** Bellini ducts are also known as papillary ducts and represent the distal parts of collecting ducts of the kidney, and play an important role in water reabsorption and electrolyte balance.

Comments: Stensen's ducts transport saliva from parotid glands into the mouth while the Wharton duct is longer and thinner and drains saliva from submandibular and sublingual glands to the floor of mouth. Bartholin's ducts are the largest among the sublingual ducts, while a similar name was given to the ducts of Bartholin glands in the vulva. The Rivinus ducts are 8–20 excretory ducts of the sublingual glands.

Case 8.10

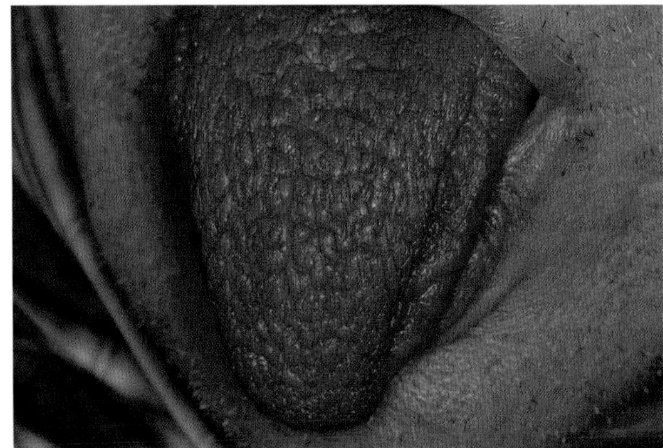

Figure 8.10

CO: A 58-year-old man was referred for an evaluation of his severe xerostomia over the last two years.

HPC: His mouth dryness started two years ago and became so constant and severe during sleeping at night that it used to wake him up.

PMH: He suffered from migraine, which partially responded to strong painkillers. These drugs were always taken together with gastro-protective drugs for an old, but healed peptic ulcer. No allergies, other drugs or harmful hobbies such as smoking or heavy drinking were recorded.

OE: The oral examination revealed a very dry, lobulated, erythematous tongue (Figure 8.10), sensitive to touch and associated with angular cheilitis and dryness in his eyes, nose and facial skin, but without enlargement of the major salivary glands or cervical lymph nodes. Lip biopsy showed evidence of atrophy of the minor salivary glands and scattered chronic inflammation. Anti-SSA and SSB but not SACE antibodies were detected in his blood.

Q1 Which is the cause of xerostomia in this patient?

- **A** Severe dehydration
- **B** Renal dialysis
- **C** Sarcoidosis
- **D** Sjogren syndrome
- **E** Drug-induced xerostomia

Answers:

- **A** No
- **B** No
- **C** No
- **D** Sjogren syndrome is the cause. This syndrome is a chronic autoimmune disease that affects salivary and lacrimal glands and other moisturizing glands,

causing mouth and eye dryness. It occurs either spontaneously (primary) or in association with other autoimmune diseases (secondary) whose symptomatology depends on the severity and organs involved.

E No

Comments: Based on the patient's medical history, his xerostomia was not related to a severe body fluid loss, kidney disease or drug-induced. The lack of non-caseating granulomas in his lip biopsy and low concentration of angiotensin converting enzyme in serum (SACE) excluded sarcoidosis from the diagnosis.

Q2 Which of the tests below are mandatory for the diagnosis of this disease?

A Biopsy
B Sialometry
C MRI
D Schirmer's test
E Sialochemistry

Answers:

A The biopsy of minor salivary glands, taken from the inner surface of the lower lip, shows an extensive lymphoid infiltration with germinal centers, interstitial fibrosis and acinar atrophy.
B No
C MRI of the parotid glands shows a salt-pepper or honeycomb-like appearance; a characteristic finding of Sjogren syndrome.
D No
E No

Comments: Sialometry and sialochemistry show a reduction of salivary flow rate and alterations in its composition, but this salivary disturbance is not exclusively seen in Sjogren syndrome, but is also found in other salivary gland diseases or induced by drugs. The Schirmer test cannot differentiate whether the cause of his eye dryness is induced by Sjogren syndrome or from other conditions such as rheumatoid arthritis, Vitamin A deficiencies, corneal infections or neoplasms.

Q3 Which of the treatments below is/are rarely used for this condition?

A Sialogogic drugs
B Interferon
C Saliva substitutes
D Steroids
E Stem cell therapy

Answers:

A No
B Interferon α is given only to patients with primary Sjogren syndrome with neurological involvement at a low dosage orally. This drugs acts by activation of their adaptive immune system with the production of autoantibodies against the RNA-binding proteins SSA/SSB and by increasing the unstimulated whole salivary flow without significant adverse effects.
C No
D No
E Allogeneic mesenchymal stem cells are given intravenously to suppress autoimmunity by acting on T cells to restore salivary gland functions in mouse models and patients with primary Sjogren syndrome.

Comments: In mild cases, sialogogic drugs like pilocarpine and cevimeline act as muscarinic agonists and increase saliva production, while saliva substitutes such as cellulose or carboxy-methylcellulose lubricate the oral mucosa. In severe cases, systemic steroids, such as prednisone and prednisolone, are widely used.

9

Swellings (Diffuse/Lumps)

Oral swellings are heterogeneous group of lesions that appear as discrete swellings (lumps) or diffused lesions with congenital, reactive, infective, autoimmune, or even neoplasmatic (benign or malignant) etiology. Some of the swellings are painful and associated with local inflammation and require treatment some others are asymptomatic and require only regular follow-up. Some swellings last only few days or weeks and some others last for more than two months (See Figure 9.0) and cause severe complications some of which can jeopardize patient's life.

Table 9 lists the most important causes of swellings (diffused or discrete lumps)

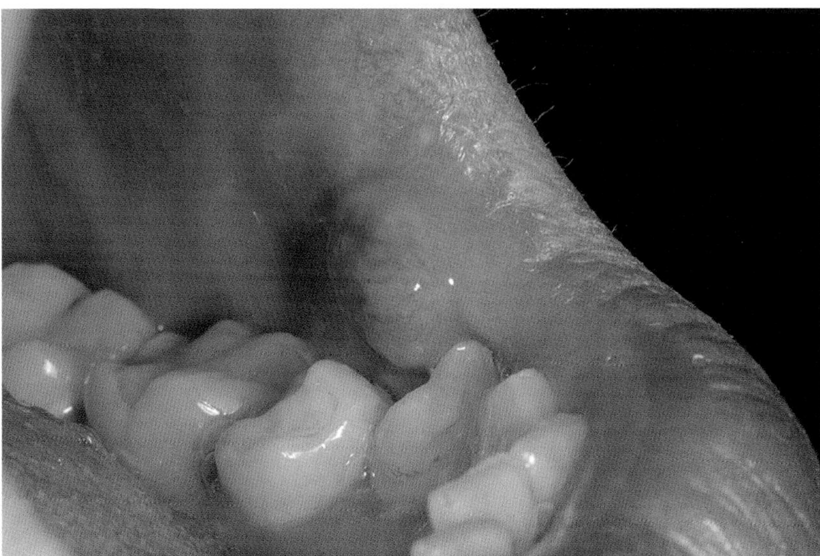

Figure 9.0 Traumatic fibroma.

Clinical Guide to Oral Diseases, First Edition. Dimitris Malamos and Crispian Scully.

Companion website: www.wiley.com/go/malamos/clinical_guide

Table 9 The most important causes of swellings and lumps.

- ◆ Congenital
  - Exostoses
  - Tori
    - Upper
      - Palatinus
    - Lower jaw
      - Mandibularis
  - Vascular
    - Angiomas
    - Lymphangiomas
- ◆ Acquired
  - Anatomical
    - Unerupted teeth
  - Reactive
    - Foreign bodies
  - Traumatic
    - Local trauma
    - Traumatic/post-traumatic edema
    - Hematoma
    - Surgical emphysema
  - Infective
    - Abscess
    - Actinomycosis
    - Lymphadenitis
    - Facial swelling (cutaneous/dental)
    - Oral infections
    - Cellulitis
    - Fascial space infections
  - Inflammatory
    - Pyogenic and other granulomas
    - Cysts
  - Immune related
    - Amyloidosis
    - Sarcoidosis
    - C1 esterase inhibitor deficiency
    - Crohn's disease and other orofacial granulomatosis
    - Melkersson-Rosenthal syndrome
    - Allergic angioedema
    - Insect bites
  - Neoplasm
    - Benign
      - Oral mucosa
        - Papilloma
        - Neurofibromas
        - Fibrous lumps
      - Bones
        - Fibrous dysplasia
        - Cherubism
        - Paget disease
    - Malignant
      - Oral mucosa
        - Carcinomas
        - Lymphomas
        - Sarcomas
        - Melanomas
      - Bones
        - Osteosarcomas
        - Lymphomas
  - Drugs

Case 9.1

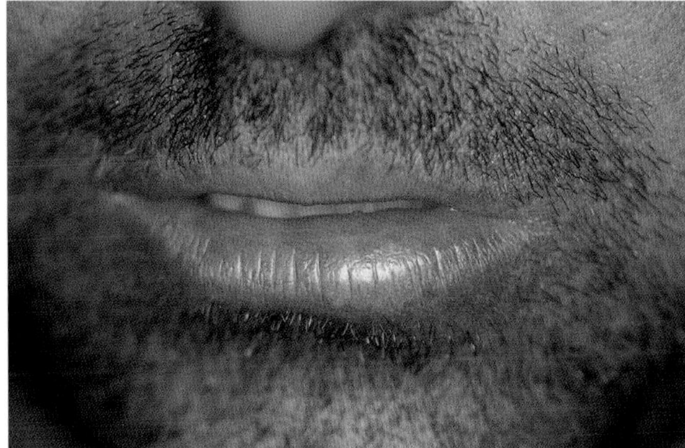

Figure 9.1

CO: A 28-year-old healthy man was presented with a diffuse swelling of his lower lip.

HPC: This lesion started two hours ago with a burning, tingling sensation on the left corner of his mouth. The lesion appeared immediately after eating his salad meal and gradually extended to the half of his lower lip. No other similar episodes of swellings had been reported by the patient or any of his close relatives in the past.

PMH: His past medical history was clear from any serious diseases or common allergies, drug use or harmful habits such as smoking or drinking. Given the fact that he was a builder, chronic exposure to solar radiation was recorded.

OE: A diffuse swelling on the lower lip was extended from the vermilion border to the adjacent skin and from the left-hand corner of the mouth to the middle line (Figure 9.1). No other similar lesions were seen on his oral and other mucosae or facial skin.

The swelling reached its biggest size within the next two hours, but started to be slow down within the next hour. The swelling was soft, painless and cause esthetic patient concern.

Q1 What is the possible cause?

- **A** Allergic cheilitis
- **B** Cheilitis granulomatosa
- **C** Traumatic injury
- **D** Hypothyroidism
- **E** Angioneurotic edema

Answers:

- **A** No
- **B** No
- **C** No
- **D** No
- **E** Angioneurotic edema is the cause and is characterized by recurrent episodes of swelling due to vascular leakage on the submucosa. This is an acute lesion on various parts of the face, mouth, respiratory or abdominal tract and genital organs, being associated with a burning sensation and mild pain without pronouncing itching or erythema.

Comments: Allergic cheilitis and traumatic injuries were excluded as both conditions are generally characterized, apart from swelling, by erythema, ulcerations, or desquamation that are related to various allergies in cosmetics, foods or drugs or recent head injury. Cheilitis granulomatosa and hypothyroidism were also exempted as their swelling is chronic and gradually reaches its biggest size over the following three to four weeks, staying the same after then, but associated with signs and symptoms from its main disease.

Q2 Which of the laboratory tests below are NOT commonly used for the diagnosis of this condition?

- **A** C1 esterase inhibitor
- **B** D-dimers
- **C** C4 levels
- **D** CH50 levels
- **E** Thyroid tests

Answers:

- **A** No
- **B** No
- **C** No
- **D** No
- **E** Thyroid tests (T3; T4; TSH, and thyroid auto-abs) are widely used for estimation of thyroid gland function and rarely used to distinguish if the swelling is due to angioedema or hypothyroidism.

Comments: C1 esterase inhibitor and complement total CH50 and C4 show alteration in both types of angioedema (hereditary or acquired). D-dimers are elevated in hereditary angioedema episodes.

Q3 C1 esterase inhibitor protein is diminished in the following types of angioedema:

- **A** Acquired idiopathic
- **B** Acquired drug-induced
- **C** Hereditary angioedema type I
- **D** Hereditary angioedema type II
- **E** Hereditary angioedema type III

Answers:

- **A** No
- **B** No
- **C** The angioneurotic edema type I is caused by a mutation in the SERPING 1 gene which diminishes the level of C1 Inhibitory protein.
- **D** No
- **E** No

Comments: Hereditary angioneurotic edema type II causes dysfunction rather than alteration of the level of C1 inhibitor protein, while type III acts only on coagulation factor XII. Drug-induced and idiopathic angioedema are the two acquired forms and their pathogenetic mechanism is not related to this protein.

Case 9.2

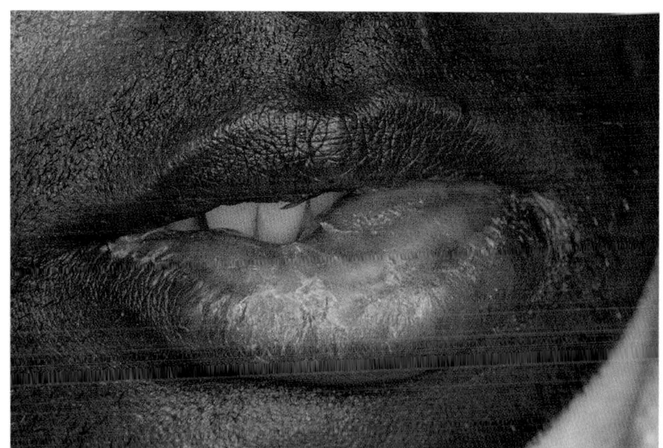

Figure 9.2a

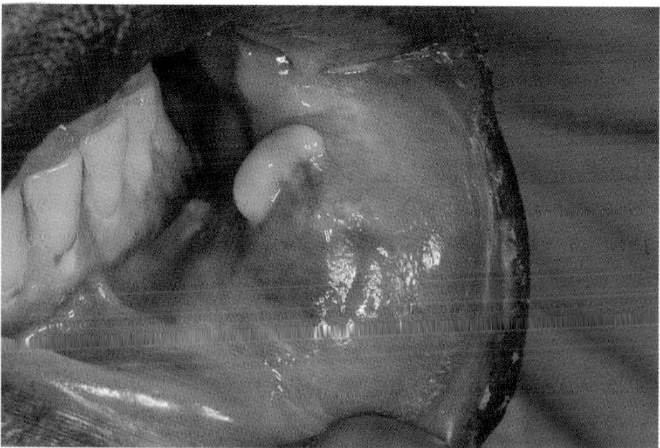

Figure 9.2b

CO: A 25-year-old Nigerian man was presented with painful swelling on his lower lip.

HPC: The swelling appeared three days ago, right after a lip bite. It started as a small traumatic ulcer followed by a small swelling which gradually increased in size and with pressure, an exudation of pus was released accompanied with throbbing pain and fever.

PMH: His medical history was clear, with no known allergies or drug use. Working as a farmer, he was daily exposed to solar radiation and rarely to pesticides, but was never a smoker or heavy drinker.

OE: A large diffuse, painful swelling on his lower lip (Figure 9.2a) which was bigger on the left half part, exuding pus with pressure (Figure 9.2b).This swelling was not associated with general symptomatology, but submandibular cervical lymphadenopathy and fever was found.

Q1 What is the possible diagnosis?

- **A** Glandular cheilitis
- **B** Lip abscess
- **C** Cold sores
- **D** Mucocele
- **E** Actinic prurigo

Answers:

- **A** No
- **B** Lip abscess is the answer and is characterized by an accumulation of pus within the submucosa of the vermilion border of the lip. A former lip injury facilitates the entrance of pathogenic germs within the lip, therefore causing local inflammation with pus production.
- **C** No
- **D** No
- **E** No

Comments: Mucoceles and cold sores can be easily excluded as their fluid content is clear and not pus. Cheilitis glandularis and actinic prurigo are also ruled out given the fact that the inflammation in cheilitis glandularis is chronic and characterized by a clear fluid excretion from numerous duct orifices, while in actinic prurigo, an itchy skin rash with numerous inflamed papules, plaques, or ulcerations are always present together with lip lesions.

Q2 Which other characteristics differentiate cold sores from lip abscesses?

- **A** Onset
- **B** Duration
- **C** Symptomatology
- **D** Treatment
- **E** Predisposing factors

Answers:

- **A** Cold sore lesions are presented within a few hours, whereas lip abscesses appear within a few days from the onset of lip symptoms.
- **B** Cold sores can be healed within 10–14 days whereas untreated abscesses persist longer.
- **C** No
- **D** In immunocompetent patients, cold sore lesions require no treatment, while abscesses need surgical drainage and a broad range of antibiotics.
- **E** No

Comments: Both conditions present with painful erythematous lip swelling along with various symptomatology following stressful events, trauma or serious diseases such as immunodeficiencies, diabetes, and infectious or malignant diseases.

Q3 Lip abscess is a complication of:
- **A** Cellulitis
- **B** Blastomycosis
- **C** Erysipelas
- **D** Tuberculosis
- **E** Furuncles

Answers:
- **A** Cellulitis is a bacterial infection on the dermis and submucosa from *Staphylococcus* and hemolytic *Streptococcus,* creating small abscesses in different places including lips.
- **B** No
- **C** Erysipelas is a bacterial infection on the upper dermis from *Streptococcus pyogenes* that extends to the superficial cutaneous lymphatics and may give rise to skin abscesses which sometimes spread to the lips.
- **D** No
- **E** A furuncle is a bacterial infection on the hair follicles from Staphylococci, creating skin boils which may extend from the chin towards the lip.

Comments: Cold abscesses lack the signs of acute inflammation (i.e. redness or pain) and are mainly found in tuberculosis and deep fungal infections such as blastomycosis.

Case 9.3

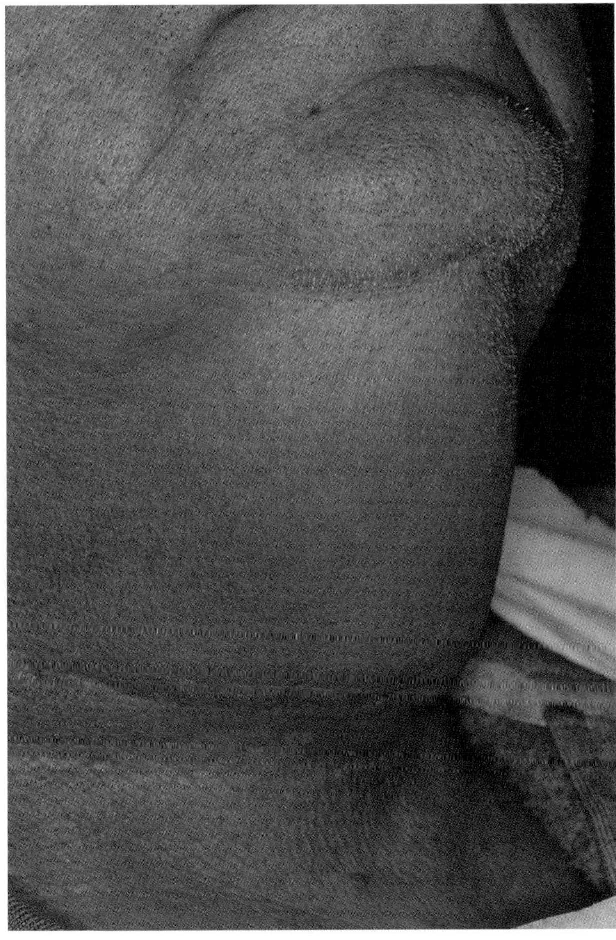

Figure 9.3

CO: A 67-year-old overweight man presented with a diffuse neck swelling at the end of his radio-chemotherapy for a tonsil carcinoma.

HPC: The swelling appeared gradually during the last sessions of chemo-radiotherapy, causing tightness and difficulties in head movement, as well as an itching sensation on his neck.

PMH: His recent medical history revealed a carcinoma on his right tonsils which had been removed two months ago and consequently treated with a course of 6 chemo (cisplatin) and 30 radiotherapy sessions. Hypertension and chronic pulmonary disease due to chronic exposure to asbestos at his work and a lung carcinoma five years ago were recorded. No allergies, alcohol use or smoking habits were reported.

OE: Extra-oral examination revealed a diffuse neck swelling extending from the lower border of the mandible to the sternal notch (Figure 9.3). The underlying skin was dark, brown, dry, and inelastic, with some exfoliated areas too, but without any signs of infection. The intra-oral examination revealed severe xerostomia, loss of taste papillae on the dorsum of the tongue, and scattered superficial ulcerations (mucositis).

Q1 What is the diagnosis?
- **A** Hygroma
- **B** Lymphedema
- **C** Hypothyroidism
- **D** Branchial cyst
- **E** Obesity

Answers:
- **A** No
- **B** Lymphedema is the cause. The lesion is characterized by an abnormal lymph drainage leading to gradual accumulation of fluid in the neck caused by the removal or inflammation and blockage of local lymph nodes during carcinoma treatment.
- **C** No
- **D** No
- **E** No

Comments: The location and the time of onset of his neck swelling leads to the exclusion of other conditions such as hygroma, branchial cysts, hypothyroidism, or obesity from the diagnosis. Hygroma is located at the left posterior triangle, while branchial cysts are at one part (left or right) of the neck and in front of sternocleidomastoid muscle. Both lesions are congenital lesions and appear at younger age while the lymphedema was present during the last sessions of radiotherapy as a diffuse swelling covering the whole neck and inside her mouth. In hypothyroidism and obesity, the swelling is also diffuse not only found in the neck, but is also extended to other parts of the face and body.

Q2 Which additional test/s could be used for estimation of neck swelling?
- **A** Measurement of swelling with tape
- **B** Neck ultrasound
- **C** Kidney function tests
- **D** Skin tests for allergy
- **E** Intravenous cholangiogram

Answers:
- **A** The measurement of the patient's neck with a tape allows us to estimate the differences in swelling through time.
- **B** Ultrasound helps to estimate the fluid accumulation within the neck tissues.
- **C** No
- **D** No
- **E** No

Comments: Intravenous cholangiogram is an unrelated X-ray procedure that is used to look at the large bile ducts within or outside the liver. The allergy skin tests can be also used by pricking or puncturing the skin with various chemicals in order to identify any possible allergens, while kidney function tests can be used to estimate the glomerular filtration rate and exclude any in kidney diseases.

Q3 Which are the recommended treatments for his neck leukedema?
- **A** Diet
- **B** Exercise
- **C** Liposuction
- **D** Laser
- **E** Antibiotics

Answers:
- **A** No
- **B** Exercise and local massage helps to relief fluid decongestion.
- **C** No
- **D** No
- **E** No

Comments: Antibiotics and low laser therapy are used to control any local or systemic infections and prevent oral mucositis rather than leukoedema. Liposuction is sometimes used for alleviating leukedema, particularly in the arms and legs, but rarely in the neck.

Case 9.4

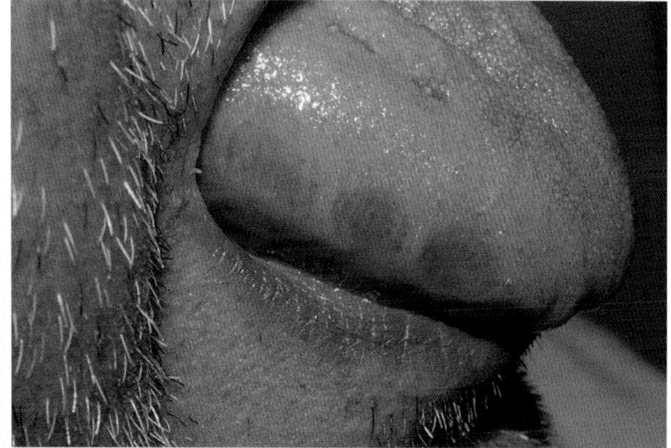

Figure 9.4

CO: A 58-year-old homosexual man presented for a swollen tongue.

HPC: The swelling appeared gradually and caused discomfort as well as difficulties in eating, swallowing or speech for the patient over the last two months.

PMH: The patient suffered from a mild hypertension and hypercholesterolemia controlled with ACE inhibitor drugs and a special diet, respectively. He had been an asymptomatic carrier of HIV infection over the last two years, but no treatment was required.

OE: Oral examination revealed a diffuse soft swelling on his whole tongue with indentations from his teeth at its lateral margins (Figure 9.4), but without any signs of local infection causing the patient discomfort. Extra-orally, no evidence of skin and other mucosae swellings, infections or allergic reactions were noted. Cervical lymphadenopathy was undetected.

Q1 What is the cause of the swelling?
- **A** HIV status
- **B** Tongue abscess
- **C** ACE-inhibitor drug-induced angioedema
- **D** Tongue lymphangioma
- **E** Tongue sarcoidosis

Answers:

A No
B No
C Angioedema is a well-known side effect of ACE inhibitor drugs, can be life-threatening in severe cases, and is presented with no pitting, swelling of the tongue, and other parts of the mouth and oropharynx.
D No
E No

Comments: The lack of any clinical signs or symptoms of an infection, like pain, erythema and malaise or presence of other lesions like erythema associated with pus exudate; well circumscribed brownish-red swellings or with easily detached pesudomembranes excludes the tongue abscess, sarcoidosis or HIV infection from the diagnosis. Lymphangioma often involves the tongue but in contrast with the patient's swelling, it appears at very early age (birth or early childhood).

Q2 Which other causes of tongue swelling can jeopardize the patient's life?

A Insect bites
B Food allergies
C Carcinomas
D Sublingual stone
E Cavernous hemangiomas

Answers:

A Insect bites can cause allergic reactions and in severe cases the tongue swelling maybe to big that interferes with breathing in such degree that could risk patient's life.
B No
C Untreated carcinomas are spread locally and via adjacent lymph nodes to distant organs (metastasis), jeopardizing the patient's life.
D No
E Ruptured cavernous hemangiomas can cause severe bleeding, and patients should ask for help at the nearest hospital to avoid hemorrhagic shock.

Comments: Sublingual stone can cause pain and swelling in the area, while food allergies can cause oral and peri-oral or orbital swellings but both conditions do not risk the patient's life.

Q3 Which of the drugs below do NOT cause tongue swelling?

A Gold salts
B Naprosyn
C Supradol
D Prednisolone
E Cisplatin

Answers:

A No
B No
C No
D Prednisolone is widely used for the treatment of tongue swelling due to allergic or autoimmune reaction.
E Cisplatin is widely used for chemotherapy of various carcinomas and rarely causes allergic reactions.

Comments: Anti-inflammatory drugs such as Naprosyn, gold salts and Supradol cause severe side-effects, including tongue swelling.

Case 9.5

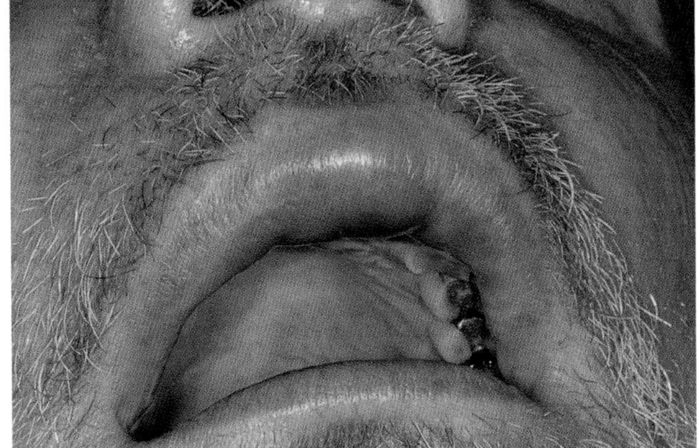

Figure 9.5

CO: A 69-year-old man presented with a swelling on his upper lip three days after a minor surgery for the removal of his anterior upper teeth by his dentist.

HPC: The swelling appeared gradually and became more intense over the last two days, being accompanied by pain and burning sensation.

PMH: His medical history was clear apart from a mild depression which was controlled with a selective serotonin reuptake inhibitor (paroxetine). He was allergic to penicillin and aspirin and therefore took a course of erythromycin and paracetamol for the extractions. His smoking and drinking habits included two packets of cigarettes per day and two bottles of beer with every meal.

OE: His gross upper lip swelling was extended from the skin close to the vermilion border to the alveolar mucosa of the extracted upper incisors (Figure 9.5). The swelling was more pronounced in the middle, below the nasal philtrum, and was present with erythema and pain on palpation. No other lesions were detected intra-orally, a diffuse swelling from the alveolar mucosa of extracted upper incisors associated with hematoma and his remaining teeth were covered with calculus due to his poor oral hygiene. Only a few submental nodes were palpable.

Q1 What is the possible cause of his lip swelling?

- **A** Iatrogenic trauma
- **B** Angioedema
- **C** Lip abscess
- **D** Granular cell cheilitis
- **E** Allergic cheilitis

Answers:

- **A** Trauma of the upper lip during tooth extraction causes tissue damage, hematoma formation leading to swelling, erythema and local pain (signs of acute inflammation).
- **B** No
- **C** No
- **D** No
- **E** No

Comments: Angioedema can sometimes be precipitated by local trauma, but is not associated with hematoma, as seen in this patient. The short onset of his swelling, the lack of other lesions or pus exudates exclude granular and allergic cheilitis or lip abscess from the diagnosis.

Q2 Which are the other causes of facial swelling among healthy people?

- **A** Diet rich in salt
- **B** Poor nutrition
- **C** Pregnancy
- **D** Sunburn
- **E** Standing for a long time

Answers:

- **A** Eating salty food causes fluid retention and edema.
- **B** A nutrition poor in proteins and electrolytes seems to affect the recovery of fluid through the lymphatic system causing, thus a nutritional facial edema which is more obvious in people in famine.
- **C** The facial swelling seen in pregnant women is a common finding, especially at their third trimester due to weight gain, and is related to the increased fluid retention during that period. Any sudden facial swelling may be an early indication of pre-eclampsia, a condition of high blood pressure and proteins detected in the urine of pregnant women.
- **D** Sunburn causes facial swelling as well as skin dryness and blisters, especially in fair complexioned people.
- **E** No

Comments: Long standing is related to swollen legs rather than the face, and is the result of fluid retention due to dysfunctional circulation.

Q3 Which other cause(s) except for trauma is or are responsible for localized soft tissue swellings?

- **A** Abscess
- **B** Insect bite
- **C** Drug allergy
- **D** Congestive heart disease
- **E** Hypothyroidism

Answers:

- **A** Infections from various pathogenic germs cause local abscess formation that is characterized by swelling, erythema and pain.
- **B** Insect bites can cause a local allergic reaction to chemicals released by insects (i.e. formic acid) and is characterized by redness, itching and swelling. The swelling is usually (<5 cm) but in severe cases is diffused and sometimes associated with breathing problems.
- **C** No
- **D** No
- **E** No

Comments: Systematic and not localized swelling is reported in allergies due to systematic drug use; in congestive heart diseases and hypothyroidism. Drug allergies are characterized by activation and degranulation of mast cells, releasing mediators (cytokines) which increase the permeability of small vessels with fluid retention sequence. Congestive heart diseases are characterized by difficulties in circulation from the periphery to the heart, while hypothyroidism is characterized by low body temperature; both diseases allow the accumulation of fluid within the body, finally causing a pitting body edema.

Case 9.6

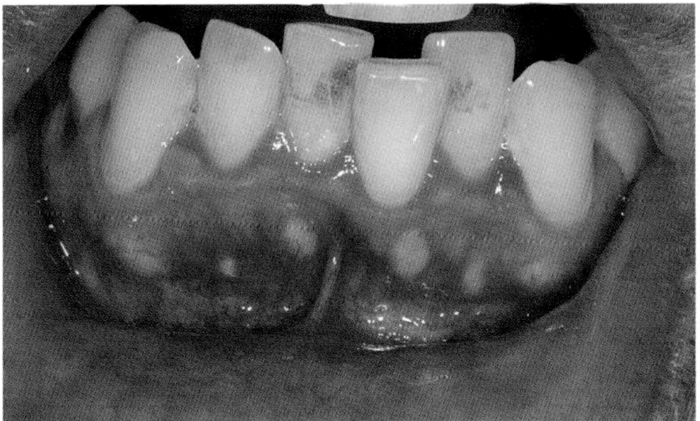

Figure 9.6

CO: A 32-year-old woman was referred by her dentist due to multiple white nodules on her lower anterior gingivae.

HPC: The nodules were asymptomatic and discovered accidentally by her new dentist during her regular dental check-up.

PMH: The patient was a healthy young woman with no history of any serious diseases, trauma or allergies and drug uptake, as well as no drinking habits. However, she smoked 10 cigarettes per day. None of her close relatives had ever reported similar lesions.

OE: The oral examination revealed multiple whitish swellings on the lower anterior gingivae, 2–5 mm in diameter. The lesions were hard in palpation, fixed with the underlying alveolar bone (Figure 9.6). No other similar lesions were found in her body. Intra-oral radiographs and routine blood tests were normal.

Q1 What is the possible diagnosis?

A Tuberous sclerosis
B Gingival cysts
C Multiple exostoses
D Cowden syndrome
E Multiple gingival fibromas

Answers:

A No
B No
C No
D No
E Multiple gingival fibromas is a variation of gingivae, seen as multiple not movable, asymptomatic whitish nodules of the anterior gingivae–alveolar mucosae of the mandible rather than the maxilla.

Comments: Oral lesions such exostoses and gingival cysts have well circumscribed gingival lesions, but with different bony or fluid content respectively, while other diseases such as tuberous sclerosis and Cowden syndrome have numerous lesions in other parts of the mouth and skin, apart from gingivae having therefore been excluded from the diagnosis.

Q2 Which test/s can be used for the diagnosis of this condition?

A Biopsy
B Intra-oral X-rays
C Vitality tests
D Diascopy
E Photography

Answers:

A The biopsy allows the examination of the lesion under routine microscopy, revealing focal accumulation of mature connective tissues within the superficial parts of the submucosa in a localized pattern.
B Intra-oral X-rays could be used to show bony, not fibrous, growths on top of the alveolar bone, thus differentiating exostoses from multiple fibromas.
C No
D No
E No

Comments: The three tests (vitality tests, photoluminescence and medical photography) are irrelevant for the diagnosis of those fibrous nodules as the dental pulp vitality tests (thermal or electrical) are used for the estimation of dental nerve function in pulp, diascopy for color alterations of the oral mucosa with pressure, and medical photography for recording the clinical appearance of the lesions at a time.

Q3 Which of the syndromes below is or are NOT related with multiple fibromas?

A Cowden syndrome
B Gardner syndrome
C Gorlin syndrome
D Apert syndrome
E Kostmann syndrome

Answers:

A No

B No

C No

D Alpert syndrome is characterized by malformations of the skull (craniosynostosis); hands and feet (syndactyly); and maxillae (high-arched palate and pseudo-mandibular prognathism) but not with multiple fibromas.

E Kostmann syndrome is a group of diseases characterized by disorders of myelopoiesis causing congenital neutropenia but not fibromas.

Comments: The Cowden, Garner and less frequently Gorlin syndromes appear with multiple hamartomas including fibromas. Cowden syndrome is characterized by numerous hamartomas on the skin, mouth and internal organs with increased risk of breast, thyroid and uterine cancers, while Gardner syndrome is characterized by polyps in the colon, osteomas and epidermal cysts. Gorlin syndrome is presented with anomalies of the nervous and endocrine systems, together with keratinocytes in the jaws.

Case 9.7

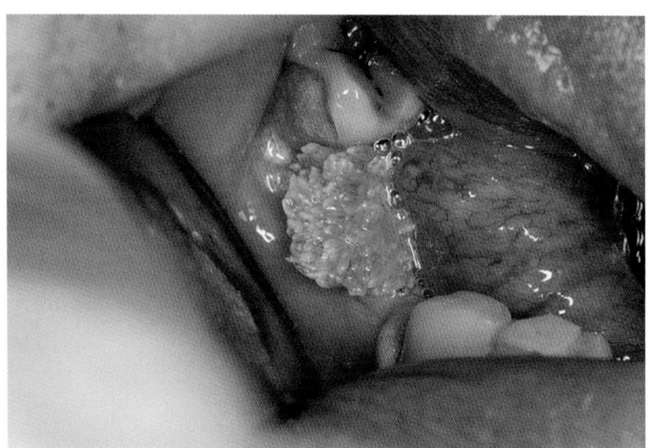

Figure 9.7

CO: A 42-year-old man was presented with a papillary lesion on his alveolar mucosa, proximal to the second lower right molar.

HPC: The lesion was first noticed one year ago as a small, asymptomatic papillary nodule which became much bigger over the last two months.

PMH: His medical history was unremarkable apart from mild hypertension and hyper-cholesterolemia that was controlled with a special diet. No skin, allergies or drug uptakes, or smoking or drinking habits were recorded.

OE: A soft white-pinkish asymptomatic lesion, maximum diameter 3.5 cm, with a papillary surface and a wide base on the alveolar mucosa of a previously extracted lower right 1st molar and 2nd premolar (Figure 9.7). The lesion was soft in consistency. No other similar lesions were found in his mouth or genitals and other mucosae.

Q1 What is the possible diagnosis?

A Papillary cystadenoma of minor salivary glands

B Papilloma

C Condyloma acuminata

D Verruca vulgaris

E Focal epithelial hyperplasia (Heck's disease)

Answers:

A No

B Papilloma is the correct diagnosis. This is a benign, exophytic, well-circumscribed lesion consisting of multiple cauliflower-like projections which are histologically epithelial outgrowths supported by a thin fibrovascular stroma.

C No

D No

E No

Comments: In the differential diagnosis of patient's papilloma other lesions with similar clinical papillary morphology like verruca vulgaris; condyloma lata and focal epithelial hyperplasia or with histological papillary elements like papillary cystic adenoma of minor salivary gland are included. Papillary cystic adenoma of minor salivary glands is also a benign tumor, but contrary to papilloma, appears as a solitary, localized, smooth swelling that is composed of cystic spaces with a few papillary projections within the lumen, at the same time surrounded with a thick fibrous capsule. Focal epithelial hyperplasia is characterized by numerous papillary growths on the oral mucosa and is caused by an HPV infection of type 13 and 32. Verruca vulgaris and condyloma acuminatum are tumors with a rough surface, but contrary to papillomas, are usually accompanied with similar lesions on the skin surface of the hands and feet or genitals respectively.

Q2 Which is /or are the differences between papillomas and fibromas?

- **A** Pathogenesis
- **B** Clinical characteristics
- **C** Symptomatology
- **D** Malignant transformation
- **E** Tendency of recurrence

Answers:

- **A** The pathogenesis is different, as chronic irritation is responsible for fibroma formation, while human papillomavirus (type 6) is responsible for the majority of papillomas.
- **B** Although both lesions have a mushroom appearance, their surface is totally different; smooth for fibroma and rough for papillomas.
- **C** No
- **D** No
- **E** No

Comments: Both fibromas and papillomas are common benign asymptomatic tumors that occur in the mouth with no tendency of recurrence or malignant transformation.

Q3 Which viruses have been associated with papillomas?

- **A** HPV 6 and 11
- **B** Coxsackie A
- **C** HSV 1 and 2
- **D** HPV 16 and 18
- **E** Rotavirus A

Answers:

- **A** HPV 6 and 11 have been isolated in 60 per cent of papilloma cases.
- **B** No
- **C** No
- **D** No
- **E** No

Comments: HPV types 16 and 18 have been isolated in genital condylomas and these viruses are responsible for cervical (mainly), oral, hypopharynx, and larynx carcinomas. Coxsackie A and HSV 1 and 2 are responsible for herpangina and herpetic lesions respectively while the rotavirus A is the most common virus among young children causing diarrhea.

Case 9.8

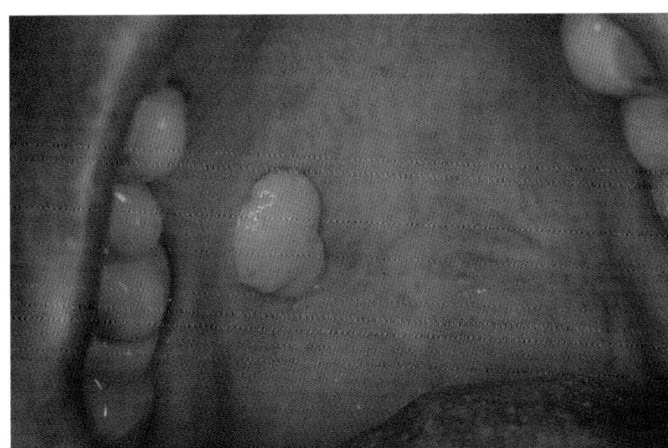

Figure 9.8

CO: A 32-year-old woman presented with a lump on her palate.

HPC: The lesion was discovered by the patient eight months ago during self-examination and had remained unchanged since then.

PMH: She was a healthy young teacher with no serious medical problems who spent her free time swimming and running. Given the fact that she had been an athlete, she had a proper diet full of vegetables and nuts, with no heavy smoking or drinking habits.

OE: A firm pedunculated lesion was found on the right side of her hard palate, close to the apex of the 2nd premolar and 1st molar, 1 × 2 cm in diameter (Figure 9.8). The lesion had a smooth surface and semi-hard consistency and normal color, but was easily detached from the palatal mucosa, painless and did not bleed during palpation. No other similar lesions were seen in the oral and other mucosae. Vitality pulp tests together with intra-oral X-rays did not reveal any tooth pathology. Excision biopsy revealed that the lesion was composed of a hyperplastic fibrous connective tissue with minimal cellularity and lack of atypia, overlain by normal thin mucosa.

Q1 What is the diagnosis?

- **A** Pleomorphic adenoma
- **B** Lipoma

C Parulis
D Traumatic fibroma
E Amelanotic melanoma

Answers:

A No
B No
C No
D Traumatic fibroma is the answer. It is the most common intra-oral benign lesion and is characterized by a firm, asymptomatic nodule with smooth and sometimes ulcerated surface, mainly noticed on the areas of lips, tongue and palate that are susceptible to chronic irritation and trauma.
E No

Comments: Lipomas and parulis are easily excluded clinically. Both lesions have a soft consistency, but parulis additionally has negative vitality tests and positive intra-oral X-rays showing a periapical radiolucency. The amelanotic melanoma is also ruled out, because of its rapid growth and absence of satellite lesions while pleomorphic adenomas has a long clinical route as patient's fibroma and requires biopsy. Biopsy is mandatory for the correct diagnosis as fibroma is characterized by hyperplasia of the connective tissue, lipoma by aggregation of fatty cells, while on the other hand amelanotic melanoma is characterized by atypical neoplastic melanocytes, while pleomorphic adenoma is characterized by neoplastic epithelial and myoepithelial cells in a myxomatous or chondroid stroma, partially lined up with an incomplete fibrous capsule.

Q2 Which other intra oral tumor(s) is or are variation(s) of a traumatic fibroma?

A Submucous fibrosis
B Giant cell fibromas
C Peripheral ossifying fibroma
D Pregnancy epulis
E Denture-induced fibrous hyperplasia

Answers:

A No
B Giant cell fibromas are tumors that are characterized by the presence of numerous multinuclear cells in a fibrous stroma.
C Peripheral ossifying fibroma is characterized by a hyperplastic vascular connective tissue intermingled with osteoid and bone formation.
D No
E Denture-induced fibrous hyperplasia is an extensive hyperplasia of connective tissue with mild to marked inflammation and appears as mucosal fibrous folds along the mucolabial and mucobuccal sulcus, due to ill-fitting dentures.

Comments: Submucous fibrosis is a condition characterized by intra-oral stiffness due to thickness of the oral mucosa. This is the result of a progressive diffuse and not localized fibrosis of the underlying submucosa due to chronic inflammation caused by chronic use of areca nut or betel quid. On the other hand, pregnancy epulis appears on pregnant women's gingivae and it is characterized by immature granuloma formation due to increased estrogen secretion, mainly in the third trimester, in combination with local irritation and bacteria.

Q3 Which is/are the difference(s) between oral fibromas and fibromatosis?

A Age of onset
B Number of lesions
C Symptomatology
D Clinical behavior
E Recurrence

Answers:

A Oral fibromas can appear at any age, but mainly in the thirties to fifties, while three-quarters of all reported cases of fibromatosis are diagnosed in patients younger than 10 years old.
B Oral fibromas are usually single lesions while fibromatosis represent a group of diseases with poorly demarcated fibrous masses of variable growth rate.
C No
D Oral fibromas are benign lesions with no tendency of malignant transformation, while some fibromatosis can be aggressive locally causing resorption of adjacent bone.
E Completely excised oral fibromas do not recur while oral fibromatosis lesions show a recurrence rate of 30 per cent, more within the first year of surgery.

Comments: Both small lesions are asymptomatic but symptoms appear when the lesions be big and interfere with mastication.

Case 9.9

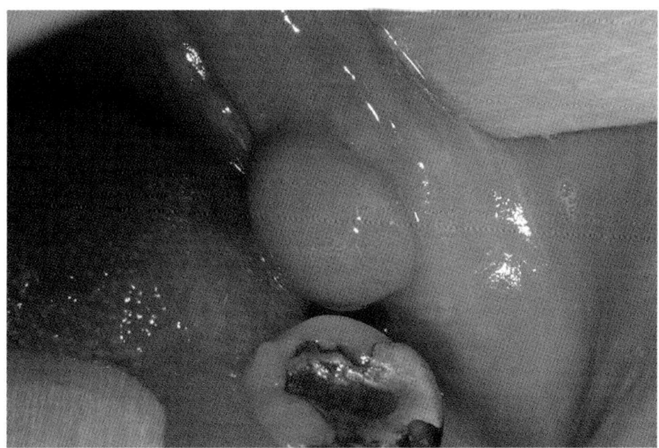

Figure 9.9

CO: A 45-year-old man was referred by his dentist for a soft nodule on his left buccal mucosa.

HPC: The lesion was asymptomatic and discovered by his dentist during a dental check-up one week ago.

PMH: He had a history of atopic dermatitis and allergic rhinitis, both having been controlled with steroids and anti-histamine drugs when needed.

OE: A soft pink to yellow colored nodule on the left buccal mucosa proximately to the lower second molar was found. The nodule was painless and covered with normal thin oral mucosa, while it was slightly fluctuant in palpation (Figure 9.9), and was not bleached with pressure. No other similar lesions were found in the mouth, skin or other mucosae.

Q1 What is the possible diagnosis?

- **A** Fibroma
- **B** Myxoma
- **C** Deep mucocele
- **D** Hemangioma
- **E** Lipoma

Answers:

- **A** No
- **B** No
- **C** No
- **D** No
- **E** Lipoma is the answer. It is a benign tumor of adipose tissue and is mainly seen on buccal mucosae, vestibules, and tongue, but rarely on the palate. Due to its mature fatty content and the thin cover of oral mucosa, the lesion has a yellow to pink color and is very soft, and fluctuant in palpation.

Comments: The clinical characteristics such as the soft consistency of the lesion and its color excluded other lesions such as fibromas having normal color, but are firm in palpation mucoceles which are translucent and fluctuant and hemangiomas which are dark red-blue in color from diagnosis. Myxoma is less frequently seen on oral mucosa than lipoma, and its diagnosis is based only on histological findings.

Q2 Which of the lesions below is/or are NOT variation(s) of a lipoma?

- **A** Fibrolipoma
- **B** Dermoid cyst
- **C** Angiolipoma
- **D** Lipoblastoma
- **E** Osteolipoma

Answers:

- **A** No
- **B** Dermoid cyst is not a variation of lipoma, despite the presence of fatty cells together with hair follicles, and glands (sweat and sebaceous) within its cystic wall.
- **C** No
- **D** No
- **E** No

Comments: What could be considered as variations of lipoma are all the tumors in which their predominant type of tissue, apart from adipose tissue, is a mature connective tissue (fibrolipoma) or consists of vascular elements (angiolipoma) or with osteoid metaplasia (osteolipoma). Lipoblastoma is a benign tumor of brown fat cells, mainly observed in children less than three years old.

Q3 Which of the syndromes below are related to multiple lipomas?

- **A** Cowden syndrome
- **B** Osler-Weber-Rendu syndrome
- **C** Magic syndrome
- **D** Proteus syndrome
- **E** Peutz-Jeghers syndrome

Answers:

- **A** Cowden syndrome is characterized by the presence of multiple hamartomas including lipomas in various parts of the body.
- **B** No
- **C** No
- **D** Proteus syndrome is a rare condition which is characterized by asymmetrical overgrowth of skin, bones and fatty tissue (lipomas) with high risk of premature death due to a deep vein thrombosis.
- **E** No

Comments: The other three syndromes do not include lipomas in their manifestations. The Osler-Weber-Rendu and the Magic syndrome are characterized by abnormal blood vessel formation and oral, genital ulcerations and polychondritis respectively while Peutz-Jeghers is characterized by hamartomatous polyps in the intestine and pigmented macules on the lips and mouth, but not lipomas.

Case 9.10

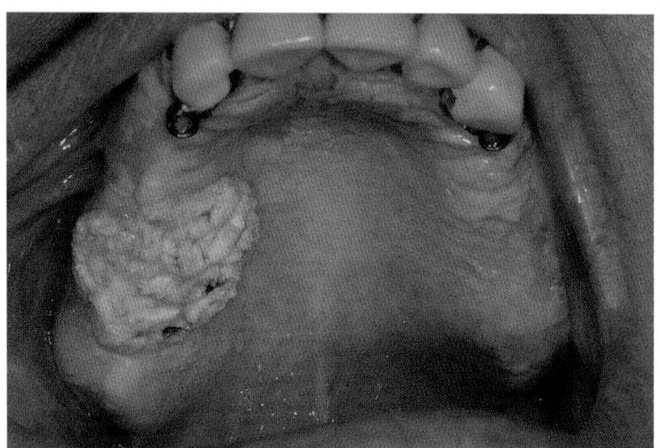

Figure 9.10

CO: A 73-year-old lady presented with a mass on her mouth.

HPC: The lesion was first noticed on the upper right alveolar mucosa by the patient two months ago, when she tried to wear her upper denture. Since then, the lesion has shown a slow gradual extension towards the palate.

PMH: Her main medical problem was a chronic lymphocytic leukemia over the last five years (Rai stage I) which had been under observation by her hematologist, but without treatment. She also suffered with mild depression and was on selective serotonin reuptake inhibitor drugs. Smoking or heavy drinking was not recorded.

OE: A white mass with a cauliflower-like surface which was located on the upper right alveolar mucosa of the premolar to molar area, extended from the buccal sulcus to the palate (Figure 9.10). The lesion was fixed to the underlying periosteum and was painless but firm in palpation. Partial biopsy from the center of the lesion revealed hyperplastic papillary acanthotic epithelium with minimal atypia invading in the superficial parts of the underlying submucosa. No similar lesions were found within the oral and other mucosae, and cervical lymphadenopathy was undetected.

Q1 What is the possible diagnosis?

- **A** Verrucous leukoplakia
- **B** Papilloma
- **C** Verrucous carcinoma
- **D** Giant verrucous vulgaris
- **E** Verrucous xanthoma

Answers:

- **A** No
- **B** No
- **C** Verrucous carcinoma is a low-grade variant of squamous cell carcinoma, and presented as an exophytic white mass with a characteristic cauliflower-like appearance, fixed in palpation, with a tendency of superficial, not deep infiltration and low risk of metastasis.
- **D** No
- **E** No

Comments: The firm consistency of the lesion and its strong fixation with the periosteum increases the clinical suspicion of being a malignancy, while the incision or complete biopsy can differentiate this lesion from other warty like-lesions such as papillomas, warts, xanthomas, or even verrucous leukoplakia. In biopsy, the presence of abundant fat laden histiocytes in the submucosa is characteristic of xanthomas while the detection of inclusion viral particles in epithelial cells is indicative of warts and verrucous vulgaris lesions. Also, the thin shape of rete pegs and the same level of "pushing border" in the underlying connective tissue is characteristic of papillomas while the presence of bulbous rete pegs with epithelial atypia but without invasion is commonly seen in verrucous leukoplakia.

Q2 Which histological feature(s) is/are NOT characteristics of this tumor?

A Epithelial atrophy
B Bulbous rete ridges
C Increased number of abnormal mitoses
D Perineural invasion of carcinoma cells
E Keratin plugs

Answers:

A Epithelial hypertrophy and not atrophy is responsible for the classical cauliflower overgrowth of this type of cancer.
B No
C The number of mitoses is low and abnormal mitoses within the hyperplastic epithelium are even rarer.
D Perineural invasion with neoplasmatic cells is characteristic of those malignancies which have a tendency of local deep invasion. Verrucous carcinoma spreads superficially and therefore perineural invasion is rarely seen.
E No

Comments: Epithelia hyperplasia is characteristic and consists of an increased granular and spinous layer forming bulbous rete ridges in which individual keratinization and squamous pearl formations are seen.

Q3 Which clinical characteristics could be indicative of verrucous carcinoma rather than leukoplakia?

A Symptomatology
B Age of predilection
C Type of lesion (solitary or multifocal)
D Immune patient status
E History of previous HPV infection

Answers:

A No
B Both conditions affect men, but verrucous carcinoma seems to affect those younger than 50 years old, while the verrucous leukoplakia affects older patients.
C Verrucous carcinoma is usually a solitary lesion while verrucous leukoplakia tends to be multifocal.
D Oral verrucous carcinomas have been found in immune-compromised patients while leukoplakias have not.
E No

Comments: Both papillary lesions are usually painless causing a roughness in the oral cavity and both have histological evidence of previous HPV infection of type 6, 11, and 18.

10

Taste Deficits

Taste or gustatory deficits are common in clinical practice and implicated in loss of appetite, malnutrition and reduced quality of the patient's life. These are classified into quantitative or qualitative deficits. The quantitative taste dysfunctions include **ageusia** (absence of the sense of taste) **hypogeusia** (decreased sensitivity of all tastants), and **hypergeusia** (enhanced taste sensitivity). The qualitative taste dysfunctions include **dysgeusia** or **parageusia** (unpleasant perception of a taste) and **phantogeusia** (a perception of a certain taste in the absence of the relevant substance). Taste disturbance can be permanent or temporal with the qualitative more frequent than quantitative (See Figure 10.0).

The most important causes of taste deficits are listed in Table 10.

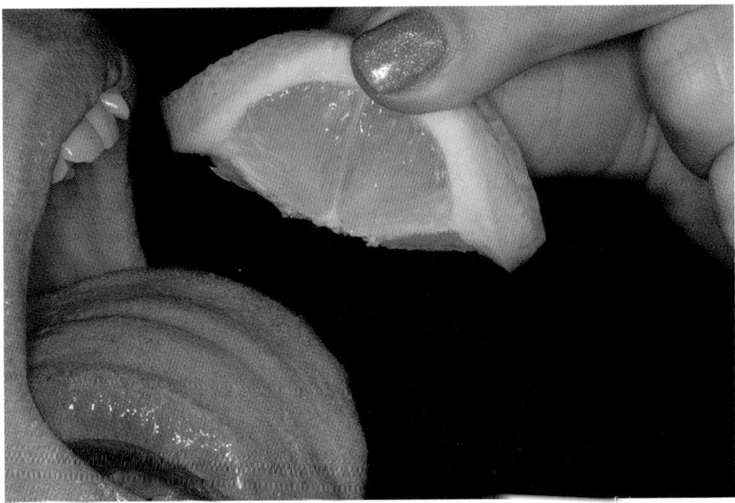

Figure 10.0 Testing sour taste with drops of lemon.

Clinical Guide to Oral Diseases, First Edition. Dimitris Malamos and Crispian Scully.

Companion website: www.wiley.com/go/malamos/clinical_guide

Table 10 The most important causes of taste changes.

- **Ageusia (complete loss of taste)**
  - Idiopathic
  - Diseases
    - Neurological
      - Bell's palsy
      - Familial dysautonomia
      - Multiple sclerosis
    - Infections
      - Primary amoebic meningoencephalitis
    - Endocrinopathies
      - Hypothyroidism
      - Diabetes mellitus
      - Cushing syndrome
    - Deficiencies
      - B3
      - B12
      - Zinc
  - Drugs
    - Antihypertensive
      - Clopidogrel
    - Antirheumatoid
      - Penicillamine
    - Antiproliferative
      - Cisplatin
    - ACE inhibitors
      - Captopril
    - Others
      - Azelastine
      - Clarithromycin
  - Habits
      - Smoking/drinking heavily
- **Hypogeusia (partial loss of taste)**
  - Aging
  - Habits
      - Smoking or drinking
  - Diseases
    - Oral
      - Herpetic stomatitis
      - Thrush
      - Carcinomas
      - Geographic tongue
      - Lichen planus
    - Neurological
      - Alzheimer's
      - Parkinson's
    - Renal
      - Renal failure
    - Liver
      - Liver failure
    - Surgery
      - Laryngectomy
      - Chorda tympani surgery

Table 10 (Continued)

    - Drugs
      - Xerostomia induced
      - Chemotherapeutic
      - Antitumor Abs
      - Bleomycin
    - Trauma
      - Craniofacial injuries
- **Dysgeusia–parageusia (distorted sense of taste)**
  - Idiopathic
  - Drugs
    - Local use
      - Chlorhexidine mouthwash
    - Systemic use
      - Antibiotics
        - Metronidazole
        - Tetracycline
      - Antihypertensive
        - Angiotensin converting enzymes
        - Calcium channel blockers
      - Antihistamines
        - Azelastine
        - Emelastine
      - Antipsychotic
        - Lithium carbonates
- **Cacogeusia (unpleasant bad taste)**
  - Local causes
    - Teeth
      - Decayed
    - Periodontium
      - Gingivitis
      - Periodontitis
    - Oral mucosa
      - Aphthous stomatitis
      - Bullous disorders
  - Systemic causes
    - Pharynx
      - Pharyngitis
    - Lung
      - Abscess
      - Bronchiectasis
      - Tuberculosis
    - Gut
      - Gastritis
    - Pancreas
      - Diabetes
    - Drugs
      - Xerostomia-induced
- **Phantogeusia (fake or phantom taste)**
  - Psychogenic
      - Epilepsy
      - Schizophrenia

Case 10.1

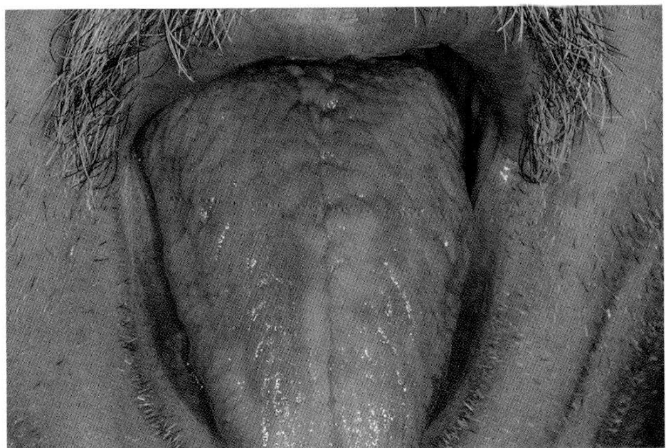

Figure 10.1

CO: A 62-year-old man was presented complaining of a total loss of taste.

HPC: The patient reported a difficulty in recognizing bitter and salty taste from foods two months ago, but gradually this sensory deficit was extended to sour, acid, and umami foods too.

PMH: His medical history revealed chronic hypertension and hypercholesterolemia both having been controlled with drugs, as well as a carcinoma of the oropharynx with cervical ipsilateral metastasis that was diagnosed three months ago. The site of the tumor did not allow any surgery and was therefore treated with a course of radiotherapy and cisplatin chemotherapy for seven weeks. He had been a heavy smoker and drinker for many years.

OE: Examination revealed a partial loss of taste papillae on the dorsum of his tongue (Figure 10.1) associated with xerostomia, erythema and some painful healing ulcerations (known as mucositis) on his soft palate-oropharynx and buccal mucosa. His neck skin was dark, anelastic, and dry with no palpable lymph nodes.

Q1 Which is the main cause of his taste deficit?

- **A** Aging
- **B** Anti-hypertensive drugs
- **C** Xerostomia
- **D** Mucositis
- **E** Radiation-chemotherapy side effect

Answers:

- **A** No
- **B** No
- **C** No
- **D** No
- **E** A transient loss of taste (partial or total) has been reported in patients undergoing chemo- or radiotherapy for head and neck tumors, due to changes in morphology and turnover time of the taste papillae. This taste deficit varies in severity and is related to the patient's health status as well as the type and duration of treatment.

Comments: Normal conditions such as aging together with other pathological conditions such as xerostomia induced by antihypertensive drugs or local inflammation (mucositis) affect the turnover of taste buds and the patient's taste procedure in a secondary and rather indirect way.

Q2 Which of the tastes below is first affected during chemo-radiotherapy?

- **A** Sweat
- **B** Salty
- **C** Sour
- **D** Bitter
- **E** Umami

Answers:

- **A** No
- **B** A sense of salt in food or drink is a common complaint after the third week of cancer treatment.
- **C** No
- **D** Bitter taste is very intense and is one of the first complaints of patients who undergo chemotherapy.
- **E** No

Comments: The sweet and umami tastes as well as the sense of fats are the last senses that are affected during radio/chemotherapy.

Q3 Which of the mechanisms below alter the taste in patients having chemo- and radiotherapy for head and neck tumors?

- **A** Reduced apoptosis of taste cells
- **B** Increased apoptosis of taste cells
- **C** Altered morphology of taste cells
- **D** Disrupted microbial flora in the mouth
- **E** Modulated pathways involved for differentiation of progenitor taste cells.

Answers:

A No

B The increased apoptosis of taste receptors is responsible for taste deficit induced during chemo- or radiotherapy.

C Radiotherapy rather than chemotherapy destroys the microvilli of taste cells and thus diminishes the recognition of various taste stimulants.

D Cancer chemo-radiotherapy changes the microbiota in mouth and gut leading to inflammation and changes in taste perception.

E Cancer therapy via modulation of the hedgehog pathway (SHH) in IV taste cells causes reduction in number of progenitor and mature taste cells.

Comments: The life of taste buds is approximately around 10–14 days and oral cancer treatment and their apoptosis is always increased.

Case 10.2

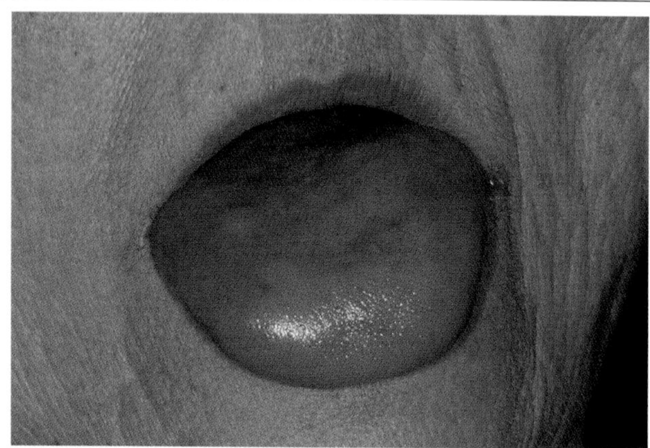

Figure 10.2

CO: A 68-year-old woman presented with a burning sensation in her mouth and loss of taste for almost five months.

HPC: Both symptoms appeared almost at the same time. The burning sensation was constant, but deteriorated during eating spicy foods, while the loss of taste started with lack of the sweet sense and gradually expanded to all of tastes.

PMH: Her medical history revealed thyroiditis of Hashimoto, asthma and an old healed peptic ulcer. She had never been a smoker or a heavy drinker, but her diet was vegetarian and her drinking water was confined to two to three glasses of water daily.

OE: The examination revealed an erythematous depapillated smooth and a shiny tongue (atrophic glossitis) that was associated with xerostomia and erythema as well as with crusting of the angles of her mouth (Figure 10.2). Her facial skin was pale but with no other skin lesions. The application of various gustatory irritants on the dorsum of her tongue revealed a significant reduction of all of tastes. Swabs taken from commissures and the tongue revealed *Candida albicans* while blood tests showed iron deficiency and vitamin B12 anemia.

Q1 Which was the most important cause of the loss of taste in this lady?

A Candida infection

B Xerostomia

C Diet

D Thyroiditis of Hashimoto

E Drugs

Answers:

A No

B No

C Diet poor in elements such as vitamin B12 and iron affects the rhythm of the turnover of taste cells and causes loss of filiform and fungiform papillae. Her B12 deficiency may also affect the function of peripheral nerves that carry the taste sensation to the CNS.

D No

E No

Comments: Various conditions such as candidosis, Hashimoto disease or drugs may alter the taste indirectly. These conditions act on taste buds by altering their function: via release of inflammatory cytokines (candidosis) or via lack of various nutritional elements (Mg, Se as seen in thyroiditis) or via chemicals (drugs). The lack of saliva hyposialia minimizes mucosal lubrication and reduces the transport of various taste stimulants to the taste buds.

Q2 Which papillae are not related to taste?

A Fungiform

B Filiform

C Circumvallate papillae

D Foliate papillae

E Taste palatal papillae

Answers:

A No

B Filiform papillae are numerous and look like small conical hairs, arranged in rows parallel to geustic lambda. These are the only papillae that do not contain taste buds, but are responsible for the sensation of touch.

C No

D No

E No

Comments: All the other taste papillae on the tongue, palate and other mucosae contain taste buds but are innervated with different nerves.

Q3 Which of the taste papillae are more susceptible to nutritional deficiencies?

A Circumvallate papillae of the tongue

B Filiform papillae of the tongue

C Taste papillae of soft the palate

D Foliate papillae of the tongue

E Fungiform papillae of the tongue

Answers:

A No

B Filiform papillae are numerous and the first of the papillae that disappear in iron or vitamin deficiencies.

C No

D No

E Fungiform papillae are the second after the filiform papillae that disappear, but are the first ones that reappear after iron or vitamin replacement therapy.

Comments: The circumvallate and foliate papillae are less affected by anemia.

Case 10.3

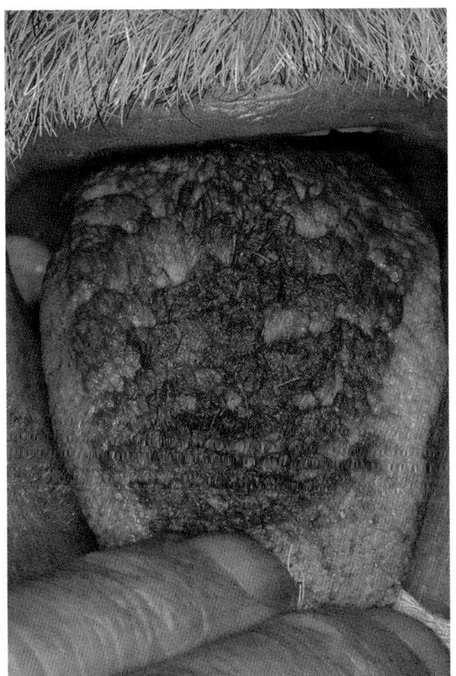

Figure 10.3

CO: An 81-year-old man presented with an unusual brown discoloration of his tongue accompanied with a partial loss of taste.

HPC: The discoloration appeared few days after a course of a broad range of antibiotics taken for his phimosis surgery one month ago. Hypogeusia was reported during the last two weeks.

PMH: The patient suffered from mild hypertension, diabetes type II, and prostate symptoms which were treated with transurethral prostatectomy. He had also been a heavy smoker of two packets of cigarettes and a drinker of more than four cups of coffee on a daily basis.

OE: The examination revealed an abnormal dark brown hairy coating on the dorsal surface of his tongue, becoming more prominent toward the middle and posterior parts. A similar brown discoloration of his fingers with which he used to hold cigarettes was noticed too (Figure 10.3). Various taste tests revealed an increased sense of bitter taste, but a reduced sense of sweet and sour.

Q1 What is the possible cause of his hypogeusia?

A Brown hairy tongue

B Candidiasis

C Diabetes

D Drug-induced

E Aging

Answers:

A Brown hairy tongue was the cause. This is a common condition in old men, rather than women, with poor oral hygiene, xerostomia or previous use of antibiotics or strong mouthwashes, as well as being related to smoking and drinking habits. It is characterized by elongation of tongue papillae causing the transport of various stimuli to the taste receptors, problematic leading to taste reduction.

B No
C No
D No
E No

Comments: Aging often comes with sensory deficits. These deficits are not restricted to one sense (i.e. only taste) and are chronic, with a tendency of being deteriorated; yet these features are not seen in this man. Candidiasis is induced by uncontrolled diabetes or drugs, and can sometimes affect taste but in this case, his clinical characteristics are irrelevant.

Q2 What is the cause of a hairy tongue?

A Elongation of foliate papillae
B Increased number of fungiform papillae
C Reduced apoptosis of filiform papillae
D Increased keratinization of circumvallate papillae
E Reduced number of filiform papillae

Answers:

A No
B No
C Hairy tongue is caused by a hypertrophy and elongation of filiform papillae. These papillae are characterized by overproduction and accumulation of keratin on the top, and reduced shedding (apoptosis) and their characteristic brown, yellow, white, or black color is rendered in the accumulation of *Candida albicans* and other chromogenic bacteria.
D No
E No

Comments: Circumvallate or fungiform papillae enlargement is often seen in various inflammatory tongue conditions (infections, allergies, smoking), but not in hairy tongue. The reduced turnover of the filiform papillae leads to an increase their number or morphological alterations.

Q3 What is the role of filiform papillae?

A Tactile sensation
B Supporting other taste buds
C Bitter sensation
D Umami sensation
E Sweet sensation

Answers:

A Filiform papillae are numerous and give a sense of touch of various foods by the tongue. Mouthfeel sensation is the sensation of foods and drinks in mouth and is not only related to their taste, but also with their texture, and here filiform papillae seem to play an important role.
B No
C No
D No
E No

Comments: Filiform papillae cannot recognize bitter, sweet and umami taste, given the fact that they do not contain taste buds.

Case 10.4

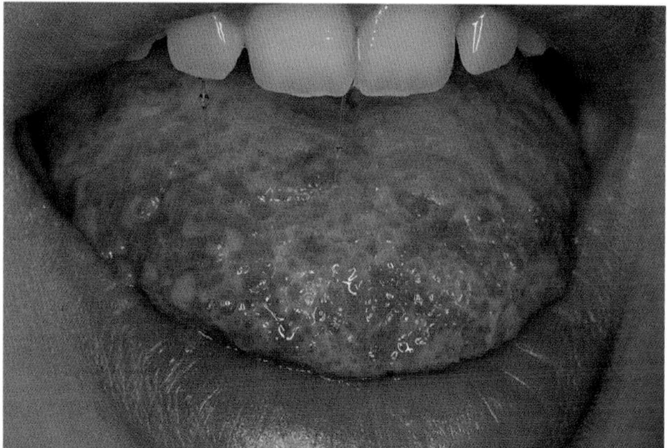

Figure 10.4

CO: A 22-year-old woman presented with painful ulcerations in her mouth associated with sialorrhea, halitosis and hypogeusia.

HPC: The ulcerations have been present over the last five days while halitosis and a partial loss of taste were noticed only for the last three days.

PMH: She was a healthy young woman with no serious skin problems, allergies or history of similar lesions in the past. She did not have any drug or drinking habits, but used to smoke five to six cigarettes per day.

OE: The examination revealed multiple painful ulcerations and small vesicles with clear fluid on the dorsum of the tongue (Figure 10.4) together with erythematous gingivae associated with sialorrhea, halitosis, and cervical lymphadenitis. High fever (>38°C) and malaise preceded the lesions, while a partial loss of taste followed two days later. Her dentition was complete with no fillings or caries.

Q1 What is the possible cause of her hypogeusia?

- **A** Smoking
- **B** Herpetic infection
- **C** Food allergy
- **D** Poor oral hygiene
- **E** Erythema multiforme

Answers:

- **A** No
- **B** Herpetic stomatitis is the cause of hypogeusia. Herpetic stomatitis is characterized by a number of painful ulcerations due to vesicle breakdown and erythematous gingivae, and is associated with general symptomatology (fever >38 C and malaise) and sometimes with taste deficits. Viruses like herpes 1 and 2, Varicella zoster, Hepatitis B,C, E,nteroviruses, HIV, mumps or even rubeola have occasionally implicated with taste alterations affecting the apoptosis of taste buds by activating various inflammatory receptors(TLRs) to produce a number of cytokines among them IFNs. These cytokines may reduce the number of taste buds and skew the presentation of different type of taste cells leading finally to taste dysfunction.
- **C** No
- **D** No
- **E** No

Comments: Erythema multiforme can be easily excluded as it does not have any serious prodromal signs or cervical lymphadenopathy which were reported in this lady. The duration of her dysgeusia did not correspond with the period of smoking or her oral hygiene status which was excellent with no caries or old fillings. Therefore, smoking and poor oral hygiene are excluded from the list of the possible causes of her taste deficits. Food allergies may appear with similar vesiculobullous oral lesions, but lack the general symptoms atology.

Q2 Which virus/es infection/s can cause taste disturbances?

- **A** Herpes virus
- **B** HIV virus
- **C** Influenza virus
- **D** Orf virus
- **E** Yellow fever virus

Answers:

- **A** Herpes virus type 1, 3 and 6 infections sometimes cause taste deficits.
- **B** Patients with AIDS often complain about alterations of taste that are sometimes related with the severity of the infection or are drug-induced.
- **C** Influenza virus causes flu, a very common human infection with high fever, muscle pains, coughing, sore throat, runny nose, and sometimes hypogeusia.
- **D** No
- **E** No

Comments: Orf virus infection causes a purulent exanthema on the fingers, arms, face, and genitals but without general symptomatology. Yellow fever disease is characterized by repeated episodes of fever, accompanied with chills, loss of appetite, nausea, abdominal pain, and liver damage leading to the characteristic yellow skin. Both viruses are transmitted from infected sheep and goats (Orf disease) and female mosquitoes (Yellow fever disease) to humans, but have never been associated with taste alterations.

Q3 What are the mechanisms for virus-induced hypogeusia?

- **A** Viral binding on taste cells
- **B** Xerostomia
- **C** Inflammation on peripheral gustatory nerve
- **D** CNS alterations induced by viruses on the temporal lobe of the brain
- **E** Paralysis of the peripheral gustatory nerves

Answers:

- **A** Taste receptors especially Toll like (TLR-3 and 4) are activated by viral particles and initiate a series of signaling-cascades, with final production of various cytokines which are capable of accelerating apoptosis and altering the turnover of taste buds.
- **B** Some viruses such as hepatitis C, mumps, cytomegalovirus, or HIV cause acinar inflammation and atrophy leading to reduced saliva secretion (xerostomia). Xerostomia reduces the lubricant and transport of taste chemicals to taste buds thus indirectly affecting taste.
- **C** Viruses such as varicella-zoster virus (VZV) infect the peripheral gustatory nerves causing inflammation along their sensory routes, with accumulation of macrophages and neutrophils. These cells release a number of factors that affect various transduction pathways responsible for taste deficits.
- **D** No
- **E** No

Comments: The gustatory cortex in the brain is located in the frontal and not in the temporal lobe, while the gustatory nerves are sensory and not motor nerves. Neurotrophic viruses, such as VZV, can cause paralysis of muscle movement and not alter their sensory function.

Case 10.5

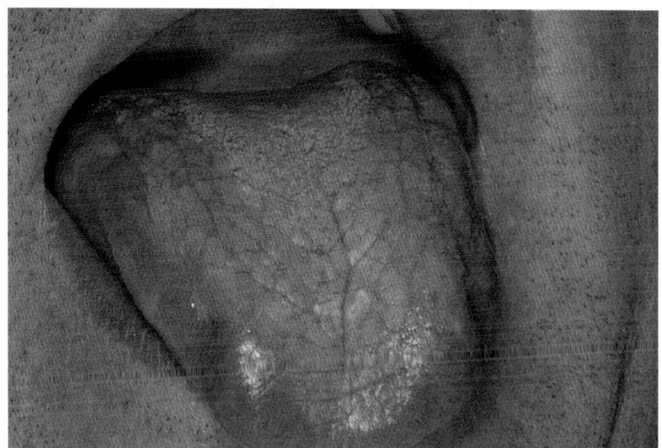

Figure 10.5

CO: A 58-year-old man was presented with soreness of his tongue over the last eight months and lack of taste.

HPC: His soreness started after an accident burning his tongue with extremely hot coffee eight months ago. His soreness has remained stable since then with few variations in intensity, and it has recently been associated with a partial loss of taste.

PMH: His medical records revealed ulcerative colitis, mild hypertension and Graves' disease, having been treated in crisis with sulfasalazine, captopril, and carbimazole respectively. Itchy skin exanthema on both his legs and elbows which was observed by a dermatologist last year, corresponded well to moisturizing and steroid creams. The patient was a chronic smoker of a packet of cigarettes since 18 years of age, and a drinker of two glasses of wine per meal.

OE: The examination revealed a mix of white shiny plaques of various sizes and depth with white atrophic areas, which covered most of the dorsum of the tongue and surrounded with fine, white striated lines (Figure 10.5). Other erythematous and ulcerated lesions intermingled with white lesions were also noted on both his buccal mucosae and the inner surface of the lower lip. The test for various taste stimulants revealed a reduced response to sweet, sour, and bitter stimuli.

Q1 What is the cause of his hypogeusia?

- **A** Leukoplakia
- **B** Candidiasis
- **C** Chronic smoking
- **D** Lichen planus
- **E** Thermal burn

Answers:

- **A** No
- **B** No
- **C** No
- **D** Lichen planus, especially its atrophic type, is the cause. This disease is characterized by atrophic oral mucosa covered with white, erythematous or ulcerated lesions, surrounded with characteristic white striated lines. When the lesions are predominantly seen on the tongue, it is associated with loss of taste buds causing taste alterations (hypogeusia).
- **E** No

Comments: Thermal burns can destroy taste buds, but their effect on this patient was temporary, and happened many months ago. The smoking-induced xerostomia may alter taste, but it would have been reported for a longer period, as the patient had been a smoker since the age of 18. Also, smoking-induced keratosis or candidosis could cause taste deficits, but their clinical characteristics are different.

Q2 Which of the treatments below is recommended for short treatment of hypogeusia?

- **A** Theophylline (intranasal or oral)
- **B** Zinc replacement
- **C** B12 injections
- **D** Antifungals
- **E** Smoking cessation

Answers:

- **A** No
- **B** No
- **C** B12 replacement treatment has been widely used for patients with pernicious anemia, which is a condition with sore, erythematous and depapillated tongue, with loss of taste buds. Replacement therapy quickly enables the normal turnover of taste buds.
- **D** Antifungals reduce *Candida* infection and tongue inflammation, and quickly restore tongue functions.
- **E** Smoking cessation reinstates saliva secretion and taste a few weeks after stopping.

Comments: Theophylline and zinc supplements improve hypogeusia if taken for a long period (>1 year)

Q3 Which is/are the possible mechanism/s attributed to hypogeusia in this patient?

- **A** Reduced number of taste buds
- **B** Alterations in saliva composition
- **C** Local inflammation
- **D** Alterations of peripheral gustatory nerve function
- **E** Perception taste alterations in the temporal lobe of the brain.

Answers:

A The reduced number of taste buds could be attributed to the atrophy of tongue mucosa and its replacement of white lesions of Lichen planus.
B No
C Lichen planus is characterized by a band dense of chronic inflammatory cells of lymphocytes and macrophages. These inflammatory cells release various cytokines that have been linked with increased apoptosis of basal cells in the epithelium and even in the taste buds.
D No
E No

Comments: Saliva components are altered through aging and in various pathologies or drugs. They are attributed to taste deficits by altering the transport of taste stimulants to the taste receptors. Although lichen planus seems to worsen during emotional disturbances (depression, stress), its induced hypogeusia seems to be unrelated to transmission and perception of taste stimulus from peripheral gustatory nerves into the brain.

Case 10.6

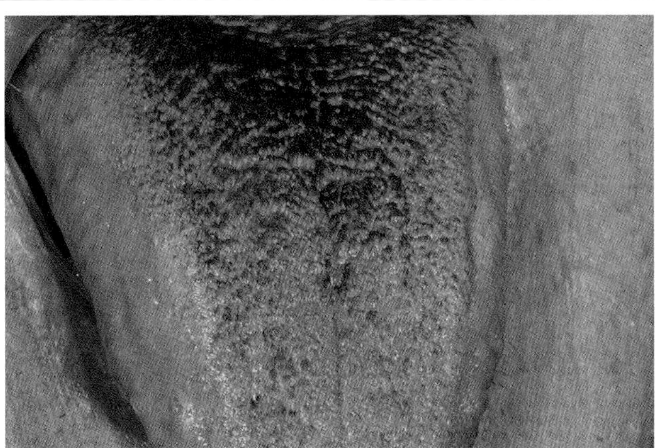

Figure 10.6

CO: A 58-year-old man presented with tongue staining and taste alterations.

HPC: The discoloration was restricted to the filiform papillae and was more prominent in the middle and posterior third of dorsum of the tongue, while it was associated with a bitter sensation over the last three weeks.

PMH: His medical history was unremarkable but his dental history revealed severe periodontitis which was initially treated with scaling and root planing and surgery. The last periodontal surgery was performed one month ago. Since then, the patient has stopped smoking and uses chlorhexidine mouthwash on a daily basis.

OE: The oral examination revealed black hairy elongation of filiform papillae on the dorsum of his tongue, mainly in the middle and posterior part (Figure 10.6). A similar dark discoloration was found on the cervical areas of the lower incisors and molars. A tingling sensation on the tip of the tongue and lips in combination with a bitter taste was reported. Taste strips revealed a reduced response to salty stimulants. No other lesions were found in the mouth, skin or other mucosae.

Q1 Which is the possible cause of dysgeusia?
A Black hairy tongue
B Chlorhexidine mouthwash use
C Periodontal surgery
D Chromogenic bacteria
E Smoking

Answers:

A No
B Chlorhexidine mouthwash used on a regular basis alters the taste in the majority of patients, hence leaving a bitter and tingling sensation in the mouth.
C No
D No
E No

Comments: The periodontal surgery involves the surgical curettage of deep pockets and does not interfere with the function of the gustatory system. Chromogenic bacteria are responsible for tongue and teeth external staining, do not influence the number or function of taste buds, while heavy smoking can cause hairy tongue and leave a bitter taste in the mouth, if the patient continues this habit.

Q2 Which tastes are affected with the chronic use of chlorhexidine mouthwash?
A Sourness
B Sweetness
C Saltiness
D Bitterness
E Savory taste

Answers:

A No
B No

C Daily use of chlorhexidine mouthwash reduces the perception of various salty foods.
D Bitter perception is progressively reduced even from the first days of chlorhexidine use, and reaches its lowest value within a week.
E No

Comments: The other three tastes (sweet, sour and umami) do not seem to be significantly affected with chlorhexidine use.

Q3 A G-protein-coupled taste receptor is activated in:
A Savory (umami)
B Sweet
C Sour
D Bitter
E Salt

Answers:
A Umami taste is initiated by the binding of various taste agents to G-protein coupled receptors (TAS1R1 and TAS1R3) in the taste bud cells. These receptors respond well to L-amino acids, especially L-glutamate and can be enhanced through the binding of inosine and guanosine monophosphate.
B Sweet taste is initiated with the activation of G-protein-coupled receptors (GPCRs) on the apical surface of the taste cells, causing an increase of c-AMP concentration, while the activation via cascade reactions results in a rise of intracellular Ca^2, which leads to a transmitter release.
C No
D Bitter-tasting compounds such as alkaloids (quinine; caffeine), urea, salts ($MgSO_4$) bind to GPCRs and activate gustducin or phospholipase C (PLC) leading to an increase in intracellular Ca^{2+} of the taste cells, and secondly to a transmitter release.
E No

Comments: Sour or salty taste is produced with free hydrogen ions or Na^+ and not related to GPCR receptors.

Case 10.7

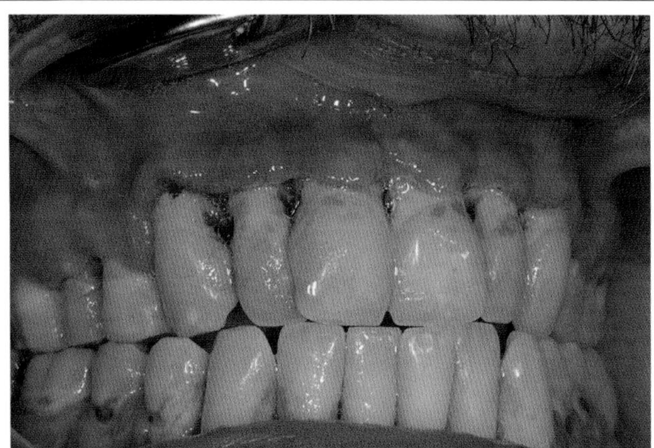

Figure 10.7

CO: A 27-year-old man was referred by his periodontist for evaluation of a bad taste.

HPC: A sharp metallic taste started two weeks ago when the patient had an episode of acute inflammation of his gingivae and visited his periodontist. The bad taste had become more intense over the last week; when his gingivae treatment started.

PMH: Severe episodes of gut pain associated with bloody diarrhea, attributed to his Crohn's disease that was diagnosed two years ago. This disease caused him weight loss and anemia despite his sulfasalazine treatment. Repeated blood tests did not show any immunodeficiencies. Smoking of two to three cannabis cigarettes daily seems to relieve the patient's intestinal symptoms.

OE: The oral examination revealed severe gum recession and destruction, and necrosis of the inter-dental papillae covered in places with necrotic slough, and associated with bad breath, sialorrhea and dysgeusia (Figure 10.7). Acute necrotizing periodontitis had been diagnosed by his periodontist and metronidazole was prescribed. Despite his treatment, the top of the interdental gingivae were lost and the metallic taste worsened.

Q1 Which is/are the cause(s) of his metallic taste?
A Acute necrotizing periodontitis
B Smoking
C Drug-induced
D Crohn's disease
E HIV infection

Answers:
A Acute necrotizing periodontitis is the main cause of his unpleasant metallic taste induced by the inflamed gingivae. The release of cytokines was capable of affecting the taste bud turnover and taste perception.

B No
C Antibiotics and especially metronidazole can cause a metallic taste which is disappears as soon as this drug is withdrawn.
D No
E No

Comments: The participation of smoking, Crohn's disease and immunodeficiencies like HIV infection are easily excluded as the period of dysgeusia did not correspond with the period of smoking and Crohn's disease, while HIV infection was not found in three repetitive blood tests.

Q2 Which other conditions are commonly related with metallic taste?
A Pregnancy
B Sinus infection
C Submucous fibrosis
D Dementia
E Candidiasis

Answers:
A Pregnancy, especially at the first trimester, is often accompanied with a metallic taste which gradually recedes with the baby's birth.
B Upper respiratory infection and especially acute or chronic sinusitis, cause changes in smell and taste.
C No
D Dementia is a group of brain diseases characterized by decreased ability of thinking and is sometimes associated with taste alterations when the taste lobe of the brain is involved.
E No

Comments: In submucous fibrosis and candidiasis, significant alterations in sweet, salt, bitter, and sour but not in metallic taste are found.

Q3 Which other drugs apart from antibiotics can cause metallic taste?
A ACE-inhibitor
B Lithium
C Antiviral
D Analgesics
E Anticonvulsants

Answers:
A ACE inhibitors such as captopril are used to reduce high blood pressure and heart failure, causing a metallic taste and sometimes partial loss of taste perception.
B Lithium is a widely used drug for bipolar disorders and can cause a metallic taste in a small group of patients (1%), especially in female ex-smoker patients taking this drug for a short period (<1 month).
C No
D No
E No

Comments: Drug side-effects such as nervousness, poor concentration, diarrhea, nausea, or vomiting are sometimes seen with various antiviral drugs and dizziness, drowsiness, tremor, and nausea, can be provoked by anticonvulsants, while stomach upset, oral ulcerations and xerostomia can be caused by analgesics. Metallic taste is rarely induced by the above drugs, and is reported only after many episodes of nausea or vomiting.

Case 10.8

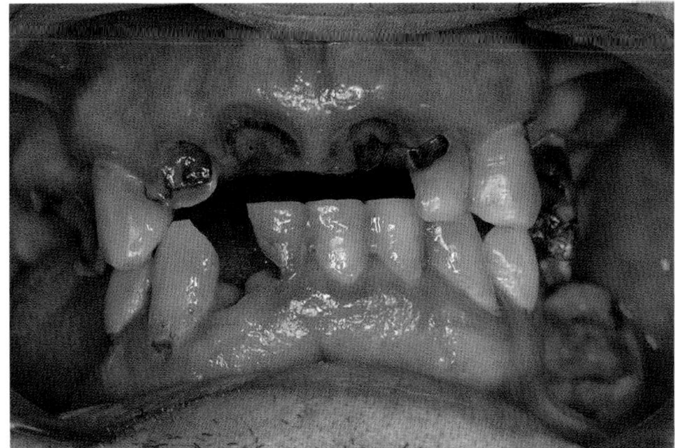

Figure 10.8

CO: A 69-year-old man presented with a bad taste over a few months.

HPC: The bad taste was a mixture of sourness and bitterness which appeared regardless of eating or drinking, being worse at night and slightly improved with teeth brushing. This bad taste appeared gradually after the return of his taste, which had been completely lost after a course of radiotherapy for a carcinoma of his tongue a year ago.

PMH: His medical history revealed severe hypertension and prostate hypertrophy, having been treated with α-blockers. A carcinoma of the posterior part of his tongue was removed last year and followed a course of 30 sessions of radiotherapy.

OE: The oral examination revealed extensive caries in the majority of his teeth; chronic gingival infection and alveolar bone exposure to the lower left molar area showing signs of sequestration (Figure 10.8). A sour smell was easily detected and associated with bad taste. Some tongue movement limitations were recorded due to partial glossectomy, and not due to tumor recurrence.

Q1 Which is/or are the cause of his bad taste?

- **A** Osteonecrosis of his mandible
- **B** Caries
- **C** Carcinoma surgery
- **D** Periodontitis
- **E** Xerostomia induced by radiation

Answers:

- **A** Osteonecrosis is a common complication of radiation treatment and is caused by the damage of small vessels within the jaw leading to a non-healing ulcer formation with necrotic bone underneath. The necrotic bone is usually infected hence causing pain, halitosis and bad taste.
- **B** Caries caused by the disintegration of food debris with various oral bacteria (*Streptococcus mutans* and lactobacilli mainly) and release of substances responsible for bad smell (halitosis) and bad taste (cacogeusia).
- **C** Glossectomy (partial or total) is widely used for the treatment of tongue carcinoma, but can cause difficulties in tongue movements. Inadequate movement eliminates the removal of foods from adjacent teeth and releases substances responsible for halitosis and bad taste.
- **D** Periodontitis is a chronic inflammatory condition that affects the periodontal tissues (gingivae and bone) and their inflammatory products activate taste receptors, causing bad taste.
- **E** Xerostomia induced by irradiation may play a role as it interferes with the transport of various taste substances to the taste receptors. The disruption of this transport could affect taste.

Comments: All the causes above participate to a greater or lesser degree in patient's cacogeusia.

Q2 Torquegeusia is a new term for cacogeusia related with:

- **A** Metallic taste
- **B** Sour taste
- **C** Salty taste
- **D** Sweet taste
- **E** Bitter taste

Answers:

- **A** Torquegeusia is a new term given for metallic taste, first described by Henkin and Frezier in 1989.
- **B** No
- **C** No
- **D** No
- **E** No

Comments: Cacogeusia is characterized by a bad taste despite the consumption of pleasant food or drinks, and can be presented as a bitter, sour, salty, and metallic taste.

Q3 Which of the taste types is mainly related with hypertension?

- **A** Sweet
- **B** Sour
- **C** Bitter
- **D** Salty
- **E** Umami

Answers:

- **A** No
- **B** No
- **C** No
- **D** Changes in salty taste sensitivity have been used to predict the onset of hypertension.
- **E** No

Comments: Other taste types such as sweet, umami or bitter have been occasionally related to blood pressure alteration.

Case 10.9

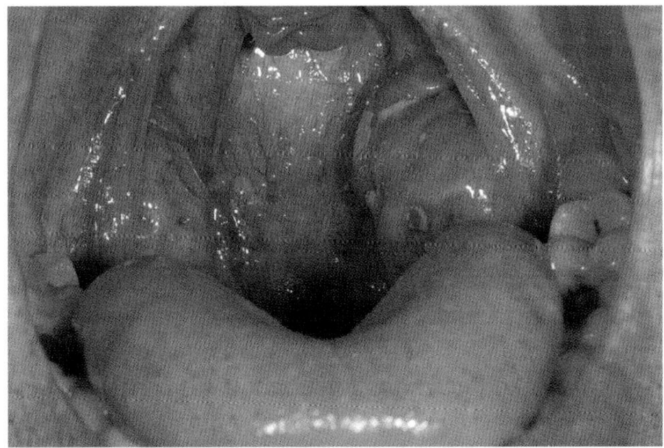

Figure 10.9

CO: A 24-year-old woman was presented with a sore throat and bad taste.

HPC: The symptoms were present for four days and referred to soreness in her throat, high fever, difficulties in speaking or eating, bad breath and taste as well as swollen lymph nodes in her neck. A constant sense of bitter taste was recorded which was worse at awakening or when drinking coffee.

PMH: Her medical history was unremarkable as it did not reveal any serious diseases, drug use or smoking and drinking habits, but her job as a kindergarten teacher often demanded close contact with children that might suffer from bacterial or viral infections regularly.

OE: Swollen tense tonsils were found with white and yellow spots (Figure 10.9) causing swallowing problems which were associated with general symptomatology such as fever, fatigue and cervical lymphadenopathy. The oropharynx was red with plenty of small inflamed minor salivary glands that appeared as small spots with clear fluid. Halitosis was easily detected and associated with the bad, bitter taste. Blood tests revealed elevated ESR, and increased white blood cell count, while *Streptococcus pyogenes* was detected in cultures, but mono test and various viral screenings were negative.

Q1 What is the possible cause of her cacogeusia?

- **A** Infectious mononucleosis
- **B** *Streptococcus* pharyngo-tonsillitis
- **C** Herpangina
- **D** Tonsillar crypts
- **E** Peritonsillar abscess

Answers:

- **A** No
- **B** *Streptococcus* pharyngo-tonsillitis or scarlet fever is a very common throat infection of young children and adults and appears with fever, runny nose, sore throat, swollen tonsils, cervical lymph node enlargement, and is also associated with halitosis and bad taste.
- **C** No
- **D** No
- **E** No

Comments: Tonsillar crypts appear as white or yellow spots within the patient's tonsils and consist of macrophages, white cells and various bacteria, but are usually asymptomatic. Throat soreness and general symptomatology is also seen in a peritonsillar abscess, infectious mononucleosis and herpangina but these conditions were excluded as the inflammation was not restricted, as seen in peritonsillar abscess; the viral and hepatic screening and mono test were negative for an EBV infection (mononucleosis) and the characteristics in herpangina oral and pharyngeal ulcerations were missing.

Q2 Which microorganism/s is/are the main cause of scarlet fever?

- **A** *Streptococcus pyogenes*
- **B** *Staphylococcus aureus*
- **C** *Mycobacterium marinum*
- **D** *Treponema pallidum*
- **E** Influenza A and B

Answers:

- **A** *Streptococcus pyogenes* is a Gram-positive bacterium which belongs to the group A of hemolytic streptococci, and is the main responsible for bacterial pharyngitis.
- **B** No
- **C** No
- **D** No
- **E** No

Comments: *Staphylococcus aureus* is also part of the normal upper respiratory flora, but is related to tracheitis rather than pharyngitis, while influenza A is responsible for viral but not bacterial pharyngitis. *Mycobacterium marinum* is implicated in skin granulomas while *Treponema pallidum* for syphilis.

Q3 Which is/are the clinical characteristic(s) that could differentiate a bacterial from viral pharyngitis?
- **A** Temperature
- **B** Swollen tonsils
- **C** Diarrhea
- **D** Fatigue
- **E** Lymph nodes

Answers:
- **A** High temperature (>38 C) is characteristic of bacterial pharyngitis.
- **B** Swollen tonsils and exudates are seen in bacterial infection.
- **C** Diarrhea is characteristic of a viral pharyngitis.
- **D** No
- **E** No

Comments: Pharyngitis (bacterial or viral) is characterized by acute soreness and erythema of the throat, as well as being associated with generalized symptoms of malaise, fatigue and cervical lymphadenopathy.

Case 10.10

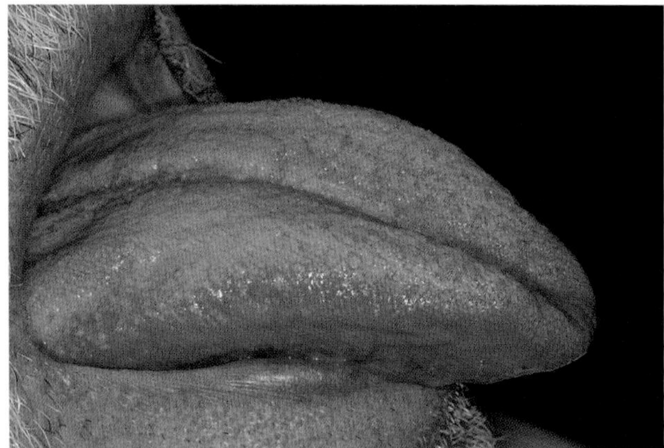

Figure 10.10

CO: A 69-year-old man presented with bad taste, regardless of his eating or drinking habits.

HPC: The bad taste appeared three years ago and was reported as a constant sense of sweet or bitter whenever he drunk water, but was worse at night.

PMH: He had suffered from deep depression since his wife's death, for which he had been on a daily 60 mg duloxetine therapy over the last year, and from mild hypotension that was controlled with diet. He was an ex-smoker and drinker and spent his free time gardening.

OE: The oral examination was not useful as his tongue was not atrophic, and showed only hyperplastic filiform papillae (Figure 10.10). No other lesions on the skin or other mucosae were recorded. Bad taste was reported and resolved spontaneously without being provoked from any taste stimuli (phantogeusia).

Q1 What is the cause of phantogeusia?
- **A** Diabetic neuropathy
- **B** Drug-induced (duloxetine)
- **C** Smoking
- **D** Depression
- **E** Hairy tongue

Answers:
- **A** No
- **B** No
- **C** No
- **D** Depression and its drug ethyl loflazepate sometimes causes phantogeusia, which is not real but a hallucination of a bad taste.
- **E** No

Comments: Phantogeusia can also be seen in patients with diabetic neuropathies, but unlike this patient, this neuropathy is always related to chronic, severe and uncontrolled disease. Other depression drugs such as duloxetine or other conditions such as hairy tongue and smoking habits can alter taste to some degree, by causing dysgeusia but never phantogeusia.

Q2 Which other neurological conditions apart from depression have been related to phantogeusia?
- **A** Schizophrenia
- **B** Parkinson's disease
- **C** Bipolar disorders
- **D** Multiple sclerosis
- **E** Epilepsy

Answers:

A Schizophrenia is a mental disorder, characterized by abnormal behavior and failure to understand reality with unclear and confusing thoughts, including false senses such as hearing voices and sometimes hallucinations of taste (phantogeusia).

B Loss of smell and taste is an early sign of Parkinson's disease. This is a progressive nervous system disease, affecting body movement and in severe CNS cases involving the orbito-frontal cortex, with phantogeusia.

C Bipolar disorders or their drugs such as lithium could cause alterations in taste ranging from the complete loss to hallucinated tastes.

D Multiple sclerosis is sometimes presents with taste deficits that are associated with MS-related lesions throughout the brain.

E An aura is often accompanied with a peculiar taste (phantogeusia) and precedes epileptic seizures.

Q3 Which alterations in taste receptors have been detected in patients with phantogeusia?

A Reduced number of taste receptors

B Increased expression of T2R taste receptor genes

C Reduced expression of T1R taste receptor gene

D Increased levels of gustducin in the taste receptors

E Reduced number of microvilli of taste cells

Answers:

A No

B In a number of patients with phantogeusia, an increased expression of T2R receptor genes was found.

C No

D No

E No

Comments: The phantogeusia is not related with alterations in the number, morphology, or gustducin release from the taste receptors.

11

Ulcerations

Oral ulcerations are very common mouth lesions caused by local trauma, infections, neoplasms, autoimmune and systemic diseases especially of gut, blood or skin as well as side-effects of various drugs. Ulcerations can be single or multiple and may affect only the masticatory oral mucosa or the whole mouth, recurrent or not, with or without general symptomatology. From a microscopic point of view, ulcerations are induced by the loss of all epithelial layers in contrast with the erosions when the loss is more superficial. Oral ulcerations appear de novo or follow the rupture of various bullae within the mouth, but only the de novo ulcerations are included in this chapter (See Figure 11.0).

The Table 11 lists the more frequent causes of oral ulcerations.

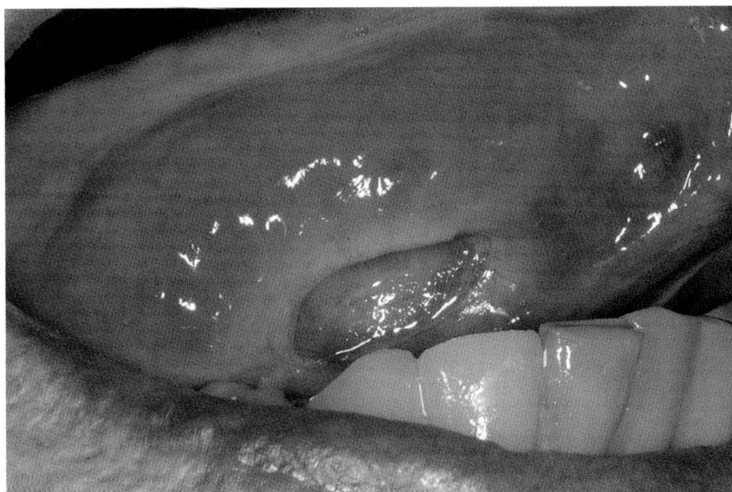

Figure 11.0 Traumatic tongue ulcer in a healing process.

Clinical Guide to Oral Diseases, First Edition. Dimitris Malamos and Crispian Scully.

Companion website: www.wiley.com/go/malamos/clinical_guide

Table 11 Ulcers: Common and important causes.

- Local causes
  - Traumatic
    - Mechanical
      - Artefactual
    - Burns
      - Chemical
      - Thermal
      - Electrical
      - Radiation
  - Neoplastic
    - Carcinoma
    - Sarcoma
    - Melanoma
  - Aphthous or aphthous like ulcerations
      - Aphthae (single)
      - Aphthae-like (part of syndromes)
        - Behcet
        - MAGIC (mouth and genital ulcers with inflamed cartilage)
        - Sweet
        - PFAPA (periodic fever, aphthous stomatitis, pharyngitis, adenitis)
- Systemic diseases
  - Cutaneous
    - Erosive lichen planus
    - Erythema multiforme
    - Epidermolysis acquisita
  - Blood
    - Anemia
    - Sideropenia
    - Neutropenia
    - Leukemia
    - Myelofibrosis
    - Myelodysplasia
    - Multiple myeloma
  - Vascular
    - Giant cell arteritis
    - Periarteritis nodosa
    - Wegener granulomatosis
    - Necrotizing sialometaplasia
    - Middle line granuloma

Table 11 (Continued)

  - Connective
    - Lupus erythematosus
    - Mixed connective tissue diseases
    - Felty syndrome
  - Autoimmune
    - Pemphigus
    - Pemphigoid
    - Dermatitis herpetiformis
    - Linear IgA disease
    - IgA pustular dermatosis
    - Chronic ulcerative stomatitis
    - Graft versus host disease
  - Infective
    - Bacterial
      - Tuberculosis
      - Atypical mycobacterial infections
      - Syphilis
      - Actinomycosis
      - Tularemia
      - Lepromatous leprosy
      - Necrotizing ulcerative gingivitis
    - Viral
      - HIV
      - Herpes simplex
      - Chickenpox
      - Herpes zoster
      - Hand foot and mouth disease
      - Herpangina
      - Infectious mononucleosis
      - Cytomegalovirus
    - Parasites
      - Leishmania
    - Fungi
      - Aspergillosis
      - Cryptococcus
      - Mucormycosis
      - Paracoccidioidomycosis
    - Neoplasmatic
      - Langerhans histiocytosis
- Drug-induced
    - Chemical burns
    - Osteonecrosis

Case 11.1

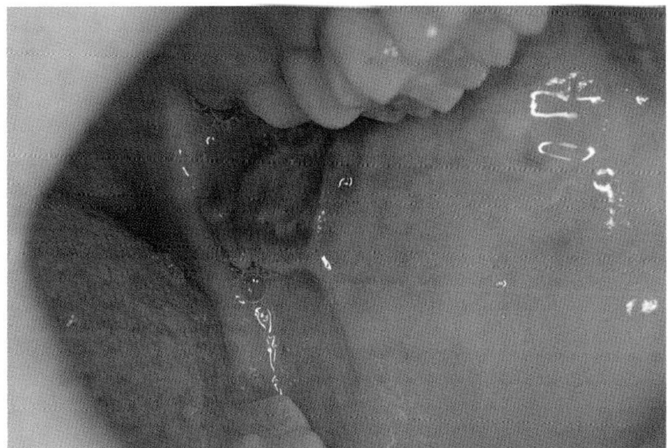

Figure 11.1

CO: A 27-year-old woman presented with a painful ulcer on her left buccal mucosa, which had appeared over the last week.

HPC: The pain appeared during eating a snack and became worse with jaw movements and the consumption of juices or spicy food. The ulcer was first noticed during a self-examination for searching for the cause of pain.

PMH: Her medical history revealed a sideropenic anemia caused by a heavy blood loss during her menstruation and allergic rhinitis that were controlled with iron tablets and antihistamine nasal spray respectively. No other serious blood, skin or gut diseases were reported while her smoking and drinking habits were restricted to social events.

OE: A large ulcer on the left buccal mucosa, opposite of the partial and ectopic upper third molar, with maximum diameter 2 cm was seen. The ulcer was painful but soft on palpation, with a granular base and raised erythematous margins (Figure 11.1). No other ulcerations, bullae or other lesions were found on her mouth, skin and other mucosae (genitals, eyes) during the examination or had ever been recorded in the past. General symptomatology like fever, malaise or topical or systemic lymphadenopathy was not reported. Extraction of his ectopic wisdom tooth caused a complete healing of the ulcer within the next 10 days.

Q1 What is the cause of her oral ulceration?

- **A** Trauma
- **B** Chancre
- **C** Large aphtha
- **D** Herpangina
- **E** Carcinoma

Answers:

- **A** Local trauma is the cause and it was induced by the biting of the buccal mucosa with the ectopic third molar during eating. Traumatic ulceration is characterized as a single painful ulcer, soft in palpation, unfixed with the underlying mucosa with minimal general symptomatology and positive history of local injury recently. This lesion appeared suddenly and disappeared without treatment, soon after the extraction of her causative tooth.
- **B** No
- **C** No
- **D** No
- **E** No

Comments: The special characteristics of this ulceration allow the exclusion of other similar conditions. Thus, its soft consistency easily excludes oral carcinomas as these tumors are usually hard in palpation and fixed into the surrounding tissues, asymptomatic at an early stage, but also associated with cervical lymphadenopathy. The lack of local lymphadenopathy and the symptomatology(pain) rules out syphilitic ulcer, while the negative history of a recent thermal burn accident or previous recurrent similar ulcerations rules out burns and aphthae from the diagnosis.

Q2 What are the other causes of an acute traumatic oral ulceration?

- **A** Mechanical injury
- **B** Chemical reaction
- **C** Thermal burn
- **D** Electrical current
- **E** Solar radiation

Answers:

- **A** Mechanical damage of oral tissues via parafunctional habits (grinding; sucking) or broken sharp teeth or ill-fitting prostheses, causes tissue necrosis leading to painful ulcerations.
- **B** Chemicals in solid or liquid form can be either strong acids or bases, and may cause coagulation and tissue necrosis leading to blister formation or ulcerations.
- **C** Thermal burns are usually caused by the close contact of oral mucosa to heated objects leading to tissue necrosis and ulcerations depending on the temperature, duration of application and patient's resistance.
- **D** Although electrical ulcerations are rare and found among special groups of patients (children, medically handicapped) which tend to be severe thus requiring special care at hospital.
- **E** No

Comments: The chronic exposure to solar radiation causes oral lesions, mostly on the vermilion border of the lower lip (actinic cheilitis; prurigo). A short exposure leads to lip dryness and hyperpigmentation, while a chronic exposure to more severe lesions such as chronic long-lasting ulcerations some of which have a malignant potential.

Q3 Traumatic ulcerations are commonly seen in babies suffering with:

- **A** Juvenile diabetes (type I)
- **B** Neurofibromatosis
- **C** Rega-Fede syndrome
- **D** Kostmann disease
- **E** Sweet syndrome

Answers:

- **A** No
- **B** No
- **C** Riga-Fede syndrome is characterized by a traumatic ulcer on the ventral surface of the tongue or inner surface of the lip caused by a constant friction of the mucosa against the prematurely erupted deciduous incisors teeth.
- **D** No
- **E** No

Comments: Patients with diabetes, Kostmann disease or Sweet's syndrome have oral ulcerations among their manifestations, but these lesions differ from traumatic ulcerations in pathogenesis as they are associated with a delay in healing (diabetes) or immunodeficiencies due to severe neutropenia (Kostmann disease) or acute neutrophilia (Sweet's syndrome). Neurofibromatosis is irrelevant as it is characterized by numerous neurofibromas, and café au lait pigmentation and Lisch nodules, but not with oral ulcerations.

Case 11.2

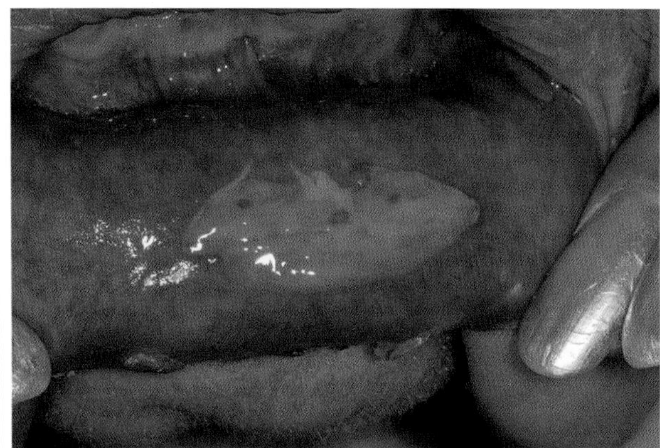

Figure 11.2

CO: A 38-year-old woman presented with pain in her mouth after trying to eat hot fried potatoes.

HPC: The problem started immediately after eating a very hot fried potato and the appearance of a superficial blister on the vermilion border and inner surface of the lips which was finally broken leaving superficial ulceration covered with whitish-yellow slough.

PMH: Her medical history was clear with no serious skin diseases, allergies or drug use. Lip biting as well as the consumption of very hot foods or drinks were her only parafunctional habits, while smoking or alcohol use were absent.

OE: The erythematous lips and tip of the tongue were found sensitive to touch and with a large superficial ulceration that was covered with a white pseudomembrane on the inner surface of the lower lip (Figure 11.2). This sloughing was easily removed leaving a hemorrhagic and painful ulceration that was superficial, soft and not associated with general symptomatology. Similar lesions were not found on the rest of her mouth, skin or other mucosae on the day of examination nor were they recorded previously.

Q1 What is the cause of ulceration?

- **A** Nail-biting induced ulceration
- **B** Mucous pemphigoid
- **C** Herpetic stomatitis
- **D** Drug-fixed reaction
- **E** Thermal burn

Answers:

- **A** No
- **B** No
- **C** No
- **D** No
- **E** Thermal burn is the cause. It is induced by the direct contact and necrosis of oral mucosa, but especially the lower lip and tip of the tongue with extremely hot food, such as fried potatoes. It is characterized by the zone of coagulation and necrosis (slough) due to vascular necrosis, surrounded by a zone of stasis which is not clearly seen in this patient, and a zone of hyperemia due

to diapedesis of blood cells towards the site of tissue damage.

Q2 Which is/are the best treatment/s for this woman?

A None
B Chemoprophylaxis
C Pain management
D Dressing
E Soft diet

Answers:

A No
B No
C Pain is always present and interferes with the patient's activities such as eating, speaking or laughing, and therefore requires early relief with acetaminophen or NSAIDs, alone or together with steroids, in oral base creams locally or systematically.
D No
E A soft diet without irritating ingredients for the oral lesion (spicy, acid or alkali), at normal temperature, is always recommended.

Comments: As the lesion is superficial and is not extended to the deep submucosa tissues like muscles or bone, and saliva has a great number of antimicrobial agents, dressing and antibiotic cover is not necessary.

Q3 Which of the factors below could determine the severity of the injury in patient's mouth?

A Patient's age
B Characteristics of causative agent
C Duration of contact
D Frequency of contact
E Patient's gender

Answers:

A Children and older patients (>65 years) have a longer reaction time due to slower reflexes to move away from the causative agent and therefore their burns tend to be more severe.
B The consistency (fluid vs. compound) and heat conduction (rapid vs. poor) characteristics of an overheated material determines the degree of oral damage.
C The longer the oral exposure, the bigger is the coagulation injury and therefore the more severe the necrosis.
D The oral injury from heat transfer is often cumulative, as it is seen in patients under radiotherapy for head and neck cancers and is presented after the second week of treatment as mucositis.
E No

Comments: Gender seems to be irrelevant in the degree of severity of burning, despite the fact that oral mucosa is more resistant in males as it is usually exposed to heavy smoking, drinking or chemicals at work.

Case 11.3

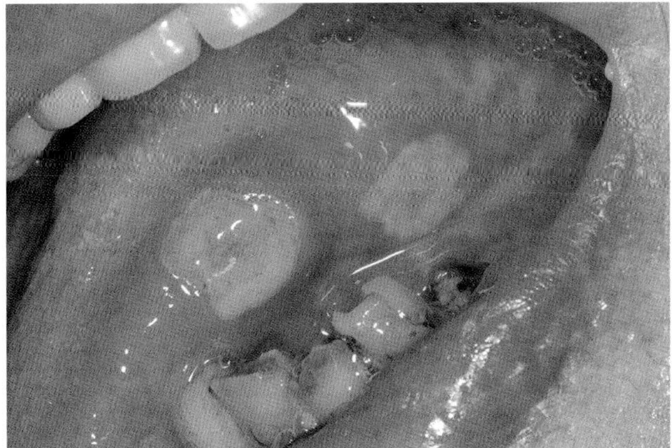

Figure 11.3

CO: A 55-year-old woman was presented with painful ulcerations on the lateral margins of her tongue and buccal mucosae over the last five days.

HPC: The lesions appeared suddenly and became associated with pain, halitosis and sialorrhea as well as difficulties in eating, swallowing or speaking. Only two small ulcerations appeared in the beginning, but had increased in number and size over the last five days.

PMH: Rheumatoid arthritis was her main medical problem since the age of 40, partially treated with immune suppressants like prednisone, methotrexate and filicine supplements. An allergy to aspirin and penicillin was reported. Other systemic diseases were not recorded for her or close relatives.

OE: A few scattered superficial painful ulcerations were noted on the margins of her tongue and buccal mucosae. The lesions were round in shape, well-demarcated with no erythematous margins and covered with white pseudomembranes (Figure 11.3), being more prominent at the left margin of her tongue opposite the broken, carious lower canine and premolars. No skin or other mucosae lesions or topical or systemic lymphadenitis were found.

Q1 What is the cause of patient's ulcerations?

- **A** Traumatic ulcers
- **B** Aphthae
- **C** Erythema multiforme
- **D** Primary herpetic stomatitis
- **E** Methotrexate induced

Answers:

- **A** No
- **B** No
- **C** No
- **D** No
- **E** The chronic use of methotrexate for treatment of rheumatoid arthritis helps the reduction of any further joint damage and preservation of joint functions, but also often (>14%) causes mouth painful ulcerations whenever the dose of this drug is abruptly increased.

Comments: The distribution of her oral ulcerations in areas irrelevant to broken teeth, as well as the absence of erythematous halo, general symptomatology or previous similar lesions in the past, easily excludes trauma, aphthae, primary herpetic stomatitis or multiple erythema from the diagnosis.

Q2 Methotrexate is widely used for the treatment of:

- **A** Psoriasis
- **B** Multiple sclerosis
- **C** Temporomandibular joint (TMJ) disorders
- **D** Leukemia
- **E** Basal cell carcinomas

Answers:

- **A** In psoriasis, it acts by attacking the rapidly divided cells and reducing the local inflammation of skin.
- **B** Methotrexate can sometimes be used as an additional therapy as it reduces relapse and progression of multiple sclerosis, but remains less useful than IFN-α.
- **C** No
- **D** This drug can be used for the treatment of acute lymphoblastic leukemia and especially for blocking the spread of this leukemia into the CNS.
- **E** No

Comments: Methotrexate has a great number of complications and therefore should not be used for the treatment of other diseases that have alternative treatments, such as the use of NSAIDs drugs in TMJ disorders or surgery in basal cell carcinomas.

Q3 What is the main mechanism of methotrexate-induced oral ulcerations?

- **A** Competes with folinic acid
- **B** Increases local ischemia
- **C** Induces apoptosis of peripheral blood cells
- **D** Changes oral microflora
- **E** Reduces local inflammation

Answers:

- **A** The mechanism of methotrexate-induced oral ulceration is based on the fact that this drug competes with folinic acid in order to enter into the cell, and blocks DNA and RNA synthesis of rapidly dividing cells, such as epithelial cells. In this way, it causes problems in tissue repair leading finally to oral necrosis-ulceration.
- **B** No
- **C** No
- **D** No
- **E** No

Comments: Methotrexate reduces local inflammation by acting on immune/inflammatory cell proliferation and apoptosis apart from the antagonist action with folinic acid, reduces local inflammation by acting on immune/inflammatory cell proliferation and apoptosis of activated T cells from the peripheral blood and affects colonization of various bacteria and increases local ischemia .

Case 11.4

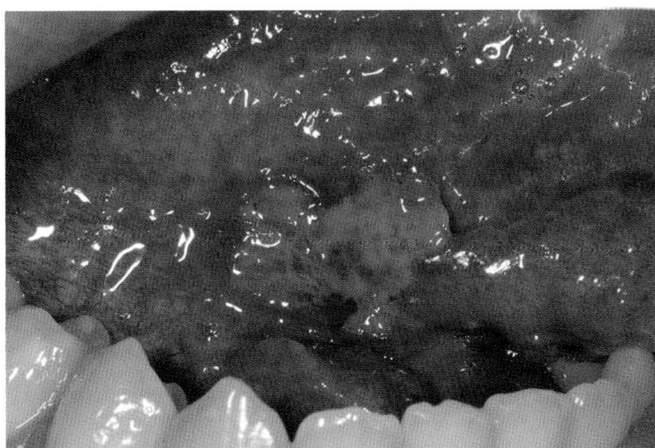

Figure 11.4

CO: A 32-year-old man was presented for an evaluation of a large ulcer on his tongue.

HPC: The ulcer was present for 10 days and caused him severe problems with eating and speaking. Similar ulcerations were reported in the past, but usually lasted only five to eight days and appeared after his smoking cessation.

PMH: His medical history did not reveal any serious diseases, allergies or drug uptakes. He was a long distance runner who had stopped smoking over the last five years.

OE: A large painful ulcer on the right lateral margin of his tongue, opposite to his normal premolars, that was associated with sialorrhea and a difficulty in tongue movements causing him problems in swallowing and speaking. The ulcer was irregular in shape, large (>2 cm), soft and covered with a thin whitish friable pseudomembrane and raised borders in places on an erythematous base (Figure 11.4). General symptomatology such as fever and fatigue was not found, apart from an ipsilateral submandibular lymphadenitis; genital or other mucosae ulcerations or bullae were not recorded. His oral hygiene was very good.

Q1 What is the cause?

- **A** Trauma
- **B** Adamantiades-Behcet's syndrome
- **C** Large aphtha
- **D** Chancre
- **E** Oral carcinoma

Answers:

- **A** No
- **B** No
- **C** Large aphtha is the cause as it is characterized by a large (>1 cm) painful recurrent oral ulceration with erythematous halo, lasting for more than two weeks and being mainly noticed anywhere in mouth, but particularly on the masticatory mucosa, occasionally causing patient concern of the possibility of a malignant tumor. The increased frequency of aphthae seems to be related with cessation of smoking, as this was happened in this patient.
- **D** No
- **E** No

Comments: The characteristics of the patient's ulceration such as the softness on palpation and association with other similar oral differentiates from other ulcerations from oral carcinomas; Adamantiades-Bechet's syndrome, syphilis or trauma. The ulcer in oral carcinomas is firm and associated with regional lymphadenopathy win Adamantiades-Bechet's syndrome is accompanied with other mouth and genital ulcerations on examination and in the past. Syphilitic ulceration is painless and always associated with systemic lynohadenopathy while a recent history of local trauma indicates traumatic ulceration. Skin lesions that were seen on the examination and in the past as well as the absence of systemic lymphadenopathy or history of local trauma, exclude oral carcinomas, Adamantiades-Behcet's syndrome, syphilis and local trauma from the diagnosis respectively.

Q2 Which characteristics are useful in the distinction of different types of aphthous stomatitis?

- **A** Location
- **B** Number
- **C** Other mucosae involvement
- **D** Complications
- **E** Size

Answers:

- **A** Large aphthae are located mainly on the palate and gingivae, while the minor, herpetiform and those associated with syndromes, on the non-masticatory oral mucosa.
- **B** Herpetiform aphthae are numerous (>10 small ulcers in clusters); 1–5 ulcers in minor aphthae, 1 or 2 in large aphthae, while those related with syndromes have a variable number.
- **C** Genital ulcerations and other mucosae lesions are characteristic in Adamantiades-Behcet's and other syndromes but not seen in simple aphthae (small; large; herpetiform).
- **D** Scarring is seen in places where repeated large aphthae occur.
- **E** The size determines the type of minor, large and herpetiform aphthae; large aphthae were bigger while small aphthae smaller than 1 cm respectively. Herpetiform are the smallest (<0.6 cm).

Q3 Which syndromes have aphthae among their characteristics?

- **A** Riga-Fede syndrome
- **B** Periodic fever, aphthous stomatitis, pharyngitis, adenitis (PFAPA) syndrome
- **C** Adamantiades-Behcet syndrome
- **D** Sjögren syndrome
- **E** Treacher Collins syndrome

Answers:

- **A** No
- **B** PFAPA syndrome is characterized by periodic fever every six to eight weeks, aphthous stomatitis, pharyngitis and cervical adenitis and is the commonest cause of periodic fever in children.
- **C** This syndrome is a rare disorder causing inflammation of blood vessels throughout the body, and is associated with aphthous stomatitis, genital ulcerations, eyes, joint and visceral inflammation and skin.
- **D** Sjögren syndrome is a chronic autoimmune disease affecting the body's moisture glands, especially salivary and lacrimal glands, and presents with dry mouth, dry eyes, skin or nose, mouth ulcerations, muscle and joint problems. Kidney, lungs, liver as well as pancreas are also involved.
- **E** No

Comments: Riga-Fede syndrome is associated with traumatic ulcerations and not aphthae, as the first lesions are constant and not recurrent, and found only on the lips and the tip of the tongue, close to prematurely erupted deciduous teeth. Treacher Collins syndrome is characterized by deformities of ears, eyes, cheek bones, and underdevelopment of the mandible with malocclusion, but not by aphthous stomatitis.

Case 11.5

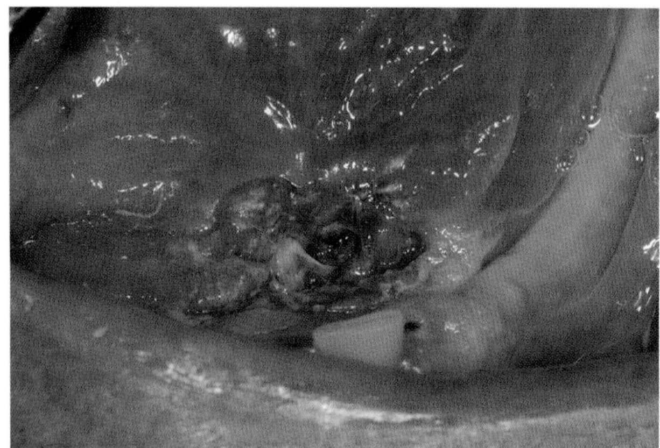

Figure 11.5

CO: A 68-year-old man was presented with an ulcer on the floor of his mouth.

HPC: His ulcer was firstly noticed by his clinician last week during a bronchoscope examination for a carcinoma of his right lung.

PMH: His medical history revealed a papillary carcinoma of his urethra which was surgically removed two months ago and a small cell carcinoma of his lower lung that was discovered last month during his routine check-up. Both tumors were associated with the patient's chronic smoking (>2 packets of cigarettes/daily) and heavy drinking (>5 glasses of wine/per meal).

OE: A large asymptomatic ulcer on the floor of his mouth was found extended from the lingual frenum to the lateral left side of his tongue with maximum diameter of 3.5 cm. The ulcer had a rubber-like consistency, irregular and raised borders, with deep granular base, being fixed in the underlying mucosa (Figure 11.5) thus causing a difficulty in tongue movements. Cervical lymph nodes were enlarged and fixed into his skin neck.

Q1 What is this ulceration?

- **A** Tuberculous ulcer
- **B** Giant cell arteritis ulceration
- **C** Oral carcinoma
- **D** Eosinophilic ulcer
- **E** Large aphthae

Answers:

- **A** No
- **B** No
- **C** Oral carcinoma is the answer. It is a long-lasting tumor with an ulceration of various size, location and symptomatology, fixed and associated with cervical ispilateral or bilateral lymphadenitis. The tumor is composed of neoplasmatic epithelial cells of various degrees of maturation and mitotic activity that infiltrate the underlying submucosa.
- **D** No
- **E** No

Comments: The hard consistency of the ulcer allows the exclusion clinically of a large aphtha and eosinophilic ulceration, while the absence of lung lesions and symptomatology rule out tuberculosis and giant cell arteritis from the diagnosis.

Q2 Which histological characteristics are indicative of an oral carcinoma?

A Increased number of mitoses
B Infiltration of submucosa with neoplastic epithelial cells
C Hyperchromatic nuclei of basal cells
D Plethora of eosinophils
E Caseous granulomas

Answers:

A No
B The breakage of basal membrane and infiltration of underlying submucosa with neoplasmatic epithelial cells differentiate an invasive carcinoma from a carcinoma in situ and a dysplastic lesion.
C No
D No
E No

Comments: The presence of an increased number of mitoses or abnormal mitoses as well as hyperchromatic nuclei is not a characteristic histological finding of oral carcinomas but can be seen in dysplastic oral mucosa. Oral carcinomas are characterized by a chronic diffuse and not in grannulomatous pattern inflammatory infiltration of lymphocytes, plasma cells and macrophages, but rarely by eosinophils which are abundant in eosinophilic ulcer.

Q3 Which are the common findings among a primary cancer and a secondary, independent, primary tumor in a patient with multiple malignancies?

A Proliferation index
B Similar risk factors
C Onset of appearance
D Hereditary predisposition
E Similar location

Answers:

A No
B Some factors such as chronic smoking, heavy drinking or long exposure to solar radiation increase the risk of growing several types of cancer throughout patient's body.
C No
D Several tumors share common tumor suppressor genes that raise the risk of development of different tumors in various anatomical unrelated organs.
E No

Comments: In patients with a history of multiple malignancies, the different primary tumors do not share the same elements. Firstly, they do not share the same time of appearance, as their onset could differ from a few months to many years; secondly, they do not share the same location as they can be found in many distant organs; and finally, the proliferation capacity and the same histological characteristics also differ.

Case 11.6

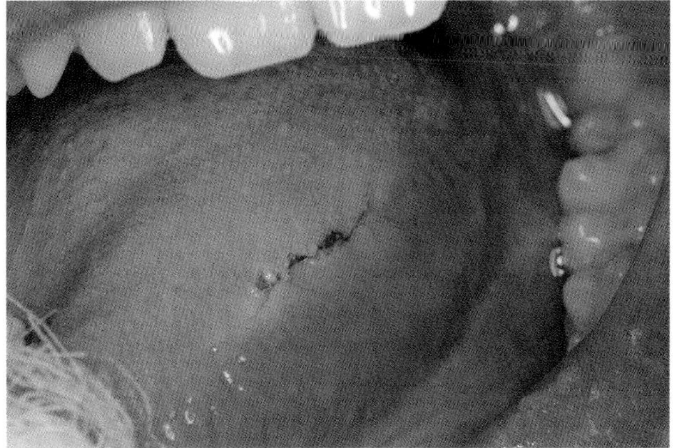

Figure 11.6

CO: An eight-year-old boy was presented with an irregular deep painful ulceration on his tongue which had lasted over a few weeks.

HPC: The ulcer was first noticed by his mother when the patient started complaining about eating problems and had remained unchanged since then.

PMH: The child's medical history was unremarkable apart from a few episodes of bedwetting since his brother's birth and grinding his teeth during sleep.

OE: A deep linear ulceration on the left side of dorsum of his tongue extended deep into tongue muscles, but without any signs of inflammation apart from the teeth imprint on his tongue (Figure 11.6). The ulcer was painful but not associated with other similar lesions in his mouth and only a mild self-induced friction keratosis on both buccal mucosae was recorded. His oral hygiene was very good and the patient's dentition was clear from caries.

Q1 What is the cause of ulceration?

- **A** Aphtha
- **B** Iatrogenic trauma
- **C** Fissured tongue
- **D** Self-induced oral ulceration
- **E** Riga-Fede syndrome

Answers:

- **A** No
- **B** No
- **C** No
- **D** Self-induced oral ulceration is the answer and is characterized by atypical oral lesions induced by patients who are under stress, depression or mental retardation via biting of their tongue, lips or buccal mucosae. The presence of friction keratosis and night teeth grinding or bedwetting reinforces the bad psychological status of this child that he was capable of harming himself.
- **E** No

Comments: Fissured tongue is a normal variation of the dorsum of tongue that is characterized by numerous grooves along its length and rarely causes symptoms such as burning sensation or pain. The lack of erythematous halo and absence of similar lesions in the past excludes aphthae from diagnosis. Iatrogenic trauma is easily excluded as the patient had a very good oral hygiene and did not require any dental intervention while the Riga-Fede syndrome is mostly found in younger children with premature erupted deciduous teeth.

Q2 Which characteristics could help clinicians to diagnose a self-induced ulcerations?

- **A** Peculiar shape
- **B** History of other self-induced lesions
- **C** Proximity of lesion with causative agent
- **D** Symptoms irrelevant of severity of injury
- **E** Unknown cause

Answers:

- **A** Self-induced ulcerations tend to be bizarre in shape as the patient traumatizes the oral mucosa many times by using different media such as teeth, fingernails, toothpicks or even a toothbrush.
- **B** The presence of other self-induced lesions during the patient's examination reinforces the clinician's initial diagnosis.
- **C** Self-induced injuries must be close to the agent that cause them; for example, biting or rubbing should be close to the teeth.
- **D** Whenever the symptomatology, like pain, does not match with the severity of the lesion, the possibility of self-induced injury should be considered.
- **E** The absence of any common cause must make clinicians consider self-induced injury as a possible cause.

Q3 Which of the oral lesions below could be self-induced?

- **A** Friction keratosis
- **B** Exfoliate cheilitis
- **C** Reactive fibromas
- **D** Gum recessions
- **E** Actinic cheilitis

Answers:

- **A** Friction keratosis is the result of a chronic biting of the oral mucosa against the teeth and appears as white hyperkeratosis lesions with a rough surface but without dysplasia.
- **B** Exfoliate cheilitis is characterized by exfoliation, crusting and desquamation of the lips that are caused by the patient's habit of licking his lips many times a day.
- **C** Reactive fibromas are induced by a chronic irritation due to rubbing or biting of the oral mucosa against broken teeth or bad prosthesis.
- **D** Gum recessions are often seen in patients with overaggressive brushing and may appear as a gum retraction from the crown of the teeth being noticed in places together with superficial traumatic ulcerations.
- **E** No

Comments: Chronic solar radiation exposure is the cause of a range of alterations in the vermilion border of the lips (actinic cheilitis) unrelated to patient's behavior. Some of them are mild like hyperpigmentation or exfoliation, but others might be more severe like chronic atrophy or ulcerations with a high risk of malignant transformation.

Case 11.7

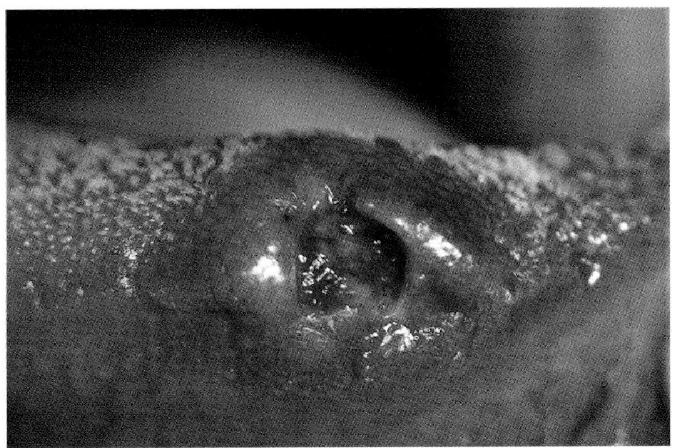

Figure 11.7

CO: A 32-year-old woman presented with an ulcer on her tongue which had lasted for almost two weeks.

HPC: The ulcerated lesion appeared after a tongue injury by accidental tongue biting during a meal. The lesion was initially small but gradually enlarged over the last 10 days causing her difficulties in tongue movements.

PMH: Her medical history was clear of any serious diseases apart from two Cesarean operations for her children's birth and with no smoking or drinking habits.

OE: A large ulcer (>2 cm max.diameter) at the right lateral margin of her tongue with normal color and consistency opposite to the lower right first molar. The lesion appeared initially as a small traumatic nodule which was gradually enlarged along with a deep ulcer in the center, which gave the impression of a chronic ulcer with raised margins (Figure 11.7). The lesion was not fixed into the underlying tissues or associated with topical lymphadenopathy, causing the patient's concern of being a cancer Its biopsy revealed the accumulation of plethora of eosinophils without atypia at the base of the ulcer whose margins were covered by hyperplatic squamous non dysplastic epithelium, while radiological examination did not reveal any bony abnormalities. The ulcer rapidly healed right after the incisional biopsy done and a topical steroid in oral balance application.

Q1 What is the lesion?

- **A** Oral carcinoma
- **B** Warty dyskeratoma
- **C** Eosinophilic ulceration
- **D** Langerhan's histiocytosis
- **E** Non-Hodgkin lymphoma

Answers:

- **A** No
- **B** No
- **C** Eosinophilic ulcer is the cause. This is a benign, self-limited painful ulcerative lesion, with raised margins and fibrinous base, the etiology of which is not clear, yet trauma may play a role. The infiltration of submucosa and mucosa with normal eosinophils is its main histological feature.
- **D** No
- **E** No

Comments: The clinical course of this lesion, negative X-ray results and a presence of eosinophils without atypia into submucosa and mucosa, where dyskeratosis was not found, excludes oral carcinomas, non-Hodgkin lymphoma, histiocytosis X and warty dyskeratosis from diagnosis.

Q2 What is/are the best treatment for an eosinophil ulceration?

- **A** None
- **B** Antibiotics
- **C** Surgical excision
- **D** Remove causative agent
- **E** Steroids

Answers:

- **A** No
- **B** No
- **C** A total surgical excision is the only treatment required for the majority of cases, although in some cases the lesion can disappear spontaneously a few days after the initial examination.
- **D** No
- **E** No

Comments: The lesion does not respond to local or systemic antibiotics, but partially responds in the withdrawal of the causative traumatic agent, such as broken teeth or fillings, as well as in topical the application of steroids in order to reduce local inflammation.

Q3 Which other oral diseases apart from eosinophilic ulcer are characterized histologically by accumulation of eosinophils?

- **A** Plasmacytoma
- **B** Chancre
- **C** Primary Langerhans histiocytosis X
- **D** Oral lichenoid reactions
- **E** Oral leukoplakia

Answers:

A No
B No
C No
D Eosinophils are predominant among chronic inflammatory cells in the lichenoid reaction rather than lichen planus.
E In leukoplakias, the increased number of eosinophils in the submucosa may be an indicator of which premalignant lesions have the potential for malignant transformation.

Comments: In plasmacytoma, the main pathological characteristic is the accumulation of plasma cells and not eosinophils at different degrees of differentiation and maturation, while mature plasma cells abundant at the base of a syphiliic ulcer. In eosinophylic granuloma the lesion is usually found in the lungs rather than mouth and closely related with smoking while the patient was never being a smoker.

Case 11.8

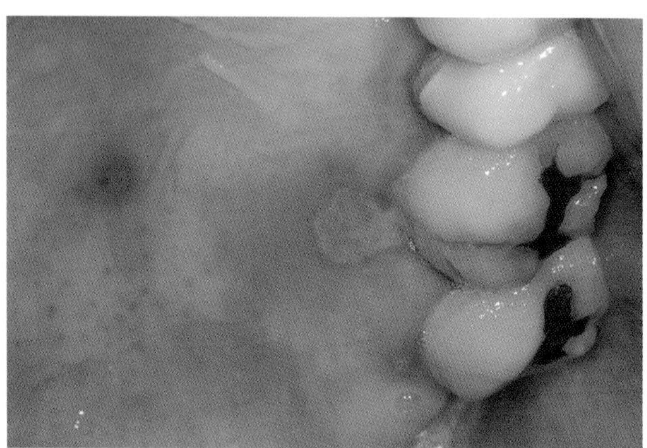

Figure 11.8

CO: A 22-year-old woman presented with a few superficial ulcerations on the hard palate.

HPC: The lesions appeared three weeks ago and were associated with pain, gingival bleeding and general symptomatology such as weight loss, general malaise and night fever as well.

PMH: Her medical history was clear apart from a few episodes of nose bleeds over the last month, and a sore throat that was relieved with antiseptic lozenges. She was not a smoker or drinker and spent her free time swimming, but she had given this up due to her constant tiredness over the last month

OE: The examination revealed a few superficial ulcerations on the buccal mucosae and hard palate near the molar gingivae. The ulcers were painful and had irregular margins with mild inflammation peripherally (Figure 11.8) and were associated with pallor of the oral mucosa and skin, as well as enlarged neck lymph nodes. Bleeding from gingivae or other parts of her mouth or skin was not found. The ulcers were restricted to oral mucosa only, and not associated with other bullous disorders. On the other hand, the blood tests revealed a partial pancytopenia and anemia, and therefore she was referred to hospital for some further evaluation of her blood problem.

Q1 What is the cause of oral ulcerations?

A Aphthous stomatitis
B Secondary herpetic stomatitis
C Mucous membrane pemphigoid
D Acute leukemia
E Erythema multiforme

Answers:

A No
B No
C No
D Acute leukemia was the cause and is generally the most common malignancy of the blood which affects young patients. This is characterized by an infiltration of premature malignant cells (blasts) within the bone marrow causing a replacement of the normal marrow cells, resulting in anemia, leucopenia and finally thrombopenia. The patient's anemia was therefore the cause of fatigue and general malaise, while the leucopenia showed an increased risk of infections (especially from oral bacterial) and the thrombopenia resulted in hemorrhages from nose and gingivae. Oral ulcerations are common and characterized as superficial, but

painful lesions with minimum local inflammation and lack marginal erythema (halo) and appear in cases of a low number of leucocytes in the peripheral blood as was seen in this woman.

E No

Comments: The clinical characteristics of an acute leukemia differentiate its atypical oral ulcerations from other conditions such as aphthae, secondary herpes infection, erythema multiforme and mucous membrane pemphigoid, as these diseases do not have a serious general symptomatology and are not associated with weight loss, fever and systemic lymphadenopathy. Additionally, the lack of bullae in oral and other mucosae as well as in the skin reinforces the idea that the patient did not have mucous membrane pemphigoid or erythema multiforme, while the presence of single isolated large ulcers in the oral mucosa and not multiple tiny ulcerations at one part of mouth ruled out the diagnosis of a secondary herpetic stomatitis.

Q2 Which are the other oral manifestations of an acute untreated leukemia?

A Gingival pigmentation
B Petechiae/ecchymoses
C Gingival enlargement
D Palatal paleness
E Hemosiderosis

Answers:

A No

B Petechiae/ecchymoses are often seen in patients with leukemia who have low platelets or liver failure due to its infiltration with neoplasmatic blast cells.

C Gingival enlargement is a common finding and is attributed initially to the gingival infiltration with leukemia cells and to gingivitis or periodontitis as sequence of reduced local immunity against plaque bacteria due to leucopenia induced secondly by leukemia.

D Palatal paleness is induced by severe anemia due to leukemia, and is often accompanied with face and skin palor.

E No

Comments: Hemosiderosis is characterized by the accumulation of hemosiderin into various tissues, including the oral mucosa of patients who take regular blood transfusions in cases of thalassemia, sickle cell anemia and even severe leukemia. Hemosiderosis appears as bluish or brown or black diffuse mucosal discoloration unlike gingival pigmentation that is usually localized and related to patient's race and smoking habits.

Q3 Which of the conditions below have an increased risk of developing acute leukemia?

A Fanconi anemia
B Neurofibromatosis (NF)
C Kostmann syndrome
D Gorlin syndrome
E Osler-Rendu-Weber syndrome

Answers:

A Fanconi anemia is a rare inherited bone marrow disorder due to the mutations of 16 genes, their proteins of which play an important role in DNA repair pathway. This anemia has an increased risk of developing myelodysplastic syndrome, aplastic anemia or acute myeloid leukemia, as well as specific tumors including oral carcinomas.

B Neurofibromatosis (NF-1) has an increased risk of developing juvenile myelomonocytic leukemia which can evolve into an acute myeloid leukemia.

C Kostmann syndrome is a group of diseases which are characterized by a congenital neutropenia that responds well to granulocyte-colony stimulating factor (G-CSF). This disease has an increased risk of developing an acute myeloid leukemia or myelodysplastic syndrome over time.

D No

E No

Comments: Both Gorlin and Osler-Rendu-Weber syndromes are irrelevant to acute leukemia induction, as both develop skin basal cell carcinomas and breast cancers respectively.

Case 11.9

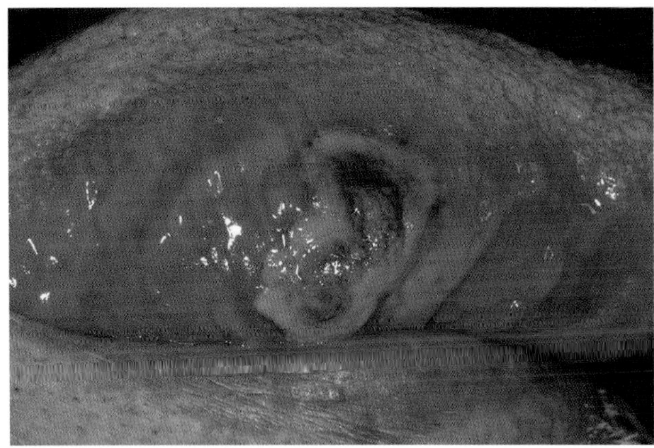

Figure 11.9

CO: A 58-year-old man was referred for a series of episodes of painful ulcerations over the last five years.

HPC: His oral ulcerations appeared for the first time five years ago after a crisis of his ulcerative colitis. Since then, 1–3 painful ulcers appeared on his tongue, lips and more rarely on his buccal mucosae, lasting approximately 10 days and causing him eating and speaking problems.

PMH: His medical history revealed mild hypertension that was treated with irbesartan and also ulcerative colitis which was also treated with a special diet and sulfasalazine and steroids (in crisis). Smoking was recorded but was limited to 15 cigarettes daily since the diagnosis of his ulcerative colitis.

OE: A painful well-defined ulceration on the right side of his tongue covered with yellow-brown pseudomembrane, 1.5 cm in diameter, associated with sialorrhea and halitosis was recorded (Figure 11.9). The general symptomatology such as abdominal pain, diarrhea and weight loss was attributed to his main illness and not to oral ulceration. Lymphadenitis (local or systemic) or other lesions on other mucosae were not reported apart from some active ulcers on his colon.

Q1 What is the cause of this oral ulceration?

- **A** Drug induced
- **B** Large aphtha
- **C** Chancre
- **D** Ulcerative colitis related
- **E** Traumatic ulcer

Answers:

- **A** No
- **B** No
- **C** No
- **D** Oral ulcerations are common manifestations in ulcerative colitis and don't differ clinically from aphthous stomatitis apart from the fact that they occur prior to or concurrently with the gastrointestinal symptoms, and also parallel to their disease activity.
- **E** No

Comments: Drugs like sulfasalazine and Irbesartan cause a number of side-effects like skin blistering, crusting, irritation and tenderness but not oral ulcerations. The patient's ulcer did not follow a head trauma, nor was it ever associated with lymphadenopathy or other oral and skin lesions. at the examination day or in the past excluding therefore, trauma, aphthae and syphilis were ruled out from the diagnosis.

Q2 What are the other oral symptoms of ulcerative colitis apart from oral ulcerations?

- **A** Burning tongue/mouth
- **B** Oral pigmentation
- **C** Tongue coating
- **D** Pyostomatitis vegetans
- **E** Taste changes

Answers:

- **A** Burning mouth and especially the tongue is an indication of anemia due to a vitamin B12 deficiency from malabsorption in patients with ulcerative colitis.
- **B** No
- **C** Tongue coating is seen in some patients with inflammatory bowel syndrome.
- **D** Pyostomatitis vegetans is characterized by erythema, edema and numerous yellowish pustules, and appears in patients with inflammatory bowel diseases (ulcerative colitis or Crohn's disease).
- **E** The reduction of olfactory and gustatory functions is seen in many patients with ulcerative colitis, regardless of the disease activity or treatment. Acid or sour taste is a common complaint too.

Q3 Which skin conditions are related with ulcerative colitis?

- **A** Erythema nodosum
- **B** Pyoderma gangrenosum
- **C** Psoriasis
- **D** Melasma
- **E** Telangiectasia

Answers:

A Erythema nodosum is the most common skin lesion in patients with ulcerative colitis and is characterized by tender red nodules on the skin of legs and arms that appear just before the beginning or a flare of the disease.

B Pyoderma gangrenosum is observed as clusters of small blisters on the patient's shin, ankles or even arms. The blisters spread and break forming painful ulcerations which are treated with various immunosuppressant drugs

C Patients with psoriasis have an increased risk of ulcerative colitis and other autoimmune gut diseases, as they all share similar pathogenic genes and therefore similar a clinical course and treatment.

D No

E No

Comments: Melasma is characterized by dark brown patches on the face that are triggered by birth control pills, pregnancy and hormone therapy, but never by ulcerative colitis. Telangectiasias are small dilated blood vessels that are seen in patients with venous malformations, systemic diseases such as cirrhosis and scleroderma but not ulcerative colitis or exposed to extreme environmental factors (cold, heat), radio-chemotherapy or steroid treatment.

Case 11.10

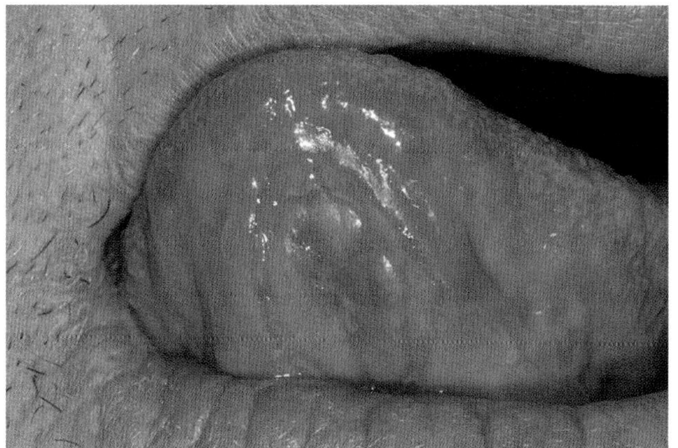

Figure 11.10a

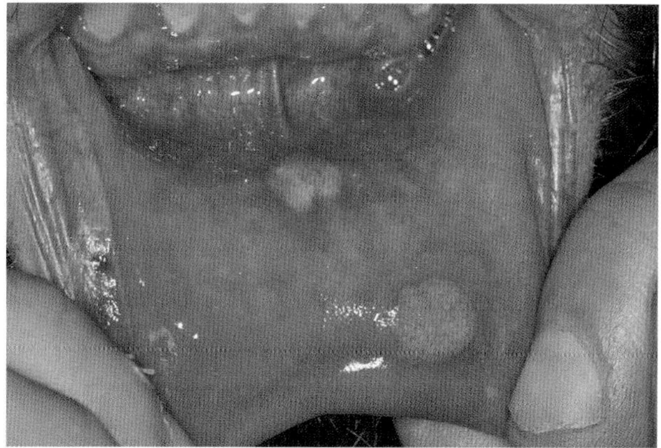

Figure 11.10b

CO: A 56-year-old homosexual man presented with a painless ulceration on the ventral surface of his tongue.

HPC: The lesion was discovered by the patient and caused him severe concern as a number of additional ulcerations in his groin were found three days previously during self-examination.

PMH: His medical history was unremarkable apart from a herpetic genital infection since adolescence, and condylomas on the skin of his penis and anus that were treated with cryotherapy and topical application of imiquimod 5% cream. He was a chronic smoker of cannabis and tobacco and drank many cups of coffee and beer on a daily basis.

OE: A large painless ulceration on the central part of the ventral surface of his tongue. The ulcer was superficial, and hemorrhagic on an erythematous and edematous base (Figure 11.10a). It was associated with soft whitish mucous patches on his lower lip (Figure 11.10b) thus causing a burning sensation during eating or smoking. Fever, malaise or other symptomatology was not recorded apart from a generalized lymphadenopathy. Small irregular asymptomatic ulcerations were also found on the skin of his groin, but his other mucosae were clear from similar lesions. Cultures taken from the lesions revealed the growth of numerous spirochetes and not *Candida albicans*.

Q1 What is the cause of this ulceration?

A Thermal burn
B Syphilis
C Large aphtha
D Candidiasis
E Drug eruption

Answers:

A No

B Syphilitic ulcer is the answer and is a manifestation of the 2nd stage of a *Treponema pallidum* infection. It appears as a large painless lesion mimicking a number of other ulcerations, but associated with general symptomatology like malaise and systemic lymphadenopathy.

C No

D No

E No

Comments: The history and clinical characteristics of this ulceration are different from other ulcerations such as burns (lack of history of a recent thermal injury from hot coffee or excessive smoking); aphtha (lack of recurrence); drug-induced (lack of drug uptake as his previous his condyloma therapy involved the skin but not his mouth) and candidiasis (negative culture).

Q2 Which is/are the other manifestation(s) of the secondary stage of this infection?

A Condyloma acuminata

B Non-pruritic skin rash

C Chancre

D Gumma

E Saddle nose

Answers:

A No

B A localized or diffuse, symmetrical non-pruritic rash on the trunk and extremities which gradually becomes maculopapular and pustular and seen at the early phase of the second stage of syphilis.

C No

D No

E No

Comments: Chancre is a manifestation of the first stage, while gumma of the third stage of syphilis. Condyloma acuminata is a sexually transmitted disease and must not be confused with condyloma lata. The first lesion was due to HPV, while the latter to *Treponema pallidum* infection. Saddle nose is a characteristic of congenital syphilis.

Q3 Which other oral conditions are related with spirochete infection?

A Facial palsy

B Acute necrotizing gingivitis

C Desquamative gingivitis

D Actinomycosis

E Pulp necrosis

Answers:

A Facial palsy has been reported in young patients after a Lyme (spirochete) infection.

B In acute necrotizing gingivitis and periodontitis, spirochetes and especially *Treponema denticola* play a crucial role in their pathogenesis.

C No

D No

E A large number of spirochetes have been isolated in necrotic pulps of deciduous and permanent teeth.

Comments: Although spirochetes are commonly seen in inflamed gingivae of various periodontal diseases, they do not play the crucial role in desquamative gingivitis pathogenesis as this gingival desquamation is not a disease but an oral manifestation of lichen planus and mucous pemphigoid as well as other autoimmune bullous conditions. Actinomyces Istraeli and Gerescenseriae and not Treponema pallidum are responsible for painful abscesses in the mouth, lungs, breast or gastrointestinal tract seen in a rare bacterial infection known as Actinomycosis.

12

Vesiculobullous Lesions

Vesiculobullous diseases are a heterogeneous group of diseases that are characterized by the formation of vesicles or bullae in the mouth only or in combination with other lesions in skin and other mucosae. Oral bullae are rather fragile lesions that break easily during mastication forming large painful superficial ulcerations. Viral infections, mucocutaneous, or immune-related conditions, autoimmune or even genetic diseases are sometimes presented with hemorrhagic or clear fluid bullae whose histological and immunofluorescence characteristics are pathognomonic. Their early diagnosis and treatment can save the patient's life (See Figure 12.0).

Table 12 lists the most common vesiculobullous diseases.

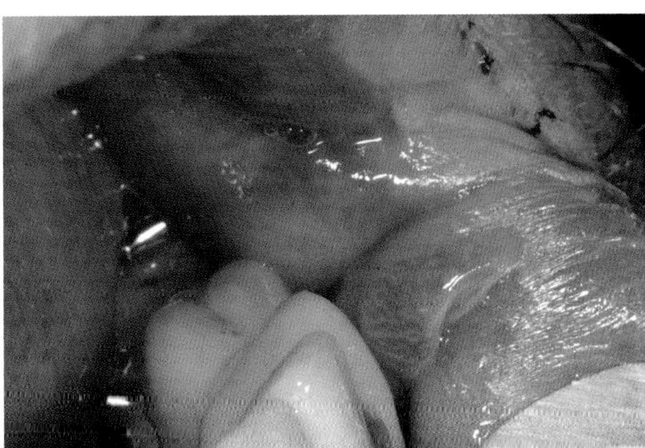

Figure 12.0 Intact bulla on the inner surface of the lower lip in a patient with mucous membrane pemphigoid.

Table 12 Common and important vesiculobullous conditions.

Vesicles–Bullae

- Real bullae
  - **Acute**
    - Related to trauma
      - Angina bullosa hemorrhagica
      - Burns
    - Related to inflammation
      - Erythema multiforme
      - Toxic epidermal necrolysis
      - Sweet syndrome
      - Steven Johnson syndrome
    - Related to infection
      - Viral
        - Herpes simplex
        - Varicella zoster
        - Enterovirus
      - Bacterial
        - Staphylococcal scalded skin syndrome
    - Related to immunity
      - Intra-epidermal IgA pustules
      - Herpes gestationis
      - Paraneoplastic pemphigus
  - **Chronic**
    - Related to heritage
      - Familiar pemphigus
      - Epidermolysis bullosa
    - Related with immunity
      - Pemphigus vulgaris
      - Pemphigus foliaceous
      - Benign MMP
      - Bullous pemphigoid
      - Dermatitis herpetiformis
      - Linear IgA disease
      - Amyloidosis
    - Related to inflammation
      - Bullous lichen planus
- False blisters
  - Abscesses
  - Cysts (soft, bony)
  - Mucoceles (single, multiple)

Clinical Guide to Oral Diseases, First Edition. Dimitris Malamos and Crispian Scully.

Companion website: www.wiley.com/go/malamos/clinical_guide

Case 12.1

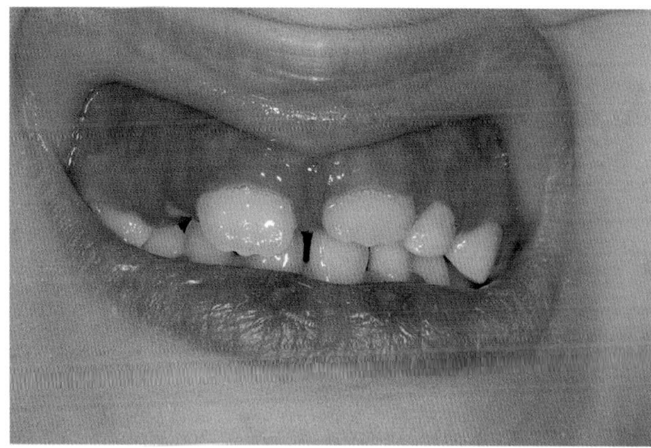

Figure 12.1

CO: A seven-year-old boy presented with painful ulcerations on his mouth and lips.

HPC: According to the patient's parents, the lesions appeared after three successive days of high fever (>38 C), malaise and sore throat followed by a gingival erythema and numerous vesicles, both spread out all over his mouth. The vesicles had clear fluid and were easily broken, leaving painful ulcerations. There was no previous medical record of similar episodes of ulcerations, but his sister recently experienced a flu-like illness and after that she developed a few itching vesicles on the corner of her lower lip two weeks ago.

PMH: His medical history was clear of any serious diseases or allergies. He spent his spare time in sporting activities such as swimming and football, but he had the habit of biting his nails since the starting his first school.

OE: The oral examination revealed a few ulcerations on the dorsum of the tongue, buccal mucosae and lower lip, which were associated with erythematous swollen gingivae where a few small vesicles were observed. The gingivae were very sensitive and bled on probing, especially on areas of partially erupted permanent teeth (Figure 12.1). Sialorrhea and halitosis were recorded. The oral ulcers were accompanied with expanded cervical lymph nodes and a dispersed erythematous rash on his body.

Q1 What is the possible diagnosis?

- **A** Traumatic ulcers due to nail biting
- **B** Erythema multiforme
- **C** Aphthous stomatitis
- **D** Chicken pox infection
- **E** Primary herpetic gingivostomatitis

Answers:

- **A** No
- **B** No
- **C** No
- **D** No
- **E** Primary herpetic stomatitis is the answer. This is an infection from herpes virus (type 1, mainly) and appears with small vesicles with clear fluid all over the mouth which are easily broken and leave painful ulcerations. These are related to erythematous gingivae and general prodromal symptomatology such as malaise, fever and cervical lymphadenopathy. Its severity varies but the initial (primary) herpetic infection, is always greater than the secondary herpes infection that is presented as herpes labialis or stomatitis.

Comments: The presence of prodromal symptoms allows the exclusion of traumatic ulcerations due to nail biting, while the detection of cervical lymphadenopathy and high fever together with the lack of history of similar lesions in the past rule out aphthous stomatitis and erythema multiforme from the diagnosis. The presence of prodromal symptomatology and similar oral lesions confuses the clinician as to whether it is a viral infection from herpes or chicken pox. However, the skin rash of chicken pox infection is rather more severe and more extensive and is characterized by a great number of red bumps, small vesicles, pustules and scabs, initially appearing on the face and trunk and later on the extremities, while the herpetic exanthema is more restricted on the trunk.

Q2 Which of the viruses below can usually cause oral lesions in young healthy patients?

- **A** Herpes simplex 1 (HSV1)
- **B** Herpes simplex 2 (HSV2)
- **C** Epstein-Barr virus (EBV or HH4)
- **D** Herpes type 6 (HH6)
- **E** Cytomegalovirus (CMV or HH5)

Answers:

- **A** Herpes simplex virus type 1 is the most common herpetic viral infection, which usually affects the mouth, head and skin above the wrist.
- **B** Herpes simplex virus type 2 affects mainly the genitals and the skin area below the wrist, but can affect the mouth via oral-genital sex.

C Epstein-Barr virus is the main cause of glandular fever in young healthy patients. It is a condition characterized by sore throat, local or systemic lymphadenopathy, gingivitis and stomatitis, liver and spleen dysfunctions and is accompanied with malaise and fatigue.
D No
E No

Comments: Although the cytomegalovirus and herpes virus 6 affect the majority of people, the mouth is rarely involved. Cytomegalovirus can only cause atypical oral ulcerations in immunocompromised patients, while the herpes virus 6 (A and B subtypes) affect patients of three to five years old and cause diarrhea, high fever and a characteristic rash (roseola) but never involve the mouth.

Q3 Which of the laboratory tests below distinguish the primary from the secondary type of infection?
A Tzanck test
B Polymerase chain reaction (PCR) technique
C Biopsy
D Culture
E Titers of Abs for herpes virus

Answers:
A No
B No
C No
D No
E The comparison of herpes Abs titers is useful. The IgG Abs for herpes 1 or 2 are negative at the early phase of this infection, but become gradually detectable two to three weeks later and persist indefinitely. Changes of IgM Abs are present at the beginning and reappear with the recurrence of this infection.

Comments: All the other tests mentioned above are useful for the detection of herpes virus from the oral lesions regardless of the infection stage. Tzanck test allows the distinction of this infection from other vesiculobullous disorders by detecting multinucleated giant epithelial cells with eosinophilic inclusion bodies in smears. Biopsy reveals an intra-epithelial blister due to acantholysis and scattered acantholytic epithelial cells with ballooning degeneration and viral inclusion particles. Viral culture is time consuming, and requires special and expensive culture media, while the PCR technique is very accurate and unique at recognizing the viral cause, but requires special and expensive techniques but does not the stage (primary or secondary) of the disease.

Case 12.2

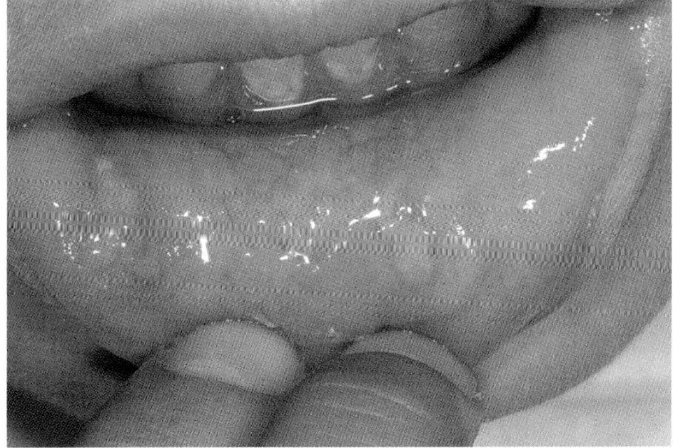

Figure 12.2a

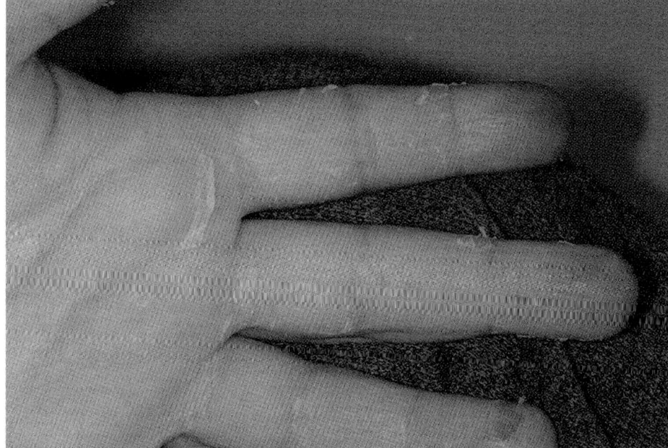

Figure 12.2b

CO: A five-year-old girl was presented with a four-day history of painful ulcerations in her mouth.

HPC: The ulcerations appeared two days after an episode of feeling unwell with fever, nausea and loss of appetite at her kindergarten, while her mother had just recovered from an upper respiratory infection.

PMH: The girl had no serious medical problems apart from a few episodes of gastrointestinal and respiratory diseases, during her daycare period at kindergarten, that were treated with a special diet and antipyretic drugs.

OE: A clinical examination revealed multiple superficial ulcerations at the inner surface of her lower lip

(Figure 12.2a), tongue and buccal mucosae being associated with erythematous throat and small pinhead vesicles, as well as skin desquamation on the tips of her hands and toes (Figure 12.2b) and fever (37.8°C). However, local or systemic lymphadenopathy or erythematous rash on her body apart from her palms and sole lesions were not recorded.

Q1 What is the possible diagnosis?
- **A** Aphthous stomatitis
- **B** Hand, foot and mouth disease
- **C** Primary herpetic gingivostomatitis
- **D** Chicken pox
- **E** Kawasaki disease

Answers:
- **A** No
- **B** Hand, foot and mouth (HFMD) disease is an acute viral infection of children (mainly) and is characterized by fever, malaise, nausea and small vesicles on the feet, hands and mouth. These vesicles are easily breakable, leaving superficial ulcerations that may cause difficulties in speaking or eating.
- **C** No
- **D** No
- **E** No

Comments: Fever is also found in children suffering from Kawasaki disease and primary herpetic stomatitis, but these diseases are different from HFMD. In Kawasaki disease the fever is higher (up to 39 C), lasts for longer, and is associated with severe conjunctivitis, cervical lymphadenitis, swollen red lips and tongue (strawberry-like), while in primary herpetic stomatitis, the lesions prevail in the oral cavity and are rarely associated with feet and hand lesions. Aphthous stomatitis and chicken pox diseases have similar oral lesions to HFMD but differ in some aspects, as the prodromal symptoms and fever are usually absent in aphthous stomatitis while in chicken pox, the skin rash appears mainly on face and trunk and rarely on the hands and feet.

Q2 Which of the pathogenic microorganisms is/are responsible for FHMD?
- **A** Papilloma virus A16
- **B** Coxsackie A16
- **C** Enterovirus 71
- **D** Influenza A
- **E** Norovirus

Answers:
- **A** No
- **B** Coxsackie A16 is the most common virus responsible for epidemics of HFMD among children.
- **C** Enterovirus 71 is the second most common virus causing HFMD with neurological problems in children.
- **D** No
- **E** No

Comments: Papilloma virus can lead to cutaneous infections in children, like warts on the skin and mucous membranes, while influenza A and norovirus are responsible for flu and gastroenteritis respectively.

Q3 Which are the complications usually seen in children with FHMD?
- **A** None
- **B** Aseptic meningitis
- **C** Encephalitis
- **D** Nail loss
- **E** Hearing loss

Answers:
- **A** FHMD is an infection which typically resolves on its own without any serious complications and therefore does not need special treatment apart from antipyretic drugs, painkillers and a soft liquid diet for symptomatic relief.
- **B** No
- **C** No
- **D** No
- **E** No

Comments: Complications such as meningitis and encephalitis are rarely seen in children with HFMD, but they must be immediately treated at the nearest children's hospital. Loss of nails, but not hearing, has been observed in children with severe forms of HFMD.

Case 12.3

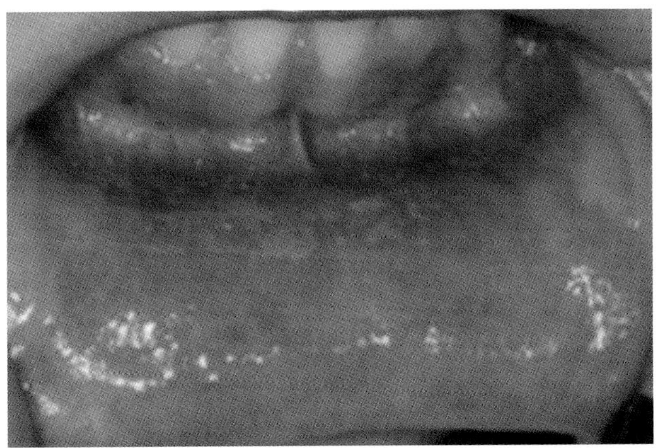

Figure 12.3

CO: A 21-year-old woman presented with a burning sensation to the inner surface of her lower lip.

HPC: The burning sensation appeared a few hours after her visit to her dentist who did a root canal treatment of her lower first right molar by using local anesthesia, a rubber dam and rinses with sodium hypochlorite. This sensation started initially as an itching sensation of her lower lip which gradually turned into a burning sensation in her whole mouth.

PMH: Her medical history was clear apart from some spring allergies that were relieved with anti-histamine drugs when needed. Her habits did not include smoking, drinking heavily or eating spicy foods, and she was a long distance runner in her free time.

OE: The oral examination revealed numerous small vesicles with clear fluid on the erythematous inner surface of her lower lip (Figure 12.3). A diffuse erythema without blisters was also detected on the top of her tongue and labial gingivae, while the rest of her oral mucosa and skin as well as other mucosae (eyes; genitals) were normal.

Q1 What is the possible cause?

- **A** Herpetic stomatitis
- **B** Erythema multiforme
- **C** Chemical burn
- **D** Benign mucous membrane pemphigoid
- **E** Contact stomatitis

Answers:

- **A** No
- **B** No
- **C** No
- **D** No
- **E** Contact stomatitis is the cause. It appears in areas within the mouth which have come into close contact with allergens. It is a delayed reaction (Type IV) to various food additives, dental and cosmetic materials, oral drugs and rubber. It appears as an erythematous burning swelling with superficial blisters or ulcerations intermingled with red or white lines or patches. The direct contact of the patient's oral mucosa with the rubber dam rather than the sodium hypochlorite, could be the cause for this allergic reaction of this patient.

Comments: Sodium hypochlorite could cause severe irritation or chemical burning but the use of the rubber dam prevented its direct contact with the oral mucosa. The restriction of oral lesions at areas of contact with the rubber dam excludes diseases like erythema multiforme cicatricial pemphigoid and herpetic stomatitis. Each of the above vesicu-lobullous diseases differentiate from each other by using clinical criteria' the presence of general symptomatology like fever and lymphadenopathy is characteristic of primary herpetic stomatitis ; the presence of acute ulcerations of various forms together with target like lesions on the skin of young patients is typical finding of erythema multiformae while the presence of chronic ulcerations intermingled with fragila bullae in the mouth and skin of middle age or older patients are commonly seen in cicatricial pemphigoid.

Q2 How could the cause of this condition be confirmed?

- **A** History
- **B** Clinical examination
- **C** Biopsy
- **D** Blood tests
- **E** Patch tests

Answers:

- **A** No
- **B** No
- **C** No
- **D** No
- **E** Patch tests are the most widely used methods by clinicians to distinguish various allergens in patients with contact or atopic dermatitis, by applying tiny quantities of the suspected allergens into the patient's upper back and interpreting the results 48 hours later.

Comments: The diagnosis of contact stomatitis is usually clinically based on a careful history and examination and rarely by biopsies or blood tests. However, the identification of the causative allergens is proved only with various allergy tests, among them the patch tests which play an important role.

Q3 Acute contact stomatitis is mainly controlled by:

- **A** Elimination of implicated allergen
- **B** Replacement of amalgam fillings
- **C** High dose of systemic steroids
- **D** Rinses with mouthwashes containing menthol or cinnamon flavor
- **E** Antifungals in oral suspension

Answers:

- **A** The elimination of the causative allergen is the most crucial step for the treatment of contact stomatitis. Patients with a history of contact stomatitis should be very careful when using unknown oral hygiene products; food rich in technical colors or flavors, drugs with known oral side effects, or dental material with a positive history of previous allergies.
- **B** No
- **C** No
- **D** No
- **E** No

Comments: Topical steroids are useful in chronic contact stomatitis while antifungals are not. Daily mouthwashes, containing cinnamon oils, are responsible, for the cinnamon induces stomatitis, while the replacement of old amalgam fillings can improve only the lichenoid reactions close to the fillings and not all contact stomatitis cases.

Case 12.4

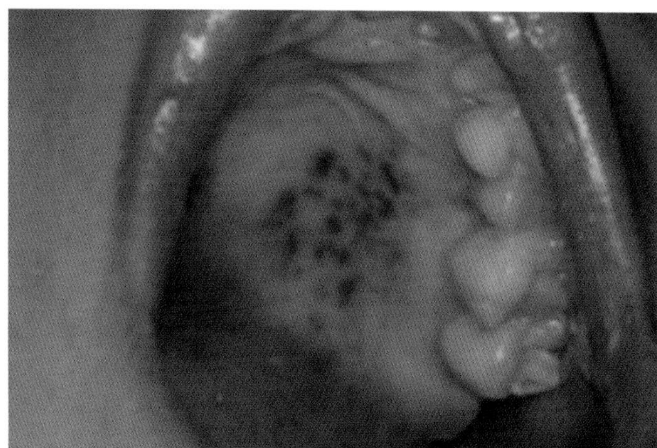

Figure 12.4

CO: A 32-year-old woman presented with a soreness on the left side of her palate over the last two days.

HPC: The symptoms appeared after her gingival scaling by an oral hygienist five days ago.

PMH: She was a patient in good health, without allergies or medicine uptake, but was a chronic smoker of 10 cigarettes per day since her twenties. She had a normal diet, but preferred hot, spicy, hard food.

OE: The oral examination revealed a group of small ulcerations on the left side of the palate from the premolars to the first molar area towards the middle line (Figure 12.4). These ulcers were covered with pseudomembranes and were intermingled with a few small vesicles with clear fluid. No other oral lesions or cervical lymphadenopathy were found.

Q1 Which is the possible cause of these oral ulcerations?

- **A** Burns from hot food
- **B** Trauma from hard tooth brushing
- **C** Syphilis (secondary)
- **D** Herpetiform aphthae
- **E** Herpetic stomatitis (secondary)

Answers:

- **A** No
- **B** No
- **C** No
- **D** No
- **E** Secondary herpetic stomatitis is the cause and characterized by numerous small ulcerations induced after the reactivation of HSV 1 or 2 on Gasserian ganglia, due to local trauma (i.e. dental procedures such as scaling or extractions), exposure to cold or hot weather, stress, and fatigue due to heavy work or illness. It is presented as a cluster of small vesicles on palate, tongue and lips which break easily, leaving tiny superficial ulcerations, associated with mild prodromal symptoms (burning or tingling sensation) but without fever, regional lymphadenopathy and other symptoms.

Comments: Thermal burns on the palate are commonly found among patients who consume very hot or spicy drinks/or food. The burn ulcerations, however, differ, as they tend to be larger and based on erythematous oral mucosae, and are close to the places where the thermal factor acts. Incorrect tooth brushing may cause similar ulcerations, but excluded due to the presence of small vesicles with clear fluid among ulcerations and a negative history of trauma during brushing. The lack of severe pain and erythematous palatal mucosa underneath the ulcerations excludes herpetiform aphthae from the diagnosis. Secondary syphilis was also excluded by the absence of snail-like painless lesions on the palate or other parts of the oral mucosa, and the lack of regional lymphadenopathy.

Q2 Which is the best treatment for this disease in immunocompromised patients?

- **A** None
- **B** Analgesics
- **C** Anti-retroviral drugs
- **D** Antibiotics
- **E** Globulin gamma

Answers:

- **A** No
- **B** No
- **C** Antiretroviral drugs such as acyclovir, ganciclovir and famciclovir are effective in immunodeficiency patients at reducing the duration, symptomatology and complications from an herpes infection. In resistant cases, foscarnet or acyclovir, intravenously dispensed, is the best choice. Acyclovir or famciclovir may be beneficial for the prophylaxis of secondary herpetic stomatitis, in dose and duration, depending on the degree of immunodeficiency.
- **D** No
- **E** No

Comments: As the oral lesions in immunocompromised patients are more aggressive, painful and long lasting, their treatment with antipyretics, analgesics or anesthetic agents including xylocaine in a spray or viscous gel, is a complementary of an antiviral therapy. Gamma globulin has been used for treatment of severe herpes zoster rather for simplex infections.

Q3 Which of the diseases below is/or are NOT related to previous herpes simplex infection?

- **A** Eczema herpeticum
- **B** Erythema multiforme
- **C** Herpetiform aphthae
- **D** Alzheimer's disease
- **E** Bell's palsy

Answers:

- **A** No
- **B** No
- **C** Herpetiform aphthae is a subtype of aphthous stomatitis, named because their lesions resemble primary herpes stomatitis, but differ from it in the fact that they are not preceded by vesicles and are more painful and larger in numbers, and have different pathogenesis.
- **D** No
- **E** No

Comments: Herpetic infections of peripheral the sensory nerves such as trigeminal nerves or parts of brain have been respectively associated with Bell's palsy and Alzheimer's disease. Upper respiratory infections, herpetic commonly, precede erythema multiforme lesions and eczema herpeticuml esions in patients with atopic dermatitis.

Case 12.5

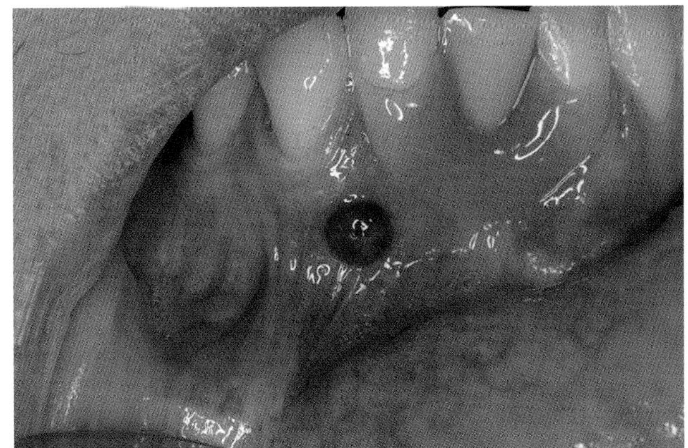

Figure 12.5

CO: A 48-year-old man presented with a hemorrhagic bulla on his anterior gingivae between the lower right lateral incisor and canine.

HPC: The lesion was first noticed by the patient and had remained at the same place, over the last four months, asymptomatic while it sometimes reduced in its size by bleeding, and became less obvious through eating.

PMH: The patient suffered from hyperlipidemia and mild hypothyroidism treated with atorvastatin and levothyroxine respectively. Blood, skin or gut disorders or allergies were not reported. He was a chronic smoker of 20 cigarettes per day.

OE: A small hemorrhagic vesicle of 3 mm max diameter was found at the attached gingivae of his lateral lower incisor and canine (Figure 12.5). Both teeth had been restored with composite fillings, but the canine did not respond to vitality tests. Although his oral hygiene was adequate, the patient had lost his ipsilateral central incisor during an accident and replaced it with a movable prosthesis. Intra-oral X-rays did not show any other teeth or jaw abnormalities. No other similar hemorrhagic lesions were noticed over his mouth, skin and other mucosae on examination day or in the past.

Q1 What is the possible diagnosis?
- **A** Gingival cyst
- **B** Thrombocytopenia
- **C** Odontogenic sinus tract
- **D** Angina bullosa hemorrhagica
- **E** Lateral periodontal cyst

Answers:
- **A** No
- **B** No
- **C** Sinus tract from the necrotic canine was the answer. The pulp necrosis gradually developed after the patient's car accident. Pulp reduce the gap inflammation induced a periapical inflammation which was finally transferred into the gingivae forming a hypertrophic sinus tract similar to a hemorrhagic vesicle.
- **D** No
- **E** No

Comments: The differential diagnosis included mainly gingival and lateral periodontal cysts. Both lesions are associated with vital teeth, but differ in the fact that the gingival cysts are exclusively located to gingivae with no serious bone involvement, while the lateral periodontal cysts are located within the alveolar bone lateral to the suspected root, and rarely perforate the bone in order to reach the adjacent gingivae. The negative medical record of serious blood dyscrasias or other hemorrhagic bullae in other parts of the mouth such as palate and tongue excludes thrombocytopenia and angina bullosa hemorrhagica from the diagnosis.

Q2 Which simple steps should a dentist do to diagnose a dental sinus?
- **A** Teeth vitality tests
- **B** Intra-oral radiographs
- **C** Biopsy of sinus
- **D** Swabs from sinus released fluid for culture
- **E** CT or MIR

Answers:
- **A** Vitality tests are always required to confirm pulp necrosis of the suspected teeth.
- **B** Inserting a gutta-percha cone in the sinus and then, by opening and pushing it until resistance, and taking X-rays, allow the clinician to clarify the sinus pathway.
- **C** No
- **D** No
- **E** No

Comments: Other techniques like swabs or biospy taken from the lesion are not regularly used and only to confirm specific bacterial infections like Actinomycoses or osteomyeltis while CT or MRI to exclude an early jaw tumor or to identify the original cause of the sinus tract.

Q3 Which other diseases are associated with dental sinuses?
- **A** Actinomycosis
- **B** Osteonecrosis due to bisphosphonates
- **C** Tuberculous osteomyelitis
- **D** Fibrous dysplasia
- **E** Acromegaly

Answers:
- **A** Actinomycosis is a bacterial infection from acid-fast anaerobic bacteria (Actinomycetes), characterized by a granulomatous inflammation and formation of multiple abscesses and sinus tracts that discharge sulfur granules that are composed of bacterial and hyaline filaments and pus cells.
- **B** Sinuses tracts are an early sign of bisphosphonate-induced osteonecrosis of jaws.
- **C** Tuberculous osteomyelitis is a very rare entity of jaws and characterized by multiple draining sinuses with minimal skin erythema and cervical lymphadenopathy.
- **D** No
- **E** No

Comments: Fibrous dysplasia (monostotic and polystotic) and acromegaly cause the proliferation of bone without signs of bony inflammation and sinus tracts formations.

Case 12.6

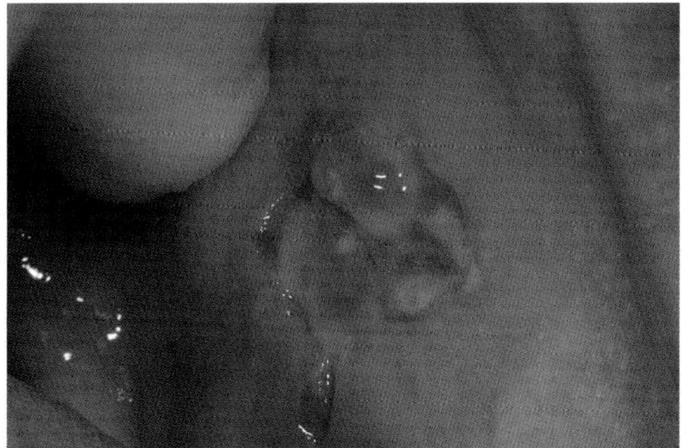

Figure 12.6a

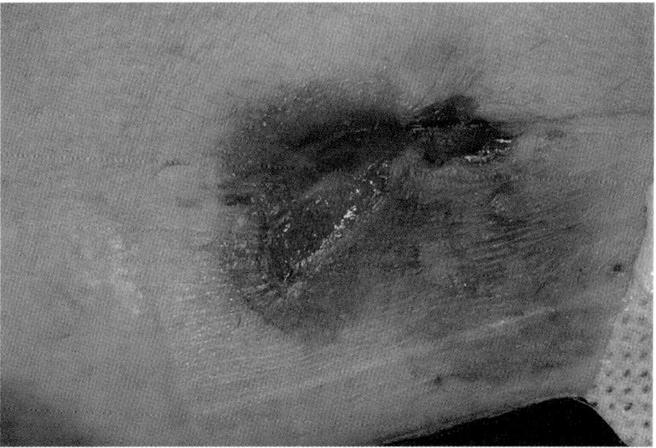

Figure 12.6b

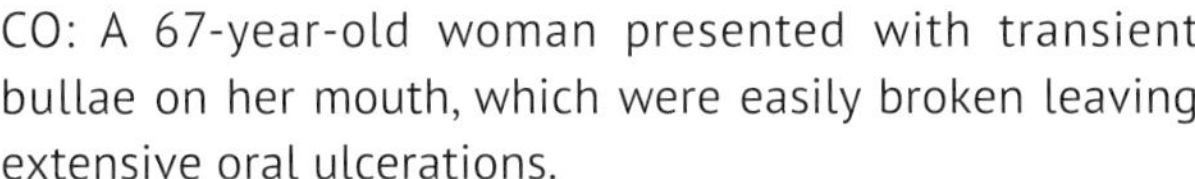

CO: A 67-year-old woman presented with transient bullae on her mouth, which were easily broken leaving extensive oral ulcerations.

HPC: Her oral ulcerations were constantly seen all over her mouth, together with skin bullae of the head, belly and legs, over the last six months. These mouth lesions had not been improved with antibiotic mouthwashes, steroids or even nystamysyn oral suspensions, but had shown a tendency for extension towards the patient's throat and floor of the mouth over the last month.

PMH: Hyperlipidemia and osteoporosis were the patient's main medical problems, which were being controlled with diet, daily walking and drugs (statins and vitamin D_3).

OE: A large superficial ulceration of her left buccal mucosa was found, (Figure 12.6a). Similar painful erosions were found on the floor of the mouth, dorsum of the tongue, and soft palate, towards the tonsillar areas and pharynx. Rubbing her normal gingivae provoked the development of a small bulla which was histologically found within the epithelium. A deep non-healing ulcer was seen on her umbilicus (Figure.12.6b) and many atrophic pigmented areas on the skin of her legs which were the result of healing of previous ulcerations.

Q1 What is the possible diagnosis?

- **A** Erythema multiforme
- **B** Cicatricial pemphigoid
- **C** Drug-induced oral ulcerations
- **D** Pemphigus vulgaris
- **E** Adamantiades-Behcet's disease

Answers:

- **A** No
- **B** No
- **C** No
- **D** Pemphigus vulgaris was the cause and is characterized by persistent painful oral ulcerations along with similar lesions on the skin and other mucosae. The ulcerations have the tendency of extending peripherally and being commonly found on the floor and roof of the mouth, skin of the head, belly, and legs. Bullae always precede the ulcerations, but are rarely kept intact on the oral mucosa as they can break easily during mastication. Systemic Steroids, at a high dose and for a long period, should be used for treatment. Untreated pemphigus vulgaris could jeopardize a patient's life.
- **E** No

Comments: The long duration of oral ulcerations, the old patient's age and the presence of fragile bullae allow clinicians to exclude Adamantiade Behcet's disease and erythema multiforme from the diagnosis, as both conditions appear at a younger age, last only a couple of weeks, and they sometimes heal without treatment. In cicatricial pemphigoid, the lesions are mainly located on the oral, eyes and genital mucosae rather than the skin, while bullae are less fragile having a thick roof which is composed of the whole epithelium while in pemphigus ithe bulla break easily as the lesion is located within the epithelium as seen in this patient.

Q2 What are the histological characteristics of pemphigus vulgaris?

- **A** Acantholysis below the stratum corneum in the epithelium
- **B** Subepithelial bulla

- **C** Basal layer intact with "row of tombstones" pattern.
- **D** IgG abs and complement C3 along the basal membrane zone at immunofluorescence
- **E** Intra-epithelial microabscess of eosinophils, plasma cells and acantholytic cells.

Answers:

- **A** No
- **B** No
- **C** Basal cells are intact and maintain their attachment to hemidesmosomes at the basal membrane zone, forming a characteristic fence line between the bulla and basement membrane zone.
- **D** No
- **E** No

Comments: In pemphigus vulgaris the bulla is intra-epithelial and mainly located at the lower part of the spinous layer, contrary to pemphigus foliaceous, which is found where the upper spinous layer and is often associated with microabscesses of eosinophils and acantholytic cells. Direct immunofluorescence shows that IgG abs are located on the cell surface of the epithelial cells in pemphigus vulgaris and along the basal membrane zone in cicatricial pemphigoid.

Q3 Intra-epithelial microabscesses are found in:

- **A** Pemphigus foliaceus
- **B** Wegener granulomatosis
- **C** Pyostomatitis vegetans
- **D** Geographic tongue
- **E** Lichen planus

Answers:

- **A** IgA pemphigus foliaceus is characterized by intra-epithelial bulla at the upper parts of the epithelium together with a number of dyskeratotic cells intermingled with neutrophils forming microabscesses.
- **B** No
- **C** Pyostomatitis vegetans is characterized histologically by intra-epithelial and/or subepithelial microabscesses of neutrophils and eosinophils combined with acantholysis and epithelial clefts.
- **D** Geographic tongue has the histological characteristics of a pustular psoriasis such as parakeratosis, acanthosis and migration of neutrophils in order to create superficial microabscesses.
- **E** No

Comments: The inflammation of chronic inflammatory cells is dense without microabscesses formation and both in lichen planus, forming a band at the upper corium, while in Wegener granulomatosis, forming granulomas deep in the corium.

Case 12.7

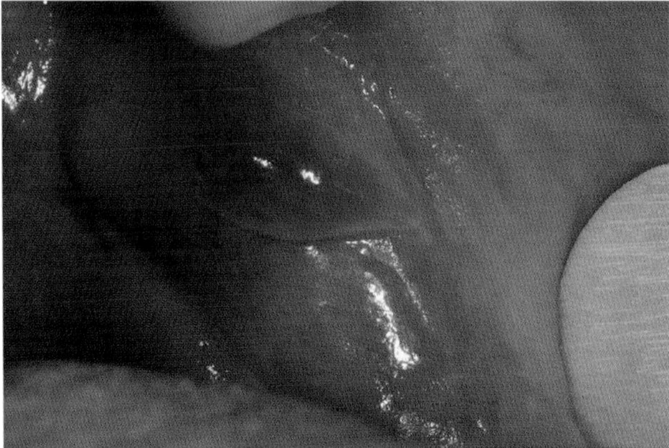

Figure 12.7a

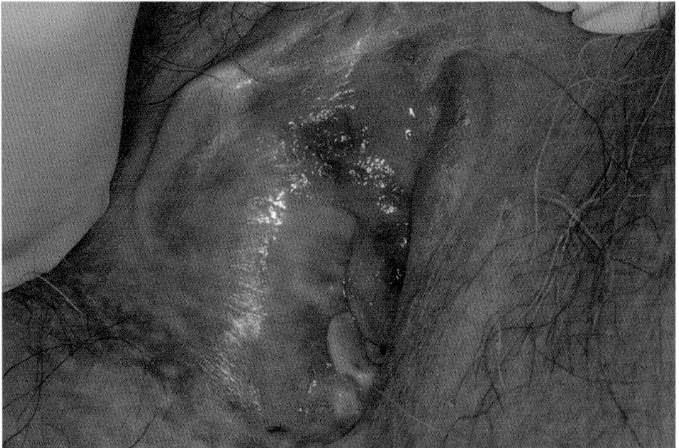

Figure 12.7b

CO: A 70-year-old woman presented with chronic ulcerations of her mouth.

HPC: The first ulcerations in her mouth appeared five years ago and disappeared without treatment in a short period, but since then, many episodes of painful ulcerations have been recorded, yet longer lasting and painful. No other members of her family have experienced similar lesions.

PMH: Her medical history revealed an episode of heart attack 10 years ago, hypertension, mild dislipidemia and diabetes II which were controlled with antihypertensive drugs and a special diet. Allergies, smoking or drinking habits were not reported. However, a recent episode of soreness on her genital area and her eyes was recorded.

OE: Multiple superficial ulcerations all over her oral mucosa with an intact bulla with clear fluid on her buccal mucosa were found (Figure 12.7a). No other lesions were noticed on the skin or other mucosae, apart from a superficial ulceration on her labia majora (Figure 12.7b) and a symblepharon in the interior formix of her left eye.

Q1 What is the possible diagnosis?

A Cicatricial pemphigoid
B Pemphigus vulgaris
C Bullous pemphigoid
D Adamantiades-Behcet's syndrome
E Syphilis (second stage)

Answers:

A Cicatricial pemphigoid or else, benign mucous membrane pemphigoid (MMP), is the cause. It is an autoimmune bullous disorder affecting mucosae such as the mouth (mainly), eyes, pharynx, larynx and genitals and less commonly, the skin. Blisters are rarely found at the oral mucosa and are finally broken with mastication leaving superficial ulcerations with a tendency of slow healing, with or without scaring.
B No
C No
D No
E No

Comments: The long duration of oral lesions, the presnce of intact bulla and their symptomatology excludes syphilis (second stage) while the patient's age and the presence of intact oral bulla exclude Adamantiades-Behcet's syndrome from the diagnosis. This syndrome has a tendency to affect young patients with characteristic aphthous-like oral lesions and eye lesions such as hypopyon, retinitis or vasculitis rather than pterygium formation. The presence of intact bullae in the patient's mouth but not on the skin, and the long course of disease without serious complications, excludes clinically other bullous diseases like pemphigus and bullous pemphigoid from diagnosis.

Q2 Which of the clinical characteristics below are hinting at mucous membrane pemphigoid?

A Intact bullae
B Ulcerations on masticatory mucosa only
C Scarring
D Prodromal symptoms
E Cervical lymphadenopathy

Answers:

A The bullae in the MMP are subepithelial and therefore, are not as fragile as they are seen in pemphigus, while sometimes, they are found intact within the oral mucosa and when they are broken, they can leave superficial painful ulcerations.
B No
C Scarring is commonly seen in chronic and severe MMP patients, hence the name cicatricial. Scarring of eyes, throat and larynx can lead to blindness, hoarseness or airway obstruction.
D No
E No

Comments: Ulcerations may be seen in any part of the oral mucosa, but especially in the gingivae, tongue, palate and buccal mucosae. These ulcerations are painful but they have no association with prodromal symptoms or cervical lymphadenopathy as seen in primary herpetic stomatitis.

Q3 What are the differences between MMP and bullous pemphigoid?

A Distribution of lesions on mucosae rather than skin
B Auto abs pattern
C Type of bullae (intra or subepithelial)
D Scarring formation
E Response in steroid treatment

Answers:

A MMP affects predominantly the oral mucosa (>80%), eyes (65%) and rarely the skin (25–30%) while on the other hand, bullous pemphigoid affects mainly the skin of the lower abdomen, upper thighs or armpits, and oral mucosa in only 30–40 per cent of cases.
B Both diseases are characterized by circulating auto abs against bullous pemphigoid Ags BP 180 and 230, but MMP has also antibodies against laminin 5, integrin a_6b_4 and type VII collagen
C No
D No
E No

Comments: Both MMP and BP are characterized as chronic subepithelial bullous diseases of autoimmune origin. Their bullae are quickly ruptured leaving superficial painful ulcerations which respond well to steroids (topical and systemic) but have a tendency of scarring.

Case 12.8

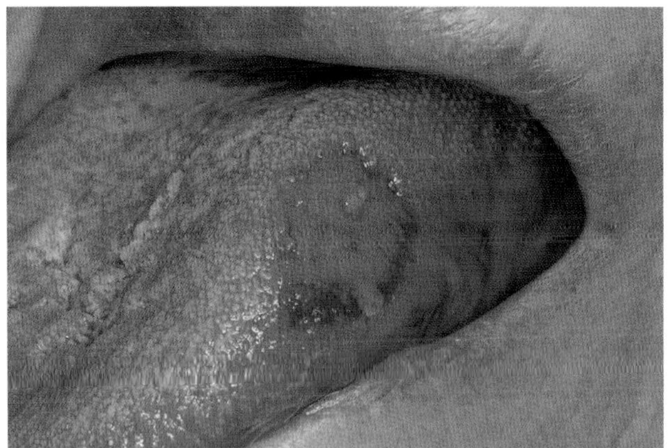

Figure 12.8a

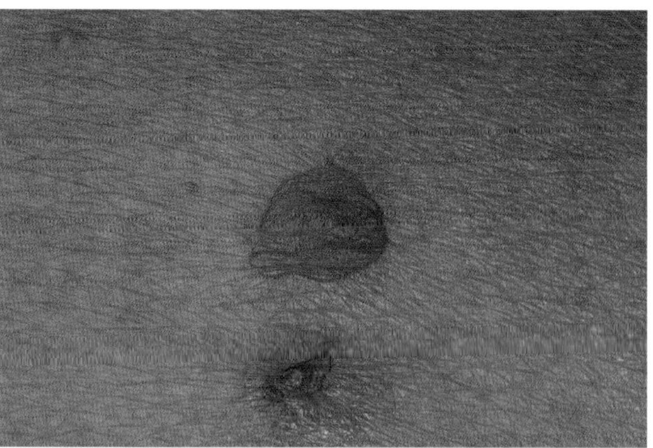

Figure 12.8b

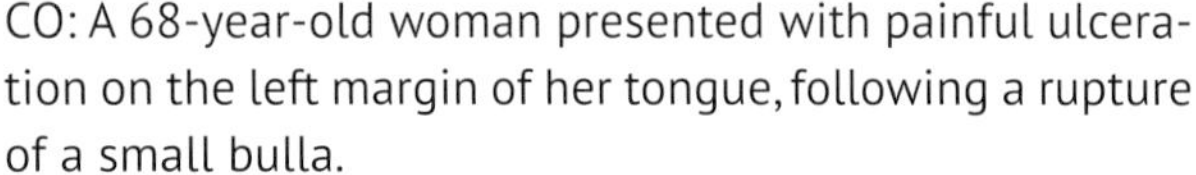

CO: A 68-year-old woman presented with painful ulceration on the left margin of her tongue, following a rupture of a small bulla.

HPC: The patient reported a few episodes of bullae formation on the skin of her abdomen and legs over the last year, being followed by pruritus alone or combined with erythematous urticarial, targetoid, lichenoid, or nodular-like lesions. Oral lesions developed together with skin lesions over the last six months, and did not respond to various antiviral or antifungal drugs. None of her close relatives had reported similar lesions.

PMH: Her medical history was clear apart from chronic osteoporosis which was controlled with Vitamin D_3 substitutes and aldronate sodium tablets; hypertension with beta blockers; and mild diabetes with a diet. In addition, over the last three years, an episode of kidney infection was recorded and treated with antibiotics while a severe herpes zoster infection on her right chest was relieved with antivirals and analgesics.

OE: The oral examination revealed an erythematous, painful ulcerated lesion on the left margin of the tongue, with an intact, small bulla at one margin (Figure 12.8a). The bulla had a clear fluid and was broken during examination. No other lesions were found apart from a vesiculobullous rash on the skin of her upper thighs and arms composed of intact or broken bullae covered with a crust (Figure 12.8b).Cervical lymphadenopathy, fever or general malaise were not recorded.

Q1 What is the possible diagnosis?

- **A** Chicken pox infection
- **B** Pemphigoid gestationis
- **C** Cicatricial pemphigoid
- **D** Pemphigus
- **E** Bullous pemphigoid

Answers:

- **A** No
- **B** No
- **C** No
- **D** No
- **E** Bullous pemphigoid is the cause. This condition affects mainly the skin and less often oral and other mucosae, and appears as multiple bullae, initially in the skin of the abdomen, upper thighs and arms and later in the mouth of patients older than 65 years old. An erythematous urticarial or psoriatic skin rash sometimes precedes the bullae formation.

Comments: Having in mind that herpes zoster virus infection requires a previous infection with varicella virus at a younger age, chicken pox infection could be easily ruled out from diagnosis as an episode of herpes zoster was diagnosed three years before his skin and mouth lesions appeared. Other pemphigoids were excluded too, such as pemphigoid gestationis, which is related to pregnancy and cicatricial pemphigoid which has a clinical preference to oral and other mucosae rather than the skin. Pemphigus lesions are more aggressive and spread out all over the body in comparison with the patient's lesions.

Q2 The differences between pemphigus vulgaris and bullous pemphigoid are found in:

- **A** Symptomatology
- **B** Distribution of lesions
- **C** Type and location of mo Abs
- **D** Location of bullae

E Course of disease in relation to serum autoantibody levels

Answers:

A No

B Both clinical entities are autoimmune diseases characterized by bullous formation which finally break, leaving superficial painful ulcerations on the oral mucosae, skin and other mucosae. In bullous pemphigoid the lesions are predominately in the skin rather than mouth while in pemphigus (>80) appear in the mouth.Intact bullaea are more often found in bullous pephigoid rather than in pemphigus.

C In pemphigus vulgaris the autoantibodies are against desmogleins (dsg 1 and 3) with dsg 3 being prominent in mucosal lesions. In bullous pemphigoid, the autoabs are against proteins of hemidesmosomes such as type XVII collagen (BP 180) and dystonin (BP 230 abs).The binding of autoabs with specific proteins causes the release of cytokines from the T cells leading to the activation of complement and recruitment of neutrophils along with the production of proteolytic enzymes which are responsible for the bullae formation.

D Intra-epithelial bullae are located in the lower part of the spinous layers and are characteristic in pemphigus vulgaris; or they appear in the upper spinous layer in pemphigus foliaceus while in pemphigoids (cicatricial or bullous are located) below the epithelium and within the upper coreum.

E The titer of serum dsg 1 and 3 correspond with the severity of pemphigus, but not with pemphigoids.

Comments: Both groups of bullous diseases (pemphigus or pemphigoids) present with painful ulcerations caused by the break of fragile bullae on oral, skin, and other mucosae.

Q3 Which of the forms below is/or are not seen in patients with bullous pemphigoid?

A Vesicullar form
B Generalized bullous form
C Pustular form
D Vegetative form
E Nodular form

Answers:

A No

B No

C Pustules are smaller than 5–10 mm lesions containing pus and seen in a number of acute skin or chronic diseases, but never seen in bullous pemphigoid.

D No

E No

Comments: The skin lesions in bullous pemphigoid can present in various forms such as (i) generalized bullous form with scattered bullae at any part of the body, mainly on flexural areas of the skin; (ii) the vesicular form with a group of small vesicles on an urticarial or erythematous base; or (iii) as nodular; and (iv) vegetative forms which are rarely seen in the axillae, groin, or neck.

Case 12.9

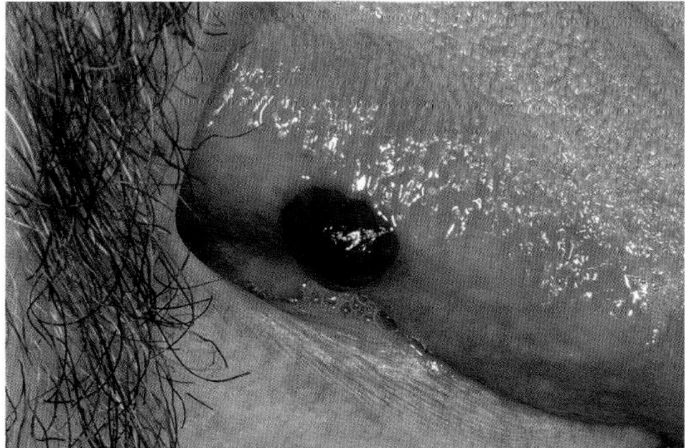

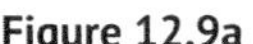

Figure 12.9a

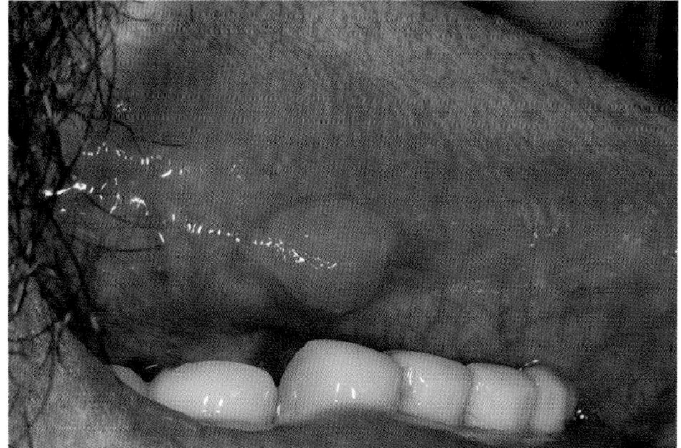

Figure 12.9b

CO: A 35-year-old man presented with a dark red bulla on the right lateral margin of his tongue.

HPC: The lesion presented last night while he was eating a meal with hot and spicy foods. None of his close relatives have a history of similar lesions.

PMH: Clear, apart from a few mild episodes of allergic asthma which were relieved with steroid inhalers. Skin and other systemic diseases or drug allergies were not reported.

OE: A large bulla of dark red-bluish color on the lateral margin of his tongue, opposite the second lower right premolar. It was asymptomatic, but was associated with two similar bullae, one on the soft palate and the other on the right buccal mucosa (Figure 12.9a). Two days later the bulla was broken during mastication leaving a superficial ulceration (Figure 12.9b). No other lesions were found on the mouth, skin or other mucosae and routine blood tests were within normal range.

Q1 What is the possible cause?

- **A** Thrombocytopenic purpura
- **B** Angina bullosa hemorrhagica
- **C** Linear IgA disease
- **D** Bullous lichen planus
- **E** Epidermolysis bullosa

Answers:

- **A** No
- **B** Angina bullosa hemorrhagica is the cause. This is a rare condition, characterized by oral mucosal blood-filled vesicles, or blisters on the soft palate, tongue, and buccal mucosae, but also on pillars of faucets, epiglottis and pharynx. It is an acute asymptomatic disease associated with trauma during food ingestion in patients with diabetes or steroid inhalers users.
- **C** No
- **D** No
- **E** No

Comments: The absence of white lesions (reticular, hyper, or atrophic) or bullae in other parts of the body excludes bullous lichen planus and linear IgA dermatoses from the diagnosis. The negative history of blood dyscracias, especially platelets, excludes thrombocytopenic purpura while the lack of bullae on the patient's extremities, rules out the epidermolysis bullosa.

Q2 Which other clinical characteristics could separate blood filled-blisters in thrombocytopenic purpura from other diseases including angina bullosa hemorrhagica?

- **A** Epistaxis
- **B** Hyperpigmentation
- **C** Ecchymoses
- **D** Gingival bleeding
- **E** Nail dystrophy

Answers:

- **A** Nose bleeding or epistaxis is a common finding of thrombocytopenic purpura, but also seen in hypertension, foreign body or neoplasms of the nose but never in angina bullosa hemorrhagica.
- **B** No
- **C** Ecchymoses or subcutaneous spots of bleeding are commonly found in patients with thrombocytopenia; coagulopathies; vascular diseases; local trauma; or drug use but never in other bullous diseases.
- **D** Gingival bleeding is a characteristic finding of periodontal diseases, bleeding disorders such as thrombocytopenia, trauma, avitaminosis and some benign and malignant tumors of the gingivae.
- **E** No

Comments: Nail dystrophies are changes in nail texture or composition caused mainly by fungal infections (>50%), trauma, congenital abnormalities or skin diseases such as lichen planus or psoriasis, but not thrombocytopenia. Hyperpigmentation is rarely seen in thrombocytopenic patients and is related with previous drugs uptake rather than disease per se.

Q3 What is the best treatment for angina bullosa hemorrhagica?

- **A** None
- **B** Steroids
- **C** Antibiotics
- **D** Imatinib
- **E** Promacta

Answers:

- **A** No treatment is needed, apart from a symptomatic relief of the discomfort, caused by the broken bulla, with chamomile or mild antiseptic mouthwash.
- **B** No
- **C** No
- **D** No
- **E** No

Comments: Steroids are used in the treatment of various bullous disorders and some forms of them (sprays) have been associated with the formation of hemorrhagic bullae in patients in angina bullosa hemorrhagica. Antibiotics, imatinib and Promacta are of no use as they are given only for the treatment of local or systemic infections, for blood disorders such as CML and ALL; and platelet production in thrombocytopenia, respectively.

Case 12.10

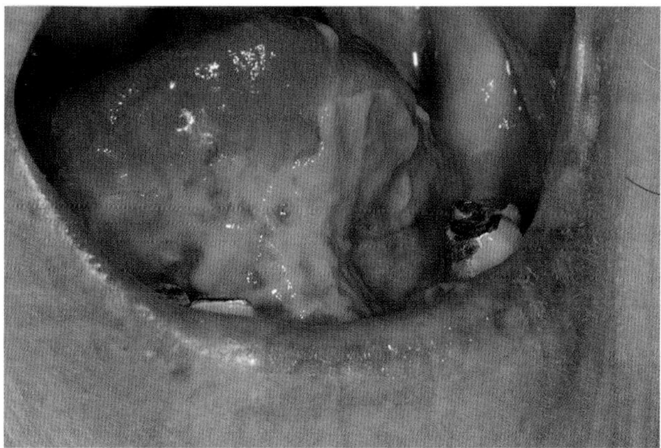

Figure 12.10

CO: A 72-year-old woman presented with extensive ulcerations on the floor of her mouth over the last two weeks, when she was taking a wide spectrum antibiotic for a deep ulcer due to thrombosis on her right leg.

HPC: A large fragile bullae preceded the ulceration and developed ten days after the beginning of antibiotic (penicillin) treatment prescribed by her surgeon for a deep leg ulcerative lesion.

PMH: Her medical history revealed a mild hypertension and diabetes insipidus which were controlled with diet and medications (ibersartan and insulin injections, respectively). No allergies or other serial diseases were recorded, apart from a deep leg thrombosis causing deep ulceration and treated with a broad spectrum antibiotics, together with anticoagulants (rivaroxaban). Smoking or drinking habits were not reported.

OE: Large painful ulcerations covered with whitish pseudomembranes were seen on the floor of the mouth (Figure 12.10), and less on the palatal and buccal mucosae. These were preceded by a large superficial bulla, together with small bullae on the skin of the face and the extremities. No nails, eyes, or genital involvement were seen.

Q1 What is the possible diagnosis?

- **A** Drug-induced bullous disease
- **B** Thermal burn
- **C** Staphylococcal scalded skin syndrome
- **D** Aphthous stomatitis
- **E** Chronic ulcerative stomatitis

Answers:

- **A** Drug-induced bullous disease is the answer. Penicillin and other antibiotics such as cephalosporins, quinolones and rifampicin can induce fragile bullae that are easily broken, leaving superficial ulcerations and erythematous scaly plaques, mainly seen on the trunk.
- **B** No
- **C** No
- **D** No
- **E** No

Comments: Although *Staphylococcus* is among the pathogenic germs that are isolated from chronic leg ulcers, *Staphylococcus* scalded skin syndrome was easily excluded, as its prodromal symptoms such as fever, malaise and irritability, were not recorded. The absent of previous similar ulcerations, erythematous halo or white lesions around the ulcerations combined with the patient's negative history of a thermal oral accident excludes aphthous, chronic ulcerative stomatitis and thermal burns from the diagnosis.

Q2 Which are the clinical indications that could indicate penicillin as the causative agent for this bullous disorder?

- **A** The onset of bullae came soon after the antibiotic intake.
- **B** The disappearance of bullae occurred immediately after the suspected antibiotic withdrawal.
- **C** The symptoms improved with antibiotic intake.
- **D** The negative patient history of previous bullous disorders.
- **E** The response of bullous disorders to steroids.

Answers:

- **A** Bullae appear after a few days of penicillin uptake and disappear after two to three weeks or more, with its attenuation.
- **B** No
- **C** No
- **D** The bullous disorders induced by drugs require a negative history of other bullous diseases in the past.
- **E** No

Comments: The bullae disappear after a few days and not immediately, as it takes some days for the circulated abs to be inactivated. The good response to steroids is observed in all autoimmune bullous disorders, and not only in drug-induced bullous disorders.

Q3 Which of the drugs below is mostly related to bullae formation?

A Steroids
B Penicillin
C Penicillamine
D Captopril
E Azathioprine

Answers:

A No
B No
C Penicillamine is widely used for the treatment of rheumatoid arthritis and its sulfhydryl (SH) groups interact with the SH parts of desmoglein 1 and 3, modifying in this way their antigenicity, which may lead to autoantibody production and bullae formation.
D No
E No

Comments: Steroids and azathioprine are widely used for treatment of various bullous diseases, whereas penicillin and captoprin may be responsible at lesser frequency than penicillamine for their induction.

13

White Lesions

White lesions are manifestations of heterogeneous groups of congenital, inflammatory, reactive, or even neoplastic diseases whose color is produced by the scattering of light through thick hyperplastic epithelium or underlying submucosa. Some of the white lesions are transient, and related to the patient's habits such as smoking, eating spicy foods or cinnamon products. Others are chronic manifestations of systemic diseases or neoplasias, and need special treatment (Figure 13.0).

Table 13 lists the most common and important oral white lesions.

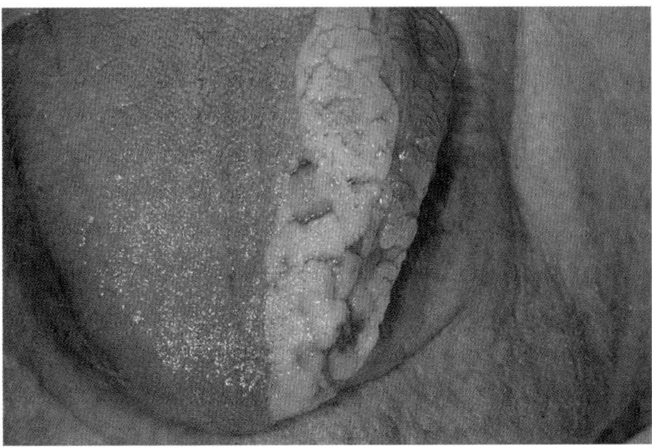

Figure 13.0 White plaque on the dorsum and lateral left margin of the tongue diagnosed as a leukoplakia.

Table 13 Common and important conditions of white lesions.

- Congenital
  - Anatomical variations
      - Fordyce spots
      - Leukodoema
  - Diseases
      - Darier's disease
      - Dyskeratosis – congenital
      - Dyskeratosis – hereditary benign intraepithelial
      - Pachonychia
      - Tylosis
      - White sponge nevus
- Acquired
  - Inflammatory
    - Infective
      - Candidosis
      - Hairy leukoplakia
      - Syphilitic leukoplakia
      - Koplic's spots
      - Papillomas
      - Uremic stomatitis
    - Traumatic
      - Frictional keratosis
      - Burns – chemicals
      - Burns – thermal
      - Scars
  - Immune-related
    - Skin
      - Lichen planus
      - Lichen sclerosus
      - Dermatomyositis
    - Gut or other organs
      - Pyostomatitis vegetans
  - Neoplastic
    - Potentially malignantss
      - Leukoplakia
    - Malignant
      - Carcinoma

Clinical Guide to Oral Diseases, First Edition. Dimitris Malamos and Crispian Scully.

Companion website: www.wiley.com/go/malamos/clinical_guide

Case 13.1

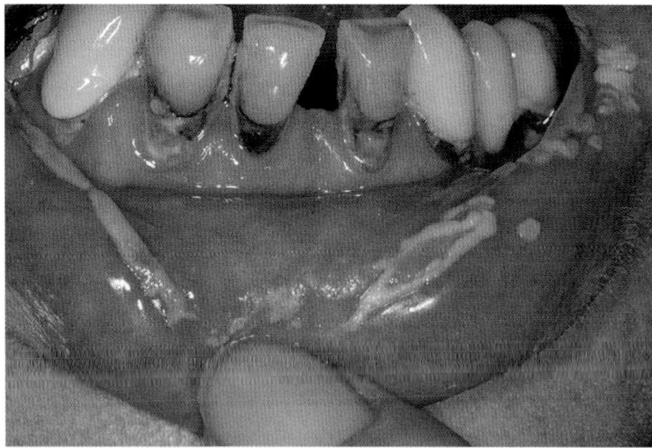

Figure 13.1

CO: A 58-year-old woman was presented with white lesions all over her mouth.

PMH: Her white lesions came together a burning sensation in her mouth plus dysphagia for one and a half week after taking a broad spectrum antibiotic for a respiratory infection.

PMH: She suffered from chronic asthma over the last five years, which had been relieved with the use of a salbutamol inhaler and corticosteroids (in crisis) and mild hypertension controlled by irbesartan 75 mg/d and moderate depression treated with mirtazapine. The patient did not have allergies and despite her lung problems she was chronic smoker (>30 cigarettes per day) for the last four decades. Over the last two weeks, she suffered from pneumonia and took antibiotics (amoxicillin and clavulanate) together with prednisolone 5 mg/os, for a short period of one week.

OE: The examination revealed white-yellow creamy plaques on her lips, tongue, buccal sulci, and soft palate that were easily removed with a wooden spatula, leaving underneath an erythematous oral mucosa (Figure 13.1). These lesions were not related with cervical or systemic lymphadenopathy, but associated with a mild burning sensation which was exacerbated with spicy foods and smoking. No other similar lesions were found in her pharynx, larynx and other part of her body. Her mouth was neglected due to poor OH and chronic periodontitis and caries in most of her remaining teeth were found.

Q1 Which is the most likely diagnosis for her white lesions?

- **A** Lichen planus
- **B** Materia alba
- **C** Candidosis
- **D** Epitheliosis
- **E** Leukoplakia

Answers:

- **A** No
- **B** No
- **C** Pseudomembranous Candosis is the cause. It is characterized by numerous white plaques that are easily removed with spatula leaving erythematous mucosa underneath.
- **D** No
- **E** No

Comments: Although White sponge nevus and lichen planus are presented with diffuse white lesions at childhood and milde age respectively both diseases are easily excluded from the diagnosis as their lesions are well fixed and not removed. Epitheliolisis has been characterized by white creamy slough, easily removable but without leaving erythematous mucosa underneath, while material alba differs from the patient's lesions as is less organized and composed of mixture of food debris, salivary proteins, dessquamative epithelial cells and bacteria located predominantly at the gumline and not scatterd in the mouth.

Q2 Which of the laboratory investigations below is/or are most likely diagnostically helpful?

- **A** Chest X-ray
- **B** Swab/culture
- **C** Biochemical tests
- **D** Oral biopsy
- **E** Pathergy test

Answers:

- **A** No
- **B** Culture from material taken with swabs from the suspected lesions demonstrates the presence of *Candida* hyphae.
- **C** No
- **D** *Candida albicans* hyphae are shown as bright red filaments with special stains like Periodic acid-Shift (PAS), within the superficial epithelial layers.
- **E** No

Comments: Oropharyngeal candidosis is a very common fungal infection is characterized the disease of diseases and its diagnosis is based on clinical characteristics and confirmed by the detection of Candida hyphae in cultures rather than biopsies. Other investigations like chest-X rays and Pathergy test provide irrelevant information about lungs and Bechet's diseases.

Q3 Which other diseases could be possibly affect the treatment for candidosis?

- **A** Atrial fibrillation
- **B** Hashimoto thyroiditis
- **C** Gout
- **D** Rickets
- **E** Hyperlipidemia

Answers:

- **A** The use of certain antifungal drugs may be problematic in patients taken warfarin anticoagulant drug for atrial fibrilation and stroke prevention as increase the action of the anticoagulant.
- **B** No
- **C** No
- **D** No
- **E** Hyperlipidemia is treated with various statins the metabolism of which takes place via the cytochrome P450 pathway. This pathway is inhibited with drugs; among them, antibiotics (macrolidia) and antifungals (azoles). Thefore, the use of various azoles require the temporal withdrawn of various statins at the period of antifungal therapy.

Comments: Hashimoto thyroiditis, gout and rickets are different diseases, but their clinical manifestations or treatments do not interfere with antifungal treatment.

Case 13.2

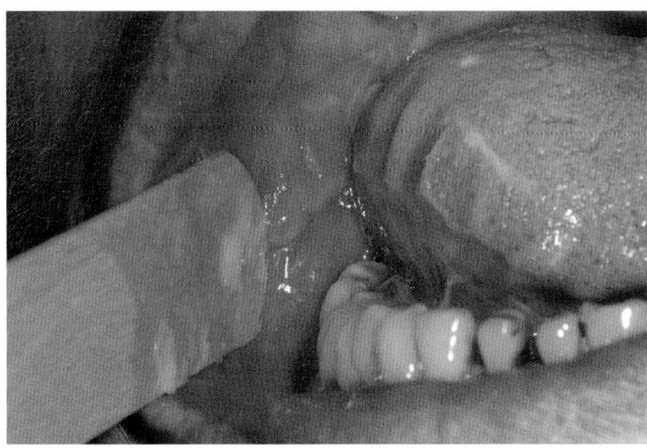

Figure 13.2

CO: A 32-year-old man presented for an oral examination as he was afraid he had caught an sexually transmitted disease (STD) three weeks ago.

HPC: He was finicky about his oral hygiene and breath, by using strong mouthwashes and cinnamon chewing gum on a regular basis, and he had an STD phobia, despite the fact that he was married and had never involved with extramarital sex.

PMH: He had no serious health problems apart from allergic rhinitis, and used to take antihistamine tablets and nasal spray in crisis. He was not a heavy smoker (up to four cigarettes per day) and drinker (up to three glasses of wine per week).

OE: His examination revealed multiple whitish sloughs which were easily removed with friction; with a spatula from his buccal mucosae-sulci and inner surface of both lips, leaving normal mucosa underneath (Figure 13.2). No other lesions were found in his mouth, his skin or genitals as well as lymph nodes (locally or systemically). Due to his phobia the patient used mouthwashes with strong alcohol flavor many times per day to eliminate oral microflora hoping to reduce the risk of STD disease .

Q1 What is the likely diagnosis?

- **A** Cinnamon-induced stomatitis
- **B** Gonorrhea
- **C** Candidiasis
- **D** Epitheliolysis
- **E** Allergic stomatitis

Answers:

- **A** No
- **B** No
- **C** No
- **D** Epitheliolysis or also known as mucosa peeling, is the sloughing of the oral mucosa due to the daily use of strong irritants such as mouthwashes, spices and extremely hot food, drinks with high alcohol content or caustic toothpastes. This is a clinical sign and not a disease.
- **E** No

Comments: Other diseases like Cinnamon-induced stomatitis, candidiasis and allergic stomatitis are presented with a burning sensation and other symptoms and signs apart from sloughing and therefore are excluded from the diagnosis. Gonorrhea is a sexually transmitted disease, usually seen in the genitals rather than the mouth, and its oral manifestation includes diffuse erythema and multiple painful superficial ulcerations, but these features were not seen in this man.

Q2 What type of cells are usually found in the smear of the epitheliolysis slough?

- **A** Epithelial cells
- **B** Inflammatory cells
- **C** Fibroblasts
- **D** *Candida* hyphae
- **E** Tzanck cells

Answers:

- **A** The smear is composed of various epithelial cells from various superficial layers.
- **B** Inflammatory cells are commonly seen and intermingled with epithelial cells.
- **C** No
- **D** Candida Albicans and various other germs are often found in the slough
- **E** No

Comments: Tzank cells are ballooning epithelial cells that are characteristically found in a viral induced lesion and not in epitheliolysis.. Fibroblast are rarely seen as the smear procedure is undergone with mild handling procedures leaving therefore intact most of the epithelial layers and the underlying submucosa

Q3 Which of the diseases below show epitheliolysis?

- **A** Lichen planus
- **B** Candidiasis
- **C** Irradiated squamous oral carcinoma
- **D** Stevens-Johnson syndrome
- **E** Darier disease

Answers:

- **A** No
- **B** No
- **C** It is commonly seen in patients receiving radio/and or chemotherapies for head and neck cancer
- **D** It is easily diagnosed as a part of toxic epidermal necrolysis (Lyell syndrome).
- **E** No

Comments: Epitheliolysis is also found in Darier disease, but there, additional histological features are shown such as grains in the stratum corneum, and corps ronds in the granular layer, acanthosis and papillomatosis, as well as heavy infiltration of lymphocytes in the upper corium. Lichen planus is characterized by hypertrophy or combination of atrophy and hypertrophy of mucosa, and candidiasis shows *Candida* hyphae and accumulation of inflammatory cells with the upper epithelium, but both diseases do not show epitheliolysis.

Case 13.3

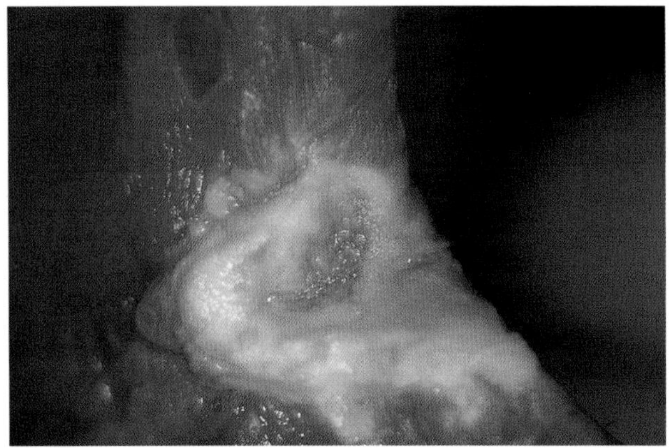

Figure 13.3

CO: A 42-year-old man presented for an evaluation of asymptomatic white plaques at the inner surfaces of both his commissures.

HPC: The white plaques had been present over last two years, and discovered accidentally by his dentist, but had remained unchanged since then.

PMH: He is a handworker with no serious medical problems apart from a fatty liver due to his heavily drinking habits that caused him increased liver enzymes (serum glutamic oxaloacetic transaminase [SGOT] and glutamic pyruvic transaminase [SGPT]). Early diabetes type 2 was diagnosed recently, partially controlled by diet. His diabetes was suspected from chronic fungal infections in his penis, and his polyuria/polydipsia symptoms over the last three months. Other skin problems or cervical lymphadenopathy or known allergies were not reported.

OE: The examination revealed thick white-yellow plaques that were fixed in the buccal mucosae near the commissures (Figure 13.3). These plaques are in some places hyperplastic and soft in palpation but were not removed with scratching or associated with other oral and skin lesions. The patient had full dentition that was heavily restored due to his poor oral hygiene.

Q1 What is the likely diagnosis?

- **A** Lichen planus (hypertrophic type)
- **B** Leukoplakia (simple)
- **C** Angular cheilitis
- **D** Candidiasis (hypertrophic)
- **E** Carcinoma

Answers:

- **A** No
- **B** No
- **C** No

D Hypertrophic candidiasis is a chronic form of fungal infection and appears usually as thick, whitish plaques almost fixed with the inflamed mucosa in patients with immuno-deficiencies or serious diseases like diabetes.
E No

Comments: The location of the lesion in the inner surfaceof buccl mucosae and not at the corners of patient's mouth easily excludes angular cheilitis from the diagnosis. The lack of other similar lesions inside patients's mouth and skin or other mucose rules out lichen planus while the differential diagnosis of leukoplakia and oral carcinoma from chronic hyperplastic candidosis require histological examination.

Q2 Which of the histological characteristics below are commonly seen in hypertrophic candidiasis?
A *Candida* hyphae in the supra-basal layers
B Hyperplasic oral epithelium
C Chronic inflammatory cells within the corium
D Basal cell degeneration
E Civatte bodies

Answers:
A No
B The epithelium is hyperplastic due to acanthosis and/or parakeratosis and appears clinically as thick white plaque at a distance from the small blood vessels of the underlying corium.
C No
D No
E No

Comments: Hyperplastic candidiasis or candida leukoplakia is a chronic fungal infection which shares some clinical characteristics with the simple leukoplakia such as its color or location, but differs from it regarding the presence of *Candida* hyphae in the superficial layers of the epithelium which cause chronic inflammation in the epithelium and corium. This lesion has a good response with various antifungals, and a higher tendency for malignancy. Basal cell degeneration and civatte bodies are characteristic of lichen planus, accumulation of inflammatory cells in the corium is a common finding in a great number of dermatoses apart from *Candida* leukoplakia.

Q3 Which syndromes are associated with hyperplastic candidiasis?
A Autoimmune polyglandular syndrome
B Asperger syndrome
C Chronic muco-cutaneous syndrome
D Down syndrome
E Cushing syndrome

Answers:
A The autoimmune polyglandular syndrome (type I) is a heterogeneous group of autoimmune diseases affecting more than one of endocrine glands that usually causes hypoparathyroidism, primary adrenal insufficiency, and chronic hyperplastic candidiasis.
B No
C This is characterized by a heterogeneous group of chronic fungal infections affecting the mouth, other mucosae and skin.
D No
E No

Comments: Syndromes like Asperger (difficulties in social activities)) Down (presence of all or part of the third copy or 21 chromosome) and Cushing syndrome (elevated cortisol levels) have an increased risk of opportunistic infections especially from Candida species. However, these infections are usually mild and respond well to antifungal and rarely deep or chronic.

Case 13.4

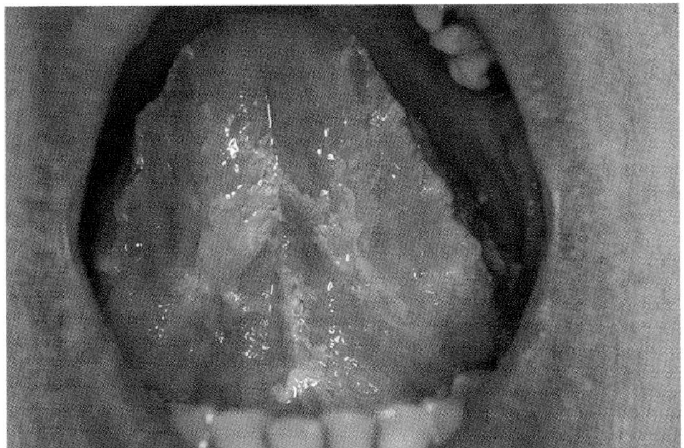

Figure 13.4

CO: A 35-year-old woman presented for evaluation of white lesions all over her mouth for the last two months.

HPC: The lesions appeared gradually initially on her tongue, and later on buccal mucosae and were associated with uremic halitosis and a burning sensation.

PMH: She had suffered from severe hypertension over the last two years due to her chronic glomerulonephritis, and took an angiotensin converting enzyme inhibitor and Vitamin D3 drugs. She was a non-smoker and not a heavy drinker, but used to rinse her mouth with various mouthwashes on a regular basis.

OE: The oral examination revealed white plaque-like fixed lesions especially on the dorsum and the ventral surface of her tongue that were not resolved with topical nystatin oral suspensions, associated with a burning sensation despite of her good OH and dysgeusia (Figure 13.4). Bad (uremic) breath was also noted. Her OH was adequate. No other similar lesions were found in other mucosae.

Q1 What is the likely diagnosis?

- **A** Stomatitis induced from mouthwash overuse
- **B** White sponge nevus
- **C** Friction keratosis
- **D** Uremic stomatitis
- **E** Hairy leukoplakia

Answers:

- **A** No
- **B** No
- **C** No
- **D** Uremic stomatitis appears in patients with severe renal failure (chronic renal failure [CRF]: creatinine >4 mg/dl) as multiple superficial ulcerations or fixed whitish plaques resembling leukoplakias and being associated with a burning sensation, uremic breath and pruritus. Uremic stomatitis is a rare complication of longstanding uremia in CRF patients. This may be considered as a chemical burn from ammonia which is released by the action of bacterial ureases into the salivary urea. There are four types of stomatitis: (i) ulcerative; (ii) hemorrhagic; (iii) non-ulcerative pseudomembranous; and (iv) the hyperkeratotic form as the last observed in this patient.
- **E** No

Comments: The location of the white lesions in areas unrelated to friction and absence of similar lesions at a younger age excludes friction keratosis and white sponge nevus from the diagnosis. Hairy leukoplakia is located mainly in the lateral rather the dorsum of the tongue and related to immunodeficiencies and not with renal failure. Stomatitis from overuse of mouthwash comes with white lesions which are easily detached (epitheliolisis) and not fixed as seen in this patient.

Q2 Which is the best treatment?

- **A** Renal dialysis
- **B** Steroids
- **C** Mouth washes containing hyperoxide
- **D** Multi-vitamins
- **E** Interferon

Answers:

- **A** Renal dialysis is required when the creatinine is over 4 mg/dl and/or glomerular filtration rate (GFR) falls below 20–25 ml/min. The oral lesions disappear over the next month after dialysis begins.
- **B** No
- **C** The use of hyperoxide mouth-wash improves the oral lesions by releasing O_2 and making an environment that is unfavorable to anaerobic bacteria, which are responsible for the ammonia production and bad breath.
- **D** No
- **E** No

Comments: Some drugs like interferon, vitamins or steroids act in different ways that are unrelated to kidney function and therefore are not used for treatment of uremic stomatitis.

Q3 Which are the cutaneous manifestations of chronic renal failure?

- **A** Skin pigmentation
- **B** Atrophy
- **C** Calciphylaxis
- **D** Nail changes
- **E** Alopecia

Answers:

- **A** The dark skin is characteristic in patiens with CRF due to the accumulation of urochromes and hemosiderin.
- **B** No
- **C** Calciphylaxis affects mainly the lower extremities, of CRF patients and characterized by multiple vascular calcifications and skin necrosis.
- **D** Nails seem to show frequent changes such as melanonychia, Beau's lines, hyperkeratosis or onychodystrophies.
- **E** No

Comments: Skin or mucosal atrophy and alopecia are features unrelated to kidney dysfunctions.

Case 13.5

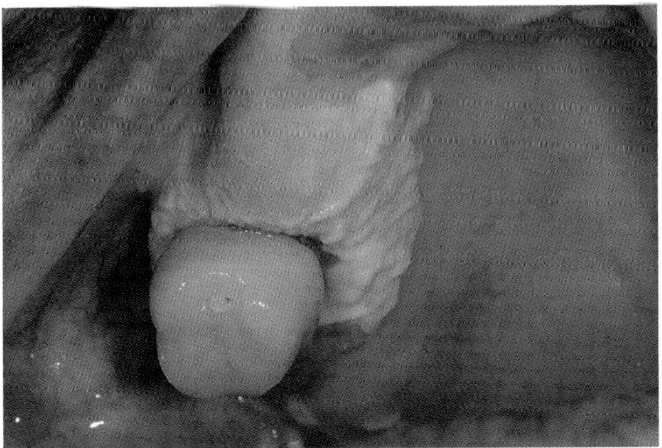

Figure 13.5

CO: A 67-year-old woman presented for an evaluation of a white lesion in her palate.

HPC: The white lesion was first noticed during a routine dental examination by her GDP for a replacement of her old upper partial denture.

PMH: She had suffered from allergic asthma since childhood and was on salbutamol and beclomethasone inhalers during crisis. She had been on a special diet to control her hyperlipidemia and hypertension, but had never been a smoker or drinker.

OE: The oral examination revealed a thick rough with furrows white plaque around the gingivae of the upper right second molar. The plaque was thick in places of friction with the clasps of an old upper denture of good stability and was extended into the buccal sulcus and hard palate (Figure 13.5). It was also asymptomatic and not associated with other lesions intra- or extra-orally.

Q1 What is the likely diagnosis?

- **A** Nicotinic stomatitis
- **B** Mucosal graft
- **C** Acute candidosis
- **D** Amelanotic melanoma
- **E** Leukoplakia

Answers:

- **A** No
- **B** No
- **C** No
- **D** No
- **E** Leukoplakia is a white patch that may not be scraped off or characterized clinically or pathologically to any other known diseases. Oral leukoplakias appear as uniform white patches (homogeneous), as white excrescences (nodular) or as a combination of white flecks on atrophic erythematous lesions (speckled). Prognosis varies, as the risk for malignant transformation varies from 5 per cent and even more with minimum potential for malignancy has been recorded in the homogeneous while the maximum in the speckled type of leukoplakia. In leukoplakia factors such as clinical characteristics, histological findings of dysplasia, biomarkers expression such as Ki-67; tumor suppressor p53, retinoblastoma (pRb) or cyclin D proteins have been used successfully as predictive markers for its possible malignant transformation.

Comments: Other oral white lesions are included in the differential diagnosis of leukoplakia such as pseudomembranous candidosis, grafts, nicotic stomatitis and even amelanotic melanoma. However, the long duration of the lesion and its failure to be removed with spatula excludes pseudomembrane Candidosis while the negative history of smoking or having previous surgery in the area rules out nicotinic stomatitis and grafts from the diagnosis. Amelanotic melanoma is presented as an irregular mass or plaque mainly in the palate with variable color (from whitish to normal), with rapid growth and presence of satelite lesions and cervical lymphadenopathy' features not seen in this lady.

Q2 Which of the histological features below are NOT seen in leukoplakias?

- **A** Acantholysis
- **B** Parakeratosis
- **C** Loss of basal cell polarity
- **D** Abnormal mitosis
- **E** Dense zone of chronic inflammatory cells in the lamina propria

Answers:

- **A** Acantholysis is the term given for the loss of intercellular connections i.e. desmosomes resulting in loss of cohesion between keratinocytes. It is a characteristic finding in pemphigus, erythema multiforme and herpetic infections.
- **B** No
- **C** No
- **D** No

E Inflammation is a common finding in lamina propria of leukoplakia but is scattered and in some places perivascular and not arranged in dense zones as seen in other white lesions such as lichen planus.

Q3 Which of the diseases below is/or are associated with leukoplakia?
- **A** Heck disease
- **B** Congenital dyskeratosis
- **C** Xeroderma pigmentosum
- **D** Hereditary hemorrhagic telangiectasias
- **E** Albright syndrome

Answers:
- **A** No
- **B** Dyskeratosis congenita is also called as Zinsser-Cole-Engmann syndrome and is characterized by abnormal skin pigmentation, nail dystrophy, and oral leukoplakias.
- **C** No
- **D** No
- **E** No

Comments: The clinical characteristics of the other diseases do not include leukoplakia as in Heck disease multiple white-pinkish hyperplastic papules or nodules and not plaques, in xeroderma pigmentosum basal cell carcinomas together with skin lesions with increased tendency of carcinoma transformation; in hereditary hemorrhagic telangiectasias vascular malformations, and in Albright syndrome fibrous dysplasia and café au lait skin lesions are found.

Case 13.6

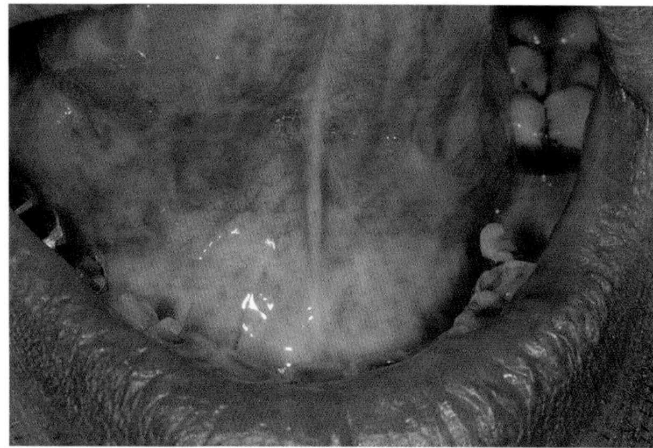

Figure 13.6

CO: A 32-year-old man presented with a burning sensation, mouth dryness and stiffness over the last year.

PMH: He was a thin, healthy man without serious medical problems or allergies. Given the fact that he comes from Southern Asia, he never drinks alcohol but has the habit of chewing pan masala and gutka betel mixture daily. His family history is clear apart from a tongue carcinoma in his brother two years ago.

OE: The oral examination revealed multiple diffused whitish plaques in the soft palate, buccal and sublingual submucosa (Figure 13.6) causing difficulties in his tongue or uvula movement. A few superficial ulcerations that were provoked by xerostomia and the consumption of hard spicy foods were noted in the inner surface of his lower lip. His teeth were heavily restored with amalgam fillings and had an external dark brown discoloration especially in the area where gutka betel chewing occurred.

Q1 What is the likely diagnosis?
- **A** Sublingual keratosis
- **B** Submucous-sublingual-fibrosis
- **C** Mucosal scarring
- **D** Mucosal tattoo
- **E** Leukedema

Answers:
- **A** No
- **B** Submucous fibrosis is a potentially malignant disorder characterized by juxta-epithelial inflammation and fibrosis of submucosa causing restrictions of movement The submucous fibrosis has four histological stages: (i) the very early (stage I) which is characterized by a finely fibrillary collagen with marked edema consisting of some congested blood vessels and inflammation in lamina propria of polymorphs and eosinophils; (ii) as seen in this patient early stage (stage II) showing early hyalinization; (iii) moderate (stage III) with moderate hyalinization and numerous constricted vessels; and (iv) late (stage IV) where the collagen is completely hyalinized, devoid of fibroblasts and with completely obstructed blood vessels.
- **C** No
- **D** No
- **E** No

Comments: In sublingual keratosis, the lesions are superficial, within the epithelium and not deep into the lamina propria and connective tissue while in leukedema disappeared with stretching. Mucosal tattoo or scarring are easily excluded, as their lesion is more restricted and a history of having tatoo or trauma was not reported in this patient.

Q2 Which of the diseases below are considered as premalignant conditions?

A Erythroplakia
B Syphilis
C Leukoplakia
D Paterson-Kelly syndrome
E Candidiasis

Answers:

A No
B Syphilitic leukoplakia is a rare manifestation of tertiary syphilis, and appears as white plaque on the dorsum of the tongue with an increased risk for oral cancer. A local inflammation from a *Treponema* infection in association with other causative factors such as malnutrition, alcohol or tobacco use often seen in these neglected patients has been implicated in malignant transformation of oral carcinomas.
C No
D Iron deficiencies have been associated with oral and pharyngeal cancer, especially in women of northern latitudes as carcinogenicity of iron has been clearly shown in animals models and in human experiments. It seems that iron deficiencies are associated with increased oxidative stress and increased risk of oral cancer.
E *Candida* leukoplakia seems to have a high potential for malignancy as the fungus may participate In initiation of carcinogenesis by; a) metabolizing various external pro-carcinogens and b) by modifying the oral -micro-environment and inducing chronic inflammation.

Comments: Leukoplakia and erythroplakia are premalig nant lesions and not conditions and considered to have the highest risk of malignant transformation.

Q3 Which is the key treatment for oral submucous fibrosis?

A Cessation of chewing habit
B Steroids
C Placental extracts
D Hyaluronidase
E Interferon gamma

Answers:

A Cessation of chewing habits of pan masala and gutka helps to stop the local irritation of various carcinogens arising from the betel mixture to the oral mucosa.
B No
C No
D No
E Submucosal injections with interferon (IFN) have a high anti-fibrotic action and may reverse submucuous fibrosis lesions.

Comments: Hyaluronidase and placental extracts have minimal effects, while steroids can be given to relieve the symptoms and accelerate the healing of superficial ulcerations in severe submucous fibrosis cases only.

Case 13.7

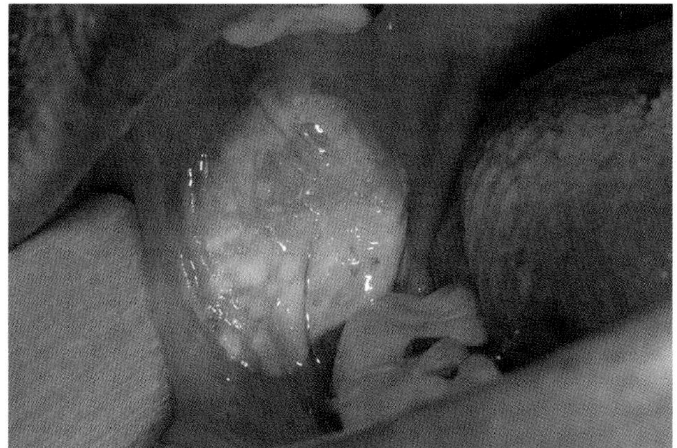

Figure 13.7

CO: A 46-year-old man presented with white lesions in his mouth over the last sixmonths.

PMH: He suffered from mild hypertension and allergic rhinitis and had a predisposition for diabetes which was controlled only with diet. He was found to have hepatitis B antibodies, but with had no serious liver problems.

OE: White lesions of different size and shape were found in his buccal mucosa, dorsum and lateral margins of the tongue, inner surface of the lower lip and in the gingivae of the upper molars. Some lesions forme a fine network at the periphery and others had an atrophic-ulcerated center, while a few formed plaques as seen here (Figure 13.7). These lesions were associated with an itchy rash in the skin, penis as well as the scrotum, which appeared two months later from his oral lesions.

Q1 What is the likely diagnosis?
- **A** Aphtha major
- **B** Lichen planus
- **C** Burn
- **D** Graft
- **E** Condyloma lata

Answers:
- **A** No
- **B** Oral lichen planus is a chronic mucocutaneous disease which is characterized by white lesions with a reticular network at the periphery, atrophy-ulcerations or even fixed thick plaques similar to those seen in this patient. The oral lesions are often associated with genital similar lesions, skin pruritic rash and/or nail involvement like nail atrophy; longitudinal ridging and fissuring, distal splitting and trachyonychia.
- **C** No
- **D** No
- **E** No

Comments: Other oral lesions share similar clinical picture regarding of the color and shape with the patient's lesion. White slough is also seen coverlying aphthaes, burns and condyloma lata but in contrary to the patient is easily removable leaving an erythematous area underneath. Graft is well fixed into the tissues but is easily excluded as this is not associated with other white oral and skin lesions or with previous surgery.

Q2 Which of the diagnostic tools is/are NOT useful for lichen planus?
- **A** Biopsy
- **B** Culture
- **C** Diascope
- **D** Skin patch test
- **E** Wood's lamp examination

Answers:
- **A** No
- **B** No
- **C** Diascope is used to distinguish whether a skin lesion is vascular, nevus or hemorrhagic by applying pressure with a glass slide on the lesion and observing color changes.
- **D** No
- **E** Wood's lamp examination is helpful for examination of pigmented and not pigmented skin lesions, teeth discoloration in erythropoietic purpura and detection of fungi as well as other skin parasites.

Comments: Biopsy is useful to exclude this skin disease from other chronic diseases including malignancy while culture is to isolate pathogenic germs capable to alter the clinical picture of the lesion while skin patch test to identify possible allergens responsible for lichenoid reactions' lesions with great similarities with patient's lesion.

Q3 Civatte bodies are diagnostic findings in histological sections from:
- **A** Lichen planus
- **B** Dermatitis herpetiformis
- **C** Discoid lupus erythematosus
- **D** Bullous pemphigoid
- **E** Graft-versus-host skin disease (GVHSD)

Answers:
- **A** Civatte bodies are numerous in lichen planus, where the inflammation is prominent, and appear as round eosinophilic PAS+ve, masses from apoptotic epithelial cells in the deeper parts of epithelium.
- **B** No
- **C** Apoptotic epithelial cells are also found in discoid erythematous lupus forming clusters in the upper part of epidermis.
- **D** No
- **E** No

Comments: GVHSDs, bullous pemphigoid and dermatitis herpetiformis are three different diseases with distinct etiopathogenesis, but with common skin and oral vesiculobullous lesions. These diseases share some histological characteristics such as vacuolar degeneration, dyskeratotic epithelial cells and diffuse inflammatory infiltration but not Civatte bodies formation.

Case 13.8

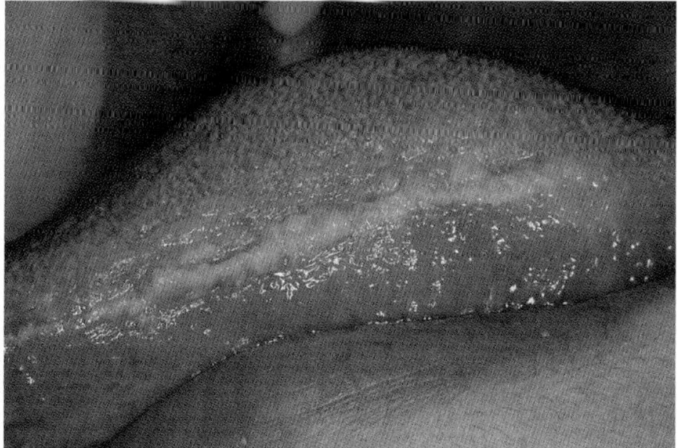

Figure 13.8

CO: A 21-year-old student presented with white lesions on the lateral margins of her tongue and buccal mucosae.

HPC: The lesions were found accidentally by her dentist during an examination for the removal of her upper right wisdom teeth.

PMH: This young patient had no serious health problems apart from common acne for which she was under antibiotics such as minocycline (50 mg/d) and topical use of benzyl peroxide gel 2 per cent. She had no known allergies, smoking or drinking habits apart from chewing her tongue and buccal mucosae. This habit was more intense during her final exams at the University. None of her close relatives had similar lesions.

OE: Thick white-yellowish linear like plaques on the lateral margins of her tongue (Figure 13.8) and buccal mucosae were partially removed with a wooden spatula, leaving a slightly irritated, itching, and burning oral mucosa. The lesions on the tongue are associated in some places with atrophy or elongation of the tongue papillae, while the buccal lesions were prominent and rough at the occlusion level. No other similar lesions were recorded in other mucosae.

Q1 What is the likely diagnosis?

- **A** Candidiasis
- **B** Lichen planus
- **C** Uremic stomatitis
- **D** White sponge nevus
- **E** Frictional keratosis

Answers:

- **A** No
- **B** No
- **C** No
- **D** No
- **E** This keratosis is a benign hyperplasia of oral mucosa as the result of a chronic and constant irritation – friction of the mucosa against sharp teeth or prosthesis.

Comments: Other diseases appear with similar to patients;s lesion but easily excluded based on the young age, the good health of the patient and lack of other similar lesions in her body or among her close relatives. Specifically, uremic stomatitis lesions and Candidosis are common in patients with serious medical problems while white sponge nevus and lichen planus have similar white lesions but with different age of onset' at childhood for nevus and adulthood for lichen planus.

Q2 Which information is the MOST useful for the clinicians to confirm the aetiology of this condition?

- **A** History
- **B** Clinical characteristics
- **C** Histopathology report
- **D** Culture results
- **E** Blood results

Answers:

- **A** Clinicians can easily diagnose this condition, having in mind the patient's habit of chewing her oral mucosae and negative family history of other familiar diseases such as white sponge nevus.
- **B** No
- **C** No
- **D** No
- **E** No

Comments: Clinical characteristics like location, color, fixation of the lesion help more than blood or culture results to differentiate this reactive keratosis from other white lesions and define thus its etiology

Q3 Which other conditions show frictional keratosis?

- **A** Lesch Nyhan syndrome
- **B** Epilepsy
- **C** Familial dysautonomia
- **D** Palmaris et plantaris keratosis
- **E** Munchausen syndrome

Answers:

- **A** Lesch Nyhan syndrome is an inherited disorder caused by a deficiency of the enzyme hypoxanthine-quanine phosphorylotransferase causing neurological disturbances such as hypotonia, dystonia and uncontrolled self-injuring (tongue biting).
- **B** No

C Familial dysautonomia is characterized by various abnormalities of the autonomic nerve system causing involuntary tongue movements that provoke friction keratosis lesions at its lateral margins.

D Papillon Lefèvre syndrome, also known as palmaris et plantaris keratosis, is a rare disease that is characterized by the development of scaly plaques in the soles and palms, and is associated with early periodontitis causing an early loss of deciduous and permanent teeth, oral keratosis and nail dystrophies.

E No

Comments: Epilepsy and Munchausen syndrome are characterized by traumatic ulcerations rather than frictional keratosis induced by unconscious or deliberate mucosa biting respectively.

Case 13.9

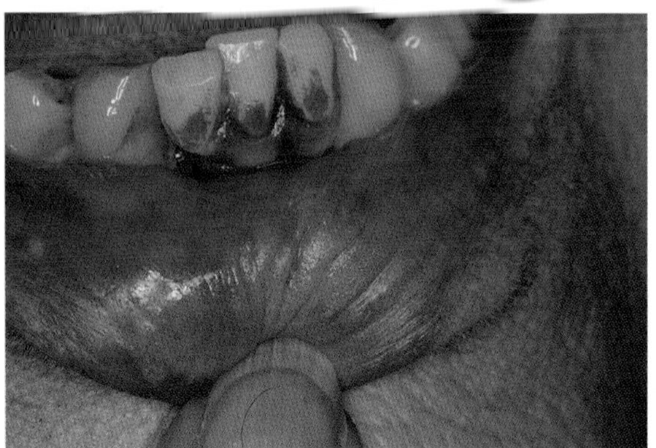

Figure 13.9

CO: A 46-year-old woman presented to check on white superficial lesions of her lips.

HPC: Her lesions seem to have appeared at the same period when the patient changed her tobacco use, and associated with a burning sensation on his mouth over the last year.

PMH: Her medical history included hyperlipidemia and chronic respiratory failure due to asbestos in her lungs due to her chronic dust exposure at work. She had been a chronic smoker and never drinker since the age of 20.

OE: The examination revealed white, fixed, superficial plaque, mostly on the inner surface of her lower lip (Figure 13.9), floor of the mouth and palate, which was exacerbated by smoking and associated with yellow discoloration of her lower anterior teeth.

Q1 Which is the possibly diagnosis?

A Lichen planus
B Tobacco keratosis
C Leukedema
D Thermal burn
E Submucous fibrosis

Answers:

A No

B Tobacco or smoker's keratosis is the diagnosis. This appears as superficial but irregular white plaques caused by a chronic irritation and inflammation of the oral mucosa, especially of the lips, floor of the mouth or palate from tobacco use. These lesions are produced by the combined action of the released heat during smoking, with the various tobacco products and/or carcinogens into the oral mucosa.

C No

D No

E No

Comments: Although tobacco is the main cause of keratosis and submucous fibrosis, their pathogenesis and clinical manifestations differ from each other. In tobacco keratosis, the changes are superficial and mainly within the epithelium (hyperplasia without dysplasia) while in submucous fibrosis they are deep within the fibrous stroma of the submucosa (fibrosis) where other etiological factors such spicy foods may contribute to it as well. Lichen planus causes white lesions, but with striated lines at the periphery while thermal burn causes an acute painful ulceration covered with necrotic slough, and leukoedema appears as a white diffuse lesion which disappears with stretching.

Q2 Which other oral lesions may often be seen in a patient with tobacco keratosis?

A Black hairy tongue
B Aphthae
C Teeth staining
D Periodontal problems
E Xerostomia

Answers:

A Smoking induces hypertrophy and elongation of filiform papillae that together with nicotinic staining and dark colored germs is responsible for the black hairy tongue.

B No

C The teeth staining induced by tobacco is external and is mainly located in the rough areas of the tooth surfaces, and can be easily removed with scaling and tooth polishing.

D Periodontal diseases such as gingivitis or periodontitis are more common in smokers than non-smokers, due to their low blood circulation locally (capillary vasoconstriction) and due to a defective immune response (reduced function of various inflammatory cells) against the gingival plaque.

E Xerostomia is a common finding and was put down to the reduced salivary flow, the released heat during smoking, and diminished fluid consumption that are often seen in heavy smokers and drinkers.

Comments: Smoking makes the oral mucosa stronger to traumatic stimuli, and this could be an explanation as to why the frequency of aphthae is lower in smokers than non-smoking patients.

Q3 Which of the body functions below are influenced by tobacco use?

A Accelerated wound healing
B Increased melanin production
C Reduced salivary flow
D Reinforced taste or smell
E Antifungal activity

Answers:

A No

B In smokers' melanosis the melanocytes that are located in the lower part of the epithelium and appear like coffee beans in histological sections. When are stimulated produce melanin, the basic element of this melanosis.

C Tobacco seems to reduce salivary flow rate causing xerostomia that leads increased cervical caries, gingival problems and halitosis.

D No

E No

Comments: The type and frequency of tobacco induced oral lesions, are mainly dependent on the type of tobacco use (conventional, reverse and smokeless tobacco), its duration alone or in combination with other risk factors such as alcohol and poor diet. All forms of tobacco accelerate the growth of pathogenic bacteria and fungi due to the reduced saliva cleansing effect and local immunity (vasoconstriction and presence lazy inflammatory cells). The local vasoconstriction may play a role in the delay of wound healing, while smoking destroys the taste and smell receptors by increasing their apoptosis.

Case 13.10

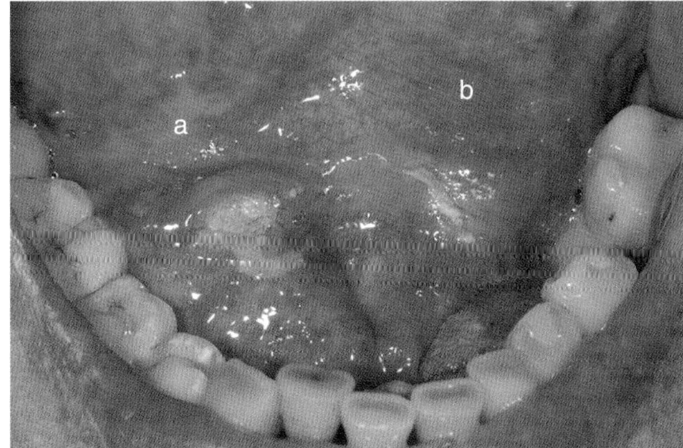

Figure 13.10

CO: A 67-year-old woman was referred by her GDP for evaluation of two white plaques in the floor of her mouth.

HPC: The lesions were discovered accidentally by the patient one month ago and had remained unchanged since then.

PMH: The patient had a clear medical history apart from a mild osteoporosis and was on Vitamin D3 supplements on a regular weekly basis. She had been a chronic smoker (<10 cigarettes/day) since the age of 17 but never an alcohol drinker.

OE: The examination revealed only two white lesions in the floor of the mouth on the other side of her lingual frenulum and above the ducts of submandibular glands (Figure 13.10). The white lesion which was located close to the right lower premolars first molars was indurated in palpation and had slight raised margins with a verrucous surface (lesion a) while the other lesion was a superficial, smooth one, located opposite the left second premolar (lesion b). Extra-orally, one lymph node was palpable, hard and fixed at the right site of the neck in front of the upper sternocleidomastoid muscle.

Q1 What is the possible clinical diagnosis for the lesions a and b?

A Carcinoma
B Leukoplakia
C Lichen planus
D Syphilis
E Psoriasis

Answers:

A Lesion a is a carcinoma with possible neck metastasis and characterized by indurated, well demarcated white ulcerated lesion with max diameter of 1,5 cm with papillary surface.

B Lesion b is a leukoplakia (sublingual keratosis). Both lesions are strongly related with the patient's smoking. Biopsy is mandatory to provide information about the presence of dysplasia or not (lesion b) and the degree of tumor differentiation and possible metastases as well (lesion a).

C No

D No

E No

Comments: The lack of other oral and skin lesions rules out lichen planus and psoriasis from diagnosis. Condyloma lata are superficial lesions without a velvety surface or indurated base as seen in this woman, and are therefore excluded.

Q2 Which of the clinical characteristics of a leukoplakia are suggestive of malignancy?

A Size

B Location

C Color intensity

D Symptomatology

E Consistency

Answers:

A A size of $\geq$ 4 cm showed to be significant predicting factor of malignant transformation in many leukoplakias as the bigger their size the more chance to be dysplastic.

B Lesions on the floor of the mouth and retromolar area have a higher risk of a malignant transformation.

C The presence of red lesions alone or mixed with the white lesions is more suspicious for malignancy than plain white lesions.

D No

E White lesions fixed into their surrounding tissues causing difficulties in movement or being hard in palpation, are suspicious.

Comments: Carcinomas or dysplastic white lesions can be presented regardless of their size or symptomatology, as symptoms appear in advanced lesions only where local nerves are compressed or invaded or secondary infection follows.

Q3 Which of the histological types of an oral carcinoma has the BEST prognosis?

A Well differentiated oral squamous cell carcinoma

B Poorly differentiated oral squamous cell carcinoma

C Basaloid oral squamous cell carcinoma

D Spindle cell oral adenocarcinoma

E Verrucous oral carcinoma

Answers:

A No

B No

C No

D No

E Verrucous oral carcinoma is characterized as a white cauliflower exophytic growth with the best prognosis, as it is composed of very well-differentiated stratified epithelium with bulbous rete ridges, consisting of minimal atypia and intact or discontinuous basement membrane.

Comments: The preference site of different histological types of oral carcinomas varies. Spindle cell and poorly differentiated carcinomas have a worse prognosis than basaloid and well-differentiated ones. The tongue and floor of the mouth are common in conventional (well, intermediate and poorly differentiated) carcinomas; the buccal mucosa and hard palate in verrucous carcinoma; while the base of tongue and floor of the mouth, are sites for the basaloid oral carcinomas.

14

Yellow Lesions

Yellow lesions are manifestations of a heterogeneous group of diseases such as developmental, metabolic, infections, or even cysts and neoplasms (benign or malignant). The yellow color is the common finding of all these diseases which appear as diffuse macular lesions (jaundice, carotenemia); papular lesions (Fordyce spots, lipoproteinemia and amyloidosis); hypertrophies (yellow hairy tongue), pustular (untreated ulcerative colitis); cysts (dermoid, lymphoepithelial) and neoplasm (lipoma/fibrolipoma/liposarcoma) (See Figure 14.0).

The Table 14 shows the most common conditions with yellow lesions.

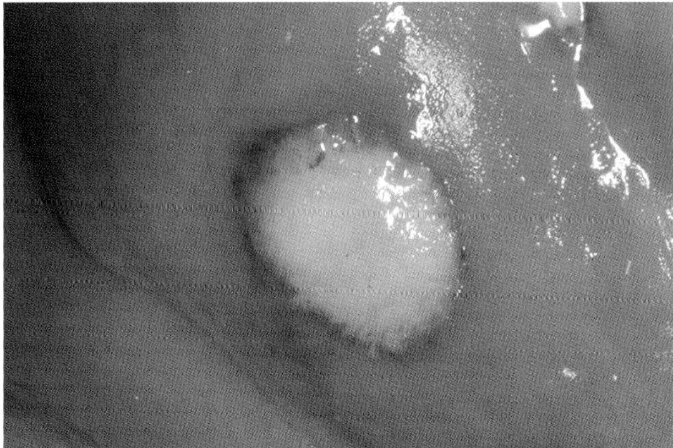

Figure 14.0 Aphtha.

Table 14 Common and important conditions of yellow lesions.

- Congenital
  - Localized
    - Fordyce spots
  - Diffused
    - Jaundice due to hemoglobulinopathies
- Acquired
  - Localized
    - Neoplasms
      - Benign
        - Lipoma
        - Xanthoma
      - Malignant
        - Liposarcoma
    - Cysts
      - Dermoid
      - Epidermoid
      - Lymphoepithelial
    - Immune-related
      - Aphthae
    - Infections
      - Pyostomatitis vegetans
    - Reactive
      - Yellow hairy tongue
  - Diffused
    - Pigment deposits
      - Jaundice due to liver diseases
      - Amyloid due to amyloidosis
      - Carotene due to carotinemia
    - Drug-induced
      - Bismuth containing

Clinical Guide to Oral Diseases, First Edition. Dimitris Malamos and Crispian Scully.

Companion website: www.wiley.com/go/malamos/clinical_guide

Case 14.1

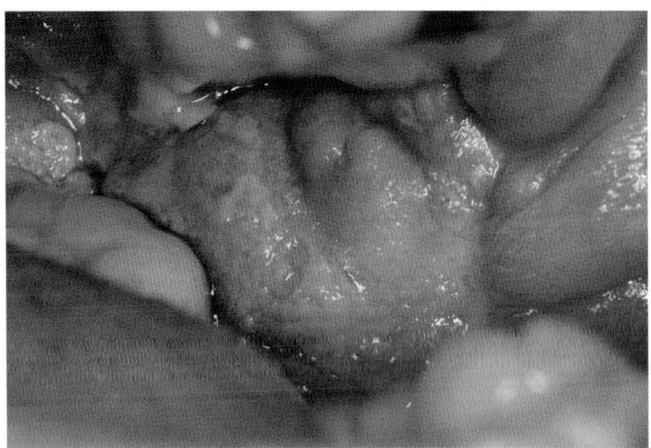

Figure 14.1

CO: A 67-year-old man was referred by his oncologist for oral examination after a course of radio-chemotherapy.

HPC: He had a large carcinoma of his left tonsil-pillar area which was surgically removed and replaced by a skin graft two months ago. He continued a course of radio-chemotherapy which ended three weeks ago.

PMH: His medical history revealed only hypertension and prostate hyperplasia controlled with drugs, while the cysts in his right kidney were under observation only.

OE: Intraoral examination revealed erythematous oral mucosa with healing superficial ulcerations, xerostomia, and reduced mouth opening. The area of his surgery was partially lobulated with normal color, apart from a large area at left retromolar and tonsillar pillar area which had smooth surface with yellow color and was asymptomatic (Figure 14.1). No other similar lesions were recorded in his mouth, skin, or other mucosae and his MRI did show complete tumor disappearance.

Q1 What is the yellow lesion in his mouth?

- **A** Radiation-induced fibrosis
- **B** Buccal fat
- **C** Healing mucositis
- **D** Carcinoma
- **E** Skin graft

Answers:

- **A** No
- **B** No
- **C** No
- **D** No
- **E** Skin graft was the answer. This graft was taken from the inner side of his arm and contained epidermis, dermis and submucosal fat, and therefore had a different color (yellow-whitish) from the rest of his oral mucosa.

Comments: Oral lesions with yellow color may be manifestation of various malignant lesions like carcinomas, or attributed to their treatment complications, such as radiation induced fibrosis and mucositis -oral ulcerations covered with yellow slough and to grafts, covering mucosal defects after surgery. Radiation-induced fibrosis appears as thick strings rather than plaque. Excessive buccal fat is present in both buccal mucosae of fat people, and differs from the brown fat of babies whose accumulation of fat is mainly on the upper half, part of the spine towards the shoulders However, yellow-white fat is not the case as the patient was very cachectic due to his previous radio-chemotherpy and did, not have, a new metastasis as his recent MRI was negative.

Q2 Which was the type of graft used in this patient?

- **A** Partial thickness graft
- **B** Local graft
- **C** Distant graft
- **D** Full thickness graft
- **E** Free graft

Answers:

- **A** Partial thickness graft was used for reconstruction of the missing part of his oral mucosa after surgery.
- **B** No
- **C** The graft was taken from the inner surface of his skin, distant to his mouth.
- **D** No
- **E** No

Comments: The missing part in his mouth was extensive and therefore could not be repaired with full thickness grafts as these can be used for small defects only. Local flaps or free grafts could also not be used, as they were not available in such large donor areas adjacent to the recipient site where the vascularirity was impaired, due to previous radiation, and microvascular surgery was not involved.

Q3 Which of the flaps below are commonly used for oral mucosa and NOT for lower jaw repair?

- **A** Buccal or fat flap
- **B** Nasolabial flap
- **C** Facial artery musculo-mucosal flap
- **D** Fibular flap
- **E** Scapular flap

Answers:

- **A** Buccal or fat flap is the commonest flap used for reconstruction of buccal mucosa/oropharyngeal; retromolar and soft palate defects.

B Nasolabial flap is used for anterior maxilla, floor of the mouth and oro-nasal defects
C Facial-artery musculo-mucosal flap is used for the anterior maxilla and foot of the mouth and lips.
D No
E No

Comments: Fibular and scapular flaps are used for mandible reconstruction.

Case 14.2

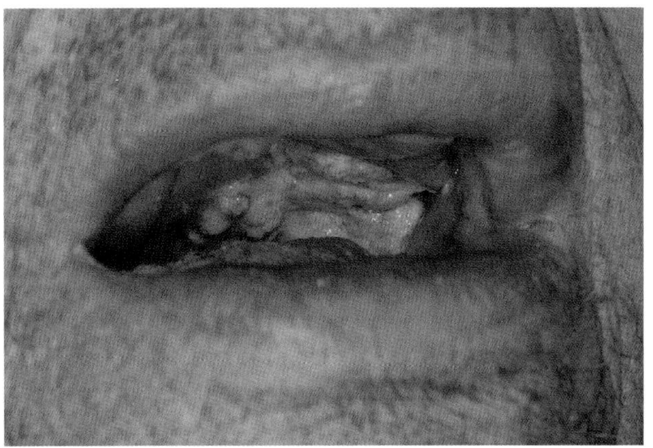

Figure 14.2a

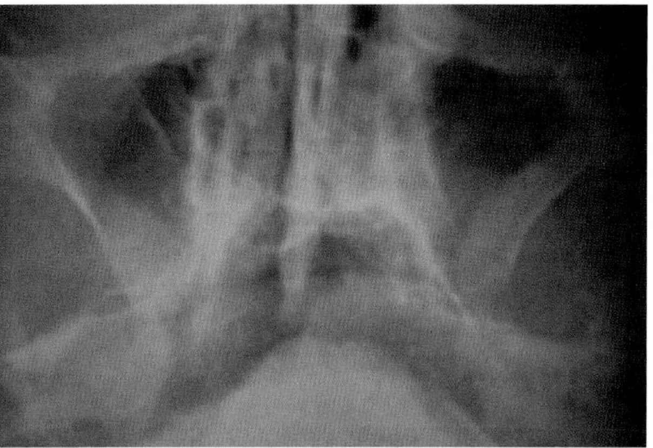

Figure 14.2b

CO: A 69-year-old man was referred for a yellow indurate lesion on his palate.

HPC: The lesion had been present for over six months, asymptomatic at the beginning but had been causing him trismus, pain and eating problems over the last two months.

PMH: He suffered from hypertension and was under ACE inhibitors, and diabetes type II controlled with diet and metformin daily. Nose bleeding was reported and associated with antral congestion which was not improved with a course of antibiotics. He was a heavy smoker and drank two to three bottles of beer with his meals daily.

OE: A large yellowish plaque with irregular margins extended from half of his palate (hard and soft) and extended to the left pillars and ipsilateral part of the oropharynx was (Figure 14.2a). The lesion was well fixed in the underlying mucosa and in some places was hard while in other soft, and bled easily with touch. Limited mouth opening was recorded (8 mm maximum) and a sharp pain appeared durinp patient's attempt to open his mouth.

No other oral lesions were found apart from a white irrigated white plaque (sublingual keratosis) in his neglected mouth and a large fixed submandibular lymph node was detected. Nose bleeding was not seen on examination, but sinus X-rays revealed thickness of the left antral mucosa (Figure 14.2b). A smear instead of biopsy was taken due to limited opening and examination under microscopy revealed numerous squamous neoplasmatic hyperchromatic epithelial cells mixed with chronic inflammatory cells, but fungi and eososinophils were absent.

Q1 What is the cause?
A Oral carcinoma
B Antral carcinoma
C Eosinophilic granuloma
D Bacterial chronic sinusitis
E Deep mucosis

Answers:
A Oral carcinoma often involves the palate and can enter into the ipsilateral antrum, causing nose congestion and bleeding, local pain and trismus and sometimes results in cervical metastases.
B No
C No
D No
E No

Comments: The absence of ciliated epithelial cells on smear test and irregular antral anatomy as seen in sinus X-rays excludes sinal neoplasia, while the failure to responsed to a course of antibiotics ruled out bacterial sinusitis from the diagnosis. The absence of fungi or a plethora of eosinophils excluded a deep fungal infection like mucormycosis and eosinophilic granuloma from the diagnosis respectively.

Q2 Which other destructive diseases apart from carcinomas affect the palate?

A Syphilis tertiary
B Tuberculosis
C Middle line granuloma
D Lymphomas
E Actinomycosis

Answers:

A Syphilitic gumma is a proliferative, indurated lesion due to vasculitis (arteritis obliterans) induced by Treponima pallidum resulting in local necrosis leading to palatal necrosis.
B Primary tuberculosis of the hard palate is a rare manifestation of life-threatening mycobacterial infection, and is presented as an irregular ulceration with slough surface and usually followed a lung TB infection.
C Lethal middle line granuloma is a midfacial necrotizing lesion causing rhinorrhea, epistaxis, nasal stiffness and obstruction.
D Extranodal lymphomas are rarely seen in the palate and appear as large painless ulcerated lesions alone or part of disseminated disease.
E Actinomycosis is a chronic infection induced by *Actinomyces* species causing granulomatous ulcerated lesions with numerous sulfur granulomas.

Q3 What are the main predisposing factors for antral mucormycosis?

A Diabetes mellitus
B Hay fever
C Malnutrition
D Viral sinusitis
E Osteomyelitis

Answers:

A Uncontrolled diabetes mellitus comes usually with with ketoacidosis and is one of predisposing factors for mucormycosis as *Rhizopus oryzae* organisms produce ketoreductase which can utilize a patient's ketone bodies.
B No
C Malnutrition reduces patient's immune system causing him vulnerable to severe infections including mucormycosis.
D No
E No

Comments: Bacterial or viral Infections in the jaws or sinuses and allergic reactions in patients with a good immune system do not allow mucormycosis spores to germinate into the oral and nasal mucosa and establish infection. In contrary, malignancies like leukemiae or lymphomas), severe diseases like AIDS. renal failure needing kidney and ,other organ transplantation requiring longterm steroid treatment, or immunosuppressants, are common predisposing factors, for antral mucormycosis.

Case 14.3

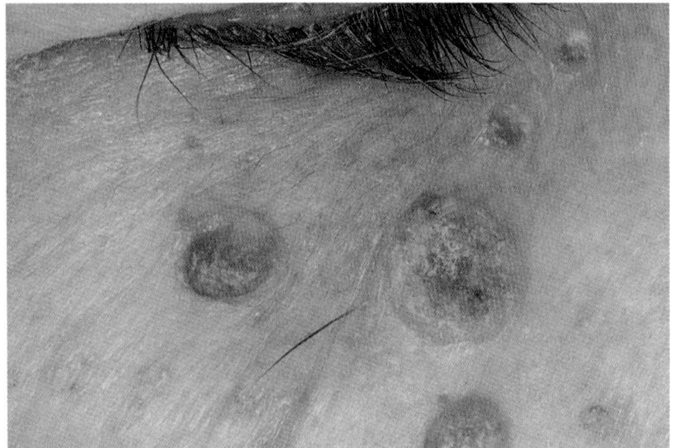

Figure 14.3

CO: A 58-year-old woman presented with multiple yellow nodulo-ulcerated lesions on her face.

HPC: The lesions were scattered on her checks and started initially as a small asymptomatic growth on the skin of her right nostril four years ago.

PMH: Her medical history was unremarkable apart from a chronic dermatitis induced by chronic exposure to solar radiation due to her work in fields. Allergies or drug use or habits like smoking or drinking were not recorded.

OE: Extra-oral examination revealed multiple yellow round nodules with central ulceration on both her checks (Figure 14.3). The lesions were asymptomatic, of various size but well fixed on the facial skin and associated with mild actinic cheilitis. No other skin or oral lesions were found.

Q1 What are the skin lesions?

A Actinic keratosis
B Keratoacanthoma
C Basal cell carcinoma
D Molluscum contagiosum
E Seborrhoeic dermatitis

Answers:

A No
B No

C Basal cell carcinoma is the most common cancer of the skin and appears as small nodule with central ulceration (nodular type); with brown or black spots (pigmented type); flat or slightly depressed (fibrosing or sclerotic type); and scaly or red spots (superficial type). This carcinoma is closely related to chronic patient's exposure to solar radiation due to her work in fields.
D No
E No

Comments: The lack of other skin lesions excludes actinic keratosis and seborrhoeic dermatitis, while the presence of multiple lesions excludes clinically keratoacanthoma from diagnosis. Molluscum contagiosum can also present with numerous bumps with a central depression, but its lesions are smaller and associated with itchy sensations not seen in this lady. The final diagnosis of the above lesions must be based on histological characteristics only. Basal cell carcinomas are characterized as, basaloid epithelial tumor of cells with mild atypia, keratoacanthomas with the pushing tongue -pike epidermal growths into dermis and a center keratin plug while the molluscum contagiosum by the presence of abundant Henderson-Peterson eosinophilic inclusion borders. Dermal elastosis is characteristic of actinic keratosis and psoriasiform hyperplasia of sebarrhoic dermatosis.

Q2 Which of the parameters below differentiate psoriatic lesions from these superficial skin lesions?
A Location
B Distribution
C Symptomatology
D Relation to solar radiation
E Response to conventional therapy

Answers:
A Psoriatic plaques are commonly seen on the extensor surface of the skin and rare on the face, while basal cell carcinomas are often seen on the face and sun-exposed skin areas.
B Basal cell carcinomas are usually single district lesions, while psoriatic lesions are multiple in a symmetrical pattern.
C Psoriaris is usually associated with itching, while superficial basal cell carcinomas are asymptomatic.
D Solar radiation exposure induces basal cell carcinoma formation, but improves psoriatic skin lesions.
F Psoriatic lesions respond well with conventional therapies (topical emollients, salicylic acids and steroids and UV light), but basal carcinomas do not.

Q3 Which of the skin diseases below has/have an increased risk of this tumor development?
A Xeroderma pigmentosus
B Gorlin syndrome
C Albinism
D Darier's disease
E Psoriasis

Answers:
A Xeroderma pigmentosum is a rare autosomal recessive photosensitive disorder with impaired ability to repair DNA damage induced by UV radiation, and with increased risk of development skin tumors such as basal cell and squamous cell carcinomas or melanomas.
B Gorlin syndrome is characterized by numerous nevoid basal cell carcinomas at adolescence or early adulthood, associated with keratocystic odontogenic tumors, heart fibromas and medulloblastomas, and sometimes with rib and skull abnormalities.
C Oculocutaneous albinism is an autosomal recessive disorder of melanocyte differentiation, and predisposes to facial skin cancers including basal and squamous carcinomas.
D No
E Psoriasis seems to have a higher risk of basal cell carcinomas among patients with a fair complexion, exposure to coal tar and solar radiation.

Comments: Darrier's disease is autosomal dominantly genodermatosis characterized by keratotic papules on face, scalp, chest and back and has not shown any link with basal cell carcinogenesis.

Case 14.4

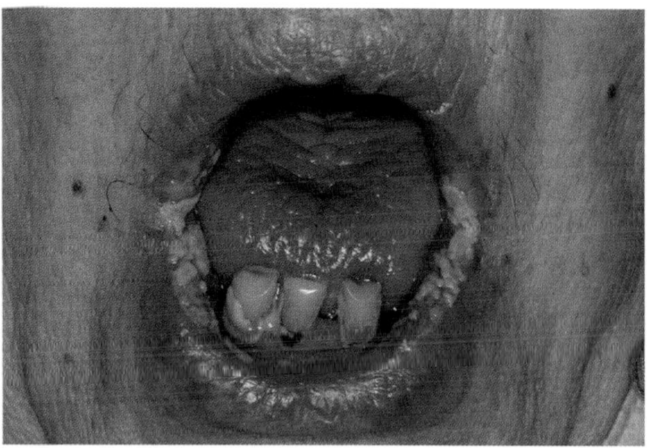

Figure 14.4

CO: A 72-year-old woman presented with yellow pseudomembranous plaques on the corners of her mouth.

HPC: The lesions began one week after a course of antibiotics taken for an episode of pneumonia.

PMH: Uncontrolled diabetes mellitus and chronic bronchitis were the only serious diseases reported. Heavy smoking of two packets of cigarettes daily since the age of 20 was reported, and her diet was poor in vegetables and fruits, but rich in meat and sweets despite her high blood sugar levels.

OE: Oral examination revealed extensive yellowish creamy lesions on both commissures. The lesions were easily detached with a wooden spatula leaving superficial ulcerations and erythema underneath, while her oral mucosa and especially the dorsum of her tongue was extremely erythematous but not atrophic (Figure 14.4) and associated with a burning sensation and a mild difficulty in swallowing. No other oral lesions were recorded while cervical lymphadenopathy was absent. Her oral hygiene was poor and she wore old, badly fitting dentures.

Q1 What is the cause?

- **A** Drug-induced candidiasis
- **B** Avitaminosis
- **C** AIDS
- **D** Diabetes
- **E** Iron deficiency anemia

Answers:

- **A** Previous use of antibiotics were the cause of her pseudomembranous at the commissures and oral mucosa.
- **B** No
- **C** No
- **D** No
- **E** No

Comments: Iron deficiency anemia, diabetes and avitaminoses cause chronic angular infection, associated with atrophic glossitis, xerostomia, and oral ulcerations respectively, and therefore these diseases were easily excluded from the diagnosis as the patient's lesions appeared one week after of course of antibiotics.

Q2 Which of the lesions below are NOT associated with *Candida* infection?

- **A** Angular cheilitis
- **B** Denture-induced stomatitis
- **C** Median rhomboid glossitis
- **D** Geographic tongue
- **E** Linear gingival erythema

Answers:

- **A** No
- **B** No
- **C** No
- **D** Geographic tongue is an inflammatory condition of the tongue with unknown etiology and characterized by focal depapillation of the dorsum of the tongue, forming circles which change over time like geographic maps.
- **E** No

Comments: *Candida* species have been implicated in the pathogenesis of inflammation of the corners of mouth (angular cheilitis) underneath dentures (denture-induced), middle of the tongue (rhomboid glossitis) or even along the gingival margins of HIV patients (linear gingival erythema).

Q3 What are the suspected mechanisms by which antibiotics increase the hazard of candidiasis?

- **A** Overgrowth of *Candida* species
- **B** Local destruction
- **C** Conversion of *Candida* to a more invasive form
- **D** Changes in saliva pH
- **E** Changes in host response

Answers:

- **A** The overgrowth of *Candida* species is commonly seen in vitro and in vivo by competing other pathogenic germs, which are destroyed by antibiotics.
- **B** Local destruction may help the entrance and growth of *Candida* into the tissues.
- **C** The antibiotics may select among *Candida* species those which are more invasive to local tissues.
- **D** No
- **E** Antibiotics may alter the host response by reduction of antibody synthesis and phagocytic activity.

Comments: The changes of pH in gastric juices rather than in saliva seem to be an important factor for germ colonization and growth.

Case 14.5

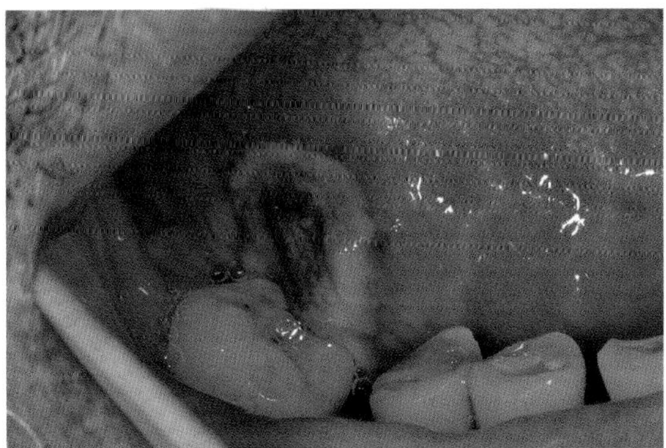

Figure 14.5

CO: A 46-year-old man came with a painful yellow lesion on the right lateral margin of his tongue.

HPC: The lesion appeared four days ago after an episode of tongue biting during a meal with lobster.

PMH: His medical history was unremarkable as no serious diseases or allergies were recorded. Lifestyle habits included smoking of two packets of cigarettes daily since the age of eighteen.

OE: A large superficial, round, well-defined soft lesion on the lateral surface of his tongue opposite his first right lower molar was found (Figure 14.5). The lesion was covered with yellow brown slough which was easily removed leaving a hemorrhagic painful ulceration associated with difficulties in eating and swallowing. No other lesions on his oral mucosa were seen on the day of examination or in the past. Cervical lymphadenopathy or other mucosae lesions were not detected.

Q1 What is the lesion?

- **A** Oral carcinoma
- **B** Major aphtha
- **C** Traumatic ulcer
- **D** Tuberculous ulcer
- **E** Chancre

Answers:

- **A** No
- **B** No
- **C** Traumatic ulceration is the answer. Characterized by a well-defined ulceration associated with a local trauma induced by biting of the oral mucosa with sharp, rough food or broken teeth, and disappears as soon as the causative agent is withdrawn.
- **D** No
- **E** No

Comments: Oral carcinomas were easily excluded due to the soft consistency of the lesion, while the absence of cervical lymphadenopathy and symptoms like pain or signs of a serious infection or similar lesions in the past excluded chancre or tuberculosis and large aphtha from the diagnosis.

Q2 Which of the characteristics below differentiate a traumatic from an eosinophilic ulcer?

- **A** Age of patients
- **B** Location of the ulcer
- **C** Pathogenesis
- **D** Symptomatology
- **E** Histological characteristics

Answers:

- **A** Traumatic ulcer can be seen in patients regardless of their age, while eosinophilic ulcers are predominantly seen in young patients.
- **B** No
- **C** No
- **D** No
- **E** The presence of a plethora of eosinophils is the pathognomonic histological finding of an eosinophilic ulceration-granuloma, but is rarely seen in simple traumatic ulcerations.

Comments: Both lesions are related with local trauma and appear on any part of the oral mucosa with mild symptomatology.

Q3 Which histological characteristics differentiate a traumatic ulcer from an aphtha?

- **A** Fibrinopurulent exudates at the top of the ulcer
- **B** Pseudoepithelial hyperplasia at the margins
- **C** Presence of germs within the ulcer
- **D** Granulation tissue at the base
- **E** Depth of inflammation

Answers:

- **A** No
- **B** No
- **C** No
- **D** No
- **E** The inflammation in aphthous stomatitis is rather superficial while in traumatic ulcer it can reach the muscle fibers, causing atrophy in places.

Comments: Both lesions are covered by fibrinopurulent exudation, which appears clinically as a yellow-white slough where various bacteria are present. Their base consists of granulation tissue with lymphocytes, histiocytes, eosinophils, and a few plasma cells, while the adjacent epithelium at their margins is hyperplastic with a few mitoses.

Case 14.6

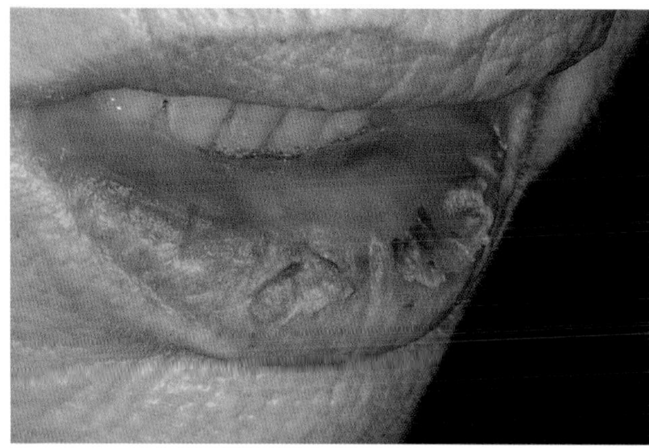

Figure 14.6

CO: A 62-year-old woman presented with yellow keratinaceous crusting and desquamation of the lower lip.

HPC: The lip crusting appeared one month ago when the patient was involved in picking olives in very cold weather. Two similar episodes of lip desquamation were recorded in the past and both episodes appeared in very stressful periods.

PMH: Her medical history revealed mild depression after her husband's death and mild late diabetes controlled with sertraline and metformin respectively. Allergies or other skin diseases were not reported. She was a smoker of 10–15 cigarettes, but did not have the habit of licking or biting her lips.

OE: Extensive scaling and yellow flaking of the lips (mainly of the lower lip) were found and associated with a tingling, burning sensation (Figure 14.6). The flakes were of different sizes, and when were removed left normal mucosa underneath. No other oral or skin lesions were noticed.

Q1 What is the cause of lip lesions?

- **A** Actinic cheilitis
- **B** Allergic cheilitis
- **C** Factitious cheilitis
- **D** Glandularis cheilitis
- **E** Exfoliative cheilitis

Answers:

- **A** No
- **B** No
- **C** No
- **D** No
- **E** Exfoliative cheilitis is an inflammation of the lips and characterized by excess keratin production on the vermilion border. It appears as flakes that are easily removed with licking or scratching, and is associated with exposure in extreme weather conditions and affect young female patients with psychological disturbances like depression or stress.

Comments: Actinic, factitious, allergic and glandular cheilitis can be easily excluded as the patient's outdoor work is short and her habits did not include lip licking or exposure to use of cosmetic lipsticks and erythematous swelling causing inflammation of minor salivary glands with purulent exudates were not seen.

Q2 Which of the diseases below is/or are associated with exfoliative cheilitis?

- **A** Psychiatric disorders
- **B** AIDS
- **C** Liver diseases
- **D** Avitaminosis
- **E** Hypothyroidism

Answers:

- **A** Young women with severe anxiety or depression often suffer with exfoliative cheilitis.
- **B** AIDS patients commonly present exfoliative cheilitis which is associated with *Candida* infection.
- **C** No
- **D** No
- **E** No

Comments: Hypothyroidism causes swollen puffy lips, but without keratin overproduction and scaling, while avitaminosis and liver failure cause angular rather than exfoliative cheilitis.

Q3 Which is/are the diagnostic test/s for exfoliative cheilitis?

- **A** Cultures
- **B** Allergy prick tests
- **C** Biopsy
- **D** None
- **E** Diascope

Answers:

- **A** No
- **B** No
- **C** No
- **D** None is the correct answer, as the diagnosis of exfoliative cheilitis is based only on its clinical characteristics and patient's history.
- **E** No

Comments: Other clinical tests (diascope; allergy prick tests) or laboratory tests (culture or biopsy) are rarely useful in exfoliative cheilitis and are used only to exclude indirectly, by other diseases such as *Candidosis*, allergic and actinic cheilitis or various pigmented lip lesions.

Case 14.7

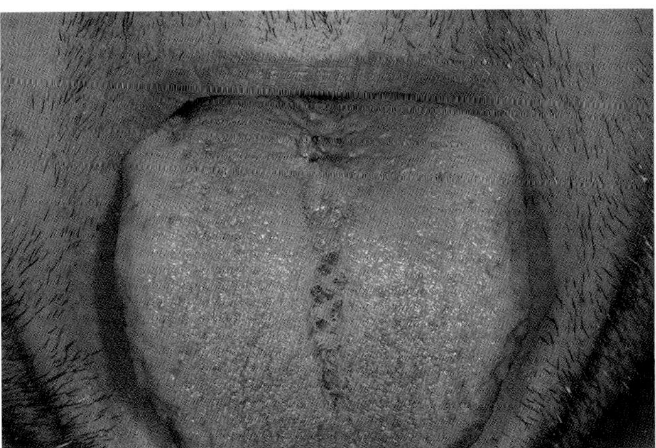

Figure 14.7

CO: A 26-year-old man presented with a yellow tongue.

HPC: His tongue's yellow color appeared three days ago, when the patient started to use lemon lozenges for relief of his sore throat.

PMH: His medical history was clear apart from a recent episode of viral pharyngitis treated symptomatically. He was not on any medications, or having known allergies, while his smoking and drinking habits were limited to social events only.

OE: A yellow thick but partially removable with spatula coat on the dorsum of his tongue (Figure 14.7) associated with mild xerostomia and halitosis. No other similar lesions were seen on his mouth, skin or eyes.

Q1 What is the cause of yellow discoloration of his tongue?

- **A** Jaundice
- **B** Yellow hairy tongue
- **C** Drugs
- **D** Smoking
- **E** Diet

Answers:

- **A** No
- **B** Yellow hairy tongue is the cause. It is characterized by an elongation of filiform papillae, which can easily trap chromogenic bacteria, producing yellow-colored pigment, dead cells and yellow food debris.
- **C** No
- **D** No
- **E** No

Comments: The fact that the patient rarely smokes and has not changed his diet or taken any drugs recently excludes smoking, diet or drugs as the possible cause of his tongue discoloration. Systemic diseases such jaundice produce colored pigments like bilirubin responsible for yellow skin, sclera and oral mucosa which are not seen in this man.

Q2 Which other diseases cause yellow mucosal discoloration?

- **A** Jaundice
- **B** Lipoproteinemia
- **C** Hemosiderosis
- **D** Carotinemia
- **E** B12 deficiency

Answers:

- **A** Jaundice is a yellowish disorder characterized by increased accumulation of bilirubin causing yellow skin and sclera.
- **B** Lipoproteinemia is characterized by increased accumulation of lipoproteins into the tissues causing numerous yellow discrete waxy lesions known as xanthomas.
- **C** No
- **D** Carotinemia is a disorder caused by excess consumption of dietary carotenoids and appears in the skin of young patients as a diffuse yellow skin discoloration that differs from jaundice as it does not affect the sclera of the patient's eyes.
- **E** No

Comments: Hemosiderosis is characterized by the deposition of hemosiderin into the tissues causing a diffuse dark blue discoloration, while the deficiency of B12 causes a diffuse erythema of oral mucosa and atrophy of tongue papillae.

Q3 Which drugs can cause mucosal yellow discoloration?

- **A** Rifampin
- **B** Gold
- **C** Colchicine
- **D** Bismuth containing drugs
- **E** Chloroquine

Answers:

- **A** Rifampin is an antibiotic used for chronic infections such as tuberculosis or leprosy, alone or in combination with other antibiotics, and causes yellow discoloration of the skin and oral mucosa.
- **B** No
- **C** No
- **D** No
- **E** No

Comments: Anti-malarials like chloroquine anti-rheumatoid like gold salts and anti-inflammatory drugs are widely used and cause (hyper rather than hypopigmentation) pigmentation changes by acting on melanocytes of the skin and mucosae but never provoke yellow discoloration. Bismuth containing drugs are used as an alternative therapy in patients with gastritis and other gut diseases, and cause black, discoloration resembling argyria.

Case 14.8

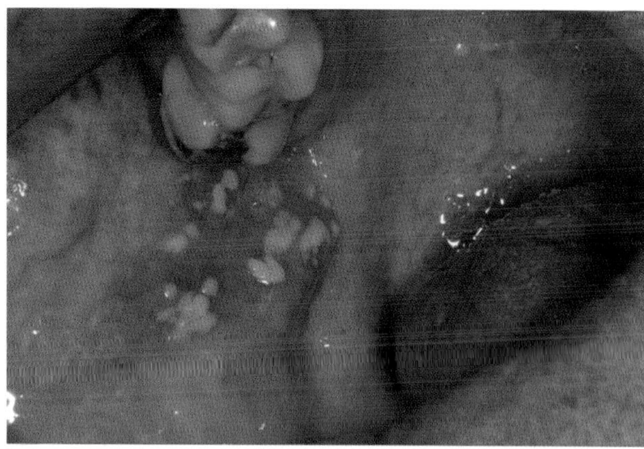

Figure 14.8

CO: A 67-year-old man presented with scattered yellow-white lesions on his mouth occurring over the last two weeks.

HPC: The lesions appeared after an upper respiratory infection three weeks ago, treated with wide spectrum antibiotics and a nasal decongestion spray. The lesions were scattered allover her mouth apart his palate where an old partial denture was lying on.

PMH: Chronic uncontrolled diabetes and chronic bronchitis treated with daily insulin injections, and bronchodilators and steroids in crisis. A recent upper respiratory infection exacerbated his chronic sinusitis and therefore he took antibiotics. He was a chronic heavy smoker, despite his respiratory problems.

OE: Multiple yellow creamy materials scattered on an erythematous oral mucosa (mainly on palate, buccal mucosae vand tongue) (Figure 14.8) associated with a burning sensation, and metallic taste. No other lesions were found in his mouth or skin, apart from an itchy, erythematous penis.

Q1 What is the main cause?

- **A** Acute pseudomembranous candidiasis
- **B** Materia alba
- **C** Lichen planus
- **D** Allergy to antibiotics
- **E** Nicotinic stomatitis

Answers:

- **A** Acute pseudomembranous candidiasis is characterized by yellow/white slough easily removed by rubbing, leaving erythematous and in places bleeding mucosa underneath. It is the most common form of candidiasis appearing in infants, people taking antibiotics or immunosuppressant medications, or immunocompromising diseases like diabetes.
- **B** No
- **C** No
- **D** No
- **E** No

Comments: Diseases like nicotinic stomatitis and lichen planus are characterized by the the presence of well fixed white yellowish lesions allover patient's mouth but these diseases are easily excluded as in nicotinic stomatitis the lesions are intermingled with red dots which are the inflammatory ducts of the minor salivary glands of palate while in, lichen planus the lesions have reticular pattern at their periphery. Materia alba was ruled out as this yellow slough should be predominately found, below his upper denture and not in places like buccal and tongue mucosae where can be easily, removed with mastication movements.

Q2 Which is/are the most serious *Candida* infections?

- **A** Fungal arthritis
- **B** Intra-abdominal candidiasis
- **C** Fungal Endocarditis
- **D** Mucocutaneous candidiasis
- **E** Candidemia

Answers:

- **A** No
- **B** No
- **C** Endocarditis is the second most serious fungal infection with a high mortality rate, as there are difficulties and delay in diagnosis from other causes of endocarditis.
- **D** No
- **E** Candidemia is the most important fungal infection that spreads anywhere in the body, causing serious complications leading to patients having a long stay in hospital, or even leading to death. This fungal infection of the blood appears with fever and kidney failure, leading gradually to shock. It is diagnosed with the isolation of the causative fungus in the blood, and treated with iv fluconazole, caspofungin, or amphotericin.

Comments: The other three fungal infections have restricted involvement like skin and mucous membranes (mucocutaneous candidiasis); abdomen (intra-abdominal candidiasis) and joints or bones (fungal arthritis) and therefore do not jeopardize the patient's life.

Q3 What are the basic steps for changing the saprophytic to pathogenic *Candida albicans*?

A Adherence to host surface
B Morphogenesis
C Escape of phagocytosis
D Degradation of host tissues
E Destruction of the immune host cells

Answers:

A The adhesion of *Candida* species with host cells is carried out via adhesins.
B In response to temperature, alkaline pH, starvation and CO_2 the fungi change their morphology from yeast to hyphae.
C The escape is done via vomomytosis, phagolysosomal neutralization, or pyroptosis.
D The degradation is done via hydrolytic enzymes like secreted aspartyl proteases (seps), lipases, other proteases.
E The secretion of cytolytic peptides (candinalysin) that damage host immune cells.

Case 14.9

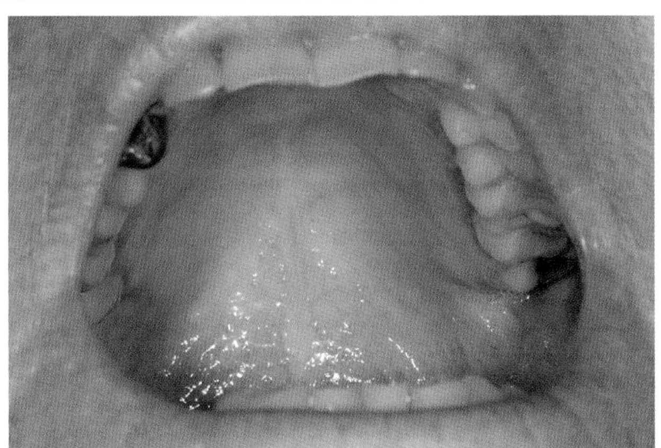

Figure 14.9

CO: A 56-year-old woman was referred by her dentist for evaluation of the yellow discoloration of her oral mucosa.

HPC: Her yellow discoloration was first noticed during a routine dental check-up three weeks ago and remained unchanged since then.

PMH: Her medical history revealed beta thalassemia causing her severe anemia, which was treated with regular blood transfusions, iron chelation and folic acid replacements. Splenectomy was done eight years ago and congestive heart disease was diagnosed last month. Smoking or drinking habits were never reported.

OE: The color of her oral mucosa (predominantly her palate) was pale yellow (Figure 14.9) while her skin was dark yellow-brown. The oral mucosa discoloration was diffuse and was not associated with other lesions in her mouth, skin and other mucosae.

Q1 What is the cause of her yellow mouth discoloration?

A Hemosiderosis
B Drug-induced
C Smoking
D Thalassemia beta
E Congestive heart disease

Answers:

A No
B No
C No
D Thalassemia beta is a group of inherited diseases characterized by reduced or absent production of beta chains of hemoglobin that results in severe hemolytic anemia. This is characterized by damage of red blood cells, decreased level of hemoglobin, but increased unconjugated bilirubin in blood up to 2–3 mg/dl, thus changing the color of oral mucosa to pale and yellow.
E No

Comments: Although hemosiderosis and congestive heart disease have different pathogenesis as hemosiderosis is characterized by increased deposition of iron into the body tissues due to chronic use of iron tablets or blood transfusion and congestive heart disease due to an inadequate heart pump, both conditions are presented with bluish discoloration of the oral mucosa. Smoking and drugs with bismuth may cause a yellow or brown discoloration due to nicotine or bismuth, but the patient had never been a chronic smoker or using those drugs.

Q2 Which is/are the main clinical characteristics of a thalassemia beta major?

A Jaundice
B Anemia
C Kidney enlargement
D Bone changes
E Mental retardation

Answers:

A Jaundice is a characteristic finding due to increased concentration of bilirubin in blood and soft tissues.
B Hypochromic anemia is the result of increased red blood cell lysis due abnormal hemoglobin synthesis.

C No
D Bony changes are seen in severe untreated cases and characterized by skull and facial bone enlargement (maxillary enlargement is common), expansion of ribs, cortical thinning and osteoporosis.
E No

Comments: Liver and spleen rather than kidney enlargement was characteristic. Kidney enlargement is a secondary complication of stones sometimes seen in patients with thalassemia. Mental retardation is rare and usually seen in patients with alpha thalassemia and related ATR-16 or -X syndromes.

Q3 Which laboratory investigations are mandatory to confirm thalassemia beta?
A Liver function tests
B Abdominal ultrasonography
C Skull X-rays
D Hemoglobin analysis
E Human leukocyte antigen (HLA) typing

Answers:
A No
B No
C No
D Hemoglobin analysis reveals the type and degree of its abnormities, as in thalassemia major the HbA is minimal or absent, HbF and HbA2 are elevated, while in intermedia the HbA is decreased and HbF and HbA2 elevated, while in trait mostly elevated are HbA, F and A2.
E No

Comments: The other laboratory investigations are indicative but are not pathognomonic for the diagnosis: the white blood cell count (WBC) reveals the presence of microcytic anemia; liver function tests, elevated lactate dehydrogenase (LDH) and bilirubin (total, unconjugated); skull X-rays widening of diploic space and facial deformity; ultrasonography enlarged spleen and skull; while HLA typing reveals the genetic associations of the patient.

Case 14.10

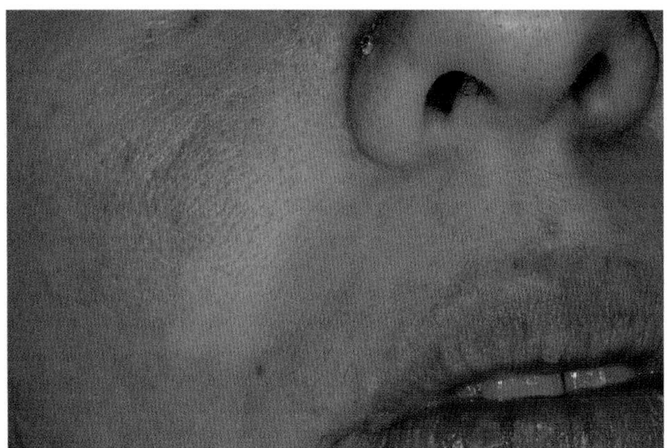

Figure 14.10

CO: An 18-year-old woman appeared with a yellow discoloration of her face in the area next to her right nostril and upper lip.

HPC: The discoloration appeared after a local anesthetic injection for removal of caries from her upper right canine.

PMH: Her medical history was unremarkable, with no allergies, serious diseases or drug use. She was a non-smoker and non-drinker and spent her free time playing volleyball.

OE: A yellow diffuse facial bleaching in the area above the upper right lip-nostril, unchanged with pressure and associated with local numbness (Figure 14.10). No other similar discolorations were found inside her mouth and other mucus membranes. This yellow discoloration was not permanent, and the skin color came back to normal within the next hour.

Q1 What is the cause of her facial discoloration?
A Angioedema
B Hematoma
C Facial bleaching
D Jaundice
E Birth mark

Answers:

- **A** No
- **B** No
- **C** Facial bleaching is a rare complication of local anesthesia, and occurs when the anesthetic containing a vasoconstriction substance like epinephrine is injected into a blood vessel like the maxillary artery as happened in this lady.
- **D** No
- **E** No

Comments: The recent onset and short duration of this discoloration and the absence of recent trauma or similar lesions on the skin or other mucosae associated with facial swelling rules out birthmarks, traumatic hematoma, jaundice and angioedema from the diagnosis respectively.

Q2 Which is/are other important complication/s apart from facial discoloration of a local anaesthesia?

- **A** Trismus
- **B** Facial palsy
- **C** Hypersalivation
- **D** Hematoma
- **E** Angioedema

Answers:

- **A** Trismus is a rare complication and appears whenever a local anesthetic injection enter into the pterygomandibular muscles and space.
- **B** Facial palsy occurs when the anesthetic blocks the facial muscles, causing paralysis and lack of facial expression.
- **C** No
- **D** Hematoma occurs after an injury of local blood vessels or soft tissues caused by the anesthetic fluid or needle used.
- **E** Angioedema is a rare complication of the trauma induced during the anesthetic procedure which provokes facial swelling together with discoloration.

Comments: Hypersalivation is a secondary, minor complication, in anxious patients who consider the numbness from anesthesia as a foreign body and try to remove it or spit it out with tongue movements.

Q3 Epinephrine reaction after a single local anesthetic intra-oral injection is characterized by:

- **A** Increase systolic/diastolic blood pressure
- **B** Tremor
- **C** Cardiac dysrhythmias
- **D** Headache
- **E** Palpitation

Answers:

- **A** No
- **B** Tremor is a common finding after anesthesia (local or general) and caused by the discomfort due to the body's thermoregulatory capability or triggered by postoperative pain.
- **C** No
- **D** Headache is more often seen in patients who have undergone general rather than local anesthesia, and appears earlier than after receiving spinous anesthesia.
- **E** Palpitations are noted when the anesthetic containing epinephrine enters into the small vessels and travels into the heart, making it beat too faster.

Comments: When the dose of anesthetic drug is large, it may cause alterations of blood pressure (increased) and arrhythmias.

Section II

15

Buccal Mucosa

Buccal mucosa lesions are a heterogeneous group of lesions located within the inner surface of the cheeks from the angles of lips to the line of attachment between the pterygomandibular raphe and the upper and lower alveolar ridge. These lesions are manifestations of various congenital, reactive, inflammatory, autoimmune, or even neoplastic diseases that need special treatment, while they sometimes can be normal anatomical variations requiring patient's reassurance only (Figure 15.0a and b).

The Table 15 lists the most common and important conditions affecting the buccal mucosae.

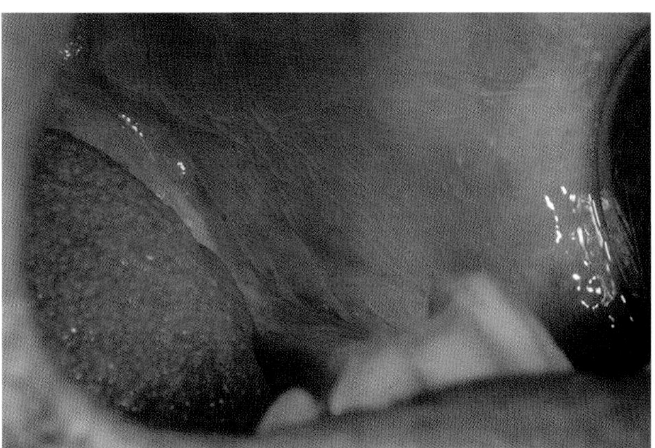

Figure 15.0a Leukoedema.

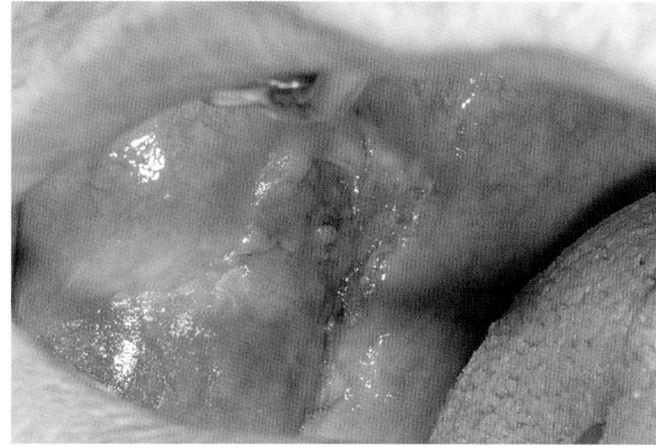

Figure 15.0b Oral carcinoma.

Clinical Guide to Oral Diseases, First Edition. Dimitris Malamos and Crispian Scully.

Companion website: www.wiley.com/go/malamos/clinical_guide

Table 15 Buccal mucosa: Common and important lesions.

- Congenital
  - White lesions
    - White sponge nevus
  - Red/blue lesions
    - Angiomas
  - Yellow lesions
    - Ectopic sebaceous glands
- Acquired
  - Traumatic
    - White alba
    - Leukoedema
    - Fibrous lumps
    - Frictional keratosis
    - Mucoceles
  - Neoplastic
    - Leukoplakia
    - Erythroplakia
    - Carcinomas
    - Lymphomas
    - Sarcomas
  - Inflammation
    - Stensens's duct papilitis
      - Stone
    - Aphthae
  - Infections
    - Bacterial
      - Noma
      - Syphilis
      - Tuberculosis

Table 15 (Continued)

- Fungal
  - Acute pseudomembranous or erythematous
  - Chronic hyperplastic or part of multifocal or mucocutaneous Candidiasis
  - Deep mucoses like Aspregillosis, mucormucosis or cyptococcosis
- Viral
  - Herpes 1 and 2
  - HPV
  - HIV
- Systemic diseases with oral involvement
  - Skin
    - Lichen planus
    - Lupus erythematosus
    - Chronic ulcerative stomatitis
    - Bullous disorders
  - Blood
    - Anemia
  - Gut
    - Granulomatous diseases
  - Hormones
    - Hyper parathyroidism (soft tissue calcifications
    - Hypo-parathyroidism (chronic Candidosis), thyroidism (oedema) and hypofunction of:
    - adrenals (Addison disease, pigmentation)
    - pancreas (Diabetes. lichen planus,deep mucoses)
- Allergies
  - Cinnamon induced stomatitis

Case 15.1

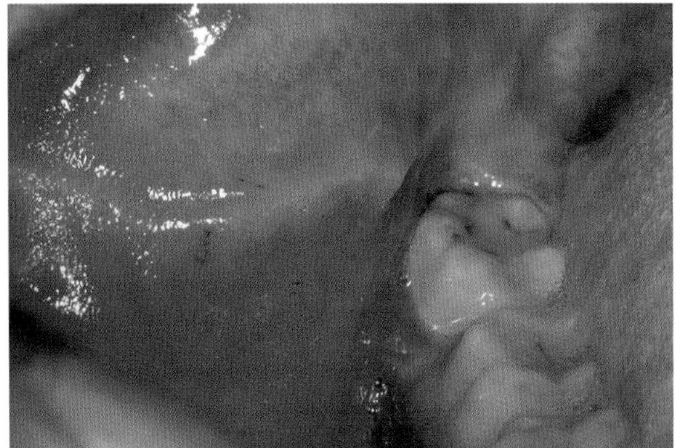

Figure 15.1

CO: A 44 year old man presented with white asymptomatic lesions on both his buccal mucosae.

HPC: The lesions were discovered, by the patient during a self-oral examination last month and remained asymptomatic and unchanged since then.

PMH: His medical history was clear apart from a mild gastritis which was treated with diet and anti-acid drugs, as well as a panic crisis that responded to psychotherapy and lorazepam drug. Moreover, no allergies, or parafunctional habits were reported, while his smoking and drinking habits were limited.

OE: A white linear string-like lesion on a diffuse opalescent white base, extended from the retromolar area to the commissures, on both buccal mucosae (Figure 15.1). The white, string-like lesion was located along the occlusion line, but was a lot more prominent at the molar area and not detached with scrubbing, while the diffuse opalescent lesion disappeared with stretching. Similar opalescent lesions were found on his labial mucosa as well. Finally, no other lesions were seen inside his mouth, skin or other mucosae.

Q1 What are these white lesions?

A Linea alba
B Morsicatio buccarum
C Lichen planus
D Leukoplakia
E Leukoedema

Answers:

- **A** Linea alba is a linear string like elevation of the oral mucosa at the level of the occlusion line, and is seen in dentulous patients or patients with dentures, as it is mostly caused by pressure, friction or sucking during smoking.
- **B** No
- **C** No
- **D** No
- **E** Leukoedema is a normal variation rather than a pathological condition and it commonly appears in Afro-Caribbeans and patients who smoke; it is characterized as a diffuse whitish plaque lesion that can disappear with stretching.

Comments: The string like appearance of the linea alba clinically differentiates this lesion from others like leukoedema that is diffuse lesion that is gone with stressing; leukoplakia and morscicario buccinatom that are white well fixed plaques with smooth or corrugated surface anywhere or in friction areas respectively. Lichen planus has a characteristic network at the periphery and is often associated with a pruritic skin rash' features are not seen in this patient.

Q2 Which is the best treatment for both white lesions?

- **A** None
- **B** Antifungal therapy
- **C** Surgery
- **D** Steroid treatment
- **E** Extraction of adjacent teeth

Answers:

- **A** Both lesions are harmless conditions and therefore no treatment is required
- **B** No
- **C** No
- **D** No
- **E** No

Comments: Having in mind that both lesions are not manifestations of a fungal infection like candidiasis or a mucocutaneous disease like lichen planus, the use of antifungals or steroids (topical or systemic) is useless. On the other hand, the benefits of the surgical removal of these lesions or extractions of adjacent teeth are minimal as their cause (suction, friction) remains.

Q3 Which of the histological characteristics below are common in both two conditions?

- **A** Increased epithelial thickness
- **B** Intraepithelial edema of spinous cells
- **C** Severe fibrous hyperplasia within the underlying submucosa
- **D** Low scattered mild inflammation of the underlying corium
- **E** Presence of *Candida* hyphae within the basal layer.

Answers:

- **A** The epithelium is hyperplastic across the occlusion line (linea alba) or covers larger area (leukoedema).
- **B** No
- **C** No
- **D** The irritation of the mucosa from friction or suction may cause a local mild inflammation within the upper parts of the corium.
- **E** No

Comments: Intracellular edema of spinous cells is a pathognomonic finding of leukoedema and not of the linea alba. In both conditions the inflammation is not severe and not extended deep into muscle while. *Candida albicans* and other pathogenic germs are easily detected with special stains within the upper parts of epithelium.

Case 15.2

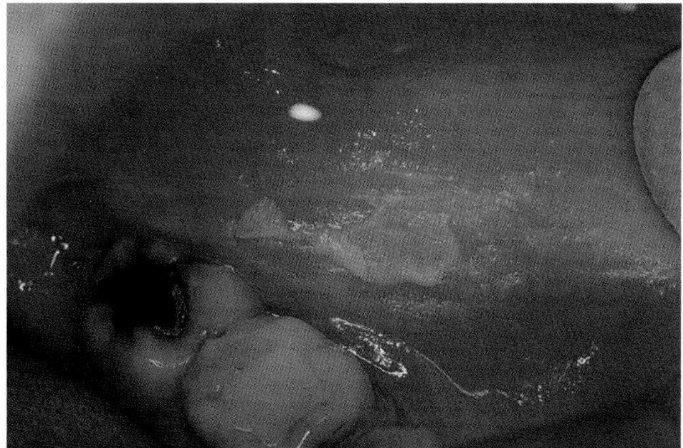

Figure 15.2

CO: A 27-year-old woman presented with desquamative yellow-white plaques on her bilateral buccal mucosae.

HPC: The lesions had been present for approximately eight years and caused her discomfort due to an alteration of the texture in her mouth. These lesions were not stable and they became exacerbated during stressful family events.

PMH: Her medical history did not reveal any serious diseases or known allergies. Smoking or drinking were not reported but the patient had the habit of chewing her cheeks.

OE: The intra-oral examination revealed distinct, diffused opaque to translucent white plaques at the occlusion line. These plaques were asymptomatic, partially removed with scratching, and caused a burning sensation.

(Figure 15.2). These lesions were accompanied with a scalloped tongue and in places with similar hyperkeratotic lesions on its lateral margins. No other lesions were seen in her mouth, skin or other mucosae and none of her close relatives had any similar lesions.

Q1 What is the possible diagnosis?

- **A** Leukoplakia
- **B** Pachyonychia congenita
- **C** Candidiasis
- **D** Lichen planus
- **E** Morsicatio buccarum

Answers:

- **A** No
- **B** No
- **C** No
- **D** No
- **E** Morsicatio buccarum is the answer. This is the result of constant teeth rubbing or chewing against adjacent oral mucosae (labial, buccal or lingual), causing hyperkeratotic plaques with no sign of malignancy known as friction keratosis.

Comments: In contrast to the patient's lesions, the white lesions in acute candidiasis are easily removed, leaving an erythematous mucosa underneath while in leukoplakia, the lesions are well fixed and have different etiology and prognosis and therefore excluded from the diagnosis. Similarly, well-fixed white lesions are also found in lichen planus and in pachyonychia congenita, but their lesions appear at very late age (lichen planus) and at childhood(pachyonichia congenta) and are rather more associated with characteristic skin and nail involvements that were not seen in this patient.

Q2 Which of the lesions below is or are related with the patient's parafunctional habits?

- **A** Linea alba
- **B** Enlargement of foliate papillae
- **C** Scalloping tongue
- **D** Erythematous tip of tongue
- **E** Hairy tongue

Answers:

- **A** Linea alba is the white string-like lesion on the buccal mucosae that is produced by chronic irritation of buccal mucosa due to its constant suction or rubbing with adjacent teeth.
- **B** Erythematous, enlarged foliate papillae are induced by the constant rubbing of lateral margins of the tongue against adjacent teeth.
- **C** Imprints of teeth on the tongue's lateral margins make crenations giving the impression of wavy indentations (scalloping).
- **D** Chronic irritation of the tip of the tongue from the constant friction against upper and lower incisors causes erythema and hypertrophy, or even loss of papillae, and is accompanied with a tingling or burning sensation.
- **E** No

Comments: Hairy tongue is characterized by the elongation of filiform papillae that gives the impression of a hairy coat and not plaque, as it is only seen on the dorsum of tongue. It is the result of poor mouth cleaning, drug use including antibiotics like metronidazole or strong mouth washes, radiotherapy as well as excessive smoking or drinking alcohol, coffee, or tea.

Q3 What is/are the histological characteristic/s of this keratosis?

- **A** Hyperparakeratosis
- **B** Colonization with fungi rather than bacteria of superficial epithelial layers
- **C** Severe inflammation within the epithelium
- **D** Epithelial atypia is always present
- **E** Presence of clefts or fissures within the keratin

Answers:

- **A** Hyperkeratosis is a common finding.
- **B** No
- **C** No
- **D** No
- **E** Clefts or fissures are common findings within the keratin layers.

Comments: The colonization of the superficial epithelial layers in friction keratosis is made of with a mixture of pathogenic germs and not only with fungi as seen in Candida leukoplakia. In frictional keratosis the inflammation is mild and located mainly in the upper part of corium. Epithelial atypia is almost missing confirming thus the benign character of this lesion.

Case 15.3

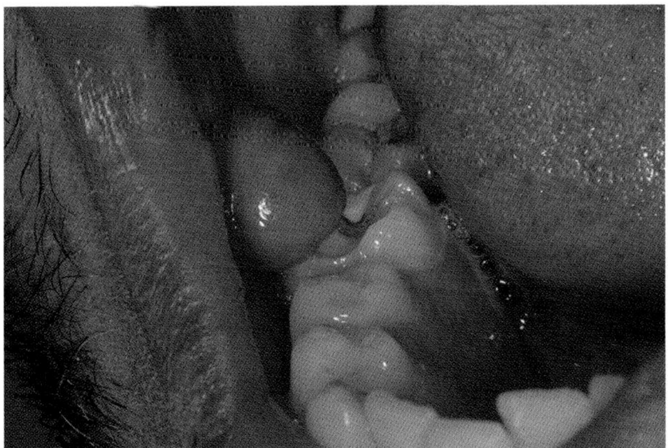

Figure 15.3

CO: A 32-year-old man was presented with a lump on his right buccal mucosa.

HPC: The lump appeared after cheek biting during a meal three months ago. It appeared as a soft, asymptomatic, swelling which obtained its maximum size within the next month and had remained unchanged since then.

PMH: He was a healthy young man with no history of any serious diseases, known allergies or any medicine uptake. Smoking or drinking or other parafunctional habits were not recorded.

OE: A soft pedunculated nodule on his right buccal mucosa, opposite the first lower molar was noticed. The lesion was asymptomatic, not fluctuant and slightly sensitive on touch, but with a normal color and a smooth, non-ulcerated surface, with a maximum size of 1.5 cm (Figure 15.3). No other similar lesions were found in his mouth, skin, or other mucosae and cervical lymphadenopathy was undetected.

Q1 What is this lesion?

- **A** Mucocele
- **B** Epulis fissuratum
- **C** Irritation fibroma
- **D** Pyogenic granuloma
- **E** Peripheral cemento-ossifying fibroma

Answers:

- **A** No
- **B** No
- **C** Irritating fibroma is the lesion. It is a benign reactive lesion which is more often seen on the buccal mucosa along the occlusion line, and appears as a round, asymptomatic lump with a smooth, normally colored surface which sometimes becomes ulcerated due to repeated trauma.
- **D** No
- **E** No

Comments: Other benign oral lesions are included in the differential diagnosis of irritating fibromas such as mucoceles, epulis fissuratum, pyogenic granulomas and peripheral cemento-ossifyng fibromas. All these lesions differ in: a) location: fibromas and pyogenic grannulomas can been all over patient's mouth while epulis fissuratum closely to the margins of ill-fitting denture and cemento-fibroma lesions exclusively on gingivae b) its consistency: soft in mucocele and pyogenic granulomas firm in fibromas and slightly harder in cemento-fibromas and c) composition: mucoceles are cystic lesions lined by thin granulation tissue within PAS +ve mucin in the lumen secreted from minor salivary glands and in pyogenic granuloma is mainly composed from granulation (neovascularization) tissues while in fibromas by fibrous connective tissue which may be mature in fibromas with less inflammation from epulis fissuratum and with spicules of cement or bone.

Q2 What is/are the clinical diagnostic criteria for this lesion?

- **A** History of trauma
- **B** Symptomatology
- **C** Rapid development
- **D** Firm consistency
- **E** Early response to antibiotics

Answers:

- **A** Trauma together with chronic irritations such as friction or suction are considered as the main causes of oral fibromas.
- **B** No
- **C** No
- **D** Fibromas are composed of dense fibrous connective tissues and are therefore firm in consistency
- **E** No

Comments: Oral fibromas are asymptomatic and pain may appear only when the lesions are ulcerated. These lesions gain their maximum size within the next couple of months, but do not respond to antibiotics as oral pathogenic bacteria do not participate in their pathogenesis.

Q3 What are the histological characteristics of this lesion?

- **A** Presence of capsule at the periphery
- **B** Epithelium hypertrophic and in places atrophic
- **C** Granulation tissues within the submucosa

D Fibrous connective tissue with variable numbers of fibrocytes
E Elastosis

Answers:
A No
B The epithelium may be hyperplastic, hyperkeratotic and in places atrophic or even ulcerated.
C No
D Fibrous dense connective tissue is the predominant element, containing numerous fibroblasts, a few mature fibrocytes and scattered mild inflammation of chronic inflammatory cells.
E No

Comments: Neovascularization (granulation) is a characteristic finding of pyogenic granulomas and the replacement of elastine with fibrous fibers occurs in actinic cheilitis while fibrous capsule in fibrolipomas but not in fibromas.

Case 15.4

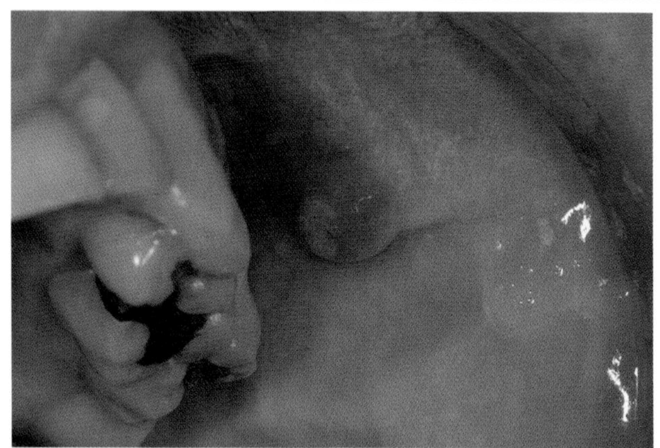

Figure 15.4

CO: A 36-year-old woman was presented with a painful lump on her left buccal mucosa.

HPC: The lump was erythematous with a central superficial ulceration and noticed over the last six days.

PMH: Allergic rhinitis and iron deficiency anemia was recorded and attributed to pollen allergy and severe blood loss due to heavy menstruation respectively. A few episodes of migraine were reported over the last years and responded well with strong painkillers. Allergies, or drugs used apart from painkillers for migraine and iron supplements for her anemia, were not recorded. Smoking, and alcohol use was restricted only to social events.

OE: The intra-oral examination revealed an erythematous nodule with a central ulceration which was covered with a yellowish pseudomembrane. The lump was soft in palpation at the area of parotid papilla (Figure 15.4), but noy associated with parotid enlargement or recent trauma. Two small painful ulcerations with yellow pseudomembrane and erythematous halo were also found on the tip of her tongue and anterior buccal sulcus near the first upper right molar. Cervical lymphadenopathy was undetected. Similar painful ulcerations had been reported in the past, but healed spontaneously within the next 10 days.

Q1 What is the cause of this lesion?
A Sialodochitis fibrinosa
B Ulcerated fibroma
C Aphtha on the parotid papilla
D Stensen's duct stone
E Sialadenitis

Answers:
A No
B No
C Aphtha located on the papilla of the left parotid gland is the answer. This aphtha causes a painful sensation and inflammation of the opening of the Stensen's duct without gland enlargement. The presence of two similar aphthae-like lesions during the examination and a positive history of recurrent, limited ulcerations in the past reinforce this diagnosis.
D No
E No

Comments: Having in mind the soft consistency of the lesion and its short duration as well as the negative history or trauma excludes Stensen's duct stone and ulcerated fibromas from the diagnosis. Sialadenitis (acute or chronic)and Sialodochitis fibrinosa come together with an inflammation of Stensen's papilla, but they are both always associated with a painful enlargement of the relevant gland with pus or mucus plug discharge, which was not seen in this woman.

Q2 Which other factor/s is/or are related to patient's lesion?

- **A** Migraine
- **B** Allergic rhinitis
- **C** Smoking
- **D** Iron deficiency anemia
- **E** Menstruation

Answers:

- **A** No
- **B** No
- **C** No
- **D** Aphthous stomatitis has been associated with various anemias, especially due to iron and B12 deficiency.
- **E** No

Comments: Migraine or allergic rhinitis does not provoke aphthous stomatitis per se, but various painkillers for migraine's relief may do so. In addition to this, smoking seems to make the oral epithelium more resistant to local trauma and aphthae formation, while hormonal alterations before the menstrual cycle seem to be related with aphthae, but their onset was not connected with the patient's menstruation cycle.

Q3 Which other factor/s can cause enlargement of the major salivary gland ducts?

- **A** Smoking
- **B** Dehydration
- **C** Poor oral hygiene
- **D** Alcoholism
- **E** Starvation

Answers:

- **A** No
- **B** Body dehydration is associated with a low flow rate of saliva leading to of bacterial sialadenitis with painful swelling of salivary glands and their ducts.
- **C** Poor oral hygiene allows the entrance of pathogenic bacteria through the main duct's opening to the duct system, and finally to salivary parenchyma, Eventually the gland becomes inflamed and swollen with pus coming out, sometimes from the enlarged inflamed duct.
- **D** No
- **E** No

Comments: Alcoholism and starvation are responsible for sialadenosis. This is a condition of the enlargement of salivary glands without any clinical evidence of infection. Smoking causes inflammation of minor but not major salivary glands openings that is widely known as nicotinic stomatitis and is mainly found in the palate.

Case 15.5

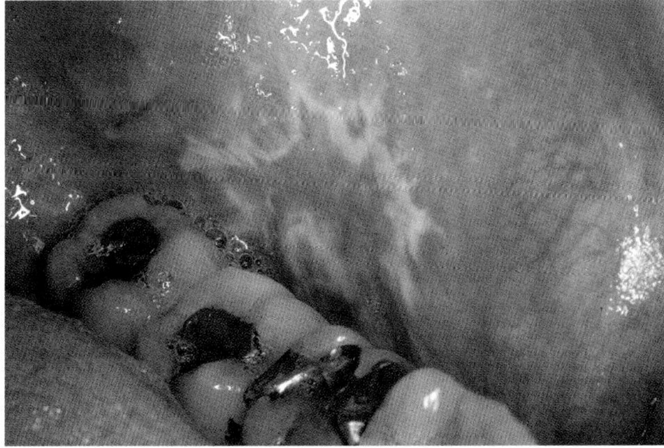

Figure 15.5

CO: A 56-year-old woman was presented with white lesions on both her buccal mucosae.

HPC: The white lesions were found during her last dental examination by her dentist three months ago and remained unchanged since then.

PMH: Her medical history included diabetes type II and mild hypertension which were controlled with diet and glucophage drugs as well as calcium channel blockers respectively. Allergies and other systemic diseases or smoking or other hazardous habits were not recorded.

OE: White patches with faint white lines forming a network at the periphery, particularly, on both buccal mucosae, dorsum of tongue and lower vermilion border were found (Figure 15.5).The white lesions were asymptomatic but caused a rough feeling on the buccal mucosae, and were not associated with other skin or genital lesions.

Q1 What is the possible diagnosis?

- **A** Reticular lichen planus
- **B** Leukoplakia
- **C** Lichenoid reaction to amalgam
- **D** Chronic candidiasis
- **E** Chronic ulcerative stomatitis

Answers:

A Reticular form of lichen planus is the diagnosis. This condition is a chronic inflammatory mucocutaneous disease which sometimes precedes or follows mouth lesions. These lesions appear as white plaques of various size, with a symmetrical, reticular pattern at their periphery and are mainly seen on both the buccal mucosae and tongue, and less on the gingivae, lips and palate.
B No
C No
D No
E No

Comments: Chronic ulcerative stomatitis is always presented with ulcerations which can look like erosive but not reticular lichen planus. In leukoplakia and hypertrophic candidiasis, the white lesions are restricted and do not have a reticular pattern at their periphery; therefore, they are ruled out from the diagnosis. Lichenoid reaction to amalgam looks similar, but differs as the distribution of the patient's lesions were scattered and unrelated with her amalgam fillings.

Q2 Which of the variations of this condition below are rarely or never seen in the oral mucosa?
A Inverse type
B Linear
C Erosive
D Hypertrophic
E Erythrodemic

Answers:

A The inverse type affects submammary, axillae, limp flexur, and inguinal regions but never oral mucosa, and is characterized by erythematous keratotic plaques with poorly defined borders and in some part, with lichenification or pigmentation.
B No
C No
D No
E The erythrodermic type is extremely rare, affecting the patient's skin, with reduced general health, and appears as pruritic red papules or plaques on the skin but never on the mouth.

Comments: The linear type is characterized by linear white lesions while the hypertrophic type is related to white plaques. The erosive type is associated with atrophic and in places ulcerated lesions of a reticular network at the periphery. All these three types are commonly seen within the oral mucosa.

Q3 Which is the major pathogenetic mechanism of oral lichen planus development?
A Accumulation of T cells
B Activation of Langerhans cells
C Cytokine production
D Apoptosis of basal cells
E Release of metalloproteinases

Answers:

A No
B No
C No
D Apoptosis of basal cells is triggered by activated CD8+ T cells is the most important mechanism for lichen planus development.
E No

Comments: All the above mechanisms participate in the pathogenesis of lichen planus like the activation of Langerhans cells, accumulation of CD4 and CD8+ cells within the epithelium and upper parts of corium aim in activating the CD 8+ cells under the presence of IL-2 and IFN γ cytokines in order to cause basal cell apoptosis. This epithelial damage is reinforced by a connective tissue matrix degradation, induced by various metalloproteins which disrupts the basement membrane and accelerates apoptosis.

16

Floor of the Mouth

The floor of the mouth is a small horseshoe-like region underneath the tongue and above the muscular diaphragm that is formed by geniohyoid and mylohyoid muscles. It contains the ducts of the submandibular and sublingual salivary glands, lingual artery, veins and nerves. The floor of the mouth is the site of various congenital and acquired diseases, some of which are very dangerous for the patient's life, like the sublingual space infections or carcinomas. Some of the lesions arise from superficial tissues and are easily diagnosed with physical examination only (See Figure 16.0), but the majority are located deep into the tissues and require additional imaging techniques (ultrasonography, X-rays, computed tomography, or magnetic resonance) to assess their extension and consistency.

Table 16 lists the more common lesions found in the floor of mouth.(Ankyloglossia)

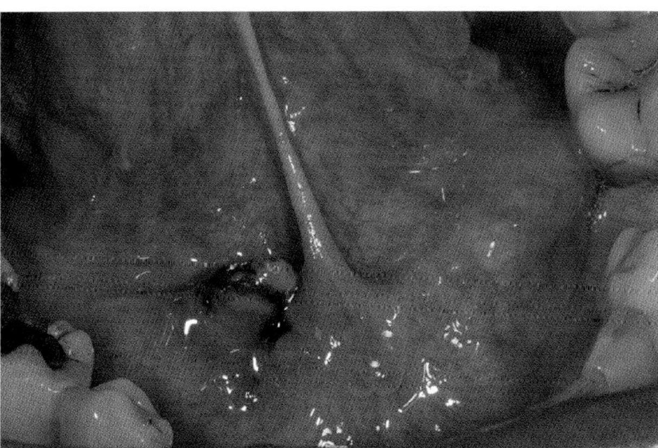

Figure 16.0 Trauma of the duct of the right sublingual gland.

Table 16 Floor of the mouth: common and important lesions and conditions.

- ◆ Congenital
  - Vascular
    - Hemangioma
    - Lymphangioma
  - Cysts
    - Dermoid
    - Epidermoid
    - Lymphoepithelial
  - Developmental
    - Tongue tie (Ankyloglossia)
  - Salivary glands
    - Aplasia salivary gland
- ◆ Acquired
  - Inflammatory
    - Abscess
      - Dental
      - Soft tissues
    - Sialadenitis
    - Sialolithiasis
    - Ranula
  - Vascular
    - Venous lakes
  - Neoplasia
    - Leukoplakia
    - Carcinomas
    - Metastatic cancers
    - Mesenchymal tumors
      - Benign
      - Malignant

Clinical Guide to Oral Diseases, First Edition. Dimitris Malamos and Crispian Scully.

Companion website: www.wiley.com/go/malamos/clinical_guide

Case 16.1

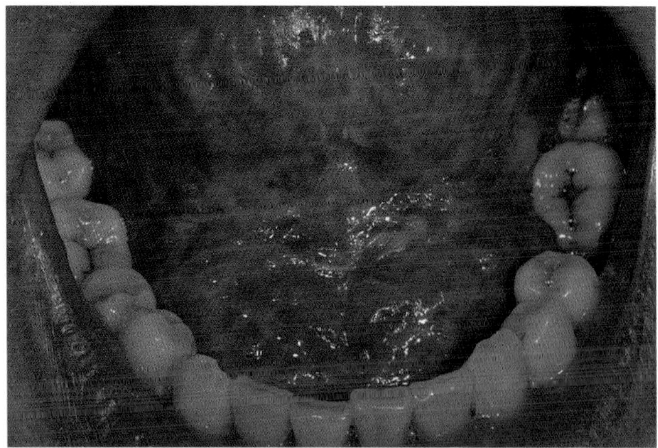

Figure 16.1

CO: A 38-year-old woman was referred for white lesions on the floor of her mouth.

HPC: The lesions were incidentally noted, three weeks ago, during a routine dental examination by her dentist who referred the patient for further investigations.

PMH: Her medical history was clear apart from chronic gastritis in which the symptoms were relieved with antiacids, and a risk of diabetes as her mother suffered from this disease. The patient liked to eat hot but not spicy foods, and smoked 15 cigarettes daily. She held chewing gum or mint flavored candies underneath her tongue to eliminate her bad breath caused by smoking. No other members of her family had similar lesions.

OE: White superficial lesions covered the whole of the floor of her mouth and intermingled with normal mucosa in places (Figure 16.1).These lesions varied in size and thickness, with no ulcerations or reticular network at the periphery. They were asymptomatic, but gave a sense of roughness underneath the tongue. The dorsum of the tongue was hairy, while her palate was white with erythematous dots, possibly related to smoking. No other white lesions were found inside her mouth, skin and other mucosae. Gingival problems and halitosis were not recorded, as her oral hygiene was adequate. Recent blood tests revealed only raised glucose levels and biopsy from the most suspicious lesion confirmed the presence of a mild hyperplastic epithelium, with a mild dysplasia and diffused chronic inflammation underneath.

Q1 What is the possible diagnosis?
- **A** White sponge nevus
- **B** Lichen planus
- **C** Sublingual keratosis
- **D** Uremic stomatitis
- **E** Congenital dyskeratosis

Answers:
- **A** No
- **B** No
- **C** Sublingual keratosis is the correct diagnosis. This condition is characterized by single or multiple white plaques with soft consistency, wrinkled surface and cover part or the whole of the floor of mouth. It is strongly related with chronic smoking, and has a high rate of malignant transformation.
- **D** No
- **E** No

Comments: The clinical characteristics such as the absence of other skin or mucosal lesions and their late onset excludes other skin diseases such as lichen planus and congenital conditions such as white sponge nevus and dyskeratosis. Also, the lack of uremic type halitosis, confirmed with the normal levels of urea and creatinine, excludes uremic stomatitis from the diagnosis.

Q2 Which of the factors below could play a role in the malignant transformation of a sublingual keratosis lesion?
- **A** Patient's health
- **B** Habits
- **C** Size
- **D** Duration
- **E** Clinical morphology of the lesion

Answers:
- **A** No
- **B** Chronic habits like smoking (especially the passive type) play an important role in malignant transformation as the floor of the mouth is a suitable area for accumulation of various carcinogens arising from smoking, drinking, or spicy foods.
- **C** No
- **D** The duration of the sublingual lesions seems to play a role in their malignant transformation, as there is enough time for these lesions to be exposed to various carcinogens.
- **E** The presence of red areas within the white lesions (speckled leukoplakia or erythroleukoplakia) is more likely to undergo malignant transformation than homogeneous leukoplakia.

Comments: The size of the lesion and patient's health status seem to be important factors for determining the treatment plan, and not the risk of malignant transformation. However the site of this leukoplakia (>4 cm) has been considered by some but not all investigators to be to be the only significant predicting factor of malignant transformation of leukoplakia general and not specifically for sublingual keratosis.

Q3 Which is/are the histological characteristics that differentiate a tongue leukoplakia from a hairy leukoplakia?

A Hyperkeratosis
B Subepithelial Inflammation
C Severe dysplasia
D Koilocytes
E Presence of *Candida*/and bacteria within the superficial epithelial layers.

Answers:

A No
B Subepithelial inflammation is never seen in hairy leukoplakia but is variable in sublingual keratosis.
C Mild atypia can been seen in both sublingual keratosis and hairy leukoplakia, but severe dysplasia in some sublingual keratoses only.
D Koilocytes are characteristic cells seen only in hairy leukoplakia. These cells are swollen with pale cytoplasm, with prominent cell borders and perinuclear vacuoles, Epstein-Barr virus (EBV) positive, seen with immunocytochemical and in situ hybridization techniques, and found predominantly in the upper part of the spinous layers.
E No

Comments: A common histological finding in both conditions is hyperkeratosis where numerous bacteria and fungi are easily demonstrated within the superficial epithelial layers.

Case 16.2

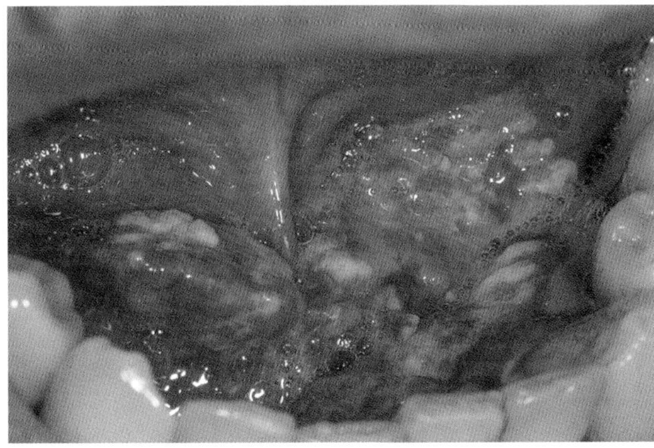

Figure 16.2

CO: A 52-year-old man was referred for a large exophytic mass on the floor of his mouth.

HPC: The lesion had been present for almost three years. Initially the lesion appeared as a small cauliflower-like growth, but had become bigger over the last six months and covered the most of his floor of mouth, causing difficulty in tongue movements during eating or speaking.

PMH: Hypercholesterolemia and mild hypertension were his main medical problems, and partially controlled with diet as the patient refused to take any medication. Allergies or other serious diseases were not recorded, but two and a half of packets cigarettes and a couple of glasses of wine or beer were consumed daily.

OE: A large, hard consistency mass with irregular margins and a papillary, and in some places ulcerated, surface covered most of the floor of the mouth (mainly the left side). The lesion was extended from the ventral surface of the tongue to the adjacent lingual aspects of the left second molar to the right second premolar (Figure 16.2). The lesion was asymptomatic, white with red areas intermingled with normal mucosa, and associated with ipsilateral cervical lymph node enlargement. The palpable nodes were of various size, well-fixed and asymptomatic. Submandibular and sublingual salivary gland enlargements were not detected. Biopsy from the main lesion revealed numerous islands of neoplastic, atypical epithelial cells invading the underlying submucosa. Fine-needle aspiration (FNA) from his biggest lymph node confirmed the biopsy results.

Q1 What is the diagnosis?

A Papillary epithelial hyperplasia
B Verrucous leukoplakia
C Verrucous xanthoma
D Oral squamous cell carcinoma
E Terminal duct carcinoma

Answers:

A No
B No
C No
D Oral squamous cell carcinoma is the answer. It appears as a chronic, indurated ulceration or swelling, with a smooth or papillary surface and white or red color, or as a combination of the above lesions. At an early stage, it is asymptomatic, well-fixed in the underlying mucosa or adjacent alveolar bone. However, in advanced stages it is accompanied with pain or earache due to local

invasion of the cranial nerves, adjacent organs and lymph nodes and with or without distant metastasis in lungs, brain, bones or other organs.
- **E** No

Comments: The detection of identical, neoplastic, atypical, epithelial cells in the biopsies from the tumor and lymph nodes rules out benign lesions such as papillary epithelial hyperplasia, verrucous xanthoma or leukoplakia from the diagnosis. Ductal carcinoma, unlike the patient's lesion, shows rapid growth accompanied with facial weakness, paralysis or even pain, and in histological sections consists of a plethora of oncocytic cells with eosinophilic cytoplasm forming cords or nests, in basaloid, micropapillary, or rabdoid arrangements which were not found in this patient and therefore this tumos, is easily excluded.

Q2 The descriptive histologic term "elephant feet" is given in:
- **A** Basal cell carcinoma
- **B** Ameloblastoma
- **C** Neurofibromas
- **D** Verrucous carcinomas
- **E** Conventional oral carcinomas

Answers:
- **A** No
- **B** No
- **C** No
- **D** Verrucous carcinomas are characterized by bulbous rete ridges that push the underlying corium and resemble elephant feet.
- **E** No

Comments: Malignant tumors, like the basal cell carcinomas of the skin, ameloblastomas of the jaws, conventional oral carcinomas and benign lesions like neurofibromas, are characterized by an arrangement of neoplastic cells within the underlying connective tissue in various patterns, unrelated to those seen in verrucous carcinoma.

Q3 Acantholytic neoplastic epithelial cells are commonly seen in:
- **A** Verrucous carcinomas
- **B** Spindle cells/sarcomatoid carcinomas
- **C** Adenoid/pseudoglandular carcinomas
- **D** Adenosquamous carcinomas
- **E** Basaloid carcinomas

Answers:
- **A** No
- **B** No
- **C** Adenoid or pseudoglandular carcinomas are rare carcinomas, usually seen in sun-exposed body areas like the lips rather than inside the mouth, and characterized by areas of conventional squamous cell carcinoma along with atypical, acantholytic, epithelial cells, forming a glandular pattern with no evidence of glandular differentiation or secretory activity.
- **D** No
- **E** No

Comments: The other histological variants of oral carcinomas have certain characteristics such as bulbous rete ridges, pushing the underlying corium and keratin plugs superficially (verrucous type); numerous spindle cells in a sarcomatoid pattern (spindle/sarcomatous type); glandular formation with secretory activity as seen in alcian blue stain (adenosquamous type); or islands of basaloid malignant epithelial cells with keratin pearls formation (basaloid type)

Case 16.3

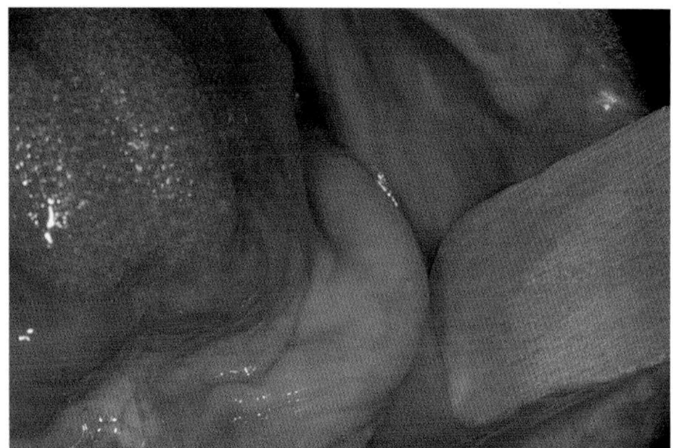

Figure 16.3

CO: A 72-year-old woman complained of a swelling in the floor of the mouth.

HPC: The swelling was found by the patient one week ago during a self-examination before seeing her dentist for construction of a new denture. The patient had all her teeth extracted due to severe periodontal problems at the age of 50, and had the same dentures since then.

PMH: The patient suffered from severe anxiety, irritable bowel syndrome, and hypertension, and smoked two packets of cigarettes daily.

OE: Oral examination revealed a soft, normal color swelling on the floor of the mouth along the sublingual fold. The swelling was soft and was more obvious when the patient moved her tongue upwards and did not wear her lower denture (Figure 16.3). No evidence of inflammation of the floor of the mouth was found and normal saliva was easily secreted from the ducts of her submandibular and sublingual glands. No other lesions were found inside her mouth, skin, and other mucous membranes. Her neck was soft without evidence of swelling (localized or diffused) or cervical lymphadenopathy.

Q1 What is the diagnosis?
- **A** Lipoma
- **B** Sublingual abscess
- **C** Sublingual emphysema
- **D** Submandibular duct occlusion
- **E** Anatomical variation of floor of the mouth

Answers:
- **A** No
- **B** No
- **C** No
- **D** No
- **E** This is an anatomical variation of the floor of the mouth and appears often in overweight, nervous patients with thin lower alveolar ridges. This "swelling" appears during lifting the floor of the mouth upwards via the contraction of the mylohyoid muscles and is not associated with pathologies like abscesses or tumors.

Comments: The secretion of normal saliva from asymptomatic submandibular or sublingual salivary glands and the lack of recent local trauma or infection exclude salivary gland stones, sublingual emphysema or abscess from the diagnosis respectively. Lipoma is also a benign, well-defined lesion that can be seen on the floor of the mouth regardless tongue movements.

Q2 Which of the muscles below participate in the formation of this "lesion"?
- **A** Palatoglossus
- **B** Geniohyoid
- **C** Hypoglossus
- **D** Mylohyoid
- **E** Genioglossus

Answers:
- **A** No
- **B** The geniohyoid muscles play a part by elevating the hyoid and depressing the mandible bone, thus making the sublingual fold more prominent.
- **C** No
- **D** The mylohyoid muscles depress the mandible and elevate the floor of mouth.
- **E** No

Comments: The other muscles affect the position of the tongue rather than the floor of the mouth; the hypoglossus depresses and retracts; the geniohyoid depresses and protrudes; while the palatinoglossus retracts and elevates the tongue.

Q3 The sublingual space is defined as the space between:
- **A** The mucosa of the floor of the mouth (superior)
- **B** Medial surface of the mandible (anterior and lateral)
- **C** Mylohyoid muscle (inferior)
- **D** Geniohyoid muscle (anterior)
- **E** Genioglossus muscle (posterior)

Answers:
- **A** The mucosa of the floor of the mouth is the upper part of this space.
- **B** The mandible acts as the anterior and lateral frontier.
- **C** The mylohyoid muscle is the base of the space.
- **D** No
- **E** The genioglossus muscle is the posterior part.

Comments: The geniohyoid muscles form together with genioglossus muscles the posterior and not the anterior part of sublingual space.

Case 16.4

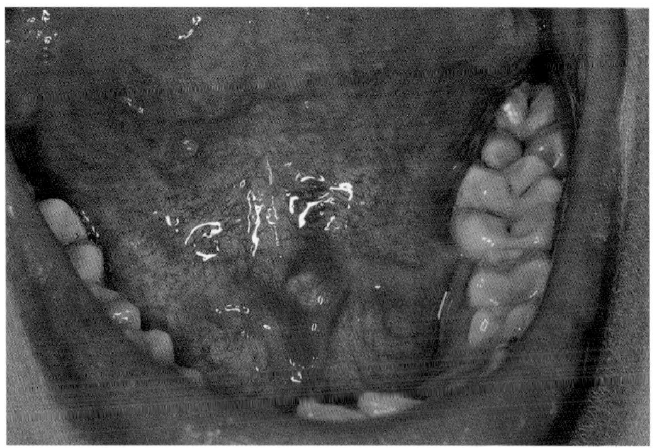

Figure 16.4

CO: A 38-year-old woman presented with a hard yellow nodule on the floor of her mouth.

HPC: The lesion was first noticed three weeks ago by the patient and associated with pain arising from a mild swelling in the left side of her neck, which became more obvious during eating or drinking.

PMH: Her medical history was irrelevant with the lesion, and did not include any serious diseases or recent trauma. Smoking or drinking habits were not recorded.

OE: A hard yellow nodule was found on the floor of the mouth and located within the left Wharton duct, where it was difficult to extract saliva during milking of the relevant gland (Figure 16.4). Xerostomia was not found, but a swelling of her right submandibular gland was detected during eating salty or sour foods. No other oral lesions or cervical lymphadenopathy were detected. Occlusal central X-rays revealed a mild radiopaque calcified mass on the floor of the patient's mouth.

Q1 What is the possible cause?
- **A** Lipoma
- **B** Submandibular duct stone
- **C** Traumatic fibroma
- **D** Foreign body
- **E** Ranula

Answers:
- **A** No
- **B** Submandibular duct stone is the cause, and characterized as a hard, palpable, yellowish nodule at the duct opening. This calcified nodule causes a partially or complete duct obstruction leading to elimination of saliva secretion, stagnation, and finally inflammation of the gland. The submandibular duct stones are often associated with intermittent pain and swelling of the affected gland, increasing prior to or during meals, but going down slowly after. The duct is sometimes swollen and erythematous material and pus may come out.
- **C** No
- **D** No
- **E** No

Comments: Lesions such as lipomas, ranulas, fibromas, and foreign bodies can affect the floor of mouth, but were easily excluded as lipomas and ranulas have a yellowish appearance similar to patient's lesion, but are soft and fluctuant while fibromas and foreign body lesions are firm and a trauma always precedes their onset.

Q2 Which of the factors below may be/or associated with the development of these lesions?
- **A** Malnutrition
- **B** Mumps
- **C** Sjogren syndrome
- **D** Gout disease
- **E** Pleomorphic adenoma

Answers:
- **A** Malnutrition seems to reduce the saliva flow rate and alters its composition of minerals and proteins to such a degree that it increases the incidence of sialolithiasis.
- **B** No
- **C** Sjogren syndrome is a chronic autoimmune disease characterized by a lymphocyte-mediated destruction of the exocrine glands like lacrimal and salivary glands, causing dry eyes and dry mouth. The reduced salivary flow rate and the high concentration of Ca^{+2} have been implicated in the pathogenesis of stone formation in parotid rather than submandibular glands.
- **D** Gout disease is characterized by deposition of urate crystals in various organs, like the kidney or salivary glands, where they act as a substrate for stone formation.
- **E** No

Comments: Mumps is an acute viral infection of the salivary glands causing severe complications such as testicular and ovarian inflammation, spontaneous abortion, and meningitis, but never salivary stones. When salivary stones exist in adult patients with mumps, the symptomatology is exacerbated. Pleomorphic adenoma is a benign, long lasting tumor of the parenchyma of the salivary glands, that is not related to stone formation.

Q3 Which of the factors below is/or are related with the predilection of the submandibular rather than parotid duct for stone formation?

- **A** pH of the secreted saliva
- **B** Viscosity of the saliva
- **C** Size of the main duct system
- **D** Size of the salivary duct opening
- **E** Concentration of inorganic elements in saliva

Answers:

- **A** The pH of the secreted saliva differs as it is alkaline from the submandibular glands and acid from the parotid. pH above 7 allows the accumulation of various inorganic elements within the duct that participate in stone formation.
- **B** The saliva from the submandibular gland is more viscous, and that allows the stagnation the saliva there and formation of mucus plugs which become the basis of stone formation.
- **C** The size of the main duct system of the submandibular is longer than that of the parotid gland and therefore has more chances for obstruction or occlusion.
- **D** No
- **E** Minerals like Ca^{+2} concentrations are higher in the submandibular rather than the parotid glands, making stone formation more likely.

Comments: The width of both ducts (orifice) is almost identical: 0.5–1.4 mm for Stensen's and 0.5–1.5 mm for the Wharton duct, but the route of saliva differs as it is almost horizontal for the parotid while uphill for the submandibular gland.

Case 16.5

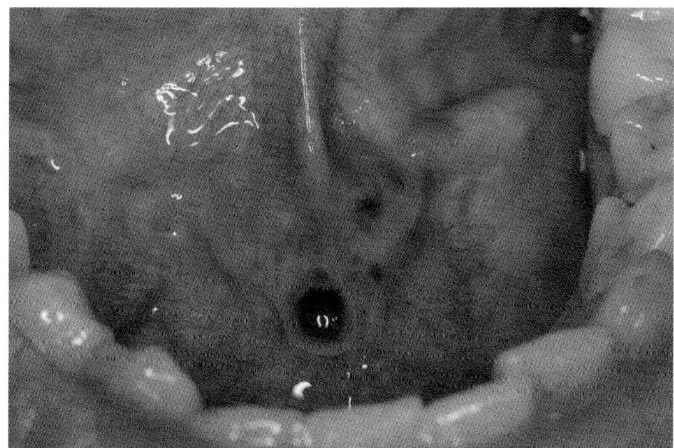

Figure 16.5

CO: A 48-year-old man presented with a dark blue lesion on the floor of his mouth.

HPC: The lesion was first found two months ago, during a deep scaling procedure, by his dentist and remained unchanged since then.

PMH: His medical history was not contributory to the lesion and trauma in the area was reported one year ago.

OE: A round nodule of bluish color with firm consistency, covered by normal mucosa on the floor of the mouth, close to the lingual frenulum was found (Figure 16.5). It was approximately 3 mm in diameter and associated with superficial vascular lesions (varicoses) and appeared shortly after a trauma in the area during eating. The lesion was examined with radiographs that showed areas of radiopacities. These were parts of a calcified thrombus in a lumen of a dilated vein, as confirmed with biopsy. No similar lesions were found in other parts of his mouth, skin, or other mucosae.

Q1 What is the lesion?

- **A** Phlebolith
- **B** Calcified lymph node
- **C** Submandibular gland stone
- **D** Melanoma
- **E** Blue nevus

Answers:

- **A** Phlebolith is a rare lesion characterized by as a small, round, hard mass of various color, depending on the location of the lesion. Superficial lesions have dark blue or black color, while deep lesions

have a normal color. The lesion reveals the formation of a calcified thrombus in the lumen of a dilated blood vessel.
- **B** No
- **C** No
- **D** No
- **E** No

Comments: Based on the histological findings only such the presence of a calcified thrombus, but not calcification of lymph nodes or ducts or the absence of abnormal melanocytes, or heavy pigmented spindle cells alternating with clear cells, excludes calcified lymph nodes; submandibular gland stones and melanoma or blue nevus from the diagnosis respectively.

Q2 Which is the best treatment for an asymptomatic head phlebolith?
- **A** Follow-up only
- **B** Surgery removal
- **C** Anticoagulant therapy
- **D** Painkillers
- **E** Laser therapy

Answers:
- **A** The asymptomatic phleboliths do not require any treatment but only regular follow-up.
- **B** No
- **C** No
- **D** No
- **E** No

Comments: The removal of a symptomatic phlebolith is done with surgery or laser together with painkillers but not anticoagulant drugs and improves patient's symptoms.

Q3 Which other diseases are presented with abnormal calcifications?
- **A** Extrapulmonary tuberculosis
- **B** Prostate metastasis
- **C** Mucinous adenocarcinoma of gut
- **D** Hyperthyroidism
- **E** Hemangiomas

Answers:
- **A** Calcifications are common findings in chronic or healed tuberculous infection.
- **B** Metastatic prostate carcinoma is often associated with osteoblastic lesions involving the skeleton and even jaws.
- **C** Mucinous adenocarcinomas are associated with raised precipitation of calcium salts; especially phosphate and carbonate, causing calcifications.
- **D** No
- **E** Hemangiomas present sometimes after trauma, local thrombosis, fibrosis, and final calcification.

Comments: The parathyroid and not the thyroid hormones influence calcium metabolism, and therefore hyperthyroidism is unrelated to tissues calcification.

17

Gingivae

The gingivae are the area where a number of legions such as neoplastic (benign or malignant) and non-neoplastic (like inflammatory, reactive, or infective from bacteria, viruses, and fungi) occur. Allergies to a variety of chemicals or cosmetic or food allergens, and autoimmune diseases, also take place in the gingivae. Some of the lesions are localized and some others are systematic and associated with variable symptomatology. Some lesions appear at birth, but the majority are acquired and present at different periods of a patient's life. Some of the lesions resolve spontaneously, but some others can jeopardize the patient's life and require immediate treatment (See Figure 17.0).

Table 17 lists the most common and important gingival lesions and conditions.

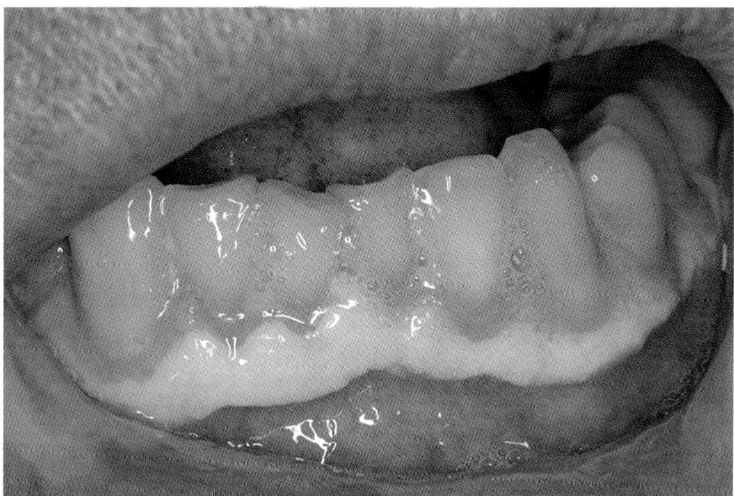

Figure 17.0 Materia alba on the anterior lower gingivae of a patient receiving chemo-radiotherapy.

Clinical Guide to Oral Diseases, First Edition. Dimitris Malamos and Crispian Scully.

Companion website: www.wiley.com/go/malamos/clinical_guide

Table 17 Gingivae lesions: common and important conditions.

- ◆ Congenital
  - Only in gingivae
    - Familial gingival fibromatosis
  - Plus other organs
    - White sponge nevus
- ◆ Acquired
  - Infections
    - Gingivitis
    - Periodontitis
    - ulcerated and part of systemic disease
    - Necrotizing gingivitis/periodontitis
    - Herpetic primary gingivitis – gingivostomatitis
    - Linear gingival erythema
  - Immune-related
    - Desquamative gingivitis
    - Granulomatous gingivitis
    - Strawberry (Wegener) gingivitis
    - Plasma cell gingivitis
  - Traumatic
    - Epulis – pyogenic granuloma
    - giant cell granuloma
    - – fissuratum

Table 17 (Continued)

  - Endocrine
    - Pregnancy gingivitis
    - Pregnancy epulis
  - Medications
    - Phenytoid
    - Nifedipine
    - Calcium antagonistics
    - Cyclosporine induced gingival enlargement
  - Avitaminoses
    - Scurvy
  - Neoplasia
    - Keratosis
    - Carcinomas
    - Sarcomas
    - Melanomas
    - Lymphomas
    - Arisen from jaw tumors
    - Metastatic
  - Skin diseases
    - lichen planus (other forms)
    - lupus erythematosus

Case 17.1

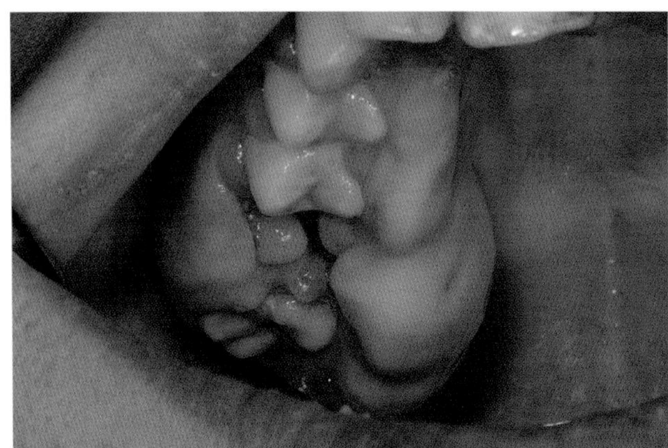

Figure 17.1a

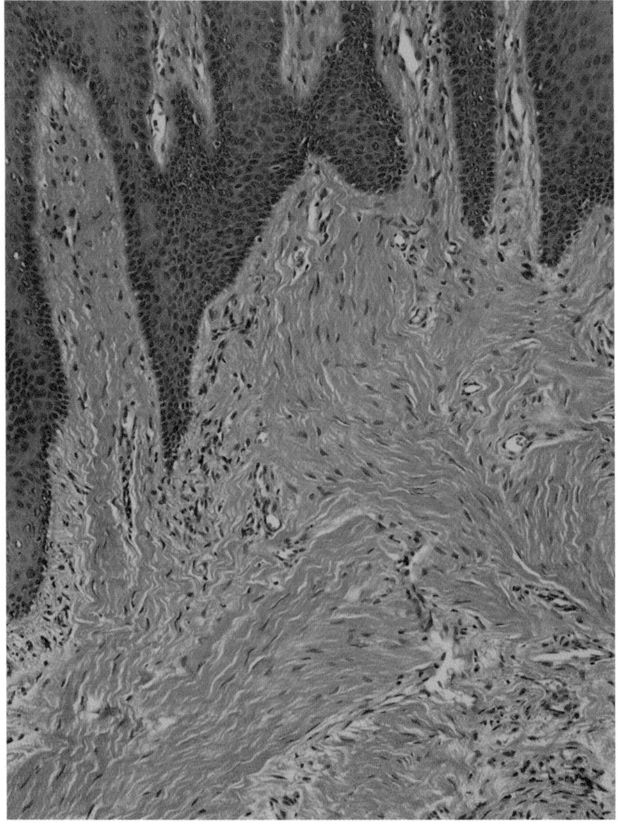

Figure 17.1b

CO: A 32-year-old woman presented for evaluation of chronic enlargement of her gingivae.

HPC: The gingival enlargement had begun from childhood, but they reached their maximum size at the beginning of adulthood.

PMH: Her medical history was negative for any serious diseases, allergies or drug use, but her father and her sister had similar lesions but with less severity.

OE: Intra-oral examination revealed gingival enlargements of all her teeth, but predominately on the upper molars (Figure 17.1a).This enlargement involved the free and attached gingival, at such degree that covered the most of their surfaces causing malocclusion, aesthetic and eating problems. No other lesions were seen in her mouth, skin or other mucus membrane. Orthopantomogram (OPG) did not reveal any alveolar bone loss. Biopsy was taken and showed that the enlarged gingivae were composed of dense collagen fiber bundles in all directions, with few fibroblasts and mild chronic inflammation that was underlying a hyperplastic epithelium with elongated rete pegs (Figure 17.1b).

Q1 What is the possible diagnosis?
- **A** Periodontitis
- **B** Mouth breathing gingivitis
- **C** Drug-induced gingival hyperplasia
- **D** Granulomatous gingivitis
- **E** Hereditary gingival hyperplasia

Answers:
- **A** No
- **B** No
- **C** No
- **D** No
- **E** Hereditary gingival fibromatosis is a rare condition of the gingivae characterized by benign, slowly progressive, non-hemorrhagic overgrowths of the gingivae. The affected gingivae were composed of diffuse bundles of fibrous connective tissue, which sometimes covers the whole crown of the teeth, causing esthetic and functional problems.

Comments: The lack of bone loss shown by OPG and absence of granulomas in the submucosa of the patient's gingivae excludes periodontitis and granulomatous gingivitis from the diagnosis. The long duration of gingival lesions, the distribution in molars rather than anterior teeth, and the absence of drug use excluded a diagnosis of drug-induced gingival hyperplasia and mouth breathing gingivitis while the presence similar but less in severity gingival lesions in her sister and father the reinforces the clinical diagnosis.

Q2 What are the differences between a localized hereditary gingival hyperplasia and gingival epulis?
- **A** Sex predilection
- **B** Composition
- **C** Symptomatology
- **D** Onset time
- **E** Heritage

Answers:
- **A** Hereditary gingival fibromatosis affects men and women equally, while gingival epulis appears exclusively in pregnant women, mainly in the last trimester of their pregnancy.
- **B** The localized hereditary gingival fibromatosis is composed of dense fibrous bundles of connective with a few small capillaries, while gingival epulis is composed mainly from granulation tissue with numerous small vessels and chronic inflammation.
- **C** No
- **D** Hereditary gingival fibromatosis appears at a very early age (around 10 years of age) while gingival epulis later and only during the reproductive phase of women's life.
- **E** Hereditary gingival fibromatosis is linked with autosomal or recessive heritage, while epulis is linked with female hormone deregulation during pregnancy.

Comments: Both gingival conditions are associated with gingival growths with hemorrhage and minor symptomatology.

Q3 This condition can be part of various syndromes such as:
- **A** Zimmermann-Laband syndrome (ZLS)
- **B** Down syndrome
- **C** Cowden syndrome
- **D** Cross syndrome
- **E** Sturge-Weber syndrome

Answers:
- **A** Zimmermann-Laband syndrome is characterized additionally by ear, nose, bone and nail defects and hepatosplenomegaly and gingival malformations.
- **B** No
- **C** No
- **D** Cross syndrome includes microphthalmia, mental retardation, athetosis, hypopigmentation and gingival fibromatosis.
- **E** No

Comments: Gingival diseases are also found in Down, Cowden and Sturge-Weber syndromes, but are associated with poor oral hygiene and local inflammation, rather than collagen overproduction as seen in this patient with fibromatosis.

Case 17.2

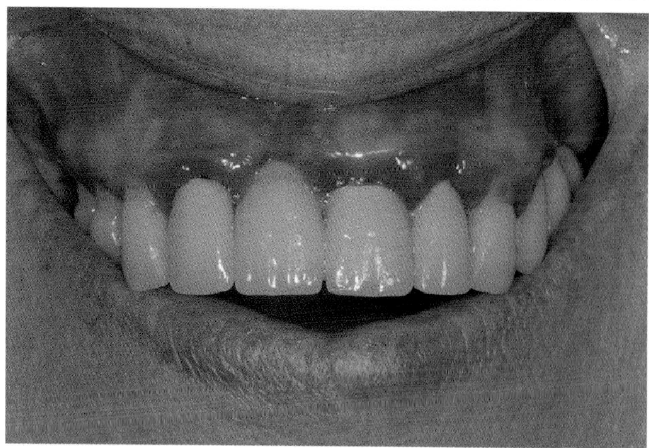

Figure 17.2

CO: A 57-year-old woman presented with swollen hemorrhagic gingivae over the last five to six months.

HPC: Her gingival problems began during her first pregnancy with mild erythema and bleeding 30 years ago, but over the last 10 years her gums became swollen and painful on brushing.

PMH: Her medical history was clear apart from mild hypertension requiring no drugs, and allergic rhinitis relieved with anti-histamine drugs when needed. She had stopped smoking recently.

OE: Oral examination revealed erythematous swollen gingivae (Figure 17.2) with deep pockets that bled easily with brushing or spontaneously, and were associated with halitosis and sialorrhea. OPG and intraoral X-rays revealed severe alveolar bone loss that was more prominent in the molar areas. No other oral, skin, gut, or other mucosae lesions were reported. Cervical or general lymphadenopathy was not detected.

Q1 What is the possible diagnosis?
- **A** Periodontitis
- **B** Ulcerative periodontitis
- **C** Plasma cell gingivitis
- **D** Leukemic gingivitis
- **E** Granulomatous gingivitis

Answers:
- **A** Periodontitis is a chronic gum disease affecting gingivae and their supporting bone-tissues. It is characterized by erythematous gingival swellings and pocket formation, loose teeth and bad breath.
- **B** No
- **C** No
- **D** No
- **E** No

Comments: The long duration of gingival inflammation and the absence of necrotic interdental papillae or other systematic lesions and lymphadenopathy exclude necrotizing periodontitis, plasma cell and granulomatous or leukemic gingivitis respectively

Q2 Which other systemic diseases are associated with this condition?
- **A** Multiple sclerosis
- **B** Stroke
- **C** Facial palsy
- **D** Glucagonoma
- **E** Heart disease

Answers:
- **A** Multiple sclerosis and chronic periodontitis both have an inflammatory origin, and it is believed that there is a link in the pathogenesis of these diseases, especially among female patients.
- **B** Periodontitis and tooth loss have been associated with the increased risk of stroke.
- **C** No
- **D** No
- **E** The inflammation seen in periodontal disease has been accused to participate in the pathogenesis of various heart diseases (heart attack; angina; atherosclerosis of blood vessels).

Comments: No association has been found between periodontal disease and facial palsy or glucagonoma. However, uncontrolled diabetes and viral infections like HIV exacerbate periodontal tissues destruction.

Q3 Which is/are the difference of a severe from an aggressive periodontitis?
- **A** Age of patients
- **B** Sex predilection
- **C** Rate of progression
- **D** Family history
- **E** Relation with local factors

Answers:

A Aggressive periodontitis usually affects younger patients (under 30 years) but chronic periodontitis is more prevalent in older adults.

B No

C The rate of progression is very fast in rapid periodontitis, with many episodes of attachment and bony loss while in chronic periodontitis it is slow.

D There is strong evidence of genetic involvement (familial) in rapid rather than chronic periodontitis.

E The degree of destruction of the periodontal tissues is strongly related with local factors (plaque; calculus; poor oral hygiene) in chronic but not in rapid periodontitis.

Comments: Men do not seem to have a higher risk for more rapid periodontal destruction than women in both chronic and rapid periodontitis.

Case 17.3

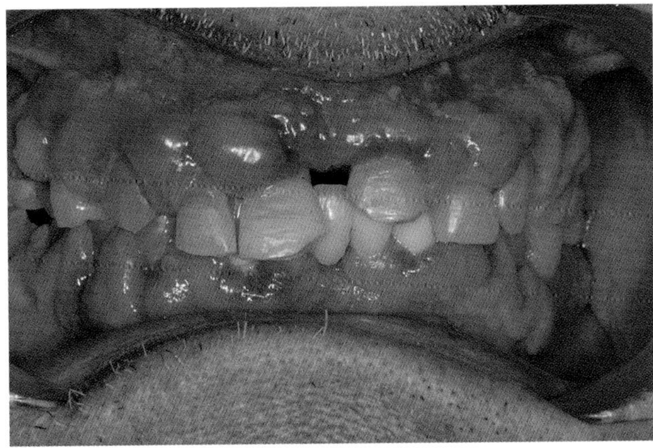

Figure 17.3

CO: A 69-year-old man, an ex-smoker, presented with diffused gingival enlargement.

HPC: His gingival enlargement started two years ago and became more pronounced over the last six months, after the patient had a hypertensive crisis and was admitted to the local hospital.

PMH: Chronic hypertension and gout were his main medical problems, partially controlled with amlodipine daily and colchicine tablets in crisis.

OE: A generalized and firm overgrowth of his gingivae was found throughout the maxilla and mandible, but particularly at the upper anterior teeth. The gingivae were pink, soft and hemorrhaged in places, forming pseudo-pockets and covered part of the teeth's surface (Figure 17.3) where mature plaque was easily detected due to his poor oral hygiene. No other lesions were found in his mouth or skin and lymph node enlargement were not detected. Blood test results were within the normal range. Gingival biopsy revealed pseudoepithelial hyperplasia overlying fibrous vascular connective tissue with chronic inflammation.

Q1 What is the main cause of his gingival hyperplasia?

A Poor oral hygiene

B Drug-induced

C Mouth breathing

D Gout complications

E Smoking

Answers:

A No

B Drugs like amlodipine for hypertension rather than colchicines for gout is responsible for his gingival hyperplasia. The mechanism of hyperplasia may start by the direct toxic effect of this drug to the crevicular fluid that causes and together with a local inflammation which leads to upregulation of several cytokine factors like TGF-β1. IL-1b and PDGF together with defective collagenase activity and upregulation of keratinocyte growth factor.

C No

D No

E No

Comments: Mouth breathing causes usually gingival enlargement of anterior maxillary and mandibular teeth rather than the posteriors. Poor oral hygiene and smoking are the main cause of severe inflammation in periodontitis, but the inflammation was not severe as seen in biopsy, and the patient had stopped smoking. Accumulation of urate crystals are often seen in the skin (tophi) but not in the gingivae in patients with uncontrolled gout.

Q2 Which is/are the best treatment/s for this hyperplasia?

A Improve oral hygiene only

B Scaling treatment

C Antibiotics (topical or systemic)

D Gingivectomy

E Drug alterations (dose/or replacement)

Answers:

A No

B No

C No

D Gingivectomy by scalpel or laser, free flap surgery or electrosurgery are various surgery techniques which are useful for the removal of gingival excess. Scalpel gingivectomy is used for the localized treatment, flap surgery for extensive lesions, while electrosurgery and laser techniques are suitable for children or mental handicapped patients as it is a very rapid procedure with good hemostasis.

E Alteration of causative drug or reducing its dose restores the gingivae within a couple of months.

Comments: Good oral hygiene is an important factor to prevent or retard the gingival overgrowths, especially after gingival surgery, but its role alone or in combination with scaling or antibiotic use topically or systemically is minimal without of the suspected drug withdrawal.

Q3 Which of the drugs below is/are related to gingival enlargement?

A Anticonvulsants

B Diuretics

C Immunosuppressive drugs

D Calcium channel blockers

E NSAIDs

Answers:

A Anticonvulsant drugs like phenytoin valproate, phenobarbitone, and lamotrigine act on fibroblasts to synthesize extracellular matrix and collagen.

B No

C Immunosuppressive drugs like cyclosporine are widely used to prevent organs rejection after transplantation, to treat chronic skin diseases such as psoriasis or atopic dermatitis and rheumatoid arthritis or nephritic syndrome.

D Calcium channel blockers like amlodipine, nifedipine, and diltiazem are widely used for hypertension treatment and cause generalized gingival enlargement.

E No

Comments: Diuretics or natriuretic drugs cause mineral imbalance, while NSAIDs cause oral ulcerations, but neither drug induces gingival hyperplasia.

Case 17.4

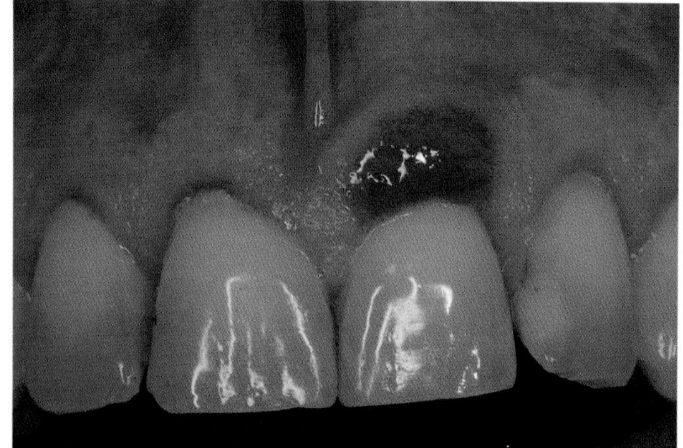

Figure 17.4

CO: A 45-year-old woman presented with a red spot in her anterior gingivae of her upper left central incisor.

HPC: Her gingival spot appeared five months ago as a small red dot that gradually extended from the free towards the attached gingivae.

PMH: Her medical history was unremarkable. No known allergies, skin or genital lesions or parafunctional habits like rubbing of gingivae or smoking and drinking were recorded. Her dental or family history was irrelevant with this lesion.

OE: A red, asymptomatic, flabby, peanut-shaped lesion in the anterior gingivae (free and attached) of upper left central incisor that bled on probing (Figure 17.4). Probing depth was normal and the patient's oral hygiene was good. No other similar lesions were found in other parts of her mouth, skin, genitals, and other mucosae. An intraoral radiograph did not show any bone loss and a complete hemogram and routine biochemical investigations were within normal values. Biopsy revealed accumulation of mature plasma cells within the corium.

Q1 What is the possible diagnosis?

- **A** Pyogenic granuloma
- **B** Hemangioma
- **C** Erythroplakia
- **D** Plasma cell gingivitis
- **E** Plasmacytoma

Answers:

- **A** No
- **B** No
- **C** No
- **D** Plasma cell gingivitis is a rare gingival condition characterized by sharply demarcated erythematous and edematous red velvety lesions, often extending to the mucogingival junction as a result of a hypersensitivity reaction that causes a diffuse accumulation of mature plasma cells into the sub-epithelial gingival tissue.
- **E** No

Comments: Having in mind the histological characteristics of this lesion such as the presence of normal epithelium without evidence of dysplasia, or the plethora accumulation of mature and not monoclonal plasma cells within the underlying corium, easily excludes erythroplakia or plasmatocytoma. The presence of newly formed vascular channels alone or in combination with the late onset and negative history of trauma, rules out hemangiomas and pyogenic granulomas from the diagnosis.

Q2 Which of the tools below is/are useful for the diagnosis of this condition?

- **A** Clinical examination
- **B** Skull X-rays
- **C** Biopsy
- **D** Allergic patch tests
- **E** Electrophoresis

Answers:

- **A** Clinical inspection helps to determine the location, size, color, and symptomatology of the lesion.
- **B** No
- **C** The biopsy should always detect mature plasma cells within the corium that are oval in shape with eosinophilic cytoplasm, along with eccentric and hyperchromatic nuclei but without atypia.
- **D** Positive allergic skin patch tests against various allergens present in toothpaste, chewing gum, mint, and certain food products could confirm the clinical diagnosis.
- **E** No

Comments: Plasma electrophoresis and skull X-rays are not useful for diagnosis of this gingival condition, which does not show a monoclonal protein (paraprotein) or bony punch-out lesions, the pathognomonic characteristics of a peripheral plasmacytoma or multiple myeloma.

Q3 Which other oral lesions show infiltrations of mature plasma cells within their submucosa?

- **A** Plasmoacanthoma
- **B** Plasma cell granuloma
- **C** Plasmacytoma peripheral
- **D** Tuberculosis ulcer
- **E** Syphilis

Answers:

- **A** Plasmoacanthoma is a verrucous tumor with mature plasma cell infiltration involving the oral mucosa, particularly oral commissures.
- **B** Plasma cell granuloma is a rare growth, seen particularly in the lungs and rarely in the mouth, and characterized microscopically by a vascular stroma with reactive inflammatory cells, mainly mature plasma cells, and usually surrounded by connective tissue septa.
- **C** No
- **D** Oral tuberculosis is a rare, secondary rather than primary manifestation of an infection from *Mycobacterium tuberculosis*. This chronic disease is characterized histologically by numerous necrotizing granulomas that consist of Langerhans type giant cells, neutrophils, lymphocytes and mature plasma cells while acid-fast bacilli that are easily detected with Ziehl-Neelsen stains.
- **E** Syphilis (primary, secondary, or tertiary) is characterized by a perivascular infiltration of mature plasma cells, but mostly seen in gingival biopsies.

Comments: Plasmacytoma is also a tumor of neoplastic but immature plasma cells capable of producing monoclonal protein.

Case 17.5

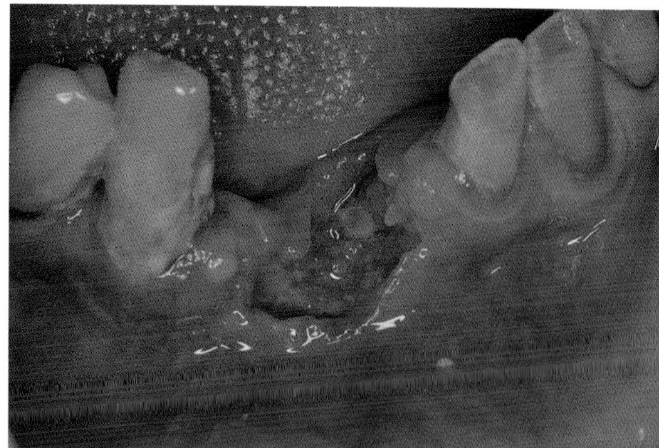

Figure 17.5

CO: An 89-year-old man presented with a chronic ulcer in his lower anterior gingivae.

HPC: The ulcer was present for almost eight months and appeared after extraction of very loose lower central incisors.

PMH: Despite his old age, no serious systematic diseases, allergies, medications or hazardous habits like smoking were recorded.

OE: A deep irregular ulcer with granular base with raised margins of normal color and hard consistency, that easily bled on palpation (Figure 17.5). This ulcer was asymptomatic but accompanied with halitosis and cervical submental lymphadenopathy. No other similar lesions were found in his mouth, skin, and other mucosae. Radiological examination revealed superficial alveolar bone loss close to the ulcer. Routine blood tests were within normal range. Biopsy from the base of the ulcer revealed of islands of epithelial cells, well-differentiated within a fibrovascular stroma with mixed chronic inflammation, while from the margins of the ulcer the epithelium was dysplastic with hyperchromatic nuclei and an increased number of mitoses.

Q1 What is the possible diagnosis?

- **A** Traumatic ulcer
- **B** Eosinophilic ulcer
- **C** Actinomycosis
- **D** Oral carcinoma
- **E** Large aphthae

Answers:

- **A** No
- **B** No
- **C** No
- **D** Oral carcinoma of gingivae is the correct diagnosis. This cancer is presented as a swelling, growth, or irregular ulcer in the gingivae sometimes causing local bone invasion and destruction, loose teeth and regional lymphadenopathy.
- **E** No

Comments: The lack of pain and long duration of the lesion easily excludes large aphtha and traumatic ulcer from diagnosis. Also, the presence of islands of neoplasmatic epithelial cells with atypia and increased mitoses and the absence of eosinophils or actinomycetomas in the underlying submucosa is an indication of that the lesion is a carcinoma rather than an eosinophilic ulcer or actinomycosis respectively.

Q2 Which of the clinical characteristics below can differentiate an ulcer of a primary oral carcinoma from a tuberculosis?

- **A** Sex predilection
- **B** Age
- **C** Clinical picture
- **D** Symptomatology
- **E** Systematic findings

Answers:

- **A** No
- **B** Age differs as oral carcinomas appear at an older age (>50 years) while the age in patients with tuberculosis is variable.
- **C** The ulcer in carcinomas looks like a crater with raised, irregular indurated margins, while in tuberculosis the ulcer is more superficial, irregular, soft, and well-circumscribed, with surrounding erythema.
- **D** No
- **E** Tubercular oral ulcer is usually a secondary rather than primary manifestation of tuberculosis, and often is associated with lungs, pleura, CNS, skin, and genitourinary involvement. The secondary tubercular oral lesions are often single, indurated, irregular, painful ulcers covered by inflammatory exudate in patients of any age group, but relatively more common in middle-aged and elderly patients. Oral cancer usually appears as a single asymptomatic lesion at initial stages without other local or distant organ involvement (metastasis).

Comments: Oral carcinomas and tubercular ulcerations have a slight predilection for males, but both conditions are asymptomatic and present with pain at later stages when local nerve involvement takes place.

Q3 Which are the common risk factors of oral carcinomas and tuberculosis?

- **A** Malnutrition
- **B** Alcoholism
- **C** Silicosis
- **D** HIV infection
- **E** Organ transplantation

Answers:

- **A** Poor diet has been liked to increased risk of oral cancer and tuberculosis as malnutrition causes a weakness of the patient's immune system against various carcinogens and pathogenic bacteria such as *Mycobacterium tuberculosis*.
- **B** Alcoholism alone or in combination with smoking and malnutrition increases the risk of oral carcinomas and tuberculosis two to three times.
- **C** No
- **D** The risk of tuberculosis is estimated to be up to 16 times higher among HIV+ patients while the risk of oral cancer is even more higher and is closely related to other additional infections from herpes simplex virus (HSV), Epstein-Barr virus (EBV), human herpes virus 8 (HHV8), and human papillomavirus (HPV).
- **E** Patients with kidney or other transplants have an increased risk of oral carcinomas (mostly of the lower lip) and tuberculosis due to life-long immunosuppressant medications that are used constantly to avoid new organ rejection.

Comments: Silicosis is a lung disease with increased risk of tuberculosis, and lung but not oral cancer.

18

Jaws

Various pathologies affect the upper jaw (maxilla) and lower jaw (mandible) regardless of the patient's age; sex and health status. Some of them appear at a very early age (congenital) but the majority appear later (acquired). A few have odontogenic origin, like cysts and odontogenic tumors but the rest are numerous and have a non-odontogenic origin like reactive (tori and inflammatory); bone remodeling (fibrous dysplasia and Paget disease); or neoplastic (benign or malignant) (Figure 18.0a and b).

Jaws are the most common site of metastases from various distant organs like prostate, breast and blood neoplasms. Some of the jaw pathologies are asymptomatic and stable for years, but others are associated with pain, teeth loosening, malocclusion eating problems and facial disfiguration, and therefore require early treatment.

Table 18 lists the most common conditions and diseases occurring in the jaws.

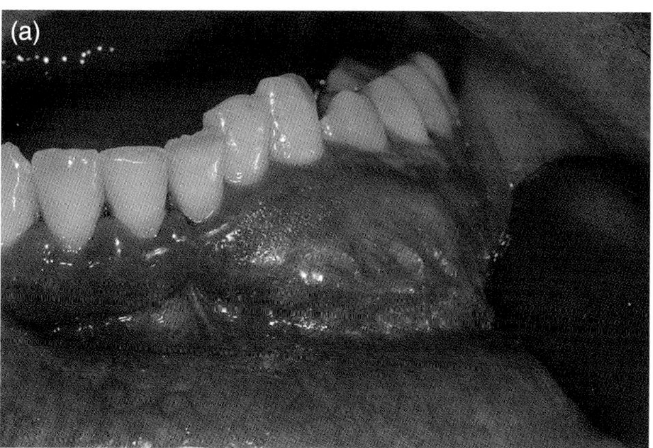

Figure 18.0a Enlargement of the mandible from an odontogenic tumor (adenomatoid odontogenic tumor).

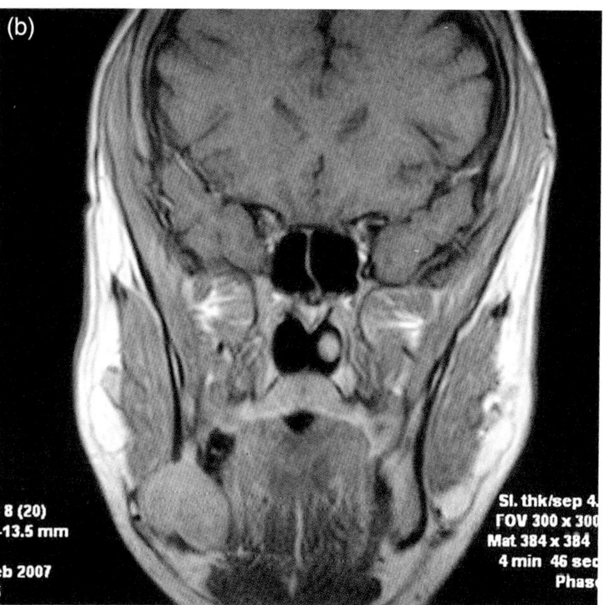

Figure 18.0b Enlargement of the mandible from non-odontogenic tumor (multiple myeloma).

Clinical Guide to Oral Diseases, First Edition. Dimitris Malamos and Crispian Scully.

Companion website: www.wiley.com/go/malamos/clinical_guide

Table 18 Common and important conditions of occurring in the jaws.

- ◆ Congenital
  - ○ Bony anomalies
    - ▪ Aplasia
    - ▪ Atrophy
    - ▪ Hyperplasia
    - ▪ torus
      - mandibularis
      - palatinus
- ◆ Acquired
  - ○ Trauma
    - ▪ Fractures
    - ▪ Injuries soft and hard tissues
  - ○ Infections
    - ▪ Osteomyelitis (acute/chronic)
    - ▪ Osteonecrosis (caused by irradiation or drugs)
  - ○ Cysts
    - ▪ Odontogenic
    - ▪ Non-odontogenic
  - ○ Tumors
    - ▪ Odontogenic

Table 18 (Continued)

    - ▪ Non-odontogenic
      - Sarcomas
      - Lymphomas
      - Myelomas
      - Metastatic
  - ○ Endocrine anomalies
    - ▪ Rickets
    - ▪ Hypo-function of endocrine glands
      - Pituitary
      - Thyroid
      - Parathyroid
  - ○ Metabolic anomalies
    - ▪ Osteopenia or osteoporosis
    - ▪ Osteomalacia
    - ▪ Paget's disease
    - ▪ Fibrous dysplasia
      - Cherubism

Case 18.1

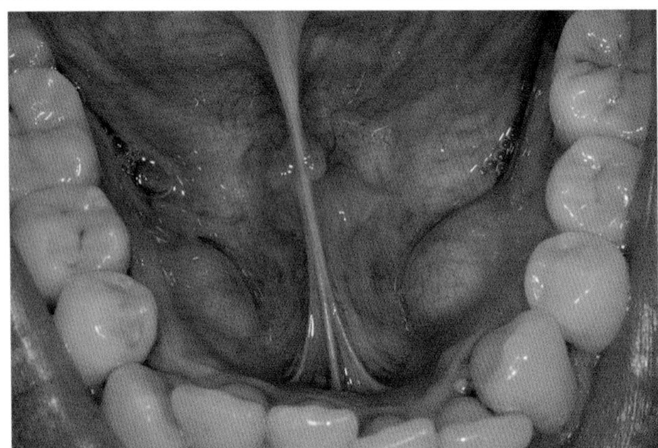

Figure 18.1

CO: A 26-year-old woman was presented with asymptomatic hard lumps in the inner surface of her mandible at premolar areas.

HPC: The lesions were found incidentally during a routine dental examination by her dentist two years ago and remained unchanged since then.

PMH: Her medical and dental records did not reveal any serious systemic diseases, local trauma, caries or periodontal diseases, while parafunctional habits like bruxism were not reported.

OE: Intra-oral examination found two hard, large lumps, well-fixed with the underlying bone in the lingual surface of the mandible and located symmetrically at the premolars area and above mylohyoid line (Figure 18.1). The lesions were covered with normal mucosa and were not fluctuant at palpation nor associated with other oral, skin and other mucosae lesions. The teeth near to the lesions responded well in vitality tests and did not show any evidence of looseness, while their underlying bone was slightly denser in radiographs (occlusals and OPG) and showed evidence of increased osteoblastic rather than osteoclastic activity.

Q1 What are these lesions?

A Multiple fibromas
B Torus palatinus
C Osteomas
D Torus mandibularis
E Osteosarcoma (blastic type)

Answers:

A No
B No
C No
D Torus mandibularis is the correct diagnosis. This torus consists of symmetrical rather than ipsilateral, asymptomatic bone overgrowths causing no to mild irritation or burning sensation. These lesions are covered by a thin normal oral mucosa and are always found in the lingual aspect of the mandible, at the canine and premolar areas.
E No

Comments: Other jaw swellings arise from the mucosa like fibromas or associated with the bone per ce like tori, osteomas or even local or metastatic tumor. Their location, duration, symtomatology as well as clinical and radiological features allow clinicians to exclude these lesions from torus mandibularis lesions. In torus palatinus the bone overgrowths are always in the palate across the middle line, while in osteomas the lesions are within the bones, giving a characteristic radiographic picture and symptomatology. The osteoblastic type of osteosarcoma appears often with similar bony overgrowths, but radiographic evidence of bony destruction is always present. Fibromas are also fibrous and not bony overgrowths, and therefore are softer on palpation and located in any parts of the body where trauma takes place.

Q2 What are the indications for surgical removal of these lesions?

A Increased risk for malignant transformation
B Implantation in thin jaws
C Reconstruction of new dentures
D Carcinophobia
E Mastication problems

Answers:

A No
B Fragments of the cortical bone taken from the tori intermingled with patient's blood have been safely used as additional bone graft in areas where the jaw is very thin, and is going to receive implants.
C During reconstruction of dentures, large torus mandibularis should be removed in order that the new dentures fit properly.
D No
E Mastication problems occur when the torus is very large and ulcerated, causing pain with eating hard foods during the mastication.

Comments: Carcinophobia is not treated with surgical intervention like removal of the tori, but is improved with patient's reassurance that the lesion is benign with no risk of malignant transformation or need for referral to specialists.

Q3 Which of the factors below is or are involved in the formation of these lesions?

A Genetic factors
B Local trauma
C Chronic periapical infections
D Starvation
E Smoking

Answers:

A Genetic factors seem to play a crucial role in the development of these tori as similar lesions have been detected among twins or close relatives, especially in Afro-Caribbeans and Eskimos, rather than in European or American white patients.
B Local trauma induced by a parafunctional habits like bruxism or during eating may cause an irritation locally leading into osteoblastic rather osteolytic activation, with finally excess bone production.
C No
D No
E No

Comments: Starvation may reduce bone growth and decrease bone mineral density causing osteopenia or osteoporosis which can be exacerbated with smoking. Chronic periapical infection usually causes bony resorption and rarely focal sclerosing osteomyelitis adjacent to the apex of the causative teeth.

Case 18.2

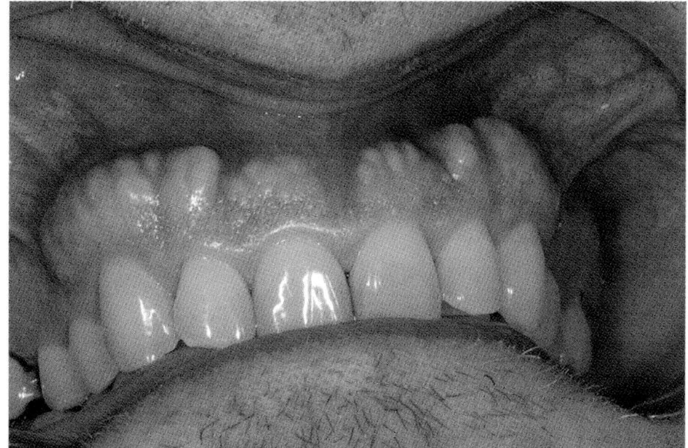

Figure 18.2

CO: A 32-year-old man presented with hard bulky masses on his upper and lower jaws.

HPC: The lesions were asymptomatic and discovered incidentally by the patient five years ago.

PMH: His medical and dental history ware clear of any local or systemic diseases. Among his habits was smoking of one packet a day, and strong teeth clenching during weight-lifting exercises in the gym.

OE: Oral examination revealed multiple hard nodules on the facial aspects of the gingivae of both jaws, but the most obvious were near to the upper anterior teeth (Figure 18.2). No other similar lesions were seen in the other bones or other parts of his body. Intra-oral radiographs revealed increased radio-opaque density in the areas of the hard lesions.

Q1 What is the possible diagnosis?

- **A** Gingival fibromatosis
- **B** Torus palatinus
- **C** Hereditary multiple exostoses
- **D** Gardner syndrome
- **E** Buccal exostoses

Answers:

- **A** No
- **B** No
- **C** No
- **D** No
- **E** These lesions were buccal exostoses, characterized by a benign overgrowth of a new bone on the buccal surface of the alveolar bone of the maxilla or mandible. These exostoses do not cause any pain or other symptoms apart from esthetic disfiguration and carcinophobia in patients under stress.

Comments: The location and the number of bony growths on the buccal surface of the mandible excludes torus palatinus lesions or hereditary multiple exostoses, as the last lesions are located in different places such as in the palate or in the long bones of the legs, upper arms or shoulder respectively. The absence of intestinal polyps or gingival hyperplasias excludes Gardner syndrome and gingival fibromatosis from the diagnosis.

Q2 Which of the clinical characteristics below can be seen in this condition?

- **A** The overlying mucosa is always erythematous and ulcerated
- **B** The lesions are symmetrical and located mainly in the anterior mandible
- **C** The lesions appear usually after the age 60
- **D** Females are more commonly affected rather than males
- **E** The lesions are always associated with pain or periapical infection of adjacent teeth

Answers:

- **A** No
- **B** No
- **C** No
- **D** No
- **E** No

Comments: Buccal exostoses appear more often in men rather than women, on the posterior part of the maxilla rather mandible and seen at early adulthood than childhood. Their adjacent teeth are normal and respond in vitality tests while the overlying mucosa is thin but not erythematous and ulcerated only with trauma.

Q3 Which other similar bony growths are seen in the head and neck region?

- **A** Footballer's lesion
- **B** Subungual lesion
- **C** Surfer's lesion
- **D** Prostate osteosclerosis
- **E** Osteophytes

Answers:

- **A** No
- **B** No
- **C** Surfer's lesion is characterized by abnormal bone growth within the ear canal as the result of a chronic ear irritation from cold wind and water exposure among cold water surfers or outdoor swimmers.
- **D** Prostate carcinoma sometimes induces osteoblastic metastases which are characterized by an increased abnormal bone formation with an elevated osteoid surface. The new bone has poor quality with reduced mechanical resistance leading to spontaneous fractures.
- **E** Osteophytes are bony spars that develop on the margins of joints like the temporomandibular joint (TMJ), secondary to chronic inflammation due to various degenerative disorders.

Comments: In footballer's and subungual exostosis, the lesions arise from the ankle and shin bone or dorsal surface of the distal pharynx of the big toe respectively.

Case 18.3

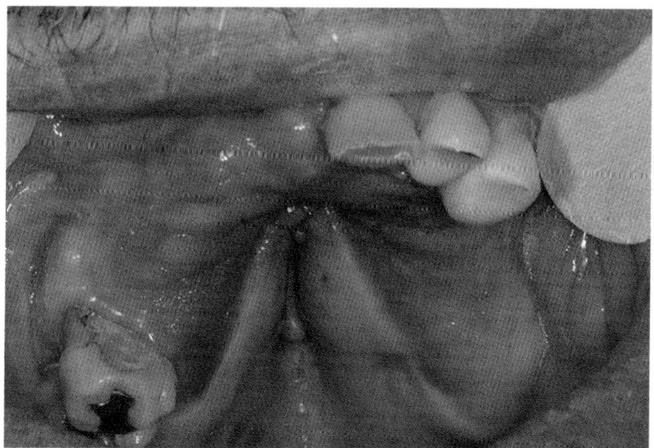

Figure 18.3

CO: A 62-year-old man came with a complaint of difficulty in wearing his upper partial denture that had caused him serious eating problems.

HPC: His complaint began one year ago after a difficult extraction of his upper left second molar, but worsened over the last four months, and since then the patient had three unsuccessful readjustments of his upper denture.

PMH: Hypercholesterolemia and diabetes type II were his main health problems and treated with low fat and sugar diet and drugs such as atorvastatin and metformin respectively.

OE: Oral examination revealed an enlarged, diffuse, asymptomatic bony expansion of his upper jaw that was particularly prominent towards the hard palate (Figure 18.3).The overlying mucosa was thin with normal color, apart from an erythematous area where the upper denture was situated. The denture's supporting teeth did not show any evidence of pulp necrosis, and their surrounding gingivae were soft, swollen but recessed, especially where the denture clasps were applied. No other growths were found in his mandible or in other bones; nor were other similar lesions reported among his close relatives. Skull X-rays revealed an enlarged maxilla with a cotton-wool like appearance. Blood tests did not reveal any anemia, and the calcium, phosphorus, urea and creatinine were within normal levels. However, increased serum alkaline phosphatase up to four times higher than normal was measured.

Q1 What is the main cause of his badly fitted denture?

A Previous extractions
B Erythematous candidiasis
C Paget's disease (monostotic)
D Hyperparathyroidism
E Thalassemia beta

Answers:

A No
B No
C The monostotic type of Paget's disease is the cause. Paget's disease of the bone is characterized by a chronic bone remodeling, leading to this deformity (enlargement) and weakness of one or more bones that is associated with pain, fractures or arthritis of associated joints.
D No
E No

Comments: The extraction of his upper left molar could affect the stability of his denture to some degree, but this has been compensated with the readjustment of his denture. Erythematous candidiasis was due to denture overpressure and caused a burning sensation only. Thalassemia beta and hyperparathyroidism may cause enlargement of the maxilla, but were excluded from diagnosis as these diseases are accompanied with reduced synthesis of beta chains of hemoglobin and increased parathyroid hormone respectively, which were not found in the patient's blood tests

Q2 What is/or are the biochemical markers for this disease?

A Reduced parathyroid hormone
B Increased alkaline phosphatase
C Reduced calcium and/or phosphorus
D Increased urinary pyridoline
E Increased thyroid hormone

Answers:

A No

B Increased alkaline phosphate is a pathognomonic finding in liver and bone diseases.

C No

D Increased pyridoline level is a better representative marker than hydroxyproline regarding of the bone activity in patients with Paget's disease.

E No

Comments: Reduced calcium and phosphorus levels and increased parathyroid hormone is characteristic of rickets or osteomalacia, while the concentration of thyroid hormones (T_3 and T_4) are both irrelevant to Paget's disease.

Q3 Which other conditions is/are NOT associated with this bone disease?

A Osteopenia

B Paresthesia

C Heart failure

D Loose teeth

E Osteomyelitis

Answers:

A Osteopenia is a distinct bone disease that sometimes comes together, with other metabolic bone diseases but not with Paget's disease.

B No

C No

D The enlargement of the mandible or maxilla leads to spacing between adjacent teeth and hypercementosis, making the affected teeth well-fixed and difficult to extract.

E No

Comments: In extensive Paget's disease (>40% of bones involved) new blood vessels are required to ensure an adequate blood supply, leading sometimes to heart failure. Compression of various nerves from the enlarged bones in Paget's disease often causes pain or paresthesias, depending on the nerves involved and the pressure applied. The enlargement of the mandible or maxilla causes malocclusion and the teeth are separated from each other. Osteomyelitis is a common complication and occurs after a recent extraction of a severely decayed tooth with periapical infection.

Case 18.4

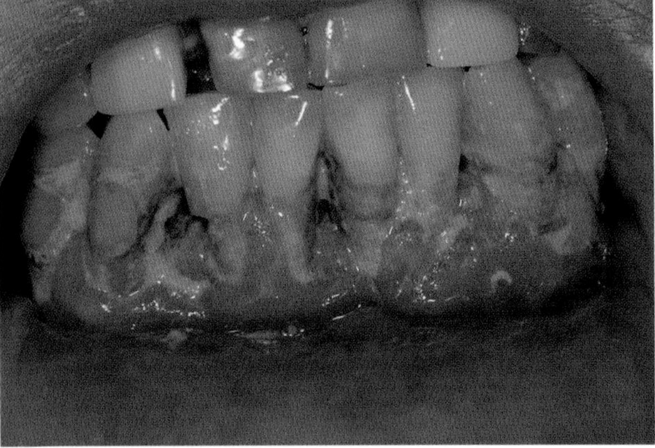

Figure 18.4a

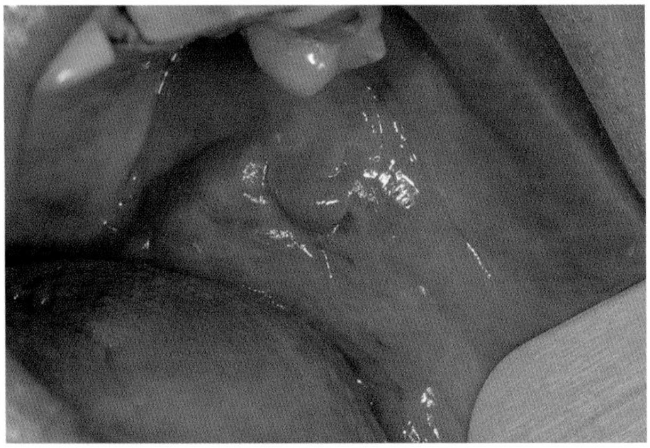

Figure 18.4b

CO: A 52-year-old woman presented with painful ulcerated gingivae and loose teeth.

HPC: The problem with her mouth started three years ago with pain from her lower anterior teeth and swollen gingivae. Despite root canal treatment of suspected teeth and scaling, no improvement was recorded.

PMH: Diabetes insipidus (mild) together with various myoskeletal problems were recorded over the last two years and partially responded to fluid uptake and NSAIDs. A few episodes of otitis were recorded and responded well to antibiotics.

OE: Oral examination revealed soft, inflamed and partially ulcerated gingivae that were very sensitive and bled on probing, while the adjacent teeth were loose and painful, despite her root canal treatment (Figure 18.4a). A few nodular-plaque lesions of both buccal mucosae were also found (Figure 18.4b) and associated with cervical lymphadenopathy. Radiological examination revealed multiple radiolucencies particularly in the mandible, skull and the right tibia (Figure 18.4c and d). Blood tests revealed reduced antidiuretic hormone (ADH), an increased white blood count but with normal pattern,

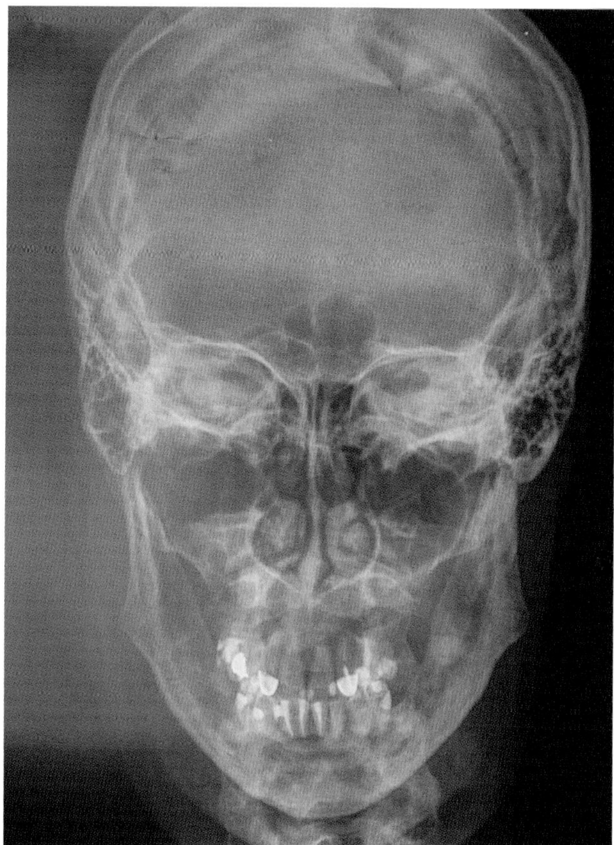

Figure 18.4c

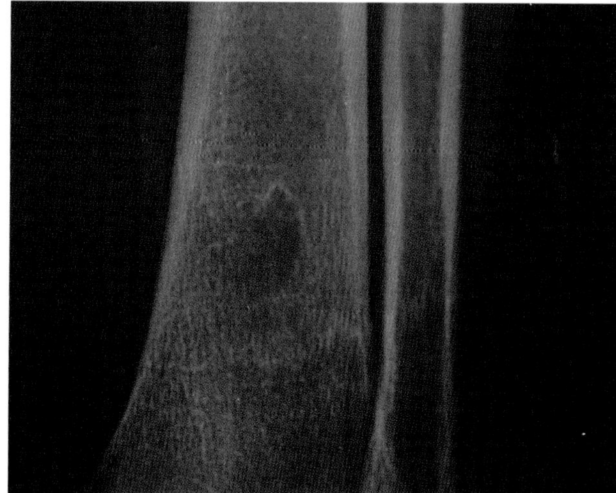

Figure 18.4d

lack of paraproteins, and calcium and phosphorus within the normal values. Gingival biopsy revealed a plethora of aggregation of Langerhans cells and eosinophils within the submucosa.

Q1 Which is the possible cause?

- **A** Multiple myeloma
- **B** Osteomyelitis of mandible
- **C** Congenital neutropenia
- **D** Severe chronic periodontitis
- **E** Histiocytosis X

Answers:

- **A** No
- **B** No
- **C** No
- **D** No
- **E** Histiocytosis X (Langerhans cell histiocytosis, LCH) is the cause. This is a group of rare diseases characterized by local or generalized proliferation of histiocyte cells arising from the monocyte macrophage lineage. It affects one (unifocal) or numerous organs (multifocal) of young children to adult patients and is characterized by numerous bony osteolyses alone or together with one or more extra-bony involvements such as in lungs, spleen or liver, lymph nodes and oral mucosa and skin, with variable prognosis. Diabetes insipidus together with bone defects and mucocutaneous lesions are characteristic of the Hand-Schuller-Christian histiocytosis (chronic multifocal type) as seen in this patient.

Comments: In chronic periodontitis the bony defects were restricted in the alveolar bone supporting the teeth, while in histiocytosis the bony lesions were punched out lesions, very often extending below the apex of the teeth, and seen additionally in other bones. The absence of paraproteinemia or neutropenia in blood tests excludes multiple myeloma and congenital neutropenia, while the lack of necrotic bony sequestra excludes osteomyelitis from diagnosis.

Q2 Which is/are the pathognomonic histological finding/s of this condition?

- **A** Eosinophil accumulation
- **B** Plasma cells
- **C** Foam cells
- **D** Birbeck granules
- **E** Coffee-bean like histiocytes

Answers:

- **A** No
- **B** No
- **C** No
- **D** Birbeck granules or bodies are rod-shaped or tennis racket-shaped cytoplasmic organelles seen in electron microscopy exclusively in Langerhans histiocytosis.
- **E** Coffee-bean like histiocytes are atypical cells that are distinguished by their eosinophilic cytoplasm and the longitudinal nuclear grooves in hematoxylin and eosin (HXE) stains, and their positive reaction in CD1a and Langerin (CD207) receptors in immunohistochemical stains.

Comments: Eosinophils, plasma and foam cell collections are often seen in histiocytosis-X, but are not pathognomonic as participants in other diseases such as atherosclerosis, diabetic nephropathies and bacterial infections.

Q3 Which is/are the recommended treatment/s for this multisystemic disease?

- **A** Surgical excision
- **B** Limited radiotherapy
- **C** Intra-lesional steroids
- **D** Chemotherapeutic agents
- **E** Antimetabolites

Answers:

- **A** No
- **B** No
- **C** No
- **D** Chemotherapy with vinblastine in combination with steroids is the first line of treatment for multisystemic LCH.
- **E** Antimetabolites like 2-chlorodeoxyadenosine and methotrexate interfere with DNA production and are widely used to stop division of abnormal Langerhans histiocytes.

Comments: Surgical excision or a low dose of radiotherapy, and sometimes intralesional injections of steroids like triamcinolone acetonide are effective only in the treatment of monostotic lesions.

Case 18.5

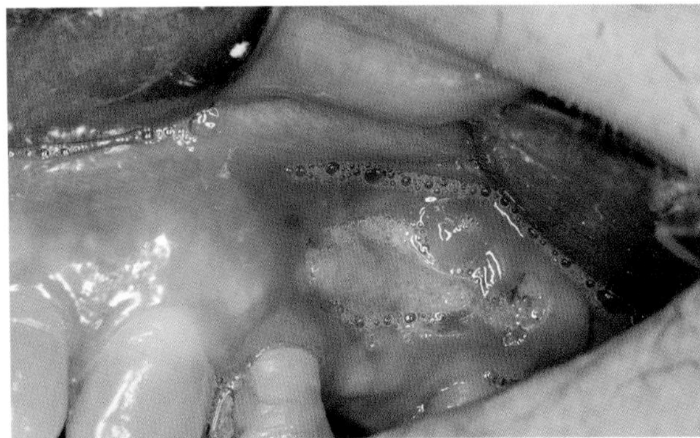

Figure 18.5a

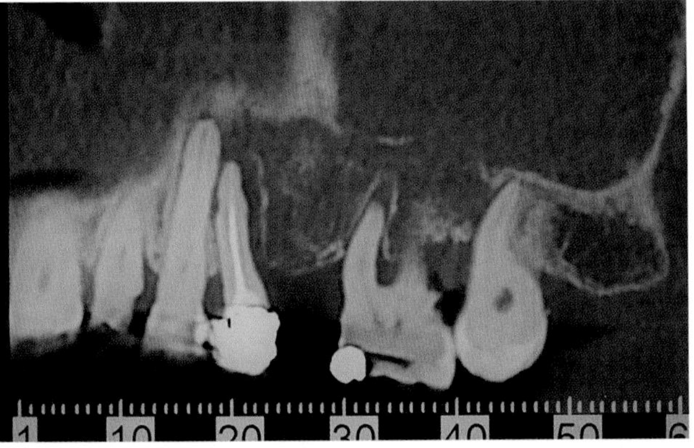

Figure 18.5b

CO: An 80-year-old woman presented with pain from her upper left gingivae over the last eight months.

HPC: The pain was constant, throbbing with exacerbations at night, and preceded a large swelling coming from the gingivae of the second upper left premolar to the molar area. The swelling was partially improved with a course of antibiotics leaving the underlying alveolar bone exposed.

PMH: From her medical records the patient used to take systematically a number of drugs such as acarbose together with metformin and pioglitazone hydrochloride for diabetes type II, amiloride for hypertension, atorvastatin for hypercholosterinemia and denosumab together with Ca and Vitamin D_3 for her chronic osteoporosis. No other serious diseases or allergies were recorded.

OE: Intra-oral examination revealed exposed bone of a yellow-gray color, roughly 2 cm in size, on the buccal aspect of the maxilla on the area of the second left premolar to molars (Figure 18.5a). This bony fragment was loose and the surrounding gingivae were red and erythematous and associated with purulent exudate, halitosis and sialorrhea. Cervical lymphadenopathy and general symptomatology like fever or malaise were not reported. Blood tests were within a normal range apart from a raised erythrocyte sedimentation ratio (ESR) and WBC. X-rays revealed a well-defined radiolucency beginning from the apex of the canine and extended toward the apex of the second molar and perforated the inferior wall of the maxillary sinus (Figure 18.5b). Histological examination of a piece of exposed bone revealed necrosis and absence of osteoblasts and osteocytes, together with a plethora of pathogenic bacteria and mixed inflammatory cells.

Q1 What is the possible diagnosis?
- **A** Alveolar osteitis
- **B** Medication-related osteonecrosis of the jaw (MRONJ)
- **C** Osteosarcoma
- **D** Bony metastasis
- **E** Osteoradionecrosis

Answers:
- **A** No
- **B** MRONJ induced by denosumab is the cause and characterized by the presence of exposed necrotic bone in the maxillofacial region that does not heal within eight weeks and is related to an anti-resorptive agent uptake and not to previous radiotherapy. The necrotic bone does not show evidence of rapid bony remodeling, as it lacks osteoblasts and osteocytes. This condition appears regardless of the patient's age, sex and race and its severity depends on the type, dose and duration of therapeutic agent used for treatment of bone metastases or osteoporosis, and on the patient's general health status.
- **C** No
- **D** No
- **E** No

Comments: Having in mind the negative history of previous radiotherapy or extractions in the area, osteo radionecrosis and alveolar osteitis are easily excluded, while the absence of neoplastic cells on biopsy rules out malignant tumors like osteosarcomas or metastasis from the diagnosis.

Q2 What is/are the available treatment/s for this condition?
- **A** Conservative treatment
- **B** Surgical debridement
- **C** Drugs like pentoxifylline
- **D** Hyperbaric O_2
- **E** Radiotherapy

Answers:
- **A** Conservative therapy includes improvement of patient's oral hygiene, elimination of active dental and periodontal diseases, and long use of topical or systemic antibiotics is effective in early stages.
- **B** Surgery is important in some cases with sequestra, and the affected necrotic bone should be removed until healthy bone is reached.
- **C** Pentoxifylline is a promising new drug, as it increases erythrocyte flexibility to optimize the microcirculatory flow, causes vasodilation, inhibits human dermal fibroblast proliferation and extracellular matrix production, and increases collagenase activity.
- **D** No
- **E** No

Comments: Hyperbaric oxygen has been used with controversial results in osteonecrosis, while radiation therapy even at a low dose worsens bony destruction.

Q3 The causative factor for this condition acts on one or more pathogenic mechanism/s such as:
- **A** Vascularity
- **B** Mucosal integrity
- **C** Micro-organism aggregations
- **D** Bone turnover
- **E** Osteoclasts functions

Answers:
- **A** No
- **B** No
- **C** No
- **D** No
- **E** Denosumab is a monoclonal antibody that binds and inhibits the cytokine RANKL which is an essential mediator in the formation, function and survival of osteoclasts and therefore reduces their osteoclastic activity.

Comments: Biphosphonates and not denosumab have delayed healing properties, and inhibitory effect on the proliferation of epithelial cells, thus reducing the mucosal barrier and allowing pathogenic bacteria to enter and aggregate into the bone.

19

Lips

Lips are the visible external parts of the mouth in humans and many animals that contribute in a number of functions such as food intake, articulation, facial expression, touch, and sexual interplay. Lips could be the place where local and systemic diseases manifest. Their pathogenesis is dependent on genetic or acquired factors like topical irritants, infections, inflammatory, autoimmune or neoplastic disorders, and those resulting from habits. The diagnosis of the majority of lip diseases is mainly based on clinical criteria, but sometimes requires histological confirmation (See Figure 19.0).

Table 19 lists the most common and important lesions or conditions that affect lips.

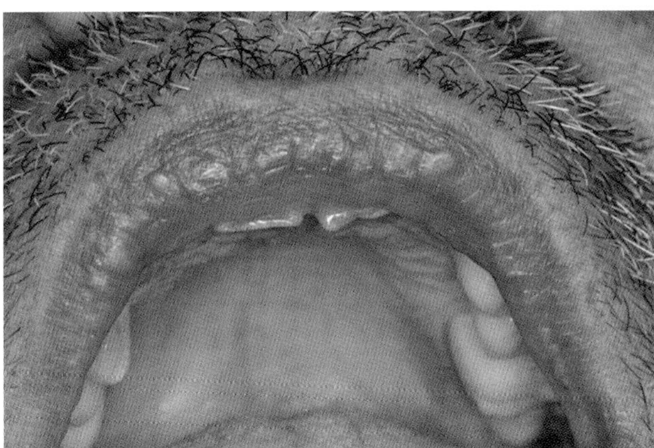

Figure 19.0 Fordyce spots on the vermilion border of the upper lip.

Table 19 Common and important conditions of the lips.

- ◆ Congenital
  - Anatomical
    - Lip pits
    - Double lip
    - Clefts
- ◆ Acquired
  - Lower lip
    - Actinic cheilitis
    - Glandular cheilitis
    - Granulomatous cheilitis (late)
    - Mucoceles
  - Upper lip
    - Minor salivary gland tumors (mainly malignant)
    - Granulomatous cheilitis (early)
  - Both lips
    - Actinic prurigo
    - Angiomas
    - Exfoliative cheilitis
    - Contact cheilitis
    - Plasma cell cheilitis
    - Lip fissures
    - Soft tissue abscess
    - Melanotic macules
    - Fordyce granules
  - Commissures
    - Angular cheilitis
  - Others
    - Perioral dermatitis

Clinical Guide to Oral Diseases, First Edition. Dimitris Malamos and Crispian Scully.

Companion website: www.wiley.com/go/malamos/clinical_guide

Case 19.1

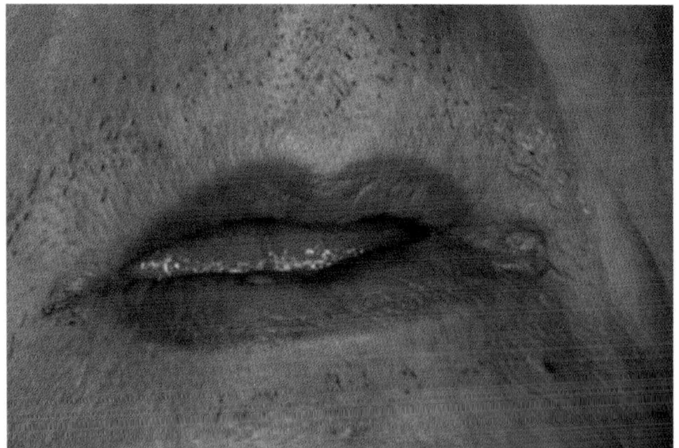

Figure 19.1a

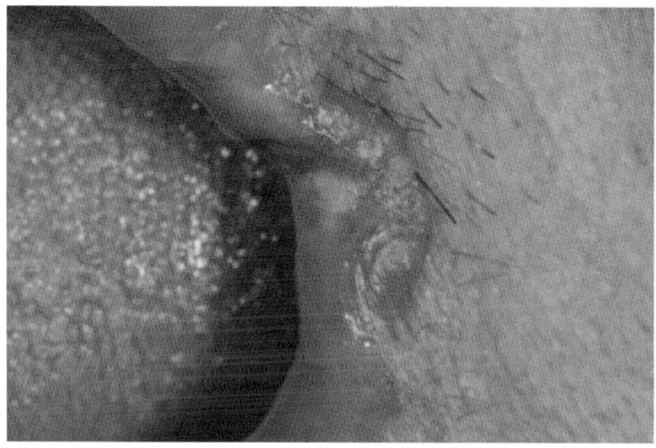

Figure 19.1b

CO: A 72-year-old woman complained about some soreness in the corners of her mouth.

HPC: The soreness was present over the last five years and according to the patient, it appeared almost at the same period of time when she was wearing a new yet unfitted lower denture. The problem became worse over the last month when the patient took a long course of antibiotics and systemic steroids for pneumonia.

PMH: Her main medical problems were hypertension and chronic bronchitis that were treated with angiotensin-converting enzyme (ACE) inhibitors on a daily basis and with steroids in crisis and anti-acids for gut protection respectively. No allergies, eczema or other skin diseases apart from hypertrichosis due to age induced hormonal changes and chronic use of steroids were recorded. Smoking or other hazardous habits were not reported, apart from the patient's habit of licking the corners of her mouth in an attempt to alleviate the itching sensation there.

OE: The extra-oral examination revealed a diffuse erythema at both commissures that was extended from the vermilion border to the adjacent facial skin (Figure 19.1a). Cracks; edema and crusting were symmetrically seen at both corners but were more prominent in the left corner where a large superficial ulceration was found. The ulcer was partially covered with a golden yellow crust and surrounded by a chronic hypertrophic granulation tissue (Figure 19.1b). These lesions were not associated with other skin, oral lesions, or cervical lymphadenopathy.

Q1 What is the possible diagnosis?

- **A** Angular cheilitis
- **B** Contact cheilitis
- **C** Herpetic cheilitis
- **D** Zinc deficiency
- **E** Granulomatous cheilitis

Answers:

- **A** Angular cheilitis is an inflammation of the mouth corners by a bacterial infection with *Staphylococcus aureus* and *beta-hemolytic streptococci* alone or in combination with a fungal infection by *Candida albicans*. It appears as a painful erythema associated with cracks, linear fissures, and superficial erosions that are partially covered with yellow crusts, especially when *Staphylococcus* is involved. The lesions are exclusively located in the corners and extended from the vermilion border to the adjacent perioral skin.
- **B** No
- **C** No
- **D** No
- **E** No

Comments: The long duration, location and type of the patient's lesions and the negative history of allergies ruled out acute diseases such as herpetic infections (herpetic cheilitis) or eczematous conditions (contact cheilitis) and chronic systematic diseases (zinc deficiencies) or granulomatous diseases (granulomatous cheilitis) from the diagnosis.

Q2 What is the best permanent treatment for a patient with this condition?

- **A** None
- **B** Photodynamic therapy
- **C** Use of anti-fungal alone or in combination with antibacterial cream
- **D** Hyaluronic acid dermal fillers
- **E** Restoring lower facial height

Answers:

- **A** No
- **B** No
- **C** No
- **D** No
- **E** The elimination of various pathogenic bacteria or fungi at the commissures remains the best treatment for angular cheilitis. This elimination comes with the improving of size reduction of the labial folds and saliva enzyme irritation by restoring the lower facial height and restricting the saliva leakage from the inner part of the mouth. As lower facial high is defined the vertical distance between anterior nasal spine (seen in x-rays) or base of nostrils (clinically) to menton. This height can be restored by Clinicians by constructing new dentures or new crowns or fillings.and altering the occlusion level. Thus, the corners of the mouth will become dry and unfriendly to the growth of various germs.

Comments: Although photodynamic therapy and the hyaluronic acid dermal fillers injections have been successfully used in isolated cases with angular cheilitis, they are not widely used nowadays as they require expert clinicians, expensive equipment and special clinics. Topical antifungals or antibacterial creams are very effective for the treatment of angular cheilitis, yet with a short-term effect and not permanent when the risk factors remain unchanged.

Q3 Which of the factors below participate in the pathogenesis of this disease?

- **A** Genetic anomalies
- **B** Malnutrition
- **C** Malabsorption
- **D** Habits
- **E** Drugs

Answers:

- **A** Genetic anomalies, as seen in the Down syndrome and in acrodermatitis enteropathica, have been implicated in the pathogenesis of this kind of cheilitis. This has been attributed to the constant drooling of the saliva in patients with Down syndrome, due to their muscular hypotonia that keeps the commissures wet. Regulatory protein defects in patients with acrodermatitis enteropathica impair the immune system, and make the angles of the mouth vulnerable to pathogenic germs.
- **B** Malnutrition is often seen in patients with a poor, inadequate and extreme diet, and in alcoholic patients. It may be associated with decreased cell mediated immunity, which thereby promotes bacteria growth.
- **C** Malabsorption of minerals and vitamins that occurs after surgery for gastrointestinal tumors or diseases like Crohn's disease, ulcerative colitis and pancreatitis seems to be related to the impaired cellular immunity of patients with this cheilitis.
- **D** Chronic licking, thumb sucking or excessive use of chewing gum are habits that constantly wet the corners of the mouth, thus causing local irritation from the digestive enzymes in the saliva, and favor the growth of *Candida albicans* and bacteria.
- **E** Several drugs, causing either xerostomia or suppression of the immune system, accelerate the growth of pathogenic bacteria and fungi in various parts of the body, including the corners of mouth.

Case 19.2

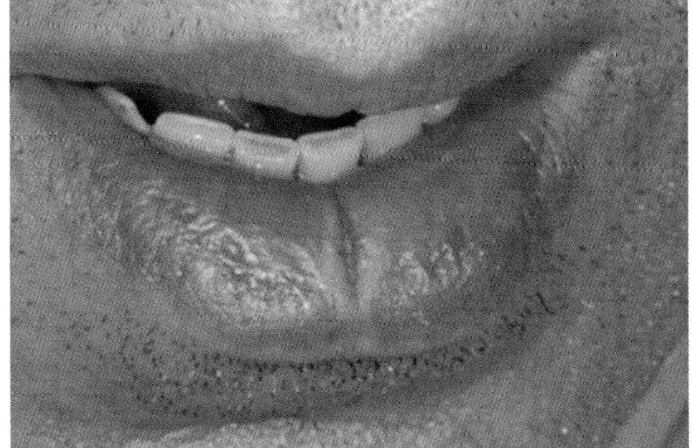

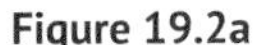

Figure 19.2a

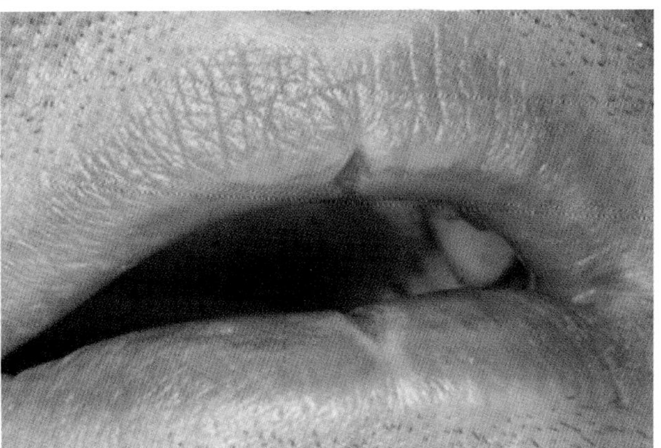

Figure 19.2b

CO: A 28-year-old man presented with a deep groove on both his lips, with a burning sensation.

HPC: The lesions had been present for two years, and were mainly asymptomatic. However, they sometimes caused pain to the patient as they were split and bled when eating.

PMH: His medical history was clear from any serious diseases or drug use, and the patient spent his free time fishing. Smoking, drinking or other parafunctional habits like lip licking or pen biting were not reported.

OE: A linear ulceration was found in the middle of the lower lip and became associated with a burning, tingling sensation and sometimes with pain during eating hard, spicy foods (Figure 19.2a). The ulcer was shallow with soft margins, and was not associated with cervical lymphadenopathy. A similar groove was found on the upper lip, but was less prominent. No other lesions were found inside his mouth.

Q1 What is the diagnosis?

- **A** Median lip fissure
- **B** Actinic cheilitis
- **C** Exfoliative cheilitis
- **D** Cleft lip
- **E** Angular cheilitis

Answers:

- **A** Median lip fissure is a rare benign lesion, characterized by a linear ulceration in the middle of the lower rather than the upper lip, possibly due to fusion weakness of the embryonic plates of the 1st brachial arch.
- **B** No
- **C** No
- **D** No
- **E** No

Comments: Lip fissures or cracks are also seen in other types of cheilitis, but differ as they are located at the angles of mouth (angular cheilitis) or scattered in the whole vermilion border of both lips, thus being associated with crusting (exfoliative) or they can be seen predominately in the lower lip and become associated with atrophic and in places hyperplastic dysplastic epithelium (actinic cheilitis). The shallow depth of this median fissure can easily exclude lip clefts from the diagnosis.

Q2 Which are the clinical characteristics of the median lip fissure?

- **A** Being an extremely rare condition
- **B** Having a male predilection
- **C** Usually affecting patients older than 45 years
- **D** Caused by chronic exposure in solar radiation
- **E** Associated with Down syndrome

Answers:

- **A** No
- **B** It is more common in males with male to female ratio (4/1).
- **C** No
- **D** No
- **E** Patients with Down syndrome show an increased frequency of fissure tongue, median lip fissures, angular cheilitis and macroglossia among their manifestations.

Comments: The median lip fissure is a rare benign lesion that affects 6 out of 1000 patients who are usually younger than 45 years. This lesion is unrelated to chronic exposure to solar radiation, smoking or other parafunctional habits.

Q3 Which is/are the recommended treatment(s) for this lesion?

- **A** Plastic surgery
- **B** Carbon dioxide laser
- **C** Zinc supplements
- **D** Systemic antibiotics
- **E** Topical antibacterial/antifungal cream

Answers:

- **A** Plastic surgery has been used for closing deep lip fissures by using the "Z technique" with very good results and minimal recurrence.
- **B** Carbon dioxide laser has been also successfully used for fissure closure by increasing the amount of collagen and elastin subepithelially.
- **C** No
- **D** No
- **E** Pathogenic bacteria like *Staphylococcus aureus* or *Candida* species have been isolated from median lip fissures, and may respond well to the topical use of antibacterial medication alone, or in combination with antifungals.

Comments: Zinc supplements are useful for the treatment of angular and exfoliative cheilitis, but not of median fissure. The super-infection of the fissure is eliminated with the use of a combination of antifungals, antibiotics and steroids topical rather than systemic antibiotics.

Case 19.3

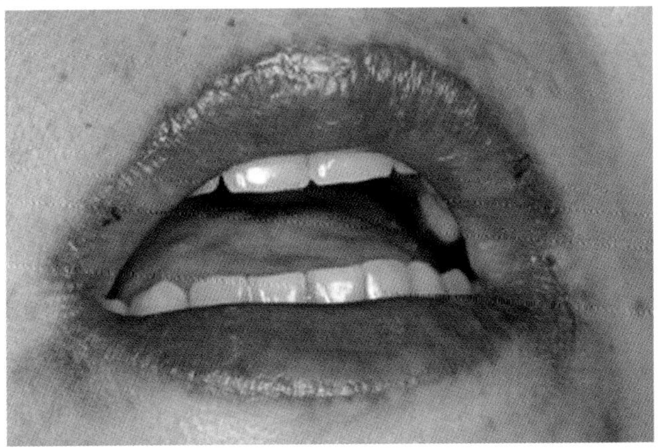

Figure 19.3

CO: A 23-year-old woman presented with a pruritic, erythematous rash involving both her lips.

HPC: This rash appeared five days ago and caused her an itching sensation which became constant over the last two days. The rash appeared, according to the patient, within a few hours after the application of a lip dryness protection lipstick with strawberry flavor, during an excursion last week.

PMH: Her medical history was clear from any serious diseases apart from atopic dermatitis and hay fever, which were treated with anti-histamine drugs and topical steroids as needed. She had never been a smoker or drinker and did not have the habit of licking her lips.

OE: The examination revealed a pruritic, erythematous rash on both her lips that were edematous, dry with superficial cracks and scales (Figure 19.3). The rash was extended to the whole vermilion border, but was more prominent on the commissures and adjacent perioral skin. No other facial skin or oral mucosa lesions were detected.

Q1 What is the possible diagnosis?

A Actinic prurigo
B Seborroheic dermatitis
C Perioral dermatitis
D Allergic contact cheilitis
E Irritant eczematous cheilitis

Answers:

A No
B No
C No
D Allergic contact cheilitis is an exogenous type of eczematous cheilitis caused by a hypersensitivity reaction type IV to topical allergens such as cosmetics, lipsticks or even toothpastes, mouthwashes and various foods. It appears as a diffuse erythema, papules, cracks, or fissures. It is associated with an itching or burning sensation on both lips, and is resolved as soon as the allergen withdraws.
E No

Comments: The lack of characteristic skin lesions can easily exclude other skin diseases like seborrheic dermatosis and actinic prurigo from the diagnosis. Also, the absence of a zone of normal skin between the vermilion border and inflamed skin, as well as a negative history of licking habits, rules out perioral dermatitis and irritant eczematous cheilitis from the diagnosis respectively.

Q2 Which of the clinical tests below can be used in the diagnosis of allergic contact cheilitis?

A Patch test
B Prick test
C Photopatch test
D Scratch test
E Rub test

Answers:

A The patch test is an accurate method to detect whether a specific substance like nickel, Peru balsam, lanolin, fragrance, drugs, exotic food or drinks and various additives or preservatives can cause inflammation on a patient's lips or skin. This test is based on the application tiny quantities of 25–150 allergens to individual square chambers on the skin of the patient's upper back in order to detect or not an allergic reaction two days later.
B No
C No
D No
E No

Comments: All the above tests are used alone or combined to check which allergens are responsible for certain diseases. Patch test is used for the confirmation of a contact dermatitis, photopatch test for photodermatitis, prick test for rhinoconjunctivitis, urticaria or atopic eczema, while scratch and rub tests are suitable for skin allergies.

Q3 Which is/are the differences between a patch and a scratch test?

A Type of reaction
B Site of application
C Methods
D Patient's age restrictions
E Complications

Answers:

A The scratch test detects an immediate allergic response (within 15 minutes) while the patch test a later one (after 24 or 48 hours).
B No
C The patch test uses patches, while the scratch test uses a small amount of allergens which enter into the skin by scratching.
D No
E No

Comments: Both tests are applied to the skin of the forearms or back, regardless of the patient's age and are not painful; they do not cause discomfort, bleeding or any serious allergic reactions.

Case 19.4

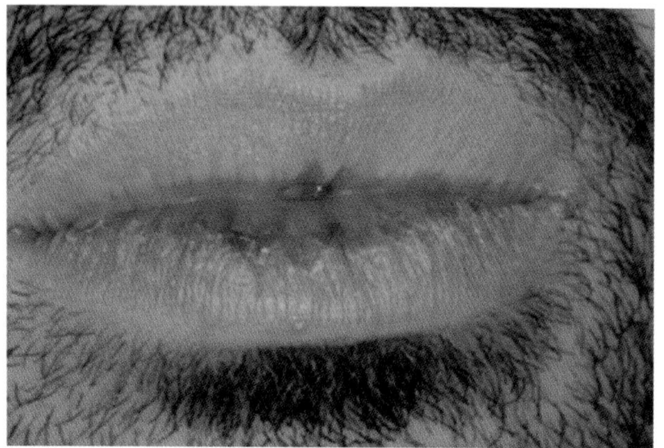

Figure 19.4a

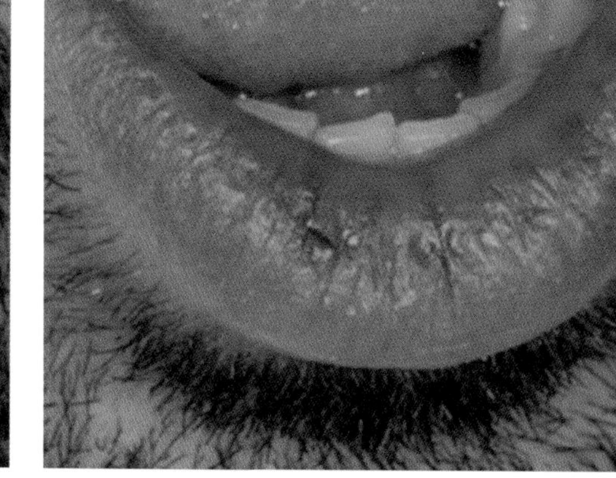

Figure 19.4b

CO: A 22-year-old university student presented with lip problems over the last two weeks.

HPC: The problem started three years ago, when the patient started his mountain sky training. His lips remained inflamed with remissions since then and occasional outbreaks. His last outbreak appeared during a local Marathon race.

PMH: He was a fit young man with no serious medical problems, drug use, allergies smoking, lip licking, or other habits.

OE: His lips were slightly edematous and dry, with numerous superficial grooves and yellow scales on the vermilion border (mainly on his lower lip) that were easily exfoliated, leaving a superficial bleeding area and causing problems on eating or smiling (Figure 19.4a and b). His lips were soft and did not release any exudates or mucus on palpation, while no other lesions were found inside his mouth or skin.

Q1 What is his problem?

A Exfoliate cheilitis
B Actinic cheilitis
C Cheilitis simplex
D Multiple erythema
E Glandular cheilitis

Answers:

A No
B No

C Cheilitis simplex or chapped lips is the cause. It appears whenever the patient is exposed to cold or hot weather, as his lips tend to become drier under these extreme situations. It is characterized by cracking, fissuring and peeling on both lips and gradually by crusting and bleeding.
D No
E No

Comments: The patient's lip lesions are different from those of multiple erythema, actinic, exfoliated and glandular cheilitis. In multiple erythema, the lips are ulcerated and covered by hemorrhagic crests, while they are also associated with a plethora of oral and/or genital ulcerations and target like skin lesions. In actinic cheilitis, the lips are dry and scaly, but have a sand-like consistency, while in glandular cheilitis they tend to be swollen, erythematous and release purulent or mucous exudates on palpation. Exfoliate cheilitis is very similar to simplex cheilitis, but it usually appears in female patients, is constant, and, though it might be worse at stressful events and to extreme wheather conditions as seen in this man.

Q2 Which is/are the difference/s of actinic cheilitis with this cheilitis?
A Location
B Age
C Symptomatology
D Course
E Cause

Answers:
A No
B In actinic cheilitis the majority of patients are older (>50 years) who have been exposed to sunlight for a long period, while in simplex cheilitis patients may be involved regardless of their age.
C No
D The lip changes in cheilitis simplex are reversible, while in actinic cheilitis they are permanent, and sometimes have a tendency for malignant transformation.
E Short lip exposure in cold or hot weather conditions is responsible for simplex while long exposure to sun is to actinic chelitis.

Comments: Simplex and actinic cheilitis affect both lips, but predominantly the lower lip, accompanied with a mild burning or itching sensation.

Q3 Which of the drugs below are mainly related with chapped lips?
A Vitamin A
B Gold salts
C D-penicillamine
D Penicillin
E Prednizone

Answers:
A Vitamin A excess is rare nowadays, and mainly seen in patients who consume high quantities of liver and yellow vegetables rich in retinol or overtake various retinoid drugs for skin problems. The acute effects of vitamin excess are nausea, vomiting and headaches, but it might also be dryness and scaling of the skin and mucous membranes, especially the nasal mucosa and lips. The lips become dry, scaly, or crack and are easily colonized with *Staphylococcus aureus*.
B No
C D-penicillamine is widely used for the treatment of rheumatoid arthritis and Wilson's disease, but comes with a number of side-effects among which are cases of cheilosis (inflammation, cracking, and scaling of lips), epigastric pain, glossitis, oral mucosa ulcer, and taste changes.
D No
E No

Comments: Among the major side effects of gold salts, penicillin and prednisone use, cheilitis is not included. Skin rash, mouth and lip swelling or ulcerations and lichenoid reactions are common side-effects of gold salts that are widely used in arthritis treatment. Penicillin is a wide broad antibiotic which sometimes causes allergic reactions causing itchy skin rash, facial and lip swelling, angular cheilitis or stomatitis, as it reinforces the growth of *Candida* species. Prednisone is mostly used to suppress the immune system and decrease inflammation, and therefore it cannot directly induce cheilitis.

Case 19.5

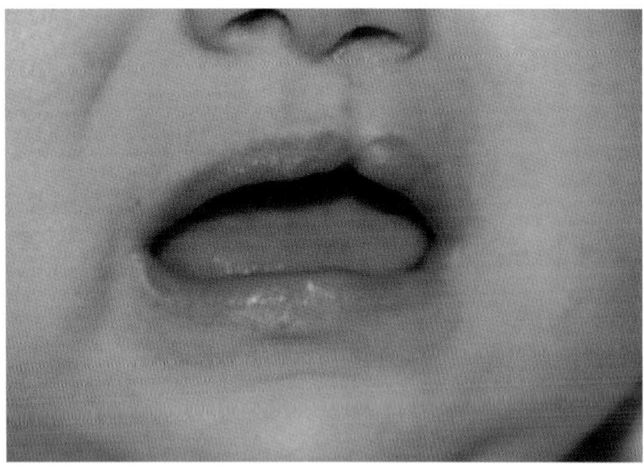

Figure 19.5

CO: A two and a half month old baby was presented with a split of his upper lip.

HPC: The split was discovered at birth, having a tendency since then to increase in size in parallel with the baby's growth so that it caused severely concerne its parents.

HPC: From his medical records, the patient did not have any other craniofacial abnormalities, serious medical problems or any kind of positive family history. The child was born full-term without complications during his mother pregnancy. His growth regarding his weight and size was average and did not show any indications of mental retardation.

OE: A healthy, good-looking baby with no head, ear, nose, and mouth lesions apart from an incomplete but deep split on the left part of his upper lip. The split covered the half of length of the upper vermilion border but did not reach the skin of his left nostrils (Figure 19.5) or extended inside his mouth into his anterior maxilla or palate.

Q1 What is the baby's lip problem?

- **A** Congenital lip hypoplasia
- **B** Lip median fissure
- **C** Double lips
- **D** Cleft lip
- **E** Congenital middle-line sinus

Answers:

- **A** No
- **B** No
- **C** No
- **D** Cleft lip is the problem and is characterized by a failure in fusion of lip tissues before birth, leaving an opening like a small split, or going deep through the lip to the nose. This cleft can be located in one or both sides or in the middle of the upper lip and often becomes associated with cleft palate or other craniofacial syndromes.
- **E** No

Comments: Congenital lip abnormalities such as hypoplasia, median fissure and fistula at such severity or pits as well as double lip do not show any failure of fusion, with that seen in clefts. Therefore, they can be easily excluded from the diagnosis. In hypoplasia, the fusion is complete, but the size of one part of the upper lip is smaller than the other due to the labial muscle hypoplasia, while in the double lip a hyperplastic soft tissue in the inner surface of lip is present, giving the impression of two lips fixed together. In median fistula or pits, the sinuses breach the orbicularis oculi muscles, but they do not communicate with the oral cavity, while in the median lip fissure the groove is very superficial and not extended into the underlying muscles.

Q2 What are the complications of this mild defect?

- **A** Feeding difficulties
- **B** Speech problems
- **C** Esthetic problems
- **D** High cost of lip repair
- **E** Dental anomalies

Answers:

- **A** No
- **B** Movements of the upper and lower lip participate in lip vowel formation, and therefore lip clefts seem to affect the speech (labialization).
- **C** The cleft lip causes facial disfiguration and serious esthetic problems, leading to the patient's isolation.
- **D** The cost of lip cleft repair is highly geographic dependent and in USA ranges from 5000$ to 10 000$ and even higher when the cleft comes together with cleft palate.
- **E** No

Comments: Feeding and tooth abnormalities are not considered as very serious problems in patients with mild cleft lip, as these babies can breast feed and their feeding and teeth anomalies seems to appear in cleft palate rather than a cleft lip and in severe cleft lips alone or parts of other craniofacial disorders.

Q3 Which of the drugs below, taken during pregnancy, is/are not associated with the cleft lip formation?

A Topiramate
B Methotrexate
C Naproxen
D Folic acid
E Hydrocodone

Answers:

A No
B No
C No
D Folic acid supplements taken regularly during pregnancy reduce the baby's chance of being born with a facial cleft at a significant rate.
E No

Comments: The use of topiramate, methotrexate, naproxen, and hydrocodone during pregnancy (especially during the first trimester) have been associated with an increased risk of oral clefts (i.e. cleft lip with or without cleft palate) in the offspring.

20

Neck

The neck is that part of the body that separates the head from the torso. It contains important structures such as lymph nodes, blood and lymphatic vessels, nerves, muscles and vertebrae, glands (salivary, thyroid, and parathyroids) and organs of the upper aerodigestive tract, larynx, hypopharynx and segments of esophagus and trachea. A plethora of congenital lesions (thyroglossal duct, branchial and dermoid cysts, lymphoangiomas, and hygromas); neoplastic benign lesions like lipomas malignant ones like lymphomas and rhabdomyosarcomas or metastatic; as well as reactive or/and infective lesions account for a significant amount of cervical masses (See Figure 20.0).

Table 20 lists the more important lesions of the neck.

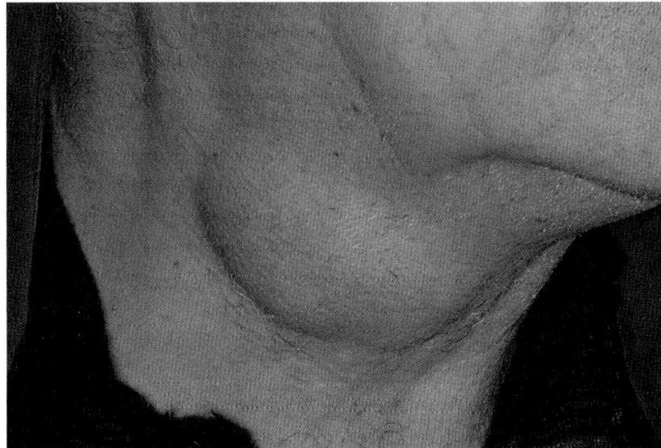

Figure 20.0 Lipoma of the neck.

Table 20 Neck: common and important lesions.

- Congenital
  - Cysts
    - Branchial
    - Cervical brochogenic
    - Dermoid
    - Thyroglossal
    - Thymic
  - Vascular
    - Lymphangioma
      - Hygroma
- Acquired
  - Infections
    - Abscesses
    - Cellulitis
      - Ludwig angina
    - Lymphadenitis
    - Scrofula (TB in skin)
  - Neoplasms
    - Lymphoma
    - Goiter
    - Thymoma
    - Squamous cell carcinoma arising from mouth
    - Glandular arising from sublingual or submandibular salivary gland
    - Metastatic
  - Vascular
    - Arteriovenous fistula
  - Glandular
    - Ranula
    - Salivary gland calculus
    - Sialadenitis

Clinical Guide to Oral Diseases, First Edition. Dimitris Malamos and Crispian Scully.

Companion website: www.wiley.com/go/malamos/clinical_guide

Case 20.1

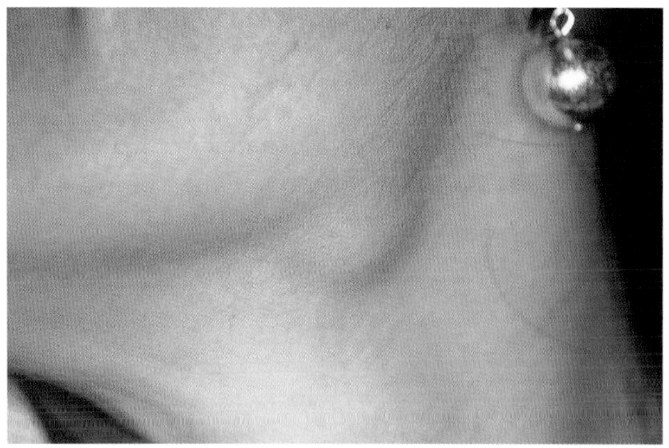

Figure 20.1

CO: A 29-year-old woman was referred for an examination of a lump in her neck, below the angle of the mandible.

HPC: The lesion appeared eight months ago and was gradually increasing, reaching its maximum size four months ago. It had remained unchanged since then.

PMH: The patient was a long-distance runner and did not have any serious diseases or allergies. Her nutrition was adapted to her hobby, and therefore was rich in proteins, vitamins, minerals, and trace elements.

OE: A small asymptomatic lump on her neck, below the left angle of her mouth, was found with a maximum diameter of 3 cm. The lump was firm, well-fixed in the underlying tissues, and covered with normal skin (Figure 20.1). It was not transferred or changed with swallowing. No other lesions were found inside her mouth, skin, and other mucous membranes. Neck X-rays were negative, but an ultrasound scan revealed a mass in the lower lobe of her left parotid gland, which histologically consisted of numerous mature lymphocytes, plasma and acinar myoepithelial cells, intermingled with normal parotid acinar cells.

Q1 What is the diagnosis?

- **A** Enlarged submandibular lymph node
- **B** Neck tuberculosis
- **C** Lipoma
- **D** Lymphoma
- **E** Benign lymphoepithelial lesion

Answers:

- **A** No
- **B** No
- **C** No
- **D** No
- **E** Benign lymphoepithelial lesion is the cause and characterized by an asymptomatic swelling of the parotid or lacrimal glands. The swelling is usually diffuse and affects middle-aged women rather than men, while it is also associated with autoimmune or neoplastic diseases. It is very unusual in young patients and/or in one gland only. Its diagnosis is based on some histological findings like the marked lymphoplasmacytic infiltration of the gland, where small clusters of ductal myoepithelial cells and hyaline deposits, or in severe cases acinar atrophy and destruction are seen.

Comments: Based on clinical and histological characteristics, diseases like lipomas, lymphomas, or reactive lymphadenitis and tuberculosis based on characteristic histological findings affecting the neck are easily excluded from the patient's lesion. Lipomas are composed of mature fatty cells, lymphomas of immature neoplasmatic lymphocytes while caseous necrosis and grannulomas with few TB bacilli are seen in tuberculosis and follicular hyperplasia with increased number of immunoblasts, plasma cells, histiocytes and fibrosis in lymphadenitis.

Q2 Which of the diseases below have been associated with this lesion?

- **A** Sialosis
- **B** Facial palsy
- **C** Sjogren syndrome
- **D** HIV infection
- **E** IgG-4 sialadenosis

Answers:

- **A** No
- **B** No
- **C** Sjogren syndrome is an autoimmune disorder characterized by the gradual destruction of salivary glands by the dense lymphocytic infiltration of activated CD4+ helper T cells and some B cells, including plasma cells and tingible-body macrophages, a process which is considered as the final termination of a lymphoepithelial lesion.
- **D** It is observed that in HIV+ve patients, whose persistent generalized lymphadenopathy and lymphoepithelial sialadenitis are common.
- **E** Lymphoepithelial parotid lesion is considered to be a part of Ig G4 related sialadenosis.

Comments: Sialosis is characterized by a bilateral swelling of major salivary glands (parotid mainly) and associated with malnutrition, alcohol or anti-hypertensive, sympathomimetic drug overuse. Facial palsy is the commonest type of facial muscle paralysis and it is caused by various infective or neoplastic agents, along the route of the facial nerve. Both diseases have different clinical picture can affect the salivary glands but do not present in their parenchymal histological characteristics of a lymphoepithelial hyperplasia or sialadenosis where accumulations of inflammatory and enlarged myoepithelial cells is seen.

Q3 Which of the lesions below have a predominant lymphoid component?

A HIV-associated salivary gland disease
B Marginal zone B cell zone lymphoma
C Warthin's tumor
D Pleomorphic adenoma
E Chronic sclerosing sialadenitis

Answers:

A Salivary gland involvement can be the first manifestation of an HIV infection and is presented as numerous lymphoepithelial cysts, lymphoepithelial lesions, or even lymphomas. It is usually bilateral and accompanied by cervical lymphadenopathy. Microscopically, the salivary glands show an extensive lymphoid follicular hyperplasia that replaces the normal glandular parenchyma. The hyperplastic lymphoid follicles are large and irregularly shaped with areas of lysis, as they also contain numerous tingible body-macrophages.

B Lymphomas are among the most common malignancies of the major salivary glands and composed mainly of neoplastic B cell lymphocytes that infiltrate and destroy salivary gland parenchyma by replacing acini, and infiltrating nerves, fat, and periglandular connective tissues.

C Warthin's tumor is a common parotid tumor, usually seen among smokers, and it is composed of numerous bilayered columnar and basaloid oncocytic epithelial cells that form numerous cysts or papillae within follicle-containing lymphoid tissue.

D No

E Chronic sclerosing sialadenitis is a chronic inflammation of the salivary glands that progresses in fibrosis and parenchymal atrophy. This condition affects submandibular rather than parotid glands, and is often related to salivary gland stones. Microscopically, it is characterized by a diffuse inflammation of lymphocyte (predominantly) plasma cells, which form small granulomas.

Comments: Pleomorphic adenoma is a slow-growing benign salivary gland tumor, most commonly arising in the parotid gland that is microscopically characterized by a great variety of neoplasmatic epithelial and mesenchymal-like tissues, but not of an inflammatory cell population.

Case 20.2

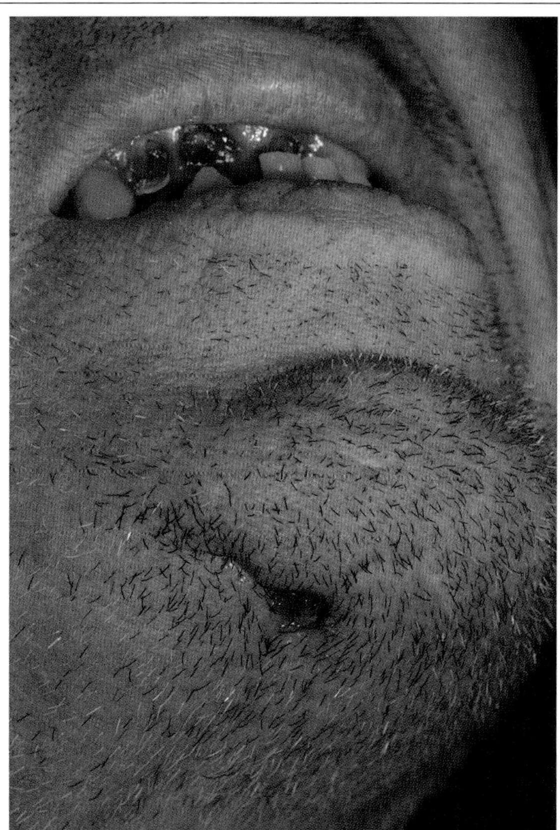

Figure 20.2

CO: A 58-year-old man presented with a hole in his chin.

HPC: The lesion appeared three weeks ago and it was associated with pain and swelling in his lower buccal sulcus, close to the carious right lower canine and first premolar teeth.

PMH: His medical history revealed severe depression and hypertension that were partially controlled with drugs such as selective serotonin reuptake inhibitors and calcium channel blockers, respectively. A carcinoma on his left tonsils was diagnosed one year ago, attributed to his heavy smoking habits, and treated with a course of chemo-radiotherapy. Allergies, lung infections or other serious diseases were not reported and his blood, and biochemical hormone tests were within the normal range.

OE: A sinus tract connecting the skin below his chin and the lower buccal sulcus adjacent to severely decayed right lower premolar-canine teeth was found (Figure 20.2). The sinus discharged a hemorrhagic exudate after milking off his buccal mucosa and sulcus, while the related teeth were carious, broken and did not respond to any vitality tests. Xerostomia was intense and caused by drugs (antihypertensive and antidepressant), previous chemo-radiotherapy, and it was also reinforced by his reduced fluid consumption. His oral hygiene was poor and responsible for the extensive caries seen in the majority of his remaining teeth and his severe periodontal disease. His intra-oral X-rays revealed a periapical lesion at the apex of the lower right canine and first premolar.

Q1 What is the possible diagnosis?
- **A** Orocutaneous fistula
- **B** Thyroglossal duct fistula
- **C** Actinomycosis sinus
- **D** Osteoradionecrosis
- **E** Scrofuloderma

Answers:
- **A** Orocutaneous fistula is the correct diagnosis and characterized by an abnormal channel arising from the inflamed alveolar bone at the apex of necrotic teeth to the patient's skin. The hemorrhagic exudate is transferred from the oral mucosa to the skin through this same channel.
- **B** No
- **C** No
- **D** No
- **E** No

Comments: The presence of thyroglossal duct or scrofuloderma sinuses was easily excluded due to the short duration of the fistula, normal blood tests and lack of active thyroid gland or lung diseases. The absence of necrotic sequestrum or severe bone destruction where sulfur granules were not detected in the sinus discharge also rules out osteoradionecrosis and actinomycosis from the diagnosis.

Q2 Which of the diagnostic tests are LESS useful for this lesion?
- **A** Vitality tests of the involved teeth
- **B** X-rays
- **C** Microbiology tests
- **D** Ultrasound scanning
- **E** Biopsy

Answers:
- **A** No
- **B** No
- **C** No
- **D** Ultrasound scanning can detect a sinus tract but cannot reveal its cause.
- **E** No

Comments: Pulp vitality tests are useful to detect any pulp necrosis, and therefore confirm a possible periapical infection which can be seen as radiolucency in plain endostomatic X-rays. A biopsy is useful for the identification of the tissues composing the fistula, while microbiology tests help to isolate and identify the pathogenic germs responsible for this infection.

Q3 The yellow purulent discharge from a fistula is an indication of:
- **A** Branchial cyst
- **B** Scrofuloderma
- **C** Actinomycosis
- **D** Dental abscess
- **E** Osteomyelitis

Answers:
- **A** No
- **B** No
- **C** No
- **D** The yellow purulent exudate comes from a dental abscess caused by *Staphylococcus* species.
- **E** No

Comments: The composition of exudate is sometimes an indicator of certain diseases such as the presence of yellow sulfur granules for actinomycosis; caseous, thin or cheesy-like exudate for tuberculosis; thin mucous fluid for branchial cysts; while bony fragments mixed with exudate account for osteomyelitis.

Case 20.3

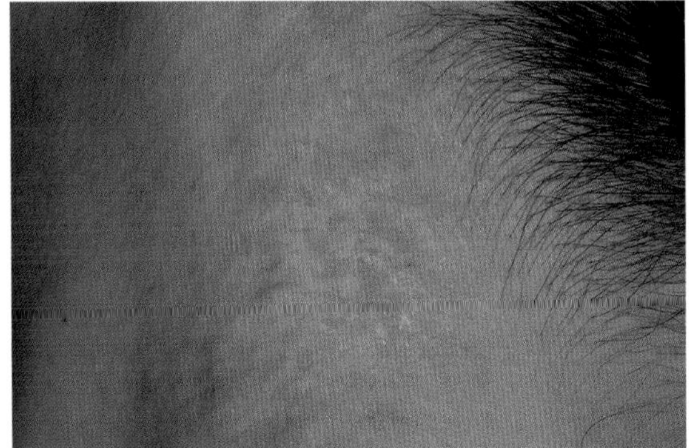

Figure 20.3

CO: A 36-year-old woman was incidentally found to have numerous yellow, soft papules and linear plaques on the right lateral aspect of her neck.

HPC: The lesion was discovered by her dermatologist during a full body examination before her scheduled plastic surgery, for the removal of a number of moles from her skin.

PMH: Her medical history was unremarkable for this lesion. Smoking or other hazardous habits were not reported.

OE: A number of yellow superficial papules or plaques along the lateral aspect of her neck were found. These yellow plaques had different size and were not painful or pruritic, nor associated with other skin, mouth, or other mucosae lesions (Figure 20.3). The lesions did not disappear with skin stretching or change their color under the pressure of a glass slide.

Q1 What is the possible diagnosis?

- **A** Xanthoma
- **B** Dermatofibrosis
- **C** Localized scleroderma
- **D** Pseudoxanthoma elasticum
- **E** Marfan syndrome

Answers:

- **A** No
- **B** No
- **C** Localized scleroderma or morphea is the cause and is characterized by yellow waxing lines on the skin of the patient's neck. These lines do not cause any serious problems apart from a mild itching sensation, and their tendency to initially appear as red or purple skin lesions that later become thickened with white color and then thinner and brown ones. Morphea may also involve the inside of the mouth, genitals, and the eyes, but when it affects the arms, legs, and the underlying bone it interferes with bony growth; when it has an impact on the head and brain or the joints it may cause seizures or limitations of movement respectively.
- **D** No
- **E** No

Comments: The negative family history and the absence of other skin, eye, and heart lesions in combination with normal levels of any or all lipids or lipoproteins in the patient's blood tests exclude dermatofibrosis, pseudoxanthoma elasticum, Marfan syndrome, and multiple xanthomas from the diagnosis.

Q2 Which are the differences between a localized and systemic scleroderma?

- **A** Patient predilection
- **B** Visceral involvement
- **C** Histological features
- **D** Autoimmune profile
- **E** Clinical course

Answers:

- **A** No
- **B** Systemic scleroderma causes fibrosis of various internal organs like kidney, lungs or heart, thus affecting their function while the localized scleroderma does not.
- **C** No
- **D** The localized scleroderma shows an increased frequency of antinuclear (antihistones) anti-centromere antibodies, while the systemic scleroderma shows increased Anti-Sci-70 Abs. Other autoantibodies like anti-Ku abs, anti-Ro, or Sm are often found in systemic sclerosis or in overlapped syndromes.
- **E** The clinical progress of morphea is very slow in contrast with systemic sclerosis, the progress of which is very aggressive and with the risk of an early visceral involvement in the disease course.

Comments: Both localized and systemic scleroderma affect patients regardless of their age, and share similar histological features such as the inflammation around blood vessels, intense subcutaneous fibrosis, and luminal narrowing and thinning of the epidermis.

Q3 Which of the syndromes below are related to the localized scleroderma lesions?

- **A** Parry-Romberg syndrome
- **B** Crest syndrome
- **C** Buschke-Ollendorff syndrome
- **D** Raynaud syndrome
- **E** Osler-Weber-Rendu syndrome

Answers:

- **A** Parry-Romberg syndrome is associated with the localized head scleroderma and characterized by a progressive degeneration of the underlying skin tissues of the face, covering the temporal and facial muscles as well as causing hemi-facial atrophy, neurological, ocular, and mouth problems.
- **B** No
- **C** No
- **D** Raynaud syndrome or phenomenon is characterized by the spasm of the arteries of the hands, fingers or toes and triggered by cold or emotional stress. It can be idiopathic or occur due to a connective tissue disorder like scleroderma or lupus erythematosus.
- **E** No

Comments: The lesions of the Osler-Weber-Rendu and Buschke-Ollendorff syndromes appear at a very early age and are related with vascular malformations or dermatofibrosis, and not with localized fibrosis. Crest syndrome is characterized by calcinosis, Raynaud's phenomenon, esophageal dysfunction, sclerodactyly and telangiectasias, and is a variation of systemic and not localized scleroderma.

Case 20.4

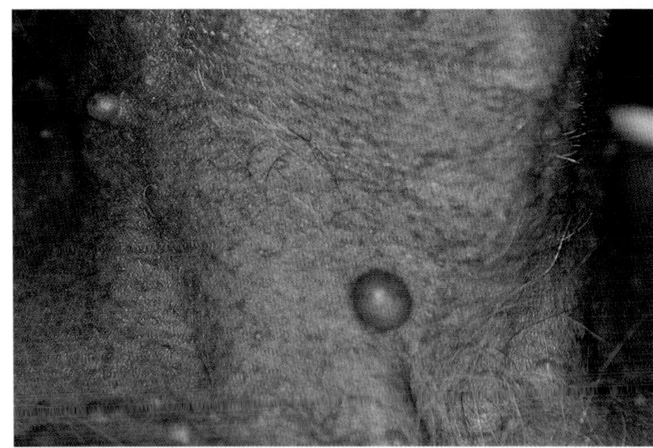

Figure 20.4

CO: A 69-year-old was presented with multiple neck nodules during a routine clinical examination.

HPC: The lesions were asymptomatic and present for more than 50 years, with a tendency of increasing both in number or size across his life time. Similar but less severe lesions were found in his daughter's skin.

PMH: His medical records revealed hypertension that was controlled with angiotensin-converting-enzyme (ACE) inhibitors and scoliosis which was relieved with working out and wearing a brace device. Allergies or other serious medical problems, apart from a few skin lesions like numerous skin lumps or pigmented spots, were not reported.

OE: The physical examination revealed a thin, healthy man of a short stature with scattered lumps on his facial, neck, and trunk skin (Figure 20.4) associated with light brown spots (café au lait) lesions. The lumps were soft in consistency and of various size (usually 0.5–1.5 mm), while they were also located in or underneath the patient's skin. Moreover, abnormal freckling on his groin areas had been reported since his puberty. Finally, the oral examination did not reveal any abnormalities but the patient had recently had a history of difficult extractions due to hypercementosis.

Q1 What is the cause of his skin problems?

- **A** Cowden syndrome
- **B** Proteus syndrome
- **C** McCune-Albright syndrome
- **D** Noonan syndrome
- **E** Neurofibromatosis 1

Answers:

- **A** No
- **B** No
- **C** No
- **D** No
- **E** Neurofibrosis (NF1) is one of the neurofibromatosis diseases and is characterized by the presence of multiple benign tumors of nerves in the skin and internal organs as well as a cutaneous brown discoloration which is known as café au lait spots, and freckling in atypical areas like axillary or inguinal regions. It is a genetic disease consisting of lesions that appear at birth and get worse through the years, having been also associated with short stature, disproportional head, and sometimes mental retardation.

Comments: The characteristic clinical features of other syndromes like Mc Cune Albright, Cowden, Proteus and Nooman syndromes are different from patient's Neurofibromatosis 1 as in McCune Albright fibrous dysplasia the lesions are located in one or mone bones and in Cowden syndrome multiple hamartomata all over patient's body are seen. In Proteus syndrome the myoskeletal anomalies prevail while in Nooman syndrome facial anomalies with heart and other organs involvement are common.

Q2 Which other pigmented lesions resemble with café au lait lesions?

- **A** Mongolian spots
- **B** Congenital nevus
- **C** Melasma
- **D** Racial pigmentation
- **E** Melanoma

Answers:

- **A** Mongolian spots are brown, blue-grey birth marks on the skin that get fainter throughout the years
- **B** Congenital nevus is a single nevus that appears at birth, but is reduced in its size or color eventually.
- **C** No
- **D** No
- **E** No

Comments: Melasma and racial pigmentation is characterized by a diffused and not localized pigmentation that appears in pregnant women and dark-skinned patients. Melanoma is an aggressive pigmented lesion characterized by color variation, satellite lesions and lymphadenopathy; these clinical features were not seen in this man.

Q3 Neurofibromatosis 1 is associated with mutations of:

- **A** ATKIN 1 gene
- **B** RUNX-2 gene
- **C** PTEN gene

D ENG gene
E NF 1 gene

Answers:
A No
B No
C No
D No
E NF1 gene encodes a protein called neurofibromin that is produced in many cells including nerve cells, oligodendrocytes and Schwann cells. It acts as a tumor suppressor protein that prevents cells from uncontrolled growing or dividing.

Comments: Genes encode proteins to participate in the pathogenesis of various genetic disorders like the Atkin 1 gene that plays a role in nuclear division, in Proteus syndrome; RUNX-2 gene provides the instructions for making a protein that is involved in the development of teeth, cartilage and bone, and the mutation of this gene is indicated with cleidocranial dysplasia. The mutations of the PTEN gene participate in various hamartomas in Cowden syndrome and cancers, and the ENG gene via endoglin protein in the development of vascular malformations in hereditary hemorrhagic telangiectasia.

Case 20.5

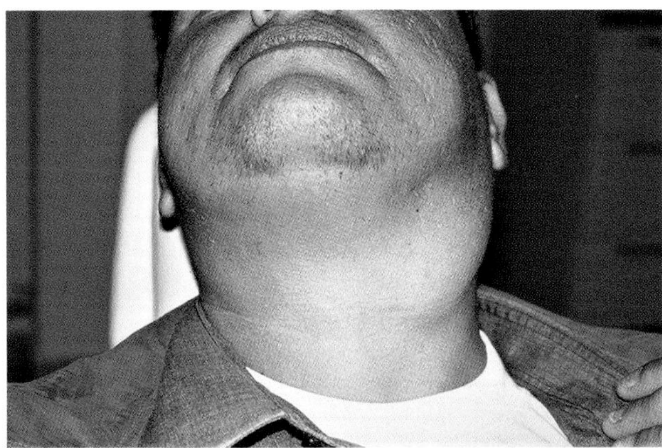

Figure 20.5

CO: A 32-year-old man was referred for an examination of a large lump in his neck.

HPC: The lesion was first noted by his parents at the age of 3, but gradually increased in size over the next 10 years and remained stable since then.

PMH: His medical and family history was unremarkable in relation to this lesion. Smoking since the age of 17 was reported and restricted to 7–10 cigarettes daily.

HPC: A large swelling on the left side of his neck was found. The swelling was located in the posterior angle of his neck and was fluctuant and covered with normal skin (Figure 20.5) causing sometimes breathing problems. CT scan confirmed the presence of a cystic lesion in the lateral side of his neck, reaching the carotid sheath, and fine needle aspiration of the "cyst-like" lesion obtained a brownish fluid material. The patient was referred to the Maxillofacial Surgery Department for surgical removal of the lesion, while its biopsy revealed loose lymphatic channels, lymph, small blood vessels, nerves and adipose tissues.

Q1 What is this neck swelling?
A Branchial cyst
B Dermoid cyst
C Lymphoepithelial cyst
D Cystic hygroma
E Neck emphysema

Answers:
A No
B No
C No
D Cystic hygroma or hygroma cysticum is a large cystic-like swelling on the neck which can be diagnosed either at birth or within the first three to five years of a patient's life. The lesion is initially small and asymptomatic, but increases in size over the following months causing esthetic disfiguration and swallowing or breathing problems. The lesion is often tender in palpation and transillumination, while it usually emits a brown fluid which is a lymph on aspiration.
E No

Comments: The histological characteristics like the presence of lymph and lymphatic channels separate this condition from other cystic lesions with stratified epithelium lining and numerous lymphocytes and germinal centers (branchial and lymphoepithelial cysts), while the soft texture and no cracking, as happens with nodules on palpation, differentiates neck hygroma from subcutaneous emphysema lesions.

Q2 Which of the treatment/s below is/are useful for a large similar lesion?
A No treatment
B Plastic surgery

C Antibiotics
D Sclerosing agent
E Drainage of lymph

Answers:

A No
B Plastic surgery is used in order to remove the lesion, and still remains the most effective treatment despite its serious complications such as the damage of adjacent nerves, vessels, and organs or local infections.
C No
D Sclerosing agents like bleomycin and picibanil (OK-432) have been more successful than doxycycline; pure ethanol and sodium tetradecyl sulfate in the treatment of hygroma.
E No

Comments: A very small number of hygromas can be resolved without any treatment by the age of four, while the drainage of lymph helps in temporarily relieving any breathing or swallowing problems. Antibiotics are sometimes used to control a secondary infection rather than to resolve the lesion.

Q3 Which of the syndromes below have cystic hygromas among their manifestations?

A Down syndrome
B Turner syndrome
C Gorlin syndrome
D Sturge-Weber syndrome
E Noonan syndrome

Answers:

A Down syndrome is known as trisomy of 21, and is rarely related with cystic hygromas, some of which are spontaneously resolved during gestation.
B Turner syndrome is a condition where a woman's partial or complete loss of an X chromosome may lead to various baby's heart defects, fertility problems and lymph malformations.
C No
D No
E Patients with Noonan syndrome usually have short stature, heart and bleeding problems, together with skeletal and occasionally lymph malformation anomalies.

Comments: Both Gorlin and Sturge-Weber syndromes affect the face and neck, but do not have an increased risk of development of neck cystic hygromas lesions. Gorlin syndrome is characterized by nevoid basal carcinomas that are associated with odontogenic keratinocysts in the jaws at an early age, and a high risk of developing medulloblastoma, while Sturge-Weber syndrome shows vascular abnormalities in the brain, skin, and eyes from birth.

21

Palate

The palate is the roof of the mouth that separates the oral from the nasal cavity and has a variety of tissues that give rise to a plethora of pathologies, some of which involve the oral mucosa and others the underlying tissues, bones, and salivary glands. Some of these diseases are congenital, like clefts and tori or various craniofacial syndromes, while others are acquired and distinguished in local and systemic diseases (See Figure 21.0).

Table 21 presents the common and important lesions seen in the palate.

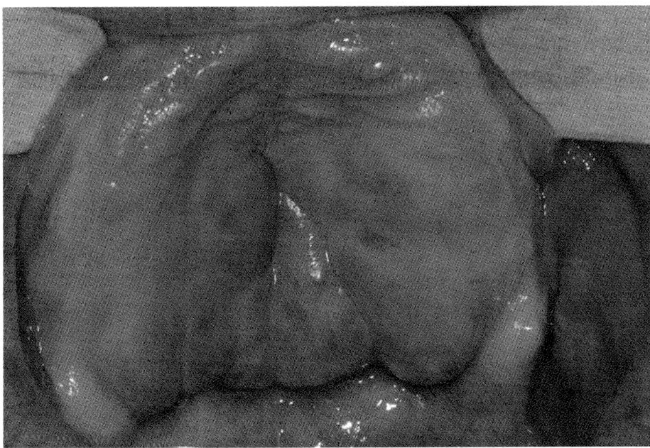

Figure 21.0 Hemangioma on the palate.

Table 21 Palate lesions.

- ◆ Congenital
  - Clefts
    - ▪ Palate (only)
    - ▪ Palate and lip
    - ▪ Part of syndromes
  - Bifid uvula
  - torus palatinus
  - vascular lesions
    - ▪ hemangioma
- ◆ Acquired
  - Infections
    - ○ Bacterial
      - ▪ Dental abscess from lat. incisors and first molar
      - ▪ Syphilis (snake-like ulcers, gumma)
      - ▪ Malignant granuloma
      - ▪ lethal middle line grannuloma
      - ▪ Tuberculosis ulcer
    - ○ Viral
      - ▪ Herpangina (soft palate mainly)
      - ▪ Herpes simplex stomatitis
      - ▪ Herpes zoster (second division of V cranial nerve)
      - ▪ Infectious mononucleosis
      - ▪ Papillomas
      - ▪ Condylomas
    - ○ Fungal
      - ▪ Deep mucosis
      - ▪ Candidosis
        - Pseudomembranous
        - Erythematous (mainly in HIV + ve)
        - Denture-induced
  - Traumatic
    - ○ Mechanical
      - ▪ Papillary hyperplasia
      - ▪ Necrotizing sialometaplasia
      - ▪ Fellatio-induced petechiae
    - ○ Thermal
      - ▪ Burns
      - ▪ Nicotinic stomatitis
      - ▪ Submucous fibrosis
      - ▪ Cocaine-induced palatal necrosis
  - Neoplastic
    - ○ Benign
      - ▪ Leukoplakia
      - ▪ Nevus
      - ▪ Odontogenic tumors
    - ○ Malignant
      - ▪ Carcinomas
      - ▪ Lymphomas
      - ▪ Melanomas
      - ▪ Odontogenic tumors
      - ▪ Sarcomas (Kaposi mainly)

Clinical Guide to Oral Diseases, First Edition. Dimitris Malamos and Crispian Scully.

Companion website: www.wiley.com/go/malamos/clinical_guide

Table 21 (Continued)

- Salivary glands
  - Adenomas
  - Carcinomas
- Cysts
  - odontogenic
    - radicular
    - keratinocyst
  - non odontogenic
    - nasopalatine
    - median palatine
    - globulomaxillary cyst

Table 21 (Continued)

- Systemic diseases
  - cutaneous
  - Lichen planus
  - Epidermolysis Aquisita
  - blood
    - Anaemia
    - Multiple myeloma
    - Leukemia
  - connective
    - Lupus erythematosus
  - autoimmune
    - Pemphigus vulgaris
    - Pemphigoid

Case 21.1

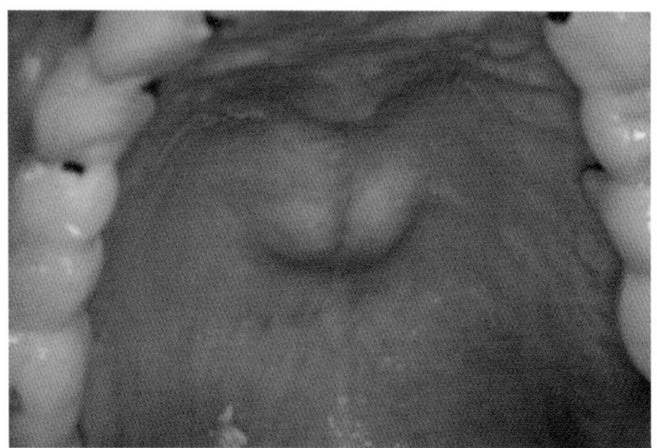

Figure 21.1

CO: A 24-year-old woman was referred for an examination of a hard mass on her palate.

HPC: The mass was asymptomatic and discovered incidentally by her new dentist one month ago.

PMH: Her medical history was unremarkable with no serious endocrinal, metabolic, gastrointestinal, bony, or skin problems.

OE: A hard, lobulated mass at the midline of her hard palate was found. The lesion was a painless growth with a broad base, well-fixed in the palate and covered with thin, normal mucosa, with a maximum diameter of 3 cm (Figure 21.1). No other similar lesions were found on the inside of the patient's mouth or in any other parts of her body or in her close relatives. Her upper teeth did not show any evidence of periapical infection clinically and radiographically, and covered with porcelain crowns.

Q1 What is the diagnosis?

A Gardner syndrome
B Median palatine cyst
C Paget disease
D Endosteal hyperostosis, Worth type
E Torus palatinus

Answers:

A No
B No
C No
D No
E Torus palatinus is the diagnosis. It's characterized by a bony protrusion on the midline of the palate. It usually appears early in life and increases its size through the years, although it might become smaller in older patients due to bony resorption. It is a harmless lesion and more often seen in women from Asia rather than Europe. The lesion can be flat, spindular, nodular, or lobular with a wide variety of sizes, and it can sometimes can cause esthetic problems and eating difficulties in hard or rough foods.

Comments: The stable morphology of the lesion through the years and the lack of other bony lesions in the patient's skull or skeleton rules out the Worth type of endosteal hyperostosis. While the lack of colonic polyps, tumors of the endocrinal glands or skin fibromas and epidermal cysts in the patient and in her relatives, excludes Garner syndrome from the diagnosis. Both the palatine cysts and torus palatinus affect the middle line of the palate, but the palatine cyst is rather soft and fluctuant; therefore is ruled out too.

Q2 Which of the histological characteristics below can be found in this lesion?

A Hyperplastic oral mucosa
B Loose lamellate cortical bone
C Scattered mature osteocytes
D Increased number of osteoclasts
E Reverse lines in bony trabeculae

Anvswers:

A No
B No
C The torus palatinus is composed of a dense mature bone with scattered osteocytes and a limited narrow space of fatty fibrovascular stroma with no evidence of osteoblastic activity.
D No
E No

Comments: The palatal mucosa is normal and sometimes very thin when it overlies large torus palatinus, while the underlying bone is dense and not loose without any histological evidence of rapid bone remodeling (absorption and formation) as this can be shown with basophilic reversal lines.

Q3 Which of the factors below may play a role in the pathogenesis of this lesion?

- **A** Hereditary factors
- **B** Chronic trauma
- **C** Periapical infection
- **D** Diet
- **E** Bony ischemia

Answers:

- **A** Inheritance seems to play an important role, as torus palatinus is commonly seen in women rather than men from certain ethnic groups like German, Norwegian, Croatian, and Thai.
- **B** No
- **C** No
- **D** A particular diet rich in calcium or fish products that is consumed by certain populations with incidents of torus palatinus, has been suspected of playing a role in the pathogenesis of this lesion.
- **E** Periosteal ischemia that is considered as secondary to the nasal septum pressure has been speculated in the formation of tori.

Comments: Torus palatinus appears regardless of the vitality or not of the adjacent upper premolars and molars. Chronic trauma like teeth grinding participate in tori development especially in the mandible (torus mandibularis).

Case 21.2

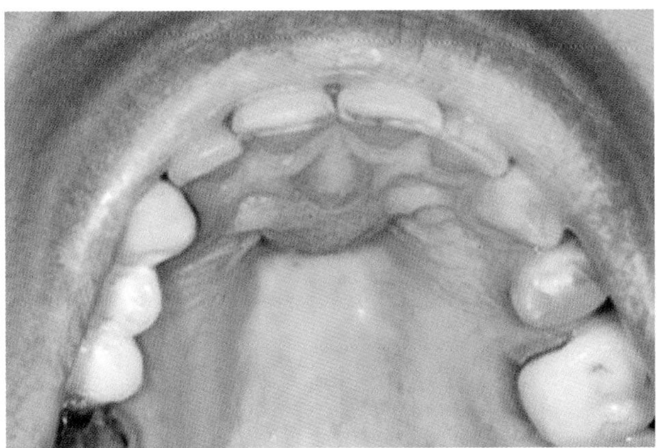

Figure 21.2a

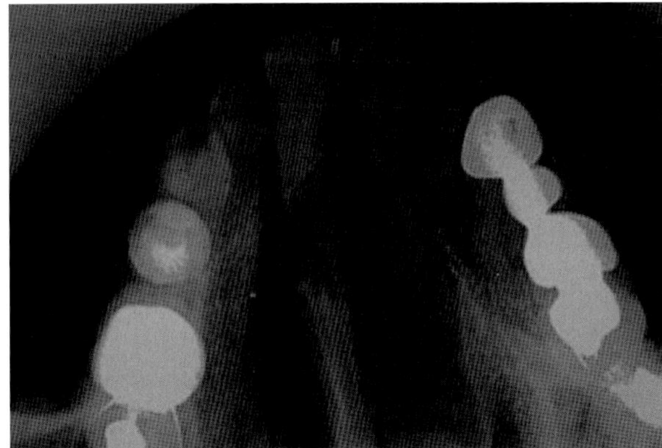

Figure 21.2b

CO: A 57-year-old woman presented with a swelling in her palate.

HPC: The swelling was observed three months ago; it was insidious at first but it gradually enlarged, finally reaching its maximum size over the past month and remaining stable since then.

PMH: Her medical history was non-contributory, while allergies or drugs were not reported. Smoking and drinking were restricted only to social events.

OE: A solitary, oval, soft swelling, measuring 1.4 cm × 2 cm was found in the midline of the palate, close to the incisive papilla. The swelling was covered with normal color mucosa, and was fluctuant and non-tender on palpation, while it was not associated with pain or pus discharge (Figure 21.2a). The occlusal radiograph showed a symmetrical oval radiolucency with well-defined borders close to the incisive canal and apices of the upper central incisors (Figure 21.2b). Her oral hygiene was good and the upper teeth had been restored, either with fillings or with porcelain caps. Last but not least, the pulp vitality tests did not reveal any pulp necrosis of her upper anterior teeth.

Q1 What is the cause of this palatal swelling?

- **A** Periapical cyst
- **B** Globulomaxillary cyst
- **C** Nasopalatine cyst
- **D** Nasolabial cyst
- **E** Lateral periodontal cyst

Answers:

- **A** No
- **B** No
- **C** Nasopalatinal cyst is a non-odontogenic cyst and appears as an oval, soft, mostly asymptomatic swelling near the incisive canal, and it is closely

related with the apices of the vital upper anterior teeth.
D No
E No

Comments: The normal vitality test of the upper anterior teeth excludes periapical cysts while the location of the lesion rules out the nasolabial, globulomaxillary, and lateral periodontal cysts, as these cysts are located in the nasal alar, between maxillary lateral incisors and the canines, or lateral to the apices of mandibular premolars respectively.

Q2 Which of the histological characteristics below are pathognomonic of this cyst?
A Squamous hyperplastic epithelium is the only cystic lining
B Loose fibrous tissue of the cystic wall
C Nerves, arteries, and veins are often seen within the cystic wall
D Primordial cysts present
E Cholesterol crystals

Answers:
A No
B No
C This cyst contains elements of incisive foramen such as the peripheral nerve, cartilaginous rests and muscular vascular channels.
D No
E No

Comments: The cystic epithelium varies from squamous, ciliary respiratory or even cuboid, and depends on the location of the cyst in relation to the incisive canal. Hyperplastic squamous epithelial lining is seen in inflamed cysts close to the palate. The cystic wall is thick, fibrous rather than loose, and it seldom contains cholesterol crystals or primordial cysts which are typical findings of keratocysts.

Q3 This cyst arises from epithelial cells from the:
A Periodontal ligament
B Nasolacrimal duct
C Rests of Malassez
D Nasopalatine duct
E Medial nasal and maxillary process

Answers:
A No
B No
C No
D Nasopalatine cyst originates from the epithelial remnants of the nasopalatine duct, which communicates the nasal cavity with the anterior maxilla in the developing fetus. These epithelial cells may be activated spontaneously during the lifetime, or are eventually stimulated by some kind of local infection, thus forming this non-odontogenic cyst of the maxilla.
E No

Comments: Epithelial cells from the periodontal ligament and the cell rests of Malassez, give rise to odontogenic cysts like the lateral periodontal and periapical cysts. Also, epithelial cells from the nasolacrimal duct or even the area between the medial nasal and maxillary process, lead to the non-odontogenic globulomaxillary and nasolabial cysts respectively.

Case 21.3

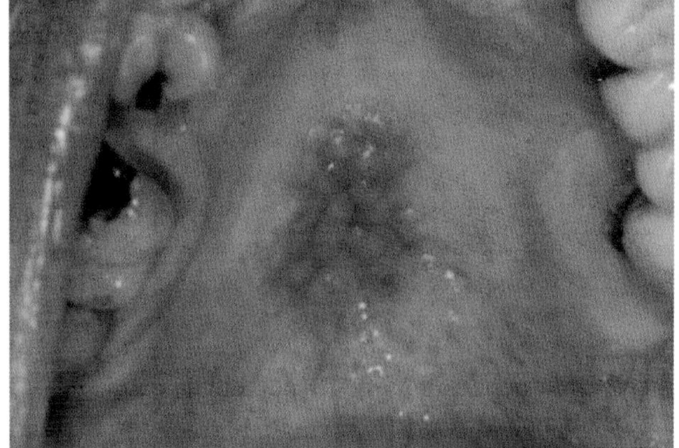

Figure 21.3

CO: A 38-year-old man was referred for an evaluation of a hard palatal nodular lesion.

HPC: The lesion was found incidentally one month ago, causing a mild itching irritation and a burning sensation on his palate.

PMH: His medical history revealed only a few episodes of gastroesophageal reflux which were controlled with H2-receptor blockers and antiacids. Diabetes or other serious diseases were not reported, while mouth breathing and smoking of 20 cigarettes a day over the last 20 years were reported.

OE: The examination revealed a healthy man with a full dentition and numerous red nodular mucosal projections of about 2 mm or less in the middle of his palate

(Figure 21.3). These nodules were soft, they did not change in color, size or secrete mucus with pressure, and were situated in the middle of his narrow, V-shaped palate. His dentition showed caries underneath old fillings and crowns and attributed to his poor oral hygiene.

Q1 What is the cause?
- **A** Denture-induced palatal candidosis
- **B** Multiple papillomas
- **C** Inflammatory papillary hyperplasia
- **D** Nicotinic stomatitis
- **E** Gastroesophageal reflux oral involvement

Answers:
- **A** No
- **B** No
- **C** Inflammatory papillary hyperplasia is a benign lesion, seen in the hard palate of middle-aged women rather than male patients, who constantly wear ill-fitting dentures, although it can also be seen among patients with a full dentition. The lesion in this case is asymptomatic, and therefore it can be incidentally found during a routine dental examination and characterized by numerous mucosal projections with variable color and a soft consistency.
- **D** No
- **E** No

Comments: Although *Candida* infection seems to play a role in the development of some but not all the papillary hyperplasia lesions, the denture – induced candidosis is not the case, as the patient did not wear dentures. Multiple papillomas can be also seen intra-orally but are usually scattered, while patient's oral lesions are different from those in nicotinic stomatitis and gastroesophageal reflux diseases. Well-defined red spots intermingled with white lesions or a diffuse erythema mainly in palate and oropharynx are seen in nicotinic stomatitis while being associated with teeth erosions on the palatal surface In gastroesophangeal reflux diseases.

Q2 What is/are the best treatment(s) for this patient?
- **A** Surgical removal of these nodules
- **B** Smoking cessation
- **C** Antifungal treatment
- **D** Photodynamic therapy
- **E** Interferon

Answers:
- **A** The removal of the large nodules can be done with a surgical blade alone or with grafting for aesthetic reasons, cryotherapy and CO_2 laser.
- **B** The cessation of smoking eliminates the local irritation of the palate which may be a predisposing factor for the papillary hyperplasia development.
- **C** Anti-fungal treatment (systemic or local) is useful in papillary lesions with *Candida* super-infection.
- **D** No
- **E** No

Comments: Photodynamic therapy is useful in the treatment of HPV-induced papillomatosis (Heck disease) while interferon may play a protective role by inducing an immune reaction against Candida infections.

Q3 Which of the factors below does NOT participate directly in the pathogenesis of these lesions?
- **A** Patient's age
- **B** Mouth breathing
- **C** Palatal morphology
- **D** Poor oral hygiene
- **E** Smoking habits

Answers:
- **A** Inflamed papillary hyperplasia occurs in patients regardless of their age, although this lesion seems to be closely related with the chronic wearing of ill-fitting dentures used by older patients.
- **B** No
- **C** No
- **D** No
- **E** No

Comments: Chronic trauma and local infection with various germs like bacteria and fungi seem to play a crucial role in the pathogenesis of this papillary hyperplasia. Specifically, in this patient, the palate was narrow and deep and it can therefore be easily traumatized with various hard foods, eventually allowing the entrance of several pathogenic bacteria there. These germs are abundant due to the xerostomia induced by the patient's habits (smoking and mouth breathing) and his poor oral hygiene.

Case 21.4

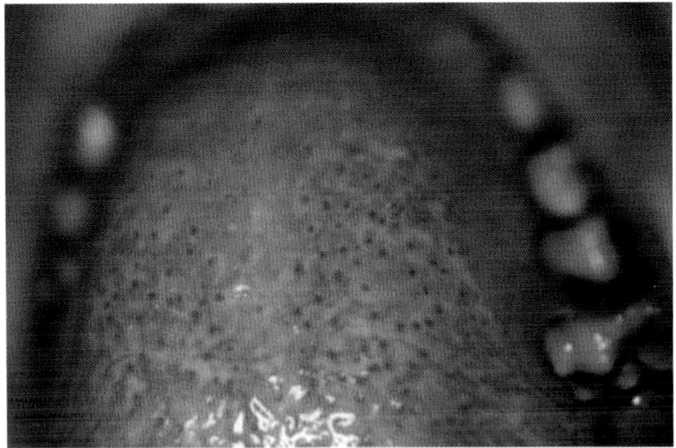

Figure 21.4

CO: A 58-year-old man was referred for an evaluation of a white lesion on his palate.

HPC: The lesion was found during a dental check-up by his new dentist one month ago, yet the onset of the lesion remained unknown.

PMH: Hypertension, mild diabetes type II and chronic bronchitis were his only serious medical problems, and were attributed to his unhealthy diet and hazardous habits of smoking and drinking. He started smoking at the age of 14, but increased over the last five years due to his financial crisis; pipe smoking was his favorite and usually come with two glasses of whisky at night.

OE: A white-gray diffuse lesion was found on his palate extending posterior to the palatal rugae and soft palate. The lesion was thick in places and was not wiped off, but was intermingled with red spots giving a speckled white and red appearance (Figure 21.4). Hyperkeratosis, mild acanthosis without atypia, but squamous metaplasia of the majority of the excretory ducts were seen microscopically. No other similar lesions were found inside the patient's or close relatives' mouth, skin, or other mucous membranes.

Q1 What is the diagnosis?

- **A** Pseudomembranous candidosis
- **B** Lichen planus
- **C** Nicotinic stomatitis
- **D** White sponge nevus
- **E** Speckled leukoplakia

Answers:

- **A** No
- **B** No
- **C** Nicotinic stomatitis affects the palate of chronic smokers (mainly pipe smoking), initially appearing as a diffuse reddened area that slowly progress to a white thickened and fissured lesion where inflamed, swollen, ducts of minor salivary glands are noted. The lesion is restricted on the posterior palate to rugae and is reversible as is disappeared with smoking cessation.
- **D** No
- **E** No

Comments: The clinical characteristics such as the location of the lesion exclusively on the patient's posterior hard and soft palate, its failure to be wiped off, together with the lack of epithelial atypia and similar lesions among his close relatives rule out other diseases like lichen planus, pseudomembranous candidosis, speckled leukoplakia and white sponge nevus from the diagnosis respectively.

Q2 The severity of this lesion is NOT dependent on:

- **A** Patient's age or gender
- **B** Duration of smoking
- **C** Intensity of smoking
- **D** Type of smoking
- **E** Combination or not with hot drinks

Answers:

- **A** The pathogenesis of nicotinic stomatitis is based on the heating irritation effect with smoking on the palatal mucosa and minor salivary glands, while it is not related to tobacco ingredients or the patient's age or gender.
- **B** No
- **C** No
- **D** No
- **E** No

Comments: The effect of the released heat during smoking on the palate depends on the duration, severity and type of smoking, and is exacerbated by the frequent consumption of hot liquids.

Q3 What is/are the differences between nicotinic stomatitis and speckled leukoplakia?

- **A** Pathogenesis
- **B** Location
- **C** Symptomatology
- **D** Histological characteristics
- **E** Risk for malignant transformation

Answers:

A Although both lesions are related to smoking, the heat released with smoking is responsible for nicotinic stomatitis, while the tobacco products (carcinogens) are responsible for speckled leukoplakia.

B Speckled leukoplakia can be seen everywhere in the mouth in contrast with nicotinic stomatitis which is exclusively found on the posterior hard and soft palate.

C No

D The red spots in nicotinic stomatitis are dilated, inflamed ducts, openings of minor salivary glands, while in speckled leukoplakia are attributed to atrophic dysplastic mucosa.

E Nicotinic stomatitis is a benign reversible reaction, while speckled leukoplakia shows dysplasia and has a high risk of malignant transformation.

Comments: Both lesions appear clinically as a combination of white plaques intermingled with red spots, and are either asymptomatic or cause some mild symptomatology like roughness or burning sensation.

Case 21.5

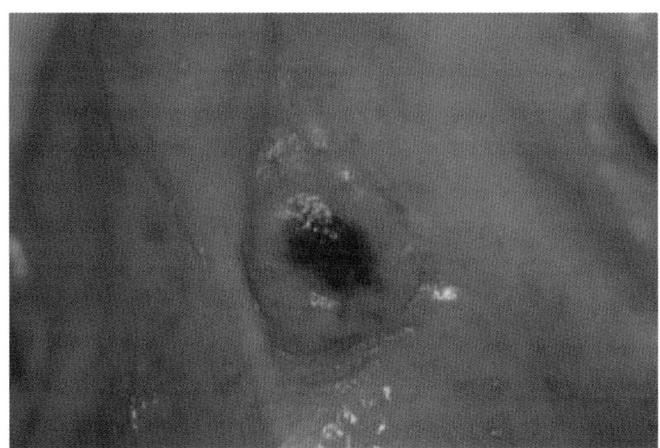

Figure 21.5

CO: A 42-year-old man presented with a non-healing ulcer on the left side of his palate over the last 10 days.

HPC: The ulcer appeared after a burning of the palate by some extremely hot food and began as a small erythematous swelling that ulcerated at the center and worsened with eating. Previous similar lesions had not been reported either by the patient nor his close relatives.

PMH: His medical history was unremarkable, and his smoking habits included tobacco and occasionally cannabis use.

OE: A large non healing ulcer with indurated margins, of 1.5 cm in diameter, being located at the left side of his palate close to the middle line. The ulcer was covered with yellowish pseudomembrane that was removed during the examination, leaving a painful lesion with an erythematous basis (Figure 21.5). No other similar lesions were seen in his mouth or other mucous membranes, while the systemic or cervical lymph nodes were not palpable and general symptomatology was absent. Incisional biopsy from the margins of the ulcer revealed necrosis and salivary duct squamous metaplasia.

Q1 Which is the cause of this ulceration?

A Large aphthae
B Syphilitic chancre
C Oral carcinoma
D Tuberculous ulcer
E Necrotizing sialometaplasia

Answers:

A No
B No
C No
D No
E Necrotizing sialometaplasia is a benign ulcerated lesion that is located at the back of hard palate. The lesion initially appears as a tender erythematous swelling that later changes into a deep, well-circumscribed ulcer covered with yellow-gray slough that is easily detached, leaving an ulcer with erythematous and granulomatous base. The ulcer is thought to be caused by an ischemic necrosis of the minor salivary glands due to local anaesthesia or burns and heals in 6 to 10 weeks, while the salivary ducts show a characteristic metaplasia.

Comments: The clinical characteristics of the ulcer like the absence of recurrence and the lack of regional or systemic lymphadenopathy exclude large aphthae and syphilis from the diagnosis. Additionally, the lack of caseous necrosis and granulomas or neoplastic epithelial islands in the biopsy excludes tuberculous ulcer and oral carcinomas from the diagnosis.

Q2 Which of the characteristics below is/or are pathognomonic of this lesion?

- **A** Pseudoepithelial hyperplasia
- **B** Ischemic necrosis
- **C** Squamous metaplasia of the ducts
- **D** Granulomas in the submucosa
- **E** Band zone of chronic inflammatory cells underneath the base of the ulcer

Answers:

- **A** Pseudoepithelial hyperplasia is seen at the margins of the ulcer.
- **B** Ischemic necrosis is characteristic and plays an important role in the pathogenesis of the ulcer.
- **C** Squamous metaplasia of the ducts of minor salivary glands is characterized by the changes of the normally cuboidal ductal epithelium to stratified squamous, and is often accompanied by local inflammation or necrosis.
- **D** No
- **E** No

Comments: Chronic inflammation with a band or granulomas pattern is characteristic of ulcerative lichen planus and tuberculous ulceration and not of the necrotizing sialometaplasia lesions.

Q3 Which is/or are the cause(s) of the ischemic necrosis seen in this lesion?

- **A** Local trauma
- **B** Smoking
- **C** Sickle cell anemia
- **D** Alcohol
- **E** Radiotherapy

Answers:

- **A** A local trauma induced by some pressure of ill-fitting dentures, hard food or after a local anesthetic injection or burns causes ischemic necrosis, due to the lack of blood supply of the minor salivary glands.
- **B** Smoking habits of tobacco or cocaine, cannabis, and other illegal drugs may cause infarctions in the salivary gland by inducing vascular stenosis in the palate. More than 10 per cent of smokers experience at least an episode of necrotizing sialometaplasia of the minor or major salivary glands.
- **C** Sickle cell anemia is sometimes accompanied with ischemic infarcts which may participate in the development of this sialometaplasia.
- **D** The excess consumption of alcohol causes avascular necrosis that may contribute to bone and salivary gland necrosis.
- **E** Radiotherapy for head and neck tumors often damages the blood supply of the salivary glands, leading to parenchymal atrophy and ischemic necrosis.

22

Salivary Glands (Minor/Major)

The salivary glands are exocrine glands that produce saliva; a fluid which mainly contains water, enzymes like lipase or amylase and antimicrobial agents like secretory IgA and lysozymes. In humans, these glands are distinguished into major glands (two pairs of parotids; sublingual and submandibular) and 800–1000 minor glands that are scattered over the oral mucosa apart from gingivae and the middle of the hard and soft palate. A variety of local and systemic diseases affect the salivary glands and alter their functions, thus causing problems in taste, mastication, swallowing, digestion and speech, and making oral mucosa-teeth vulnerable to local bacterial and fungal infections as well as caries. These diseases can be congenital like the aplasia of the salivary glands, but the majority of them are acquired and range from local innocent lesions such as mucoceles to malignant or systemic autoimmune ones like adenocarcinomas or Sjogren's syndrome respectively (Figure 22.0).

Table 22 lists the more common and important lesions and diseases of the salivary glands.

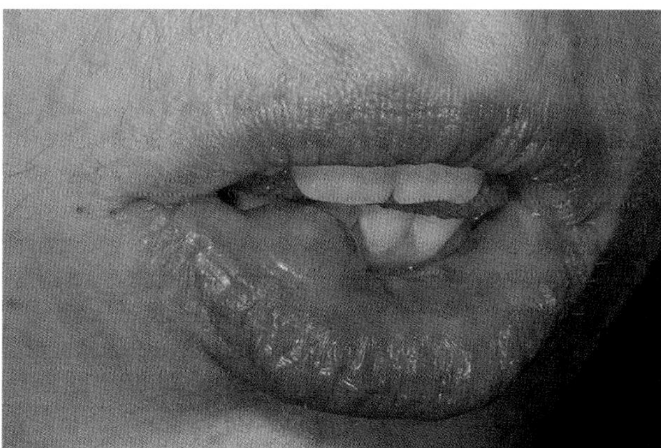

Figure 22.0 Mucocele of the lower lip.

Table 22 Common and important salivary gland lesions and diseases.

- Congenital
  - Aplasia of glands
    - Alone or
    - Part of ectodermal syndromes
- Acquired
  - Traumatic
    - Mucoceles
    - Ranula
  - Mechanical duct obstruction
    - Duct stenosis
    - Duct calculus
  - Infections
    - Siladenitis (bacterial)
    - Mumps (viral)
  - Inflammatory
    - Sialosis
  - Autoimmune
    - Sjogren syndrome
  - Neoplasms
    - Adenomas
    - Adenocarcinomas
    - Others (like lymphomas)
  - Cysts
    - Lymphoepithelial cyst

Clinical Guide to Oral Diseases, First Edition. Dimitris Malamos and Crispian Scully.

Companion website: www.wiley.com/go/malamos/clinical_guide

Case 22.1

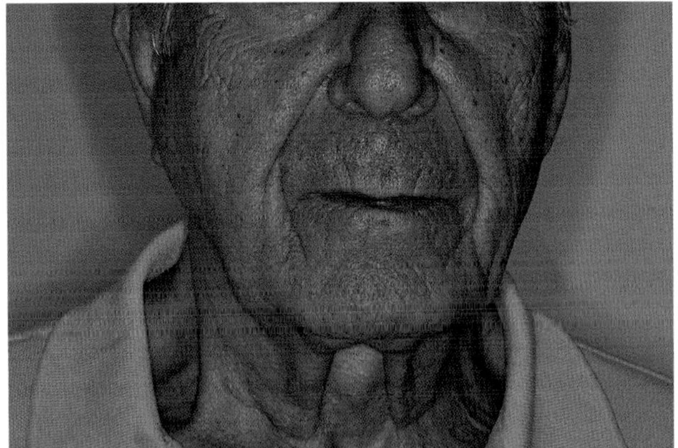

Figure 22.1a

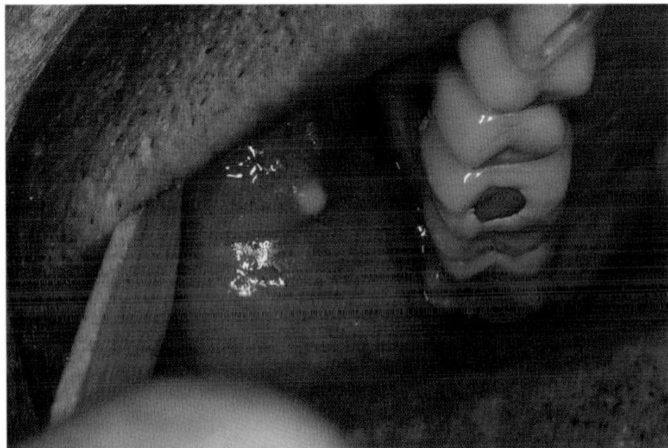

Figure 22.1b

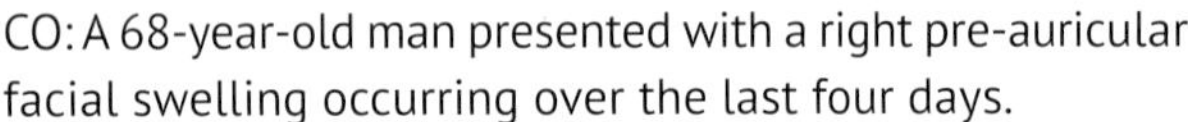

CO: A 68-year-old man presented with a right pre-auricular facial swelling occurring over the last four days.

HPC: The swelling appeared suddenly and became associated with pain and generalized malaise and fever. No similar episodes were ever recorded in his or his close relatives' medical history.

PMH: Chronic hypertension and hypertrophic prostate were his only medical problems and they were treated with angiotensin-converting enzyme (ACE) inhibitors and alpha blockers respectively. He also quit smoking five years ago after an episode of severe pneumonia.

OE: The examination revealed a swelling of his right parotid gland that was associated with erythema and edema of the overlying skin (Figure 22.1a). The gland showed a diffuse, painful swelling which released pus from his swollen Stensen duct during milking (Figure 22.1b). Xerostomia and other oral lesions were not recorded and cervical lymphadenopathy was absent. His oral hygiene was adequate and his dentition was heavily restored, yet with no evidence of infection.

Q1 What is the cause of this swelling?

- **A** Acute sialadenitis
- **B** Heerfordt syndrome
- **C** Chronic sialadenitis
- **D** Sarcoidosis of the parotid glands
- **E** Pleomophic adenoma

Answers:

- **A** Acute sialadenitis is the cause and characterized by an infection of the major salivary glands (mainly parotid) from bacteria or viruses. The swelling is painful, accompanied with purulent exudate from the duct papilla and associated with general malaise, low-grade fever and occasionally, cervical lymphadenopathy.
- **B** No
- **C** No
- **D** No
- **E** No

Comments: The short duration and the type of the swelling (diffuse rather than localized) as well as the absence of similar lesions in the past excludes diseases such as chronic sialadenitis, pleomorphic adenoma and sarcoidosis alone or combined with facial palsy (Heerfordt syndrome) from the diagnosis.

Q2 Which is/are the predisposing factor(s) for this patient's condition?

- **A** Sialolithiasis
- **B** Dehydration
- **C** Drug-induced sialorrhea
- **D** Sjogren syndrome
- **E** Neglected mouth

Answers:

- **A** Sialolithiasis usually causes the obstruction of the excretory salivary gland's duct from calculus, thus leading to stasis of saliva within the duct and glandular parenchyma, making the affected gland vulnerable to pathogenic bacteria and viruses.
- **B** Acute dehydration due to reduced fluid consumption or increased fluid loss (hemorrhage; diarrhea; burns; drugs) causes xerostomia that accelerates the growth of pathogenic bacteria. These germs enter via the salivary duct into the major glands, causing an infection that is known as sialadenitis.
- **C** No

D No
E Poor oral hygiene, allows the growth of a plethora of pathogenic bacteria being responsible for caries, gingival diseases, halitosis and oral infections including of salivary glands leading to acute or chronic sialadenitis.

Comments: Drugs that increase saliva secretion impede the growth of pathogenic germs via the antibacterial action of various elements (secretory IgA and lysozymes) and the flushing–cleaning action of saliva and therefore reduce the risk of a local infection. Sjogren's syndrome is an autoimmune disease that causes atrophy of the salivary parenchyma and eventually, chronic hyposalivation that is the major cause of chronic and not acute sialadenitis.

Q3 Which of the pathogenic germs below are commonly related to this acute bacterial infection?
A *Mumps*
B *Staphylococcus aureus*
C *Coxsackie type A*
D *Actinomycosis israelii*
E *Mycobacterium tuberculosis*

Answers:
A No
B *Staphylococcocus aureus* is the commonest of the pathogenic bacteria responsible for acute sialadenitis.
C No
D No
E No

Comments: All the germs mentioned above are responsible for acute sialadenitis, but mumps and Coxsackie are viruses, while *Actinomycosis israelii* and *Mycobacterium tuberculosis* are bacteria that rarely affect the salivary glands of the immunocompromised patients only.

Case 22.2

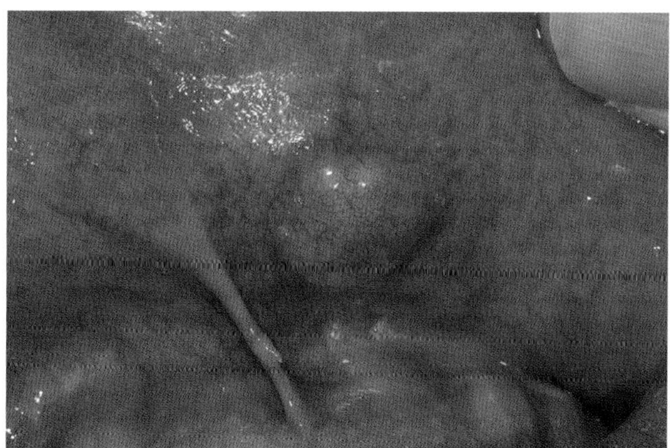

Figure 22.2

CO: A 42-year-old man presented with a swelling on the inner surface of his upper lip closely to the sulcus.

HPC: The swelling was present for more than eight months and was asymptomatic, but was gradually progressing thus causing the patient concern over the past month.

PMH: His medical history was irrelevant to the lesion, while any history of recent trauma or other similar lesions were not recorded, both for the patient or his close relatives. His smoking habit was limited to five to six cigarettes a day, while his drinking habits to one to two glasses of wine on social occasions.

OE: A firm nodule of maximum diameter of 1.2 cm, which was located in the middle of the inner surface of the upper lip, left to the labial frenulum and close to the labial sulcus (Figure 22.2). The lesion was asymptomatic, well-defined, firm on palpation and covered with normal intact oral mucosa. The lesion was more prominent intra-orally causing the patient concern that it might be malignant. No other similar lesions were found inside his mouth, skin and other mucosae, nor was cervical lymphadenopathy detected. The lesion was removed under local anesthesia and the histology revealed a partially encapsulated tumor consisting of a variety of neoplastic epithelial and myoepithelial cells of glandular origin, with minimal mitosis under a myxoid and hyaline stroma.

Q1 What is the possible diagnosis?
A Soft tissue abscess
B Deep mucocele
C Periapical abscess from incisor teeth

D Pleomorphic adenoma
E Traumatic fibroma

Answers:

A No
B No
C No
D Pleomorphic adenoma is the diagnosis and is characterized as a slow, painless, well-defined, benign tumor of both the major and minor salivary glands. It has a very low risk for malignant transformation, but an increased risk of recurrence in cases of incomplete removal. It consists of numerous epithelial and myoepithelial cells in variable stoma of a myxoid, hyaline, adipose or even osteoid source that are surrounded in places with a thick fibrous capsule.
E No

Comments: The firm consistency of the lesion can easily exclude mucocele and abscess (soft tissue or periapical) as these lesions are very soft and fluctuant and being related to trauma and local infection respectively. Trauma can also cause fibromas, but these lesions are also firm and characterized by an overproduction of collagen in fibrous and not glandular tissues; and therefore be easily excluded.

Q2 What are the clinical characteristics that differentiate a benign from a malignant salivary gland tumor?

A Growth rate
B Consistency
C Margins
D Ulceration of the overlying mucosa
E Local nerve deficits signs

Answers:

A Benign salivary tumors develop slowly, while the malignant ones grow faster.
B The malignant salivary gland tumors have a hard, firm consistency while the benign tumors are rather soft or rubbery.
C Benign tumors have well-defined margins, while the malignant lesions are irregular with no clear margins.
D In benign salivary gland tumors, the rate of growth is slow allowing the overlying mucosa to become thin but not ulcerated, in contrast with the malignant tumors, the rate of which is fast and the invasion of the surrounding tissues easily leads to ulcerated oral mucosa.
E Nerve deficits are commonly reported among malignant salivary gland tumors and they are associated with the perineural infiltration from neoplastic cells, rather than the pressure of the tumor on the local nerve. Adenocystic carcinoma can cause multiple cranial palsies, especially to the lingual, facial or hypoglossal nerves, while the pleomorphic adenomas rarely cause a facial palsy which usually appears after surgical removal of the tumor.

Comments: Malignant salivary gland tumors are rare, tend to occur in older patients and arise more frequently from the minor salivary glands, while the benign tumors are more common and arise from the major salivary glands in which pleomorphic adenoma is predominant.

Q3 Which is the most common malignant tumor of the minor salivary glands of the upper lip?

A Pleomorphic adenoma
B Warthin tumor
C Basal cell adenocarcinoma
D Adenoid cystic carcinoma
E Oncocytoma

Answers:

A No
B No
C No
D Adenoid cystic carcinoma is a rare malignant neoplasm that occurs more often in minor salivary glands of the upper lip and rarely in submandibular glands and parotids.
E No

Comments: Pleomorphic adenoma, Warthin tumors and oncocytomas are benign salivary gland tumors and are, therefore, easily excluded while the basal cell adenocarcinomas are malignant lesions that rarely affect the minor salivary glands of the upper lip.

Case 22.3

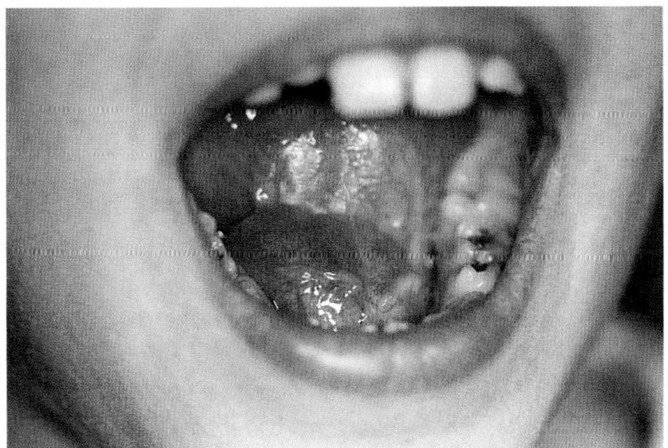

Figure 22.3a

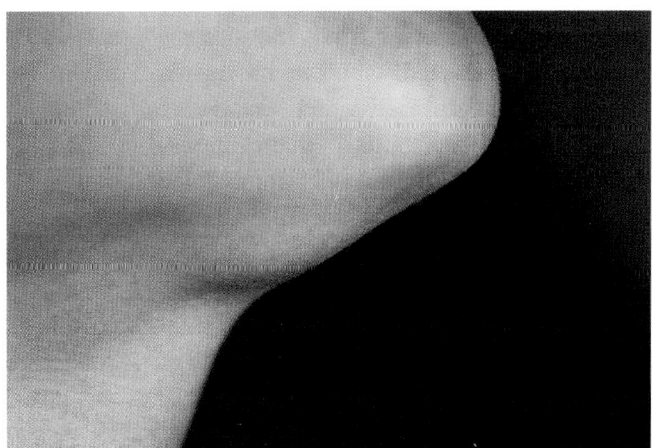

Figure 22.3b

CO: A nine-year-old boy came with his parents for an evaluation of a persistent swelling in the floor of his mouth and his chin.

HPC: The swelling was incidentally discovered by his mother three weeks ago. In the beginning, she observed a small lump within her boy's chin that was more prominent during eating. An additional examination revealed a large "cystic lesion" inside his mouth.

PMH: The boy had no medical history of any serious local or systemic diseases or recent trauma in the area, but used to bite his nails in stressful situations.

OE: A large bluish to translucent hemispherical cystic lesion was seen covering the whole right side and half of the left side on the floor of his mouth (Figure 22.3a). The lesion was approximately 3.5 cm and as it was slightly pushing the tongue upwards, it caused some difficulties during eating, swallowing and speaking. It was also deeply extended to the mylohyoid muscle, causing a small protuberance in the skin (Figure 22.3b).No other similar lesions were found inside his mouth, skin or other mucosae. Occlusal radiographs did not reveal any calculus deposition along right submandibular – sublongual duct system.

Q1 What is the cause of the swellings?

- **A** Dermoid cyst
- **B** Periapical infection of the lower anterior teeth
- **C** Sialolith of the sublingual gland
- **D** Branchial cyst
- **E** Ranula

Answers:

- **A** No
- **B** No
- **C** No
- **D** No
- **E** Ranula is the correct answer. It is considered as a bluish translucent cystic lesion in the floor of mouth, with no evidence of a calculus duct obstruction or local infection arising from adjacent teeth, tongue or floor of the mouth. It can be located either in the floor of the mouth (simple ranula) or be extended posteriorly beyond the free edge of the mylohyoid muscles and protrude into the chin (plunging ranula) as it is exactly seen in this boy.

Comments: The location of the lesion mainly at the right lateral side of the floor of mouth excludes other cystic lesions that are located in the middle of the floor, like the midline dermoid cyst or in the neck (branchial cyst). The negative for calculus occlusal X-rays together with the absence of purulent discharge from the sublingualr ducts or periapical lower anterior teeth area rule out sialolith or tooth abscess from the diagnosis.

Q2 Which is/are the best treatment(s) for this boy?

- **A** Observation only
- **B** Surgical excision of the cyst
- **C** Surgical excision of the cyst together with the affected gland
- **D** Laser
- **E** Marsupialization

Answers:

- **A** No
- **B** No

C The surgical excision of the cyst and related gland is highly recommended when the ranula is extended to the neck, especially in the parapharyngeal space, due to any possible complications like injuring the mandibular, lingual or hypoglossal nerves or forming an orocervical fistula.
D No
E No

Comments: A six-month observation is recommended in congenital ranulas in the hope that these cysts will be absorbed. Marsupialization is not recommended as this technique has a high recurrence rate and serves as a precursor for a new plunging ranula. On the other hand, enucleation of the cyst with surgery or CO_2 laser is useful when the lesion is small and solely located in the floor of the mouth.

Q3 What are the histological differences between a ranula and a dermoid cyst?
A Lumen fluid conent
B Thickness of the cystic wall
C Contents of the cystic wall
D Capsule
E Inflammatory reaction

Answers:
A The cystic lumen material is composed of keratin in dermoid–epidermoid cysts, while an amorphous eosinophilic material from amylase and other salivary proteins in ranulas.
B The wall is a thin, loose, vasculated connective tissue in ranulas, while it is thicker and more fibrous in dermoid cysts.
C The cystic wall contains salivary glands acini in ranulas, while hair and other skin appendages exist in dermoid cysts.
D Fibrous capsule surrounds the dermoid cyst but was not seen the ranula.
E Both cysts can be infected, but the type of inflammation differs. A diffused accumulation of mixed inflammatory cells, predominately of foam macrophages is seen in ranulas, while numerous granulomas with giant cells occur in dermoid cysts.

Case 22.4

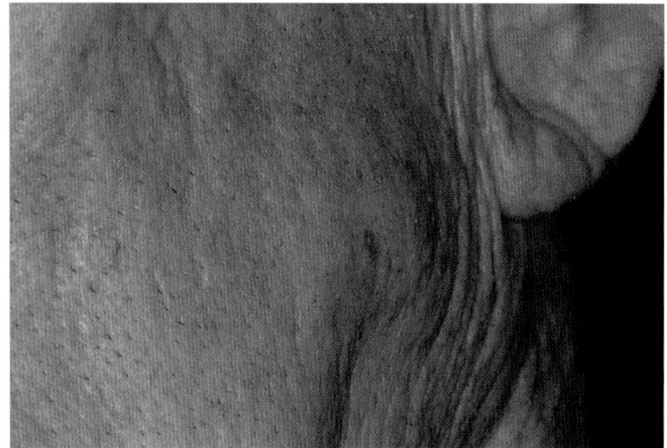

Figure 22.4a

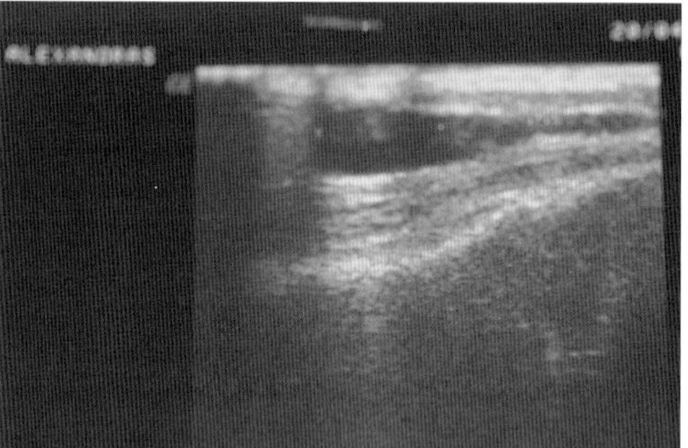

Figure 22.4b

CO: A 68-year-old man presented with a recurrent swelling of his face along the route of his left parotid duct.

HPC: The swelling appeared suddenly six months ago and automatically resolved within one week. In addition to this, two episodes of similar swellings were recorded within the last four months. However, all episodes were painless, without any fever, general symptomatology or any connection to previous trauma, local surgery, sialoliths or use of drugs that might induce xerostomia.

PMH: Hypertension and chronic bronchitis were his only medical problems; they were controlled with ACE Inhibitors and bronchodilators as well as systemic steroids (in crisis). Despite his lungs problems, smoking of 20–30 cigarettes was his daily habit.

OE: A small swelling was noted on the external left cheek, at the left parotid gland region anterior to the masseter muscle and along the route of the Stensen's duct. This swelling was soft, 2 cm, and caused some discomfort which was relieved with aggressive massage and compresses (Figure 22.4a). The ultrasound examination did not reveal a parotid gland stone or inflammation apart from a small dilation of the duct (Figure 22.4b). Intra-oral examination, revealed the adjacent buccal mucosa to be slightly raised, but the rest of oral mucosa normal. Cervical lymphadenopathy was absent.

Q1 What is the possible cause of this facial swelling?

A Sialolith
B Sialocele
C Duct stenosis
D Sialectasis
E Sjogren syndrome

Answers:

A No
B No
C No
D Sialectasis is an uncommon condition of the salivary glands characterized by a recurrent painful swelling due to the dilation of the salivary duct (partial or total). When the dilation is small, it causes a mild symptomatology but when it happens to be extensive, it is accompanied with severe pain and swelling across the duct. The fine needle aspiration (FNA) biopsy did not reveal any inflammation or neoplasia of the parenchyma, and sialogram was normal, while the ultrasonography and magnetic resonance imaging (MRI) showed some degree of dilation with no evidence of obstruction
E No

Comments: The negative history of a previous trauma or surgery at the left parotid area; the absence of anatomical strictures or calcified mass within the duct with ultrasound, or chronic xerostomia–xerophthalmia exclude sialoceles, sialoliths, anatomical duct variation (stricture) and Sjogren's syndrome from the diagnosis.

Q2 Which of the diagnostic tools below can be used for this condition?

A History
B Clinical findings
C Imaging techniques
D No
E Culture

Answers:

A The history of a recurrent painful or not painful swelling along the duct of the suspected gland is indicative of sialectasis.
B The clinical examination may reveal a swollen gland with or without parenchyma or duct infection.
C The imaging techniques like ultrasound, sialogram, MRI and computed tomography (CT) scans provide information about the structure of the parenchyma, intra-ductal architecture, presence of tumors or lymph node metastasis respectively.
D Blood immunological tests for the detection of autoantibodies like rheumatoid factor (RF), antinuclear antibodies (ANA), SSa and SSba can be used for excluding other diseases like Sjogren's syndrome.
E No

Comments: The culture of the secreted saliva can be used to isolate and identify the pathogenic bacteria that are responsible for acute or chronic sialadenitis and not for sialectasis while blood immunological tests for the detection of autoantibodies like rheumatoid factor (RF), antinuclear antibodies (ANA), SSa and SSba can be used for excluding other diseases like Sjogren's syndrome but not sialectasis.

Q3 Which of the treatments below are NOT routinely used for this condition?

A Botulinum toxin type A
B Marsupialization of the duct
C Duct papillae dilation
D Gland compression
E Antibiotics

Answers:

A No
B No
C No
D No
E No

Comments: All the above techniques have been occasionally used with promising results. Some of these are conservative like botulinum toxin and antibiotic use or gland compression, while the rest require surgery using complicated procedures dependent on the severity of each lesion.

Case 22.5

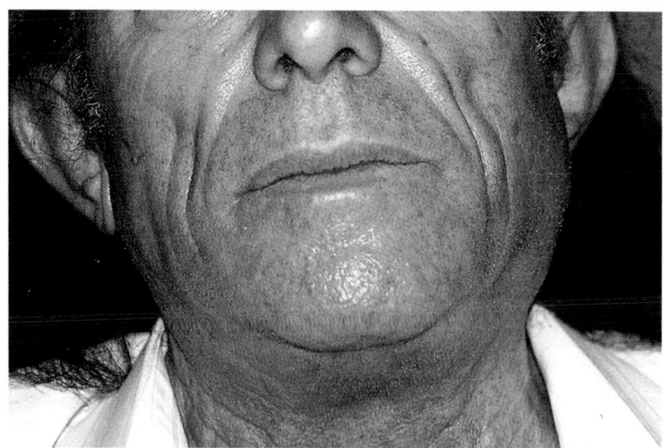

Figure 22.5

CO: A 65-year-old man presented with a three-year facial swelling.

HPC: The swelling gradually increased in size over the last three years and reached its maximum size over the last eight months.

PMH: His main medical problems were chronic diabetes and hypercholesterolemia that were diagnosed at the age of 45, but remained uncontrolled since then due to his unhealthy fatty diet, heavy drinking of beer and whisky and smoking one to two packets of cigarettes on a daily basis.

OE: Extra-orally, a diffuse swelling was mainly found at the left preauricular region of his face. The swelling was 3 cm × 3.5 cm, soft, asymptomatic, and arose from his parotid glands, while the overlying skin was normal (Figure 22.5). His right parotid was slightly enlarged while his submandibular and sublingual salivary glands had normal size and consistency. Intra-orally, xerostomia or pus coming out from the Stensen's papillae or other areas was not recorded. Cervical lymphadenopathy was absent. Ultrasonography did not reveal any cystic lesion, calculus or abnormal growth but only a diffuse swelling. FNA was undertaken and smears revealed numerous acinar epithelial cells in clusters or glandular pattern, and fibrovascular elements, yet inflammatory cells were missing.

Q1 What is the cause?

- **A** Warthin tumor
- **B** Hypertrophy of the masseter muscle
- **C** Sjogren syndrome
- **D** Infective parotitis
- **E** Sialosis

Answers:

- **A** No
- **B** No
- **C** No
- **D** No
- **E** Sialosis or sialadenosis is a chronic, diffuse, non-inflammatory and non-neoplastic enlargement of the parotids and sometimes of the submandibular, sublingual or minor salivary glands. Sialosis affects middle-aged patients with serious systemic diseases like diabetes, that may change the salivary aquaporin water channels. Correction of the underlying disorder and eliminating predisposing factors like heavy drinking may be the most successful treatment as in this case, surgery is unsatisfactory.

Comments: Having in mind that ultrasonography revealed an asymptomatic swelling within the parotid gland and not in the masseter with no general malaise, fever and other symptoms or lymphadenopathy, masseter hypertrophy and infective parotitis (bacterial or viral) are easily excluded from the diagnosis. The presence of numerous acinar epithelial cells without centrally pyknotic nuclei in fibrovascular stroma or atrophy and the lack of inflammatory cells in smears also rule out Warthin tumor and Sjogren syndrome from the diagnosis.

Q2 Which other systemic factors apart from diabetes could play a role in the pathogenesis of this condition?

- **A** Endocrine diseases
- **B** Metabolic disturbances
- **C** Gastrointestinal factors
- **D** Drugs
- **E** Autoimmunity

Answers:

- **A** Endocrine diseases such as like diabetes insipidus, acromegaly and hypothyroidism have been also associated with this condition.
- **B** Metabolic disturbances due to malnutrition, alcoholism, anorexia or bulimia seem to cause deficiencies in vitamins, basic proteins and minerals causing glandular enlargements, as these elements participate in the normal functions of salivary glands.
- **C** Liver diseases (alcoholic or non-alcoholic) like cirrhosis or celiac disease may play together with nutritional deficiencies, a role in sialodenosis.

D The chronic use of anti-hypertensive, anti-cholinergic and psychotropic drugs have been linked with this condition too.
E No

Comments: Autoimmune diseases can affect the salivary glands as in Sjogren syndrome and sarcoidosis causing diffuse bilateral swelling, but both diseases have different pathogenesis from sialodenosis.

Q3 Which of the investigations below is/are pathognomonic for this condition?
A Blood biochemistry
B Sialography
C MRI/US
D FNA biopsy
E Sialochemistry

Answers:
A No
B No
C MRI or US help the clinician to differentiate sialosis from other occupying lesions within the gland.
D FNA biopsy is a simple technique that allows the isolation of normal acinar epithelial cells and lack of inflammatory cell and this finding is pathognomonic for sialosis.
E No

Comments: Biochemical tests may reveal increased blood glucose or abnormal liver function tests; sialochemistry increases the concentration of potassium and calcium in the saliva; while sialography shows sparse peripheral ducts, but these findings are not pathognomonic for sialosis as they can be also found in other diseases.

23

Teeth

Teeth are a specialized part of the human body that participate actively in collecting, eating, mastication and speech procedures. Their successful development depends on a complex interaction of the dental epithelium with the underlying ectomesenchyme. Disruption of this interaction by local and systemic factors leads into developmental anomalies such as deviations of normal color, contour, size number, and degree of teeth development before or after birth.

This chapter has three parts:

Part A includes teeth anomalies related to the number, size, and shape (Figure 23.A).

Part B includes the diseases affecting the teeth and their structures (Figure 23.B).

Part C includes the diseases affecting the teeth's components in relation to the adjacent tissues (Figure 23.C).

Table 23 lists the more common and important conditions affecting the teeth and adjacent tissues.

Table 23 Teeth: common and important changes.

- Number of teeth
  - Anodontia
  - Hypodontia
    - Anhidrotic ectodermal dysplasia
    - Down syndrome
    - Clefts
  - Hyperodontia
    - Cleidocranial dysplasia
- Morphology of teeth
  - Size
    - Microdontia
    - Macrodontia
  - Structure
    - Amelogenesis imperfecta
    - Dentinogenesis imperfecta
    - Rickets
    - Hypoparathyroidism
    - Chemo therapy during tooth formation
- Shape
  - Anomalies within the same teeth
    - Dens invaginatus
    - Dens evaginatus
    - Taurodontism
    - Moon molars/screwdriver incisors
  - Additional tooth structures
    - Cusps
    - Odontomas
    - Hypercementosis and cementinoma
    - Dentinoma
    - Enamel clefts
    - Enamel pearls
  - Loss of tooth structure
    - Abfraction
    - Abrasion
    - Attrition
    - Caries
    - Erosion
    - Fracture
    - Trauma (mild to severe) of teeth during enamel formation
    - Periapical infection of primary tooth predecessor
  - Relation with other teeth
    - Malocclusion
- Time of teeth loss
  - Early
    - Down syndrome
    - Immunodeficiencies
    - Papillon-Lefèvre syndrome

Clinical Guide to Oral Diseases, First Edition. Dimitris Malamos and Crispian Scully.

Companion website: www.wiley.com/go/malamos/clinical_guide

Table 23 (Continued)

- Trauma
- Malignancies
- Delayed
  - Ankyloses
  - Gingival fibromatosis
- Teeth esthetics
  - Stains
    - Extrinsic
      - Chromogenic bacteria
      - Mouthwashes with chlorhexidine or iodine
      - Soft drinks (coffee or tea)
      - Beverages
      - Tobacco products
      - Drugs
      - Iron and other metals
    - Intrinsic
      - Doxycycline
      - Fluorosis (mild to severe)
      - Caries
      - Pulp hemorrhage
      - Filling material (amalgam, composite)
  - Resorption
    - Internal
    - External
  - Man's interference
    - Body art

23.1 Part A: Teeth Anomalies Related to their Number, Size, and Shape

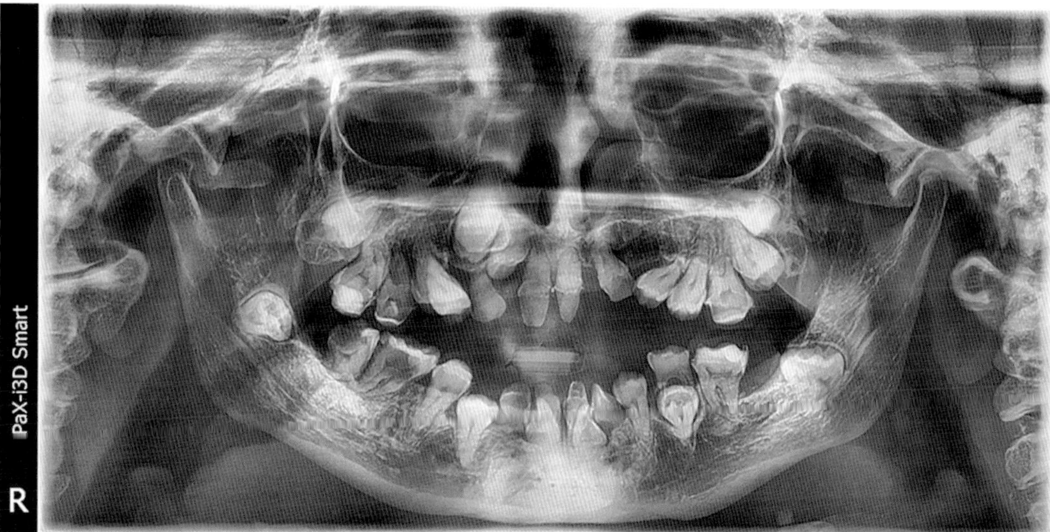

Figure 23.A Teeth anomalies in a patient with pituitary dwarfism.

Case 23.1

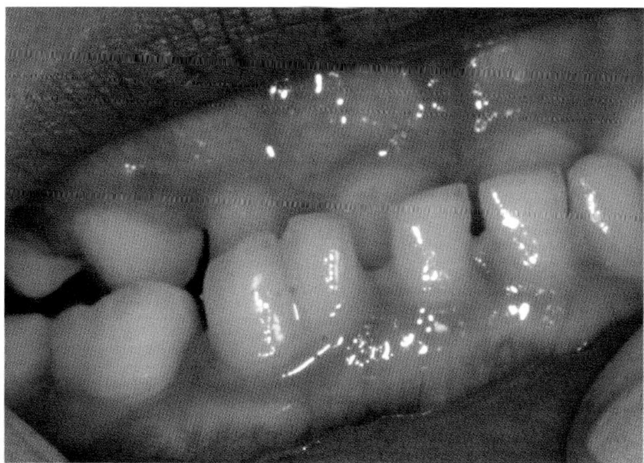

Figure 23.1

CO: A seven-year-old boy was referred for a regular dental check-up and found to have abnormal morphology in one of his lower right anterior teeth.

HPC: His teeth anomaly was discovered incidentally and did not cause any serious esthetic or eating problems.

PMH: His medical history was clear from any serious diseases and his family history did not reveal any dental anomalies; consanguinity was not reported.

CO: Physical examination revealed no stature and skin anomalies while intra-oral examination showed a fusion of the crowns of the lower right deciduous lateral incisor and canine (Figure 23.1), leading to a fewer number on measuring his teeth in the dental arch. These two teeth had a normal shape and fused along their crown and roots with complete union of their pulp chambers and canals as shown in periapical X-rays.

Q1 What is this dental anomaly?

- **A** Fusion
- **B** Germination
- **C** Concrescence
- **D** Taurodontism
- **E** Ghost teeth

Answers:

- **A** Fusion is a rare developmental anomaly of the shape of the teeth, characterized by the union (complete or not) of two adjacent teeth leading to a reduced number on counting. This anomaly is seen in both dentitions and affects more often the anterior teeth than the molars, and a number of factors such as local pressure, previous viral inflammation during pregnancy, environmental factors, clefts, vitamin deficiencies and chemotherapeutic agents like thalidomide have been implicated with this anomaly.
- **B** No
- **C** No
- **D** No
- **E** No

Comments: The other dental anomalies are easily excluded, based on clinical characteristics such as the normal number of teeth (germination), the irregular crown morphology and pattern of cementum union (concrescence)and lack of constriction at the cement–enamel junction, together with radiological characteristics such as enlarged pulp chamber (taurodontism) or ghost-like appearance (ghost teeth).

Q2 Which is the most important complication of fusion of deciduous incisors?

- **A** Increased risk of caries
- **B** Occlusal disturbances
- **C** Delayed root resorption of deciduous teeth
- **D** Pulp exposure
- **E** Descendent teeth missing

Answers:

- **A** No
- **B** No
- **C** No
- **D** No
- **E** The absence of permanent descendant teeth is the most important complication.

Comments: All the other complications such as increased risk of caries, pulp exposure delay, loss of deciduous teeth, and malocclusion may easily be prevented, detected and treated.

Q3 What is/are differences between fusion and germination?

- **A** Dentition (deciduous or permanent)
- **B** Location (upper or lower teeth)
- **C** Teeth predilection (incisors or molars)
- **D** Two tooth rule (positive or negative)
- **E** Pathogenesis

Answers:

A No

B Fusion is more common in lower teeth while germination is more common in upper teeth.

C No

D The "tooth rule" shows a reduced number of teeth (minus one) in fusion and normal number in germination.

E Fusion arises from the union of two normally separated tooth germs, while germination shows two teeth arisen from one tooth germ.

Comments: Fusion and germination affect both dentitions and usually the incisors, regardless of the patient's gender.

Case 23.2

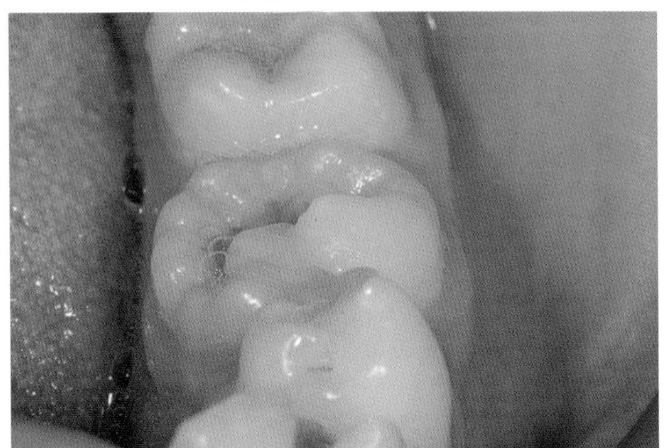

Figure 23.2a

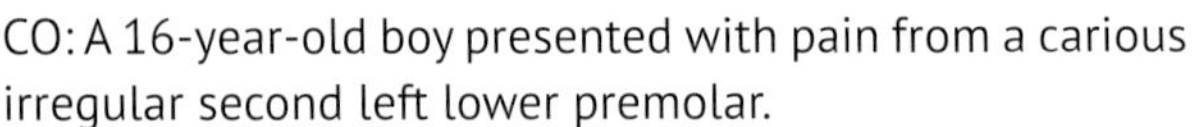

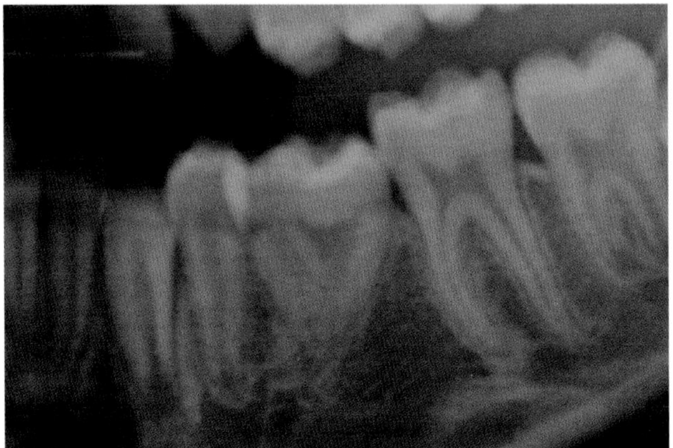

Figure 23.2b

CO: A 16-year-old boy presented with pain from a carious irregular second left lower premolar.

HPC: The pain was acute, sharp and exacerbated with sweets and cold drinks over the last two weeks. It arose from the irregular second lower left carious premolar.

PMH: His medical and family history was irrelevant and previous trauma was not reported, while his diet was full of sugar found in sweets or drinks.

OE: Oral examination revealed large bulbous lower second premolars, with central fissure and an extra cusp buccal lingually (Figure 23.2) but with enlarged and elongated pulp chambers as seen in the periapical radiograph (Figure 23.2b). Caries were detected on the occlusal surface of his left second premolar, causing pain with cold and sweet stimuli. No other dental anomalies were detected in both dentitions and his oral hygiene was adequate.

Q1 What is the cause of his premolar disfiguration?

A Congenital syphilis

B Amelogenesis imperfecta

C Taurodontism

D Macrodontia

E Dens evaginatus

Answers:

A No

B No

C No

D No

E Dens evaginatus is a rare tooth abnormality in shape, seen mainly in premolars and resembling teeth with extra cusps. This extra cusp could be easily worn down, leaving exposed pulp which can finally lead to necrosis and periapical infections. It is usually seen in premolars of the mandible rather maxilla, and in males from Asia rather than other continents.

Comments: The characteristic crown morphology without any pits, grooves but with extra cusps and irregular pulp restricted only to the premolars exclude amelogenesis imperfecta, congenital syphilis, macrodontia and taurodism from the diagnosis. In amelogenesis imperfecta changes in color(yelow, brown or grey) and tooth morphology with extra grooves and pits and enamel of various thickness and prone to wear off in agroup of teeth are detected. In congenital syphils facial deformities are accompanied with triangular (incisors) or peglike appearance(molar) permanent teeth. In taurodism, the molar teeth are enlarged vertically by pushing the floor of the pulp and the furcation of the tooth apically while in macrodontia the size of the affected teeth is more than 2 standard deviation from the average.

Q2 What is/are the main difference/s between dens evaginatus and taurodontism?

A Cause
B Location
C Pulp chamber size or location
D Race predilection
E Gender predilection

Answers:

A Taurodontism is caused by failure of Hertwig's epithelial sheath diaphragm to invaginate at the proper horizontal level while in dens evaginatus occur as a result of an unusual growth and folding of the inner enamel epithelium and ectomesenchymal cells of the dental papillae into the stellate reticulum of the enamel organ.
B Premolars are commonly affected in dens evaginatus while molars in taurodontism.
C The proportion of the pulp to tooth surface is higher in taurodontism as it is moved apically, while in dens evaginatus it is normal.
D Dens evaginatus is seen more frequently in patients with Asian rather than American or European origin while taurodontism is common in Eskimos.
E No

Comments: Both teeth abnormalities are more often seen in males.

Q3 Which of the syndromes below is/are NOT associated with this tooth abnormality?

A Klinefelter syndrome
B Down syndrome
C Sturge-Weber syndrome
D Ascher syndrome
E Marfan syndrome

Answers:

A Klinefelter syndrome has an increased incidence of taurodontism and not dens evaginatus.
B Down syndrome has a high incidence of taurodontism as seen in Klinefelter syndrome.
C Sturge-Weber syndrome is associated with gingival overgrowths rather than dental anomalies.
D Ascher syndrome causes blepharoptosis, double lip and goiter, but does not affect teeth size or morphology.
E Marfan syndrome causes malocclusion due to a narrow palate, but has never been associated with this dental anomaly.

Case 23.3

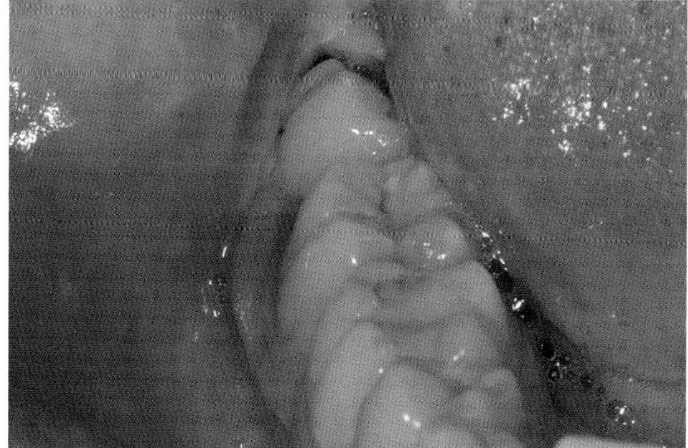

Figure 23.3a

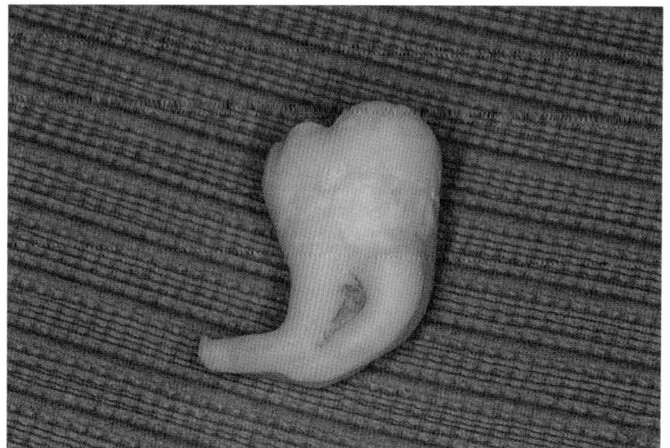

Figure 23.3b

CO: A 21-year-old man was referred for extraction of his lower right third molar.

HPC: His third molar was partially impacted and covered with inflamed gingivae and therefore was extracted and revealed a deviation of its long axis to its roots.

PMH: His medical and family history was irrelevant to wisdom tooth malformation.

OE: A partially erupted lower right third molar covered with swollen inflamed gingivae was found, causing slight trismus and pain, and pressure to the adjacent teeth (Figure 23a). The tooth was removed under local anesthesia and revealed an irregular distal deviation of its roots (Figure 23b). The rest of his teeth were free of caries or fillings. No other lesions were found inside his mouth, skin or other mucosae.

Q1 Which was the dental anomaly of the extracted molar?

- **A** Dilaceration
- **B** Taurodontism
- **C** Flexion
- **D** Hypophosphatasemia
- **E** Dentin dysplasia type I

Answers:

- **A** Dilaceration is the abrupt deviation of the long axis of the crown or root portion of the tooth (>90°) leading to a sharp bend or curve and this may be related to caused trauma during odontogenesis.
- **B** No
- **C** No
- **D** No
- **E** No

Comments: In flexion the affected roots deviate less than 90° while in taurodontism, dentin dysplasia type 1, or hyposphatasemia the affected teeth are short or hypoplastic with crown abnormalities and could be lost the age of 30–40.

Q2 Which is/are the difference/s between dilacerations and flexions?

- **A** Cause
- **B** Location
- **C** Degree of root deviation
- **D** Teeth affected
- **E** Crown morphology

Answers:

- **A** No
- **B** In flexion the deviation is restricted on roots while in dilacerations on roots or crowns.
- **C** In flexion the degree of root deviation is less than in dilacerations (< 90°)
- **D** No
- **E** No

Comments: Both dental anomalies are mainly seen in permanent teeth with normal crown and have been possibly associated with history of previous trauma, altered germ position and delayed tooth eruption.

Q3 Which is the cause of this dental anomaly?

- **A** Trauma
- **B** Idiopathic
- **C** Scars
- **D** Lesions causing delays in teeth eruption
- **E** Heritage

Answers:

- **A** Local trauma to the primary predecessor tooth due to accident or iatrogenic procedures (laryngoscopy or endotracheal intubation) is the most common cause of the crown In the absence of trauma, dilaceration may be dilacerations of the succedaneum permanent teeth.
- **B** Idiopathic it is based on the fact that there is low frequency of dilacerations contrary to the high frequency of local trauma among children. This idea is reinforced by the observation that trauma involves more than one tooth and dilacerations affect isolated teeth.
- **C** Scars are formed easily after a local injury or infections affecting the development of permanent teeth, causing alterations in their morphology.
- **D** Congenital lesions like hemangiomas or facial clefts and cysts or even tumors may cause ectopic development of permanent tooth germs and delay of primary tooth resorption that leads to longer retention of primary teeth and morphological anomalies of permanent teeth.
- **E** Heritage seems to play a role as there are a number of dilacerations have been seen among twins or close relatives of certain races.

Case 23.4

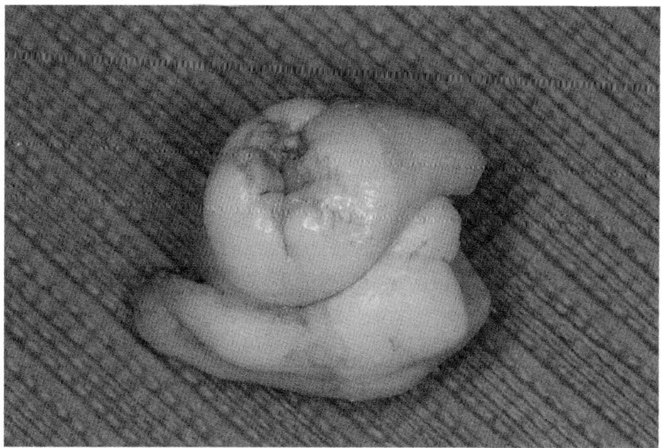

Figure 23.4

CO: A 32-year-old man came for the removal of his lower left third molar. His gingivae were inflamed around the crown, and this had caused him eating problems many times over the past three years.

HPC: His left third molar was partially erupted and had caused many episodes of pericoronitis leading to pain, dysphagia trismus, pyrexia and cervical lymphadenitis, which had resolved with broad-spectrum antibiotics.

PMH: His medical history was irrelevant.

OE: Intra-oral examination revealed a lower, left third molar with inflammation of surrounding gingivae, and was associated with ipsilateral lymphadenopathy. This tooth was surgically removed and found to be in close contact with another supernumerary but well-formed fourth molar tooth (Figure 23.4) with cementum. A class I molar relation and chronic gingivitis were recorded.

Q1 What is this dental anomaly?

- **A** Dens invaginatus
- **B** Dens evaginatus
- **C** Odontoma
- **D** Concrescence
- **E** Gemination

Answers:

- **A** No
- **B** No
- **C** No
- **D** Concrescence is a rare dental anomaly characterized by a fusion of two fully formed teeth which are joined along the root surfaces by cementum.
- **E** No

Comments: The union of two fully complete teeth with independent roots excludes odontomas, dens invaginatum and evaginatum, and gemination from the diagnosis. In gemination there are two crowns but one root, in dens in dente there is one tooth within another two, in evaginatum there is an extra cusp in one tooth, while in odontomas the dental tissues are not demarcated completely.

Q2 Which of the clinical characteristics below are NOT related with this anomaly?

- **A** Enamel fuses the joined teeth
- **B** The union is limited to a small root area
- **C** Both dentitions are affected
- **D** Lower molars predominate in this anomaly
- **E** Both sexes are equally affected

Answers:

- **A** The cementum and not enamel participates in the fusion of the two adjacent teeth.
- **B** The union varies from a small contact to full root surface.
- **C** No
- **D** The upper molars are predominantly affected.
- **E** No

Comments: Concrescence affects teeth of both dentitions regardless of the patient's age or sex.

Q3 What is the best treatment for asymptomatic teeth with this anomaly?

- **A** None
- **B** Surgical division of concrescent teeth
- **C** Root canal treatment
- **D** Extraction of both teeth
- **E** Prosthetic repair

Answers:

- **A** No treatment is required in asymptomatic concrescent teeth.
- **B** No
- **C** No
- **D** No
- **E** No

Comments: The presence of pain or esthetic problems can lead clinicians to extract these teeth. Only in selected cases, division and removal of one of the teeth and prosthetic repair with the other crown is recommended.

Case 23.5

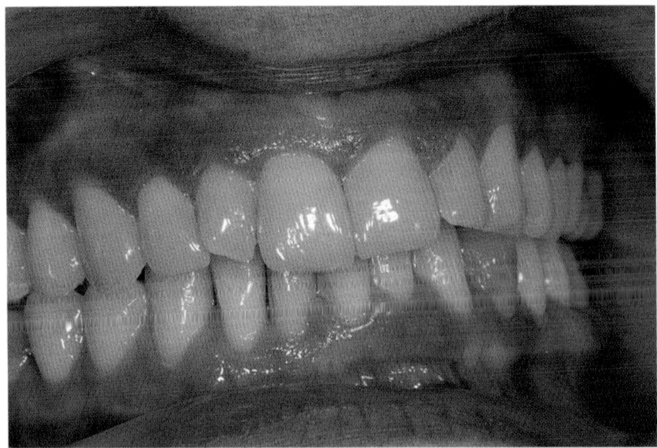

Figure 23.5

CO: A 32-year-old woman came for her annual dental check-up and during the examination a few teeth and gingival problems were recorded by her new dentist.

HPC: As the patient was unfamiliar with these problems, their duration or relation with other diseases was unknown.

PMH: Her medical and family history did not reveal any serious diseases or drug use. Her diet was rich in vegetables and fruits and low in animal products, while smoking or drinking habits were absent.

OE: A healthy young woman with dark complexion showed, intra-orally, swollen gingivae, some tooth staining, especially in the lower anterior teeth, and a complete dentition. Her teeth had normal morphology, composition and were free of caries or periapical infections or malocclusion (Figure 23.5), but were increased in number. No other oral lesions were recorded apart from a diffuse brown pigmentation, especially of her anterior gingivae.

Q1 What is her main dental problem?
- **A** Chronic gingivitis
- **B** Racial gingival pigmentation
- **C** Hyperplastic labial frenulum
- **D** Tooth discoloration
- **E** Supplemental supernumerary upper right lateral incisor

Answers:
- **A** No
- **B** No
- **C** No
- **D** No
- **E** The supplemental right lateral incisor is her main dental problem and characterized by an additional tooth presence (supernumerary) with normal morphology, fully erupted and causing crowding of the upper anterior teeth but not malocclusion.

Comments: Chronic gingivitis and racial gingival pigmentation are very common, innocent lesions. Gingivitis is the second in frequency of oral diseases in young patients after caries, while racial gingival pigmentation is seen mainly in dark skinned patients and characterized by increased melanin deposition in normal melanocytes. The labial frenum is not hyperplastic, and had not caused any central incisor displacement, while the tooth discoloration is exogenous and together with plaque, is responsible for patient's gingivitis.

Q2 Which are the morphological variants of supernumerary teeth?
- **A** Conical
- **B** Tuberculate
- **C** Supplemental
- **D** Mesiodens
- **E** Odontoma

Answers:
- **A** Conical teeth are supernumerary, peg-shaped teeth and usually found inverted or horizontal in the anterior maxilla and cause rotation or displacement of permanent teeth.
- **B** The tuberculate type of supernumerary teeth are characterized by a barrel-shaped structure with delayed root formation and located in pairs on the palatal surface of central incisors causing delay of their eruption.
- **C** Supplemental supernumerary teeth are duplicated normal teeth, commonly seen among the maxillary lateral incisors (mainly) and premolars and molars of both dentitions (but especially in primary).
- **D** Mesiodens are supernumerary teeth that have a characteristic location and morphology. These teeth are small, conical and always located in the mid line between the two central incisors.
- **E** Odontoma especially the compound type, has been considered as a morphological variation of supernumerary teeth that has similarities with a normal tooth.

Q3 Which of the diseases below are commonly associated with this dental anomaly?

- **A** Lip or palatal clefts
- **B** Cleidocranial dysostosis
- **C** Gardner syndrome
- **D** Ehlers-Danlos syndrome
- **E** Down syndrome

Answers:

- **A** Clefts (lip or palate) are associated with high incidence of supernumerary teeth, especially at the anterior maxilla, and are the result of fragmentation of the dental lamina during cleft formation.
- **B** Cleidocranial dysostosis is an autosomal disorder affecting the bones and teeth. The maxilla is characteristically hypoplastic and the mandible is normal, but sometimes shows a delay in union of the mandibular symphyses, while a prolonged retention of the primary teeth and multiple unerupted permanent and supernumerary teeth is seen.
- **C** Gardner syndrome or hereditary intestinal polyposis is characterized by colonic ployps, sebaceous cysts, jaw osteomas, and dental anomalies such as supernumerary teeth, hypodontia, compound odontomas, and impacted teeth with abnormal morphology.
- **D** No
- **E** No

Comments: Syndromes like Ehlers-Danlos (type III) and Down syndromes usually present dental anomalies like enamel hypoplasia, microdontia and hypodontia but very rarely supernumerary teeth.

23.2 Part B: Disorders of Teeth Structures

Teeth are composed of enamel, dentin, cementum, and pulp tissue. Enamel is the hardest body tissue covering the surface of the dental crown while dentin is the inner part of the tooth and covered by enamel in crowns and cementum in roots. Cementum connects the alveolar bone with the tooth via the periodontal ligaments, while the pulp via its blood vessels provides nutrients to the dentin and via nerve fibers sensory functions. A number of congenital diseases, environmental and local or systemic diseases affect the formation, mineralization and maturation of teeth structures leading to a number of conditions affecting the clinical appearance, morphology and resistance to external harmful stimuli (See Figure 23.B).

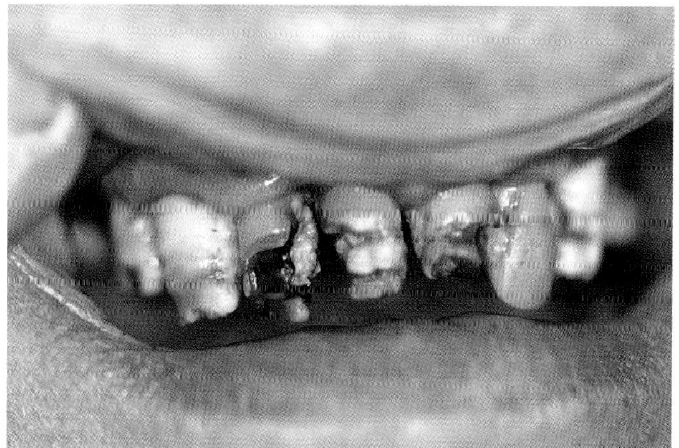

Figure 23.B Amelogenesis imperfecta in permanent teeth.

Case 23.6

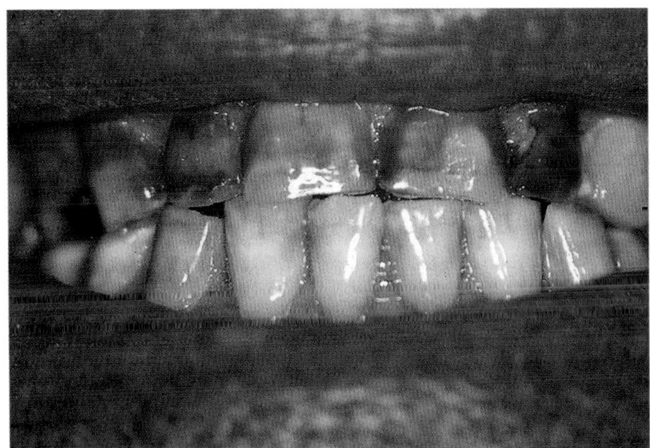

Figure 23.6

CO: A 46-year-old male presented complaining about a brown discoloration of the majority of his teeth.

HPC: The brown discoloration had been noticed earlier in life, even in his primary dentition and in dentitions of his close relatives and in several residents of his town.

PMH: Apart from joint stiffness and back pain, possibly due to his heavy work duties as a manual worker in a paint factory, he had no other serious medical problems. The patient was not on any medication and could not recall any tetracycline use by his mother while she was pregnant to him, nor by himself up to the age of eight years. He smoked a packet of 20 cigarettes per day and drank three glasses of wine per day.

OE: Extra-oral examination revealed nothing of note. Oral examination showed all his teeth to be of normal size and shape with minimal tooth surface loss, but with a brown discoloration and also pits and grooves in the enamel (Figure 23.6). This discoloration was in his anterior maxillary teeth, and lighter in his mandibular teeth, where there were white or yellow or slightly brown enamel zones. Despite his poor oral hygiene, most of his teeth were caries free.

Q1 What is the possible cause of his teeth discoloration?

- **A** Amelogenesis imperfecta
- **B** Habits
- **C** Alkopyonuria
- **D** Tetracycline staining
- **E** Fluorosis

Answers:

- **A** No
- **B** No
- **C** No
- **D** No
- **E** Fluorosis is the cause of the discoloration. It is a developmental disturbance of the dental enamel caused by fluoride overexposure during the first eight years of life and characterized by white striations in the enamel (mild form) to a deep permanent diffuse brown discoloration (severe form). This is in agreement with the fact that the patient had lived all his life in a town where the natural fluoride concentration in the drinking water exceeded 3.8 mg/l. Similar teeth discoloration were also recorded in other residents of his town. This fluoride excess interacted with the mineralized tissues, such as teeth or bones, increasing their resistance to demineralization and to caries.

Comments: Amelogenesis imperfecta shares some clinical characteristics like pits and grooves and a white-brown zone of discoloration with fluorosis, but is excluded due to the presence of attrition. Habits like heavy smoking or drinking of wine, tea or coffee, together with the patient's workplace could contribute to his teeth discoloration, but is not the main cause as had also been seen in his primary dentition and in the dentition of several non-smokers resident in his town. Alkaptonuria is accompanied with black urine, dark skin and pigmented sclera, not seen in this patient and therefore is easily excluded from the diagnosis. Tetracycline staining is also excluded, as it requires a positive history of this drug use by the patient up to eight years of age, or by his mother during the second or third trimesters of pregnancy or during breastfeeding.

Q2 What is the most common cause of this condition?

- **A** Drinking water
- **B** Toothpaste with fluoride
- **C** Mouthwash with fluoride
- **D** Fluoride tablets in excess
- **E** Over-consumption of foods rich in fluoride

Answers:

- **A** Drinking water with fluoride at a concentration of >2 mg/l is the main cause of fluorosis among residents of the same region who had drunk this type of water since birth.
- **B** No
- **C** No
- **D** No
- **E** No

Comments: Fluorosis induced by of mouthwashes, tablets or toothpastes is very rare and requires overuse for many months or years. Foods like pickles, cucumber, beans or peas have never been associated with fluorosis as their fluoride concentration is low and their consumption is not on a daily basis.

Q3 Which other organs apart from teeth are affected from this condition?

- **A** Nerves
- **B** Bones
- **C** Endocrine glands
- **D** Heart
- **E** Brain

Answers:

- **A** No
- **B** Bones are very often affected by fluorosis. Initially a damage of ligaments, tendons and joints capsules are seen, and at later stage osteoporosis of long bones, fusion of vertebrae, particularly in the spine, narrowing of spinal canal, and finally kyphosis are recorded.
- **C** Fluoride toxicity affects a number of endocrine glands such the thyroid and parathyroid glands. It directly or indirectly stimulates the parathyroid glands causing secondary hyperparathyroidism leading to bone loss, while it also induces structural changes and dysfunctions in the thyroid gland leading to hypothyroidism.
- **D** Heart rhythm is abnormal and raised with signs of myocardial damage in many patients with chronic fluorosis.
- **E** Fluoride has an adverse effect on the human brain, as there may be a risk of impaired development intelligence. Fluoride may also be the cause of demyelination and a decreased number of Purkinje cells, which are similar to the findings of Alzheimer's disease.

Comments: Fluoride does not directly cause neurotoxicity, but the neurological complaints of patients with fluorosis are rather attributed to mechanical compression of the spinal cord, due to the reduction of the anterio-posterior diameter of the spinal canal.

Case 23.7

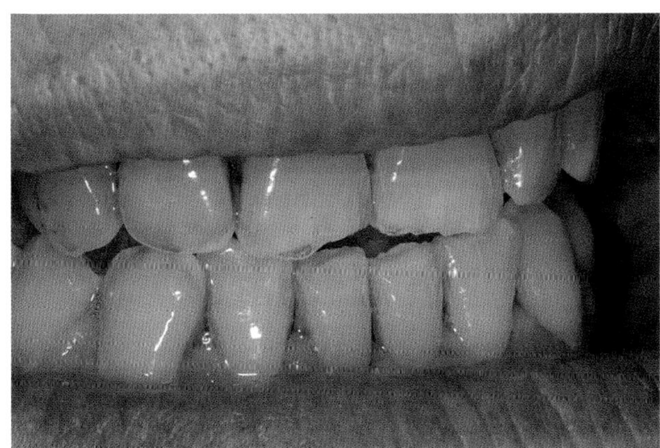

Figure 23.7

CO: A 38-year-old woman complained of pain from her anterior teeth when biting or chewing hard food.

HPC: The pain started three weeks ago when the patient tried to eat a very hard crispbread and damaged her upper central incisors.

PMH: Her medical history was clear of any serious diseases or drug use or hazardous habits, apart from grinding her teeth and chewing hard food and ice cubes.

OE: Examination revealed an extensive loss of the incisal edge of the upper central incisors with no evidence of dental caries, pulpal or periodontal pathology (Figure 23.7).These teeth responded well in the vitality test, and did not show any evidence of root fracture in the periapical X-rays. Visual examination with a magnified loupe with LED light revealed a loss of the central and distal lobe of the right central and mesial lobe of the left incisor, and to a lesser degree of the cutting edge of the lower incisors and canines.

Q1 What is the dental problem?

- **A** Cracks or chips off the incisors
- **B** Attrition
- **C** Erosion
- **D** Abrasion
- **E** Enamel hypoplasia

Answers:

- **A** The cracks or chips of the central incisors are the cause of her dental pain. This is the most frequent dental trauma, caused by chewing on hard foods, teeth grinding or following a facial injury, and is a natural aging event also.

B No
C No
D No
E No

Comments: Tooth wear is also found in other conditions like attrition, abrasion, erosion or even due to enamel hypoplasia, but differs and therefore these are excluded from the diagnosis. In attrition, the tooth loss is chronic and affects the occlusion surface of most teeth; abrasion is located along the cement–enamel junction, and erosions mainly occur on the lingual and palatal surface of anterior teeth, while enamel hypoplasia is usually located in a group of teeth and associated with white spots, pits or even grooves.

Q2 Which is/are the recommended treatment/s for this patient?
- **A** None
- **B** Resin bonding
- **C** Crowns
- **D** Root canal treatment
- **E** Extraction

Answers:
- **A** No
- **B** Resin bonding is helpful to fill the crack and missing tooth part, and to restore its appearance and function, and reduce sensitivity.
- **C** Crowns can be used in cases of resin filling failure.
- **D** No
- **E** No

Comments: Having in mind the mild symptomatology, clinicians should recommend simple ways to restore cracks like fillings or crowns, and not drastic treatments such as root canal treatments or even extraction.

Q3 Which is the type of crack found in this patient?
- **A** Crazy lines
- **B** Fractured cusps
- **C** Cracks extended into gingivae
- **D** Split teeth
- **E** Vertical root zones

Answers:
- **A** No
- **B** The cracks were restricted in the incisive lobes of the central incisors, and do not reach the pulp or gingivae.
- **C** No
- **D** No
- **E** No

Comments: The other types of teeth cracks were easily excluded as they were superficial within the enamel (crazy lines), or deep and split the crown, or moved from the occlusal surface to the gingivae and vice versa.

Case 23.8

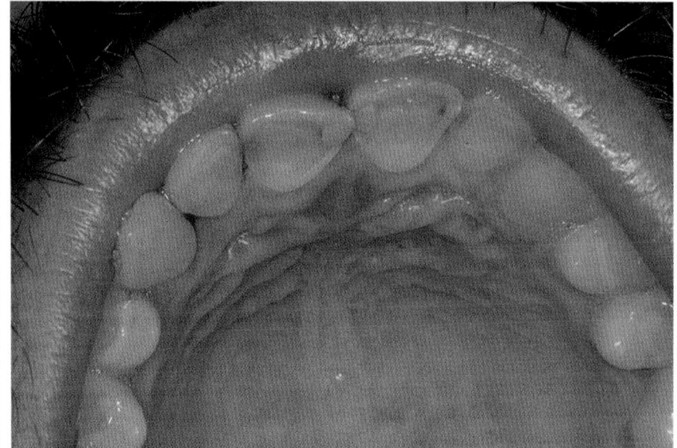

Figure 23.8

CO: A 26-year-old male was referred for an evaluation of his sensitivity from the anterior upper teeth.

HPC: This sensitivity appeared three months ago, but worsened gradually with eating acid fruits or drinks.

PMH: His medical history was clear of any serious diseases apart from bulimia nervosa, a chronic eating disorder, where by the patient used to overeat and compensated his problem with self-induced vomiting, laxatives and prolonged periods of starvation, but without any psychiatric therapy. Despite his problem, he used to work regularly as a cook. Smoking and alcohol was limited to social events, and diet cola was consumed on daily basis.

OE: A thin young man with a full dentition and good oral hygiene, and with no gingival or oral problems apart from loss of enamel of the palatal surface of the anterior teeth and occlusal surface of the molars (Figure 23.8). The affected teeth had normal size and color, but were sensitive to cold stimuli with no evidence of caries of fractures and did not show any periapical lesions on intra-oral X-rays. His lower molar teeth had been heavily restored with big resin fillings since the age of 15. No similar tooth problems were recorded among his close relatives.

Q1 What is his dental problem?

- **A** Palatal caries
- **B** Abrasion
- **C** Attrition
- **D** Dentinogenesis imperfecta
- **E** Erosions

Answers:

- **A** No
- **B** No
- **C** No
- **D** No
- **E** Dental erosions is the cause of his teeth sensitivity, characterized by an irreversible loss of the hard dental tissues (enamel, dentin, or both) to acid dissolution due to his regular surreptitious vomiting and not due to bacterial plaque. They occur initially on the occlusal surface of the mandibular first molars, followed by the palatal surfaces of the anterior maxillary teeth as seen in this patient.

Comments: Caries are the result of teeth tissue demineralization from the acids produced from cariogenic bacteria in patients with poor oral hygiene and a diet rich in carbohydrates, but this not the case as the patient had very good oral hygiene and a diet poor in carbohydrates. Caries appear with various symptomatology . location and color and depended on the hard dental tissue involvement. The normal size and color of the affected teeth rules out dentinogenesis imperfecta while the absence of total enamel wear-off from all crowns or from occlusal or cervical teeth surfaces (occlusal or cervical) excludes attrition or abrasion from the diagnosis respectively.

Q2 Which other factors participate in this dental condition?

- **A** Excessive tooth brushing
- **B** Acidic drink use
- **C** Occupation
- **D** Medication
- **E** Heritage

Answers:

- **A** Excessive tooth brushing is characteristic in patients with bulimla nervosa, and sometimes causes abrasion that accelerates tooth erosions.
- **B** Regular use of acidic drinks like diet cola accelerates the teeth dissolution due to their low pH.
- **C** Cooking requires tasting food during meal preparation many times, leading to constant tooth exposure to various acids produced by cariogenic bacteria during fragmentation of the foods tested.
- **D** No
- **E** No

Comments: The absence of similar dental lesions among patient's close relatives and any kind of medications uptake from this patients exclude these factors for the pathogenesis.

Q3 Which of the clinical characteristics below are indicative of an intrinsic rather than an extrinsic cause of this dental defect?

- **A** Dentition (primary or secondary)
- **B** Symptomatology
- **C** Location
- **D** Association with other teeth anomalies
- **E** Progression

Answers:

- **A** No
- **B** No
- **C** The location of the erosions seems to be dependent on the cause as the dental erosions are typically localized on the palatal surfaces of the upper anterior teeth in patients with vomiting or regurgitation (Intrinsic acids), while erosions on the buccal or facial surfaces may be a result of a high consumption of highly acidic foods and drinks (extrinsic acids).
- **D** No
- **E** No

Comments: Tooth erosions caused by acids (intrinsic or extrinsic) are found in both dentitions (primary and secondary) and are not related with the progression rate of dental demineralization or associated with other teeth anomalies or symptomatology.

Case 23.9

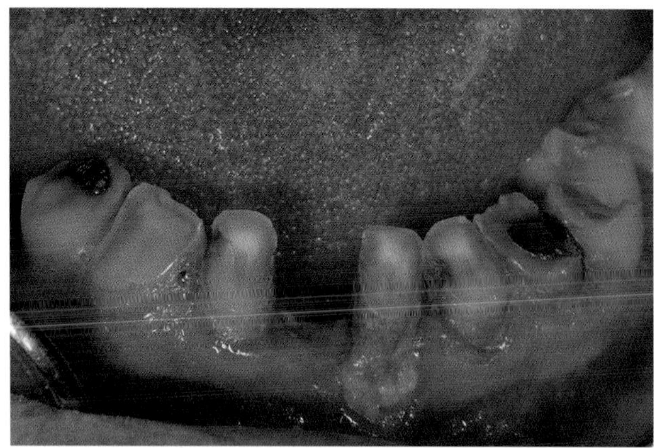

Figure 23.9

CO: A 48-year-old man was concerned about the esthetics of his teeth (mainly lower) over the last three years.

HPC: The problem with his teeth started four years ago when the patient had a car accident and began the habit of clenching and grinding his teeth. Gradually, part of his cusps were chipped off, leaving a smooth occlusal surface which was more prominent in his lower teeth.

PMH: Chronic bronchitis and hypertension were his main medical problems and controlled with drugs (steroids; antihypertensives). Among his hazardous habits were pipe smoking since the age of 30 and a diet rich in hard foods, rich in fat and carbohydrates, and drinking one to two bottles of beer with his meal daily.

OE: Oral examination revealed an extensive loss of tooth tissues from all his remaining teeth. The loss was more prominent at the occlusal-incisal surface of his lower teeth leaving dentin exposed closely to the pulp chambers, giving a yellowish color (Figure 23.9) and a mild sensitivity to cold stimuli. The fillings in the second lower left premolar and first right molar were loose and caries were found underneath. No other lesions were found inside his mouth, skin and other mucosae.

Q1 What is the main cause of his dental wear?

A Caries
B Abrasion
C Crown fracture
D Attrition
E Abfraction

Answers:

A No
B No
C No
D Dental attrition is a type of dental wear caused by tooth to tooth contact and can be a physiological process in old people, or a pathological wear due to clenching and grinding of the teeth (bruxism). In severe attrition the enamel can be completely worn away leaving dentin exposed.
E No

Comments: The location of dental wear at the occlusal surface excludes abrasion and abfraction, as both these lesions are seen in the cervical part of the affected teeth. Crown fracture is commonly seen after an accident, and is restricted in one or a group of teeth, but the lines of fracture are rather oblique and irregular and not horizontal as seen in this patient. Caries are found under ill-fitted fillings, and seen in only two teeth and are therefore not the main dental problem for this patient.

Q2 Which is/are the difference/s between attrition and crown fracture?

A Duration of dental wear
B Dentition affected
C Cause
D Symptomatology
E Association with other dental wear defects

Answers:

A In attrition the wear loss of dental tissues happens slowly, while in fracture it is abrupt and fast.
B Both dentitions are affected, but crown fractures rather than attrition occur more often in children whose number of facial injuries is high. Normal attrition increases with age, and pathological attrition is also seen in adults rather than children as bruxism is common there.
C The cause of broken crown is the extreme force applied suddenly on teeth during mastication of hard foods or foreign bodies, while attrition is the result of a constant pressure induced by teeth grinding.
D Acute pain comes together with crown fractures, while a dull ache or sensitivity to cold or sweet stimuli appear with deep attrition.
E No

Comments: Other dental defects like abrasion, abfraction or erosion weaken the strength of the teeth and therefore a strong pressure could cause enamel or dentin wear off, leaving attrition or crown fracture lesions.

Q3 Which of the syndromes below is the commonest cause of tooth attrition?
- **A** Emanuel syndrome
- **B** Down syndrome
- **C** Costello syndrome
- **D** Prader-Willi syndrome (PWS)
- **E** Rett syndrome

Answers:
- **A** No
- **B** Down syndrome accounts for approximately 8 per cent of all congenital anomalies in the European Union ,and shows severe wear loss of dental tissues (attrition and/or erosions) with a multifactorial etiology in which bruxism (mainly), gastric reflux and vomiting play an important role.
- **C** No
- **D** No
- **E** No

Comments: Attrition is a common finding in all the above syndromes but Emanuel, Costello, Prader-Willi and Rett syndromes are extremely rare. Emmanuel and Costello syndromes are characterized by multiple congenital anomalies with dental anomalies while Prader-Willi syndrome is associated with mental retardation and Rett syndrome with progressive neuropathies occurring mainly in females.

Case 23.10

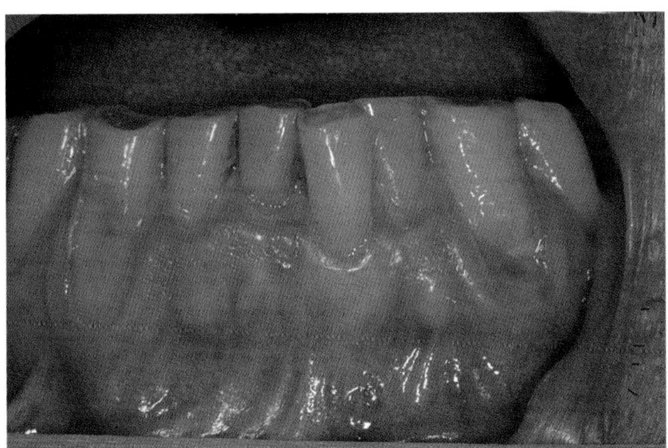

Figure 23.10

CO: A 42-year-old male was presented with tooth wear at the base of his lower canines over a period of 2 years.

HPC: His dental defects were first noticed by his dentist during an evaluation of pain coming from both temporomandibular joints (TMJ) during mastication two years ago, and had remained unchanged since then.

PMH: His medical history was unremarkable. Smoking or drinking habits were not reported apart from bruxism of his teeth during weight training and on stressful days.

OE: Oral examination revealed a wearing down of the buccal cervical surface of the lower canines (Figure 23.10) associated with sensitivity in cold stimuli. The defect was supragingival and had a smooth base, well-defined margins and a V-shape. Similarly, horizontal wear off the incisal-occlusal surface was noted and attributed to the patient's chronic bruxism and strong bite during weight-lifting. Caries or gingival problems were not found, as his oral hygiene was adequate. Extra-oral examination did not reveal any abnormalities.

Q1 What is/are his lower canine defects?
- **A** Attrition
- **B** Abrasion
- **C** Erosion
- **D** Abfraction
- **E** Cervical caries

Answers:
- **A** Attrition is the type of wear loss caused by tooth-to-tooth contact resulting in loss of tooth tissue, usually starting at the incisal surface of the lower anterior teeth and canines as seen in this patient.
- **B** No
- **C** No
- **D** Abfraction is the cervical non-caries tooth loss, observed primarily on the buccal surfaces and are typically wedge, V or C-shaped lesions with clearly well-defined margins. Its cause is multifactorial and includes tensile stress from malocclusion and masticatory forces; friction and biocorrosion due to chemical and biochemical factors, and electrochemical degradation.
- **E** No

Comments: Cervical caries are easily excluded as the cervical defect is soft with a dark brown or black color, with irregular shape features not seen in this patient. Buccal erosions are a common side-effect of acid foods or fruit overeating, and abrasion is often associated with hard brushing, but both defects are usually seen in a group and not in isolated teeth.

Q2 Which are other pathological causes of tooth wear?

- **A** Ankylosis
- **B** Attrition
- **C** Abrasion
- **D** Erosion
- **E** Resorption

Answers:

- **A** No
- **B** Attrition is defined as the loss of enamel, dentin, or restoration by tooth-to-tooth contact.
- **C** Abrasion is the loss of tooth substance from factors other than tooth contact such as hard tooth brushing, or overuse of whitening toothpastes.
- **D** Erosion is the loss of dental hard tissues (enamel; dentin) by chemical action (acids) not involving bacteria.
- **E** Resorption (internal or external) is the progressive loss of dentin and cementum by the action of osteoclasts, and cementoclasts due to inflammation induced by pulp necrosis, trauma, periodontal and orthodontic treatment, ectopic teeth, cysts, and tumors.

Comments: Ankylosis is the pathological fusion of a root via its components (cementum or dentin) to the adjacent alveolar bone.

Q3 Which is/are the differences between an abfraction and abrasion?

- **A** Location
- **B** Cause
- **C** Number of teeth involved
- **D** Shape of defect from tooth wear
- **E** Symptomatology

Answers:

- **A** Abfraction affects the cervical part of the teeth only, while abrasion affects any part.
- **B** Abrasion is provoked by excessive and strong tooth brushing, while abfraction is due to abnormal load from bruxism leading to flaking off the enamel from the neck of the tooth where the enamel is at its weakest.
- **C** Abfraction affects single teeth while abrasion affects a group of teeth.
- **D** Abrasion has a smooth round defect, while abfraction has a V-shaped defect.
- **E** No

Comments: The symptomatology of both abrasion and abfraction is dependent on the extent of dental tissue wear, and ranges from none to mild sensitivity in cold or hot stimuli, and in severe cases to constant pain due to irreversible pulpitis.

23.3 Part C: Diseases Affecting the Teeth's Components in Relation to the Adjacent Tissues

A number of Gram-positive and negative aerobic and anaerobic bacteria such as *Streptococcus* mutants, *Staphylococcus aureus* and *S. epidermidis*, *Porphyromonas*, *Actinomycoses*, *Bacteroides* and *Fusobacterium* species are responsible for a great number of dental and periodontal infections. Some of these infections affect only the teeth and/or adjacent periodontal tissues; some others spread diffusely in distant organs with a severe impact on the patient's life (See Figure 23.C).

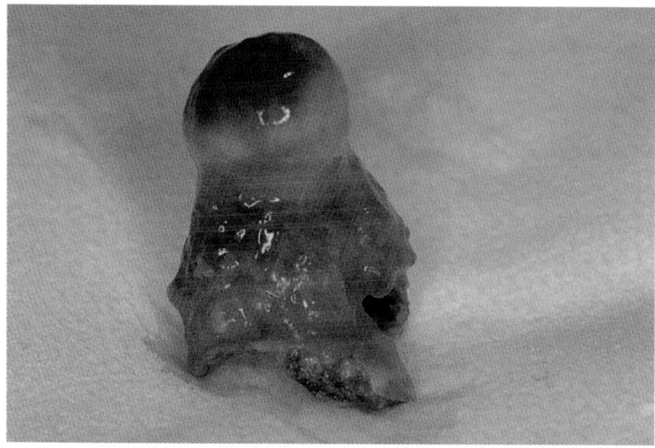

Figure 23.C Periapical cyst of a severed decayed upper molar.

Case 23.11

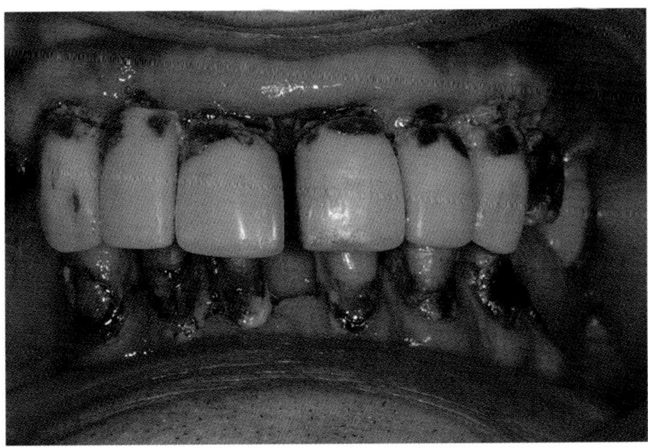

Figure 23.11

CO: A 42-year-old man presented with multiple dark brown-black discoloration of all his teeth.

HPC: His teeth had become discolored gradually over the last 10 years, causing occasional toothache and gingival swelling, relieved with painkillers and broad-spectrum antibiotics.

PMH: He suffered from severe depression which made him lose sleep and interest in living, and he became reluctant to clean his teeth and have a healthy diet.

OE: Multiple brown to dark discolored defects of all teeth surfaces of his lower teeth and at cervical areas of his upper teeth, as these had been restored with ill-fitting porcelain crowns (Figure 23.11). These defects were in some parts soft, and the enamel and underlying dentin were easily removed with excavators only. His oral hygiene was poor and food debris and plaque were stacked on his teeth; his gingivae were receded and inflamed. No other similar teeth or mucosae lesions were detected among his close relatives and residents of his own town.

Q1 What is the cause of this tooth defect?

A Rampant caries
B Amelogenesis imperfecta
C Tetracycline teeth staining
D Fluorosis
E Congenital erythropoietic porphyria

Answers:

A Rampant caries are characterized by numerous irreversible demineralization defects of the inorganic component and destruction of the organic component, leading to cavitations on multiple surfaces of many teeth. This demineralization is the effect of acids produced from cariogenic bacteria during fragmentation of carbohydrates. These caries may be seen in patients with neglected oral hygiene, a sugar-rich diet, drug-induced xerostomia, or after irradiation of head and neck tumors
B No
C No
D No
E No

Comments: The soft consistency of discolored defects easily excludes amelogenesis imperfecta; fluorosis and tetracycline staining while the absence of other skin and mucosae lesions together with the red internal stain of the teeth excludes congenital erythropoietic porphyria from diagnosis.

Q2 Which is/are the difference/s between caries and erosions?

A Dental tissues involved
B Primary cause
C Type of process
D Status of process
E Sodium fluoride action

Answers:

A No
B In caries the pathogenesis is based on an imbalance of mineral changes (Ca with Fl) while in erosions it is based on mineral loss.
C In erosions the causative acids are from foods, drugs, and vomiting, while caries originate from bacteria.
D At the initial stages of caries the defect is reversible, while in erosions it is always irreversible.
E Sodium fluoride use helps the prevention of caries, but has a minimal effects on erosions.

Comments: In both conditions (erosions and caries) the wear involves enamel and dentin.

Q3 Which is the most useful and practical caries index that can be used for this patient?

A DMFT index (mean number of decayed, missing, and filled permanent teeth)
B Caries severity index
C Caries susceptibility index

D DEF index (decayed, extracted, and filled teeth)
E Moller index

Answers:

A DMFT index is well-established as the key measure of caries experience in dental epidemiology. The DMF Index is applied to the permanent dentition and is expressed as the total number of teeth or surfaces that are decayed (D), missing (M), or filled (F) in an individual.
B No
C No
D No
E No

Comments: The other caries indices have been excluded as the DEF index is about the decayed, extracted and filled teeth in the primary dentition; the caries severity and susceptibility indices require clinical and radiographic records; and the Moller index is more complicated and requires a series of measurements by expert investigators.

Case 23.12

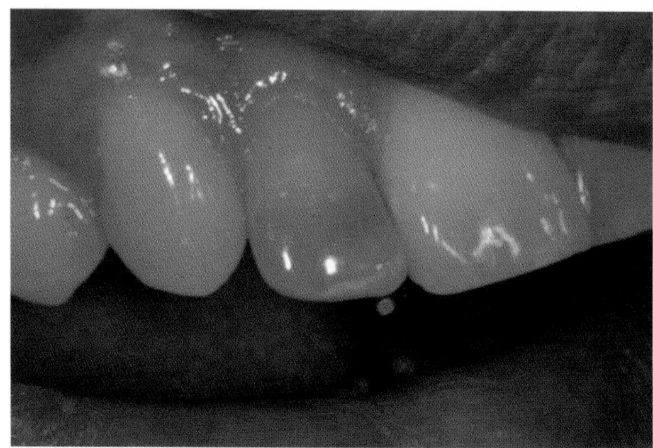

Figure 23.12

CO: A 32-year-old man complained of a discoloration of his upper right lateral incisor.

HPC: The discoloration was asymptomatic and discovered three months ago during his visit to his family dentist.

PMH: His medical and family history was clear from any serious diseases or drug use. Trauma to the upper anterior teeth was reported a year back after a fall from his bicycle. History of drugs taken by his mother during her pregnancy or by himself at age < 8 years was not reported.

OE: On examination an upper right lateral incisor was discolored (pinkish) in the upper middle of his crown in the mesio-distal direction (Figure 23.12). This tooth was non-tender to percussion and vital as it had a normal response to hot gutta percha and cold ice sticks. Caries or restorative material like amalgam was not found clinically and intra-oral X-rays revealed an oval radiolucency within the pulp chamber only with no evidence of any periapical lesions. No other discolored teeth were detected. As the tooth was asymptomatic, the patient refused to have root canal treatment.

Q1 What is the cause of this pinkish discoloration of his lateral incisor?

A Amalgam filling of its palatal pit
B Necrotic pulp
C Intracoronal resorption
D Tetracycline staining
E Hyperbilirubinemia

Answers:

A No
B No
C Intracoronal resorption is the cause, and characterized by a pinkish discoloration of a single tooth following an injury due to physical trauma with a radiological characteristic of a round to oval radiolucent enlargement of the pulp space. It is a relatively rare anomaly and affects males predominantly.
D No
E No

Comments: Clinical examination and history easily excludes other causes of internal teeth discoloration. The normal vitality tests and absence of amalgam filling in the discolored incisor easily excludes necrotic pulp and amalgam induced staining. As the discoloration is pink and restricted to one tooth only, together with a negative history of increased bilirubin blood levels or tetracycline use by his mother or by himself, hyperbilirubinemia and tetracycline staining were eliminated from the diagnosis.

Q2 Which of the diagnostic tools below are useful and practical for dentists to detect this condition?

- **A** Visual examination
- **B** Radiological examination
- **C** Vitality tests
- **D** Microscopy of involved tooth
- **E** Estimation of cytokine levels

Answers:

- **A** Visual examination reveals a pinkish discoloration of a single rather than a group of teeth (Mummery tooth).
- **B** Periapical X-rays and rarely cone beam computed tomography (CBCT) are used to detect an oval radiolucent lesion caused by the resorption within the pulp chamber.
- **C** No
- **D** No
- **E** No

Comments: Vitality tests are not useful, as the teeth with resorption (internal or external) do not always show necrotic pulp, while light and electron microscopy and estimation of IL-1α and β, IL-6, TNF-α, INF-γ, and TGF-β cytokines are expensive time-consuming techniques, requiring special skills.

Q3 Which of the characteristics below differentiate this condition from external resorption with periapical X-rays?

- **A** Location
- **B** Shape of lesion
- **C** Movement of the lesion as seen with different angled X-rays
- **D** Overproduction of root cementum
- **E** Adjacent bone structure

Answers:

- **A** In internal resorption the lesion is located within the pulp chamber while in the external it is outside.
- **B** In external resorption, the shape of the defect is irregular, while in internal it is oval and within the canal space.
- **C** In internal resorption, the radiolucent lesion "moves" within the canal while in external resorption it is outside the canal when X-rays are taken at different angles.
- **D** No
- **E** The adjacent alveolar bone has normal structure in internal but not in external resorption.

Comments: Hypercementosis is a characteristic lesion in response to local factors such as trauma or systemic factors such as gigantism, Paget's disease, or calcinosis, but it is not seen in resorption (internal or external).

Case 23.13

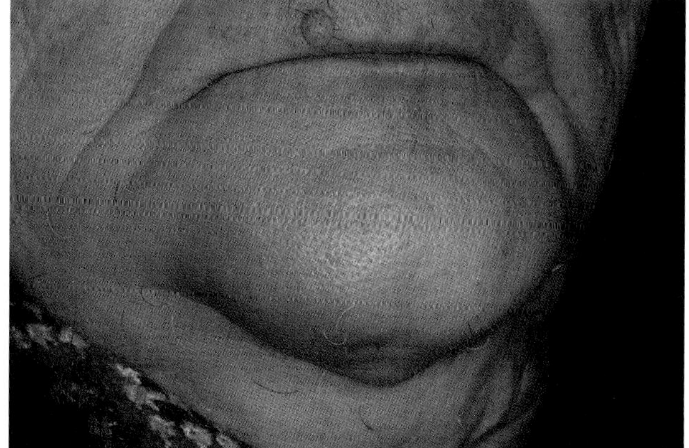

Figure 23.13a

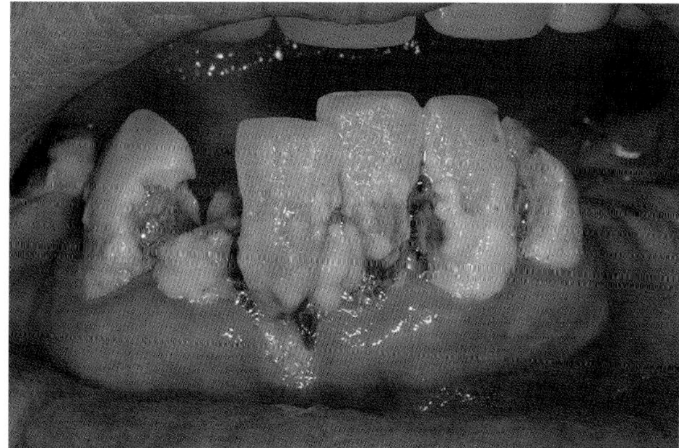

Figure 23.13b

CO: A 65-year-old woman presented with a diffuse painful swelling of her chin.

HPC: The swelling appeared suddenly four days ago, initially as a painful small lump which gradually became bigger and erythematous and extended into the whole chin and towards the neck below.

PMH: Diabetes type II, hypertension and mild depression were her main medical problems controlled with drugs like metformin, ACE inhibitors and cognitive behavioral therapy respectively. Her depression caused her to be reluctant to perform basic activities such as washing her face, or brushing her teeth.

CO: On examination, an erythematous swelling of her whole chin and below in her neck was found (Figure 23.13a). The swelling was soft and not fluctuant in palpation and was associated with general malaise, fever (38°C) and cervical lymphadenopathy. Intra-oral examination revealed a neglected mouth with excessive accumulation of calculus, plaque and food debris among her remaining lower teeth (Figure 23.13b). A swelling at the lower labial sulcus was detected and associated with decayed and necrotic lower incisors. The swelling caused her eating and esthetic problems, but her swallowing and breathing were unaffected.

Q1 What is the cause of her swelling?

- **A** Lymphedema
- **B** Sublingual sialadenitis
- **C** Allergic angiodema
- **D** Ludwig's angina
- **E** Dental abscess

Answers:

- **A** No
- **B** No
- **C** No
- **D** No
- **E** Dental abscess is the cause and characterized by a suppurative collection into soft tissues or alveolar bone due to a local infection from decayed teeth. This abscess may remain localized or extended into adjacent structures and develop a diffuse inflammation (cellulitis) as seen in this patient. This swelling is more likely seen in patients with poor oral hygiene, a weak immune system due to diabetes, Sjogren's syndrome, post-radiation/chemotherapy and use of immunosuppressive drugs.

Comments: Swellings like angioedema, lymphedema, sublingual sialadentitis and Lugwig's angina are excluded as in allergic angioedema there is an acute swelling with no general symptomatology (fever, nausea or general malaise and cervical lymphadenopathy); in lymphedema the swelling is chronic with no signs of infection and appears after a local trauma, serious surgery or radiotherapy. The severity and location of the swelling (in the chin and not in the floor of mouth or within sublingual glands) and lack of breathing problems ruled out Ludwig's angina and sublingual sialadentitis from the diagnosis.

Q2 Which of the X-rays below is the most useful diagnostic tool for this patient?

- **A** Periapical
- **B** Orhopantomograph
- **C** Lateral oblique of mandible (R/L)
- **D** Bite wing (R/L)
- **E** Occlusal

Answers:

- **A** Intra-oral periapical X-rays are the most useful to detect carious cavities, roots morphology, and anomalies and changes of the bone around the decayed teeth.
- **B** No
- **C** No
- **D** No
- **E** No

Comments: All the other X-rays may give some information about the cause of the patient's swelling, but have some serious handicaps. Intra-oral bite-wing (R or L) X-rays detect the presence or not of caries in the crowns of molars and bicuspids and not the anterior teeth, while the occlusal X-rays highlight the relation of developing teeth in the maxilla or mandible, and the presence of stone within the sublingual-submandibular glands. Extra-oral X-rays such as lateral oblique of the mandible examine the body and ramus of the mandible, and not the anterior teeth while panoramic X-rays create a gross image of all the teeth and jaws, but this image is not always clear, as it can be blocked with cervical vertebrae.

Q3 Which of the laboratory investigations below is/or are mandatory to be done in a patient with acute, severe chin swelling?

- **A** Blood tests
- **B** Ultrasonography
- **C** Culture of obtained pus
- **D** Periapical X-rays
- **E** CT scanning with intravenous contrast

Answers:

- **A** Blood tests are useful to detect leukocytosis, with neutrophils to be predominant.
- **B** No
- **C** Culture of the pus, taken with swabs or needle aspirate, is mandatory to isolate and confirm the pathogenic aerobic and anaerobic bacteria before starting the correct antibiotic therapy.
- **D** No
- **E** CT scanning with contrast is the most accurate method to determine the location, size, extent and relation of the swelling to the surrounding tissues and organs.

Comments: In severe facial swelling, the panoramic rather than periapical X-rays should be used, as the latter X-rays cover a small area of the jaw and adjacent teeth, and ultrasonography shows gross information only.

Case 23.14

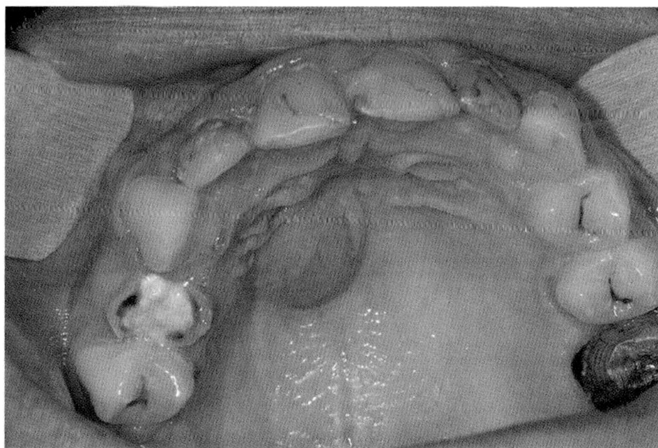

Figure 23.14

CO: A 32-year-old farmer presented with a painful swelling in his hard palate with one week's duration (Figure 23.14).

HPC: The swelling appeared two days after an episode of severe toothache from his upper right lateral incisor and gradually enlarged to reach its maximum size by the examination day.

PMH: His medical and family history was unremarkable, while his dental history revealed sporadic visits to his dentist for pain relief and fillings.

OE: A large round swelling in his hard palate close to the apex of the heavily restored with composite filling lateral right incisor. The swelling was well-fixed, fluctuant and sensitive on palpation and covered with normal mucosa, with a maximum size of 1.5 cm. Intra-oral periapical X-rays did not reveal any well-defined radiolucency apart from a widening of the periodontal ligament. Despite his poor oral hygiene and heavy restoration in the majority of his upper teeth, his gingivae did not show severe periodontal disease with deep pocket formation.

Q1 What is the cause of his palatal swelling?

A Periapical abscess
B Periodontal abscess
C Globulomaxillary cyst
D Palatal cyst
E Pleomorphic adenoma

Answers:

A Periapical abscess is the cause and characterized by a well-defined accumulation of pus at the apex of a necrotic pulp, with no bony involvement in the early stages. The abscess initially caused throbbing or constant pain which settled down as soon the pus was drained into the oral mucosa by perforating the adjacent alveolar bone.
B No
C No
D No
E No

Comments: The palatal location of the patient's swelling, close to the apex of the right lateral incisor, excludes palatal and globulomaxillary cysts from the diagnosis. The swelling in the palatal cyst is found along the incisive canal, while in globulomaxillary teeth, buccally between the lateral incisor and the canine but in both cysts, the adjacent teeth are vital. The lack of periodontal pockets of the related upper anterior teeth and the soft, fluctuant on palpation lesion with a short duration, excluded periodontal cysts and pleomorphic adenoma from diagnosis.

Q2 Which of the factors below determine the intra-oral location of this swelling?

A Alveolar bone strength
B Periodontal status
C Teeth involved
D Size of lesion
E Duration of lesion

Answers:

A The strength of the alveolar bone is the most important factor for the way a dental infection is spread. The alveolar bone is weakest on the buccal site of the maxilla, though in the mandible is the lingual region distal to the molars and the buccal side of the incisors and the canine teeth.
B No
C The roots of the lateral incisors and the palatal roots of 1st and 2nd upper molars with necrotic pulp drain easily into the palatal mucosa as their palatal alveolar bone is very thin.
D No
E No

Comments: The size and duration of the lesion seem to play a role in the destruction of tissues close to the apex of the necrotic tooth, and not in the buccal or palatal spread of the infection. Deep pockets facilitate the spread of dental infection locally in any direction, but along planes of least resistance.

Q3 Which is/are the difference/s between a periapical and periodontal abscess?
- **A** Teeth vitality status
- **B** Pocket formation
- **C** Symptomatology
- **D** Location of abscess
- **E** Radiological findings

Answers:
- **A** In periapical abscess the involved teeth are non-vital, while in periodontal abscess they are vital.
- **B** Deep pockets were measured in periodontal and not in periapical abscess.
- **C** No
- **D** In periapical abscess the swelling is located closely to the apex of a necrotic tooth, while in periodontal it is higher and lateral to a vital tooth.
- **E** In periodontal abscess, the bone destruction, as seen in intra-oral X-ray, is located laterally, while in chronic periapical abscess apical to the responsible tooth,

Comments: Pain, general malaise, fever and lymphadenitis together with eating difficulties are commonly recorded in both abscesses.

Case 23.15

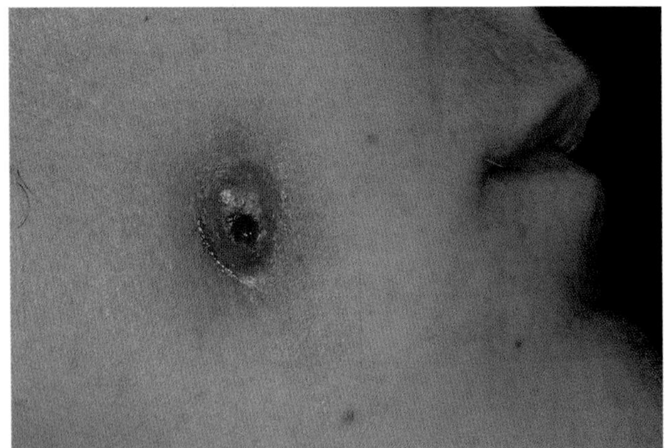

Figure 23.15a

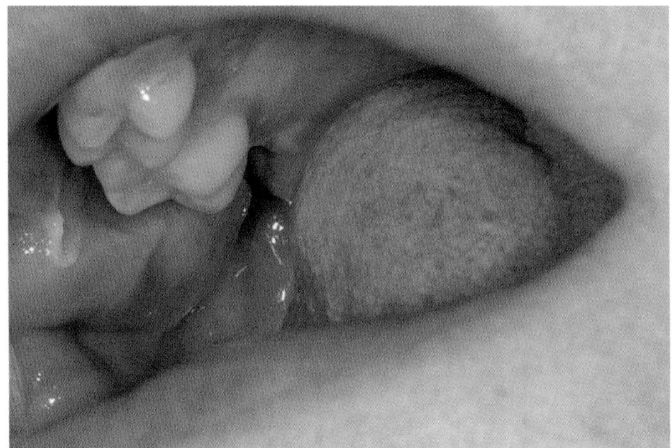

Figure 23.15b

CO: A 22-year-old woman came with an ulcerated lesion in her right cheek, present over the last two months.

HPC: The lesion appeared as a small nodule in her right check three weeks after extraction of her partially erupted upper right third molar. Her wisdom tooth was extracted under local anesthesia without antibiotic cover and within the next week pain and buccal swelling appeared and partially controlled with penicillin.

PMH: Her medical history was unremarkable, but her recent dental history referred to a difficult extraction of her upper 3rd molar due to many episodes of pericoronitis. Her smoking habits were limited to five cigarettes per day and her drinking to one glass of wine on occasions.

OE: Extra-oral examination revealed a firm painful nodule, of 1 cm in diameter, centrally ulcerated, on erythematous skin with minimal swelling of her right cheek (Figure 23.15a). Gentle pressure on the surrounding tissues elicited a scanty purulent-hemorrhagic discharge from the center of the nodule, where a cord-like palpable tract extending from the cutaneous lesion to the oral cavity inside was detected. Ipsilateral facial and cervical lymph nodes were palpable. Intra-oral examination revealed a swelling of the right buccal mucosa along the occlusal surface, ending in the area of extracted molar where healing was incomplete and halitosis was noticed (Figure 23.15b). Panoramic X-rays showed a diffuse radiolucency at the area of the extracted wisdom tooth, while biopsy of the lesion confirmed the presence of granulation tissue with a plethora of bacteria.

Q1 What is this cheek lesion?
- **A** Furuncle
- **B** Epidermal cyst
- **C** Basal cell carcinoma

D Oral cutaneous fistula
E Scrofula

Answers:

A No
B No
C No
D Oral cutaneous fistula is the lesion and characterized by a pathologic communication between the cutaneous surface of the face and the oral cavity, as sequelae to bacterial invasion into the alveolar bone after the extraction. This invasion causes local inflammation, bone resorption and drainage into the facial skin following the path of least resistance.
E No

Comments: Scrofula is characterized by mycobacterial infection of the lymph nodes of the neck and therefore is excluded. The absence of neoplastic cells, cystic lining cavity or granulomas reinforces the idea that the lesion could not be a basal cell carcinoma, epidermal cyst or tuberculous ulcer, while the presence of a cord-like palpable tract extending from the cutaneous lesion to the oral cavity indicates that the lesion is not a superficial skin infection like a furuncle.

Q2 Which of the factors below is/are related with the pathogenesis of oral cutaneous fistulas?

A Trauma
B Medication induced osteonecrosis
C Periapical actinomycosis
D Metabolic bone diseases
E Oral carcinomas invading the skin

Answers:

A Traumatic fistulas may be the result of injury or surgical repair. Head and neck reconstructive surgery, tumor removals, fracture repair, and implantation are often accompanied with fistula formations as a combination of a dental infection with host inflammatory responses.
B Osteonecrosis induced by drugs like biphosphonates and other anti-resorptive medications is characterized by necrotic bone and numerous intra- and extra-oral fistulae. These medications are widely used in the treatment of lytic bone diseases like tumor metastases, malignant hypercalcemia, multiple myeloma and osteoporosis.
C Periapical actinomycosis is one of the most common infections in the maxillofacial region that results in an orocutaneous fistula, from which a hemorrhagic exudates, with yellow granules rich in actinomycetes.
D Metabolic bone diseases such as osteitis deformans ("Paget disease"), or osteopetrosis are often associated with intra-oral and oral-cutaneous fistulae.
E Oral carcinomas invading the facial skin via numerous fistulas are very rare but aggressive tumors, and by the time of their diagnosis metastasis via lymphatic drainage has most likely taken place.

Q3 Which part of the head has the highest frequency of odontogenic oral-cutaneous fistulae formation?

A Mandible (body, mentum and angle)
B Buccal-cheek
C Nasolabial fold
D Submandibular region
E Infra-orbital region

Answers:

A The majority of oral-cutaneous fistulae originate from the teeth and adjacent mandible (especially from the body and less from the mentum or the angle of the jaw).
B No
C No
D No
E No

Comments: In decreasing order of occurrence, after the fistulae from the mandible, is the buccal-cheek fistula from infection of the maxillae from the 1st and 2nd premolars and from the 1st to 3rd molar; followed by nasolabial fistulae from incisors and canines, and last by infra-orbital fistula from the maxillary canines.

24

Tongue

The tongue is the most important muscular organ of the oral cavity as it contributes in the basic human functions of taste, chewing, swallowing, and speaking. The tongue has been considered to be the site of manifestations of several systemic diseases or diseases arisen de novo from the epithelium or the underlying connective tissues and blood vessels, but less from the muscles. Tongue lesions are manifestations of a range of disorders like developmental, infectious, nutritional deficiencies, injuries, autoimmune and inflammatory, idiopathic and premalignant and malignant tumors. Most tongue lesions are resolved shortly and spontaneously or by simple treatments, while others require special medical center treatment (See Figure 24.0a and b).

Table 24 lists the most common and important tongue lesions.

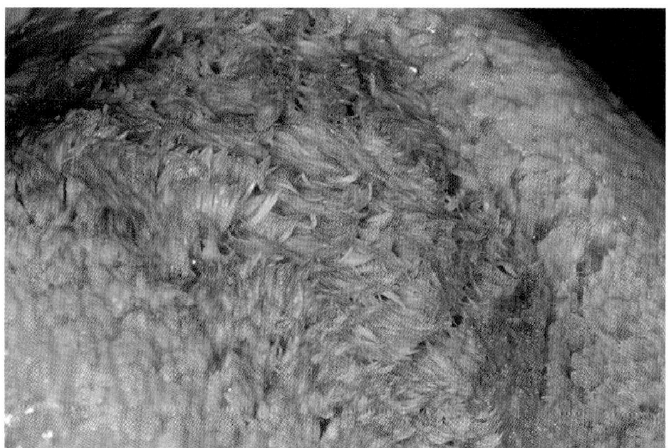

Figure 24.0a Hairy tongue (close-up photo).

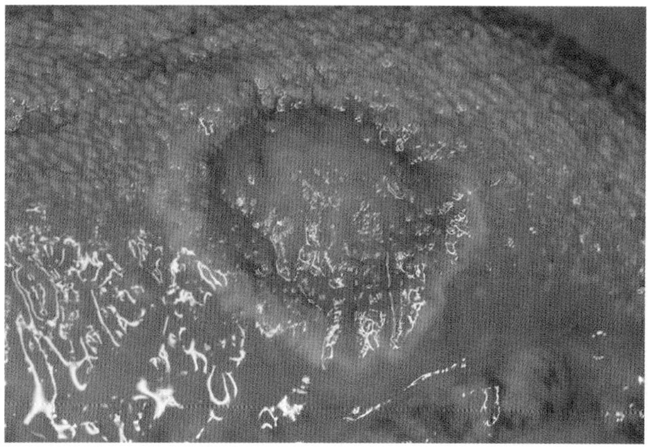

Figure 24.0b Geographic tongue (close-up photo).

Clinical Guide to Oral Diseases, First Edition. Dimitris Malamos and Crispian Scully.

Companion website: www.wiley.com/go/malamos/clinical_guide

Table 24 Common and important lesions of the tongue.

- Congenital
  - Anatomical
    - Bifid tongue
    - Tongue tie
  - Developmental
    - Fissured tongue
    - Scalloped tongue
    - Geographic tongue
  - Vascular
    - Hemangiomas
    - Lymphangiomas
- Acquired
  - Traumatic
    - Mechanical
    - Burns
  - Reactive
    - Friction keratosis
  - Infections
    - Bacterial
      - Soft tissue abscess
      - Syphilis
      - Tuberculosis
- Viral
      - Herpes
      - HIV atypical ulcerations/swellings
      - Hairy leukoplakia
- Fungal
      - Candidosis (acute/chronic)
      - Median rhomboid glossitis
      - Deep fungal infections

Table 24 (Continued)

  - Inflammatory
    - Aphthae
    - Giant cell arteritis
    - Lichen planus
  - Autoimmune
    - Bullous disorders
    - Amyloidosis
  - Allergic
    - Angioedema
    - Stomatitis induced by cinnamon
  - Neoplasma
    - Benign
      - Granular cell tumor
      - Fibromas
      - Lipomas
      - Neurofibromas
      - Schwannoma
    - Premalignant
      - Leukoplakia
      - Erythroplakia
    - Malignant
      - Oral carcinomas
      - Sarcomas
      - Lymphomas
      - Melanomas
  - Vitamin deficiencies
    - Atrophic glossitis
      - Iron deficiency
      - B12 deficiency
      - B2 deficiency

Case 24.1

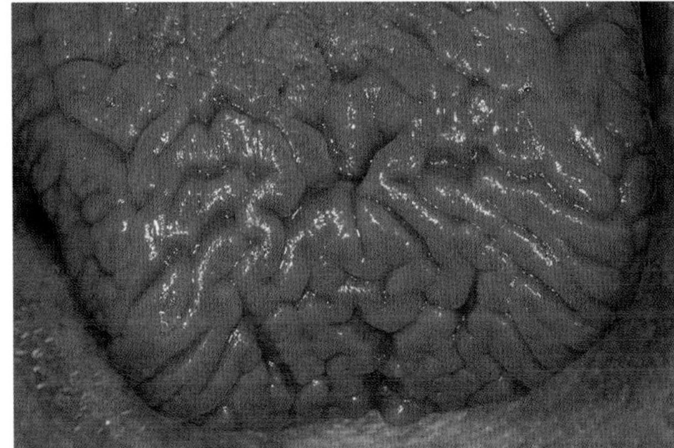

Figure 24.1

CO: A 48-year-old man presented complaining about a burning sensation on his tongue.

HPC: The burning sensation started many years ago when the patient burned his tongue with some extremely hot coffee. Throughout the years, the burning sensation had been always irritated by extremely hot and spicy foods or liquids and worsened with smoking.

PMH: His medical history revealed a mild hypertension and allergy to penicillin. No drugs were taken while the patient tried to control his blood pressure with diet and daily physical exercise.

OE: The oral examination did not reveal any oral lesions apart from a scrotal tongue. The dorsum of tongue had numerous grooves at various directions from the middle to the lateral margins (Figure 24.1) that became more prominent when the patient pushed his tongue against his anterior lower teeth. The tongue was covered with normal papillae and did not show any evidence of a local infection, despite some food debris found in a few grooves. On the other hand, the extra-oral examination did not reveal any abnormalities, cervical lymphadenopathy or facial nerve paralysis.

Q1 What is the cause of his burning sensation?
- **A** Atrophic glossitis
- **B** Geographic glossitis
- **C** Smoking-induced
- **D** Plicated tongue
- **E** Melkersson–Rosenthal syndrome

Answers:
- **A** No
- **B** No
- **C** No
- **D** Fissured, scrotal or plicated tongue is a benign developmental tongue lesion characterized by numerous fissures at various patterns. The grooves have variable depth and are seen over the dorsum and lateral margins of the tongue while they are sometimes associated with well-depapillated areas surrounded with white lines (geographic tongue).
- **E** No

Comments: Despite the fact that fissure tongue is part of the Melkersson-Rosenthal syndrome, the lack of facial paralysis (Bell's palsy) in this patient excludes this syndrome from the diagnosis. Smoking is not the main cause as the sensation preceded this habit. The presence of normal papillae also excludes other tongue lesions with lingual papillae atrophy, well-defined or diffused, as seen in geographic and atrophic glossitis respectively.

Q2 Which other oral lesions have fissures among their clinical manifestations?
- **A** Major aphthae
- **B** Angular cheilitis
- **C** Actinic cheilitis
- **D** Pemphigus
- **E** Median split of lip

Answers:
- **A** No
- **B** Angular cheilitis is an infection of one or both corners of the mouth by fungi (*Candida albicans*) or/and bacteria (*Staphylococcus aureus*; beta-hemolytic streptococci) and is characterized by an erythema, edema, fissures, ulcerations covered with yellowish crusts.
- **C** Actinic cheilitis is a reaction of the vermilion border of the lips (mainly of the lower) to chronic exposure to solar radiation, and appearing with dryness, hyperpigmentation, scaling, fissures, superficial ulcerations, and white plaques.
- **D** No
- **E** Median split of lip is characterized by a deep groove in the middle of the upper, lower or both lips, associated with pain and spontaneous bleeding.

Comments: Major aphthae and pemphigus which are characterized by large irregular shaped ulcerations, and not by narrow, long linear mucosal splits, as they are seen in oral fissures.

Q3 Which other condition/s apart from the Melkersson-Rosenthal syndrome is/are associated with this tongue lesion?
- **A** Discoid lupus erythematosus
- **B** Median rhomboid glossitis
- **C** Gardner syndrome
- **D** Osler-Weber-Rendu syndrome
- **E** Scleroderma

Answers:
- **A** No
- **B** In patients with fissured tongue, median rhomboid glossitis lesions are commonly seen.
- **C** No
- **D** No
- **E** No

Comments: Fissured tongue is a common condition with prevalence occurring in up to 30 per cent of the general population, and has been therefore noticed in patients with skin diseases like scleroderma and lupus erythematosus, as well as syndromes like Gardner and Osler-Weber-Rendu at such a frequency that no relationship could be confirmed.

Case 24.2

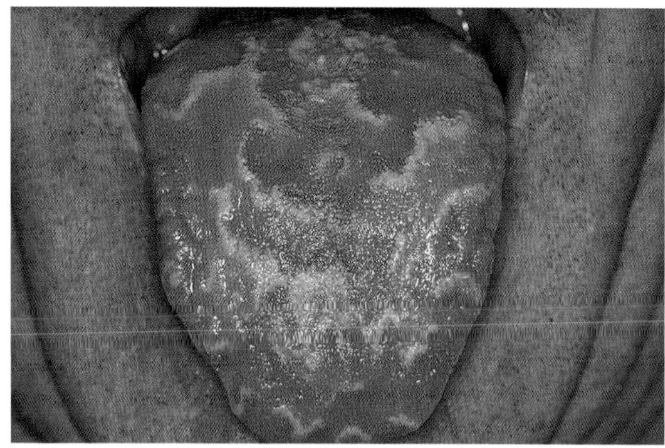

Figure 24.2

CO: A 29-year-old man presented for an evaluation of peculiar lesions on his tongue.

HPC: His tongue lesions were first noticed by his dentist at the age of 15 and remained stable since then through periods of intensification and amelioration. They were mostly asymptomatic, but a burning sensation appeared with spicy foods or strong drinks and smoking.

PMH: Serious diseases like anemias, skin diseases, drug use or allergies were not recorded. Smoking or drinking habits were minimal and only restricted to social events.

OE: The oral examination revealed irregular white patches with central erythematous areas, intermingled with normal oral mucosae. The lesions had an abnormal size and shape, and covered the whole dorsum, while they were occasionally extended to the lateral margins of the tongue, giving a map-like appearance with the patches resembling the islands or waves of a sea (Figure 24.2). The lesions were mostly asymptomatic on probing and according to the patient, they tend to change in shape and size and migrate to other areas even within hours or days. No other similar lesions were found inside his mouth, other mucosae and skin or in his close relatives.

Q1 What are these tongue lesions?

- **A** Lichen planus
- **B** Erythematous candidiasis
- **C** Speckled leukoplakia
- **D** Atrophic glossitis
- **E** Geographic tongue

Answers:

- **A** No
- **B** No
- **C** No
- **D** No
- **E** Geographic tongue is the cause. It is a common, harmless, inflammatory tongue lesion characterized by areas of smooth, red depapillation surrounded by serpiginous white or yellow white lines which migrate spontaneously over time.

Comments: The geographic tongue is easily distinguishable from other similar clinical lesions like atrophic glossitis and erythematous candidiasis by the presence of white lesions in the periphery and its migratory character, as well as the long and early onset of the lesions. Lichen planus and speckled leukoplakia are distinguished from geographic tongue by the changeable shape of the lesions, and the presence of remissions and relapses in a generally short period.

Q2 Which of the histological characteristics below are commonly seen in both psoriasis and this condition?

- **A** Orthokeratosis
- **B** Acanthosis
- **C** Loss of basal cell polarity
- **D** Mixture of neutrophils with chronic inflammatory cells
- **E** Degeneration of elastic fibers in submucosa

Answers:

- **A** No
- **B** Acanthosis is a common characteristic of both conditions.
- **C** No
- **D** Neutrophils together with lymphocytes are scattered in numbers in the corium in both conditions. Some of these neutrophils enter the superficial layers and form microabscesses.
- **E** No

Comments: The tongue mucosa belongs to the moving part of the oral mucosa and is therefore covered with parakeratin and not with orthokeratin. Moreover, the loss of the basal cell polarity is characteristically seen in the majority of dysplastic oral lesions and in some lichen planus, but not in geographic tongue. While the degeneration of elastic fibers in the submucosa is a characteristic finding in solar-induced dermatosis and actinic cheilitis.

Q3 In histological sections, the white margins of the lesions represent:

- **A** Accumulation of *Candida* species

B Loss of filiform papillae
C Restriction of small vessels
D Subepithelial infiltrates of eosinophils
E Microepithelial abscesses

Answers:

A No
B No
C No
D No
E The white margins of geographic tongue are associated with the accumulation of inflammatory cells in the submucosa, as well as the migration and accumulation of neutrophils within the superficial epithelial layers of the tongue where they create a number of superficial microabscesses.

Comments: The accumulation of *Candida* and other infections is commonly seen in geographic tongue lesions, but this is rather a secondary event as it does not participate in its pathogenesis. The loss of the filiform papillae are related to the erythematous parts of geographic lesions where vascular ectasia is present while the accumulation of neutrophils, and not eosinophils, are associated with their white borders.

Case 24.3

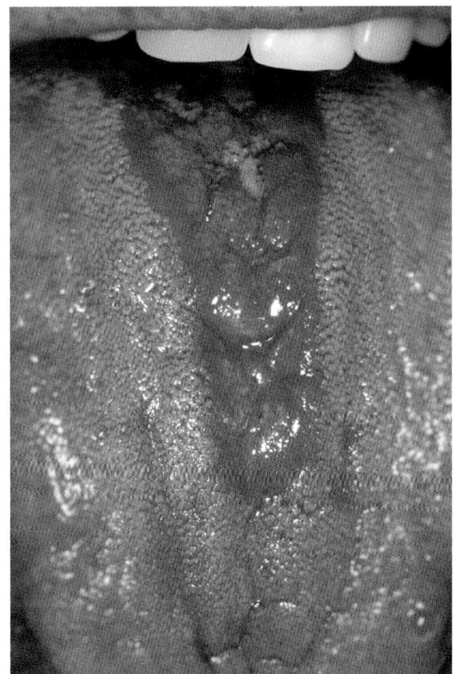

Figure 24.3

CO: A 32-year-old woman presented with a burning sensation of her tongue.

HPC: The burning sensation had been present over the last eight months after an abortion at six weeks of pregnancy. The burning sensation affected the whole tongue initially, but was eventually restricted to the middle and posterior part over the last couple months.

PMH: Her medical history was clear from any serious diseases apart from sideropenic anemia and chronic eczema, that were worse over last few months, due to her heavy blood loss during menstruation, and stress provoked by her recent abortion. Smoking and drinking habits were limited to two to five cigarettes on stressful days and one to two glasses of wine on social occasions only.

OE: A red, rhomboid, depapillated lesion on the dorsum of the tongue from the geustic lambda towards the anterior part. The lesion had a maximum size of 3.5 cm in longest diameter, it was soft, red, shiny with a lobulated surface (Figure 24.3) and did not bleed or bleach on manipulation. A few narrow grooves were occasionally seen while the rest of her tongue had a normal color and was covered with normal papillae. The lesion did not interfere with tongue movements, but caused her mild discomfort, a burning sensation, and fear of cancer. No other similar lesions were found in the rest of her mouth, skin, and other mucosae.

Q1 What is the possible diagnosis?

A Atrophic glossitis due to anemia
B Erythroplakia
C Oral carcinoma
D Hemangioma
E Median rhomboid glossitis

Answers:

A No
B No

C No
D No
E Median rhomboid glossitis is the correct diagnosis. It is a common, inflammatory lesion of the dorsum of the tongue with an unknown etiology. From a clinical point of view, it appears as a well-demarcated red, depapillated, rhomboid-shaped lesion, located in the middle of the tongue close to the geustic lambda with a maximum diameter of 1.5–2 cm. The case of median rhomboid glossitis has a smooth surface which occasionally becomes lobulated or more rarely, resembles a malignancy. More often than not, a "kissing lesion" on the palate opposite the tongue lesion is found, and may be associated with immunodeficiencies.

Comments: Depapillated tongue is also seen in atrophic glossitis due to iron deficiency, but this is not the case as this depapillation covers the whole tongue and is associated with other oral lesions like aphthous like ulcerations or angular cheilitis that are not seen in this patient. The lack of bleaching with pressure excludes vascular lesions like hemangioma from the diagnosis. Knowing that the lesion is superficial, soft and not interfering with tongue movements, yet associated with a burning sensation and not severe symptomatology, like pain or cervical lymphadenopathy, excludes erythroplasia or carcinoma from this woman's diagnosis.

Q2 The diagnosis of this lesion is mainly based on:
A History
B Clinical characteristics
C Symptomatology
D Culture
E Biopsy

Answers:
A No
B The clinical characteristics such as the location in the middle of the tongue, the lack of filiform papillae, leaving an atrophic, shiny, erythematous, well-defined lesion, along with the absence of other oral lesions allow clinicians to diagnose this lesion.
C No
D No
E No

Comments: The diagnosis could not be based only on the patient's history of any serious diseases or drug use that affect the patient's immune system and allow the growth of *Candida albicans* that this fungus can be isolated in cultures or biopsies. Biopsies are rarely used and only when the lesion resembles a malignancy, or does not respond to previous antifungal treatment.

Q3 What are the predisposing factors for this condition?
A Gender
B Vitamin B deficiency
C Immune deficiencies
D Chronic use of steroid inhalers
E Heavy drinking

Answers:
A No
B No
C Immunodeficiencies, seen in patients with an HIV infection or after a transplantation, allow the growth of fungi especially of *Candida albicans* in the median rhomboid glossitis and its opponent kissing lesion in the palate to such a degree that these lesions might be considered as a type of atrophic chronic candidiasis.
D The chronic use of steroid inhalers are attributed to the increased growth of *Candida albicans* via the anti-inflammatory and immunosuppressive effect of steroids, leading to a low salivary flow rate and higher salivary glucose concentration.
E Heavy drinkers are often dehydrated due to reduced water consumption and increased fluid loss from their kidneys, leading to xerostomia; a condition that allows the growth of pathogenic bacteria and fungi within the oral mucosa.

Comments: Median rhomboid glossitis is seen in patients regardless of their age, sex, and B12 status in the blood. B12 deficiency causes diffused erythematous depapillated areas in the anterior and lateral margins of the tongue, and not restricted closely to the sulcus terminalis where median rhomboid glossitis is located.

Case 24.4

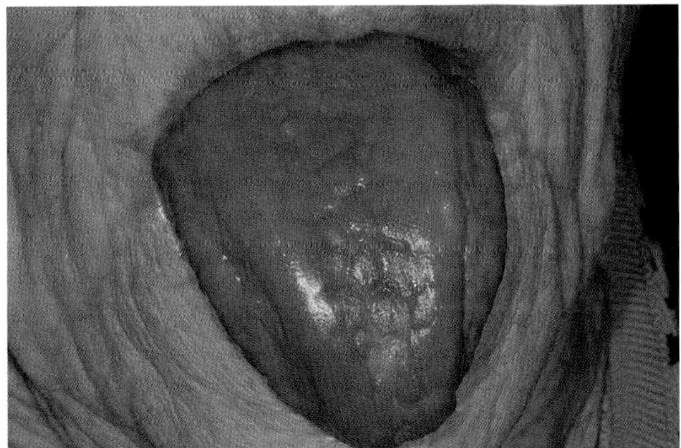

Figure 24.4

CO: A 72-year-old woman presented with an erythematous, depapillated, tongue.

HPC: The problem started one year ago when the patient had a minor heart attack and changed her diet by avoiding any meat products since then.

PMH: Hypercholesterolenemia and hypertension for many years had led to a heart attack and were treated with statins, angiotensin converting enzyme (ACE) inhibitors, diuretics, anti-coagulants after her angioplasty, diet, and smoking cessation.

OE: The examination revealed an erythematous, smooth, shiny tongue which was caused by the loss of lingual papillae. The tongue had lost its normal pinkish color, had a central groove and smaller fissures branching perpendicular and towards its lateral borders (Figure 24.4). The tongue was dry and sensitive to touch, and associated with a mild infection of the patient's commissures. No other lesions were found. Blood tests were undertaken and shown an increased serum l cholesterol and reduced B12 levels.

Q1 What is the main problem with the patient's tongue?

A Erythematous candidiasis
B Allergic reaction to acrylic resin of her dentures
C Drug side effects
D Burning mouth syndrome
E Atrophic glossitis

Answers:

A No
B No
C No
D No
E Atrophic glossitis or Hunter's glossitis was her main problem, as it was characterized by a smooth depapillated tongue associated with a burning sensation or pain and erythema. It was induced by the patient's own diet which was poor in meat and animal products, causing a gradual loss of minerals and vitamins. The absence of skin or oral pallor in combination with the red tongue leads to the conclusion that a B12 rather than an iron deficiency is responsible for the patient's atrophic glossitis and confirmed by the low B12 found in blood tests.

Comments: Burning sensation is a common finding in other conditions such as oral allergies, drugs side-effects or infections, but it is differentiated. For the allergic reaction to dentures, the erythema should be mainly restricted to the exposure of the alveolar mucosae and less in the adjacent buccal mucosae and tongue; in drug reactions the erythema should be associated with tongue swelling or ulcerations rather than depapillation, and finally, in infections like erythematous candidosis, other manifestations of immunodeficiency should be recorded.

Q2 Which are the common causes of a total tongue depapillation?

A Anemias
B Burns
C Radiotherapy
D Habits
E Aging

Answers:

A Anemias due to deficiencies of iron or B vitamins are the most common causes of atrophic glossitis.
B No
C The use of radiotherapy in the treatment of head and neck cancers causes the destruction of lingual papillae by altering their rhythm of apoptosis and renewal.

D No
E No

Comments: Aging does affect the number of taste buds but this can not be the cause of total loss of lingual papillae in both humans and animals, while burns (thermal or chemical) and habits such as smoking, spicy food eating or clenching the tongue against adjacent teeth may cause a temporal loss of lingual papillae that is solely restricted to the applied stimuli area.

Q3 What are the other forms of glossitis apart from the atrophic ones?

A Median rhomboid
B Syphilitic
C Benign migratory
D Geometric
E Transient papillitis

Answers:

A Median rhomboid glossitis is characterized by a rhomboid depapillated lesion in the middle of the tongue.
B Syphilitic glossitis is a rare complication of untreated syphilis nowadays, and is a predisposing factor for tongue oral cancer development.
C Benign migratory glossitis is characterized by transient depapillated areas surrounded with white lines of irregular shape and size on the dorsum and lateral borders of the tongue.
D Geometric glossitis is a kind of painful ulcerated, fissured glossitis due to herpes virus infections in immunocompromised patients.
E Transient papillitis is characterized by enlarged painful lingual papillae due to chronic trauma, local irritation from spicy foods, chewing-gum or candy, and is resolved within three to four days after the removal of the causative irritant.

Case 24.5

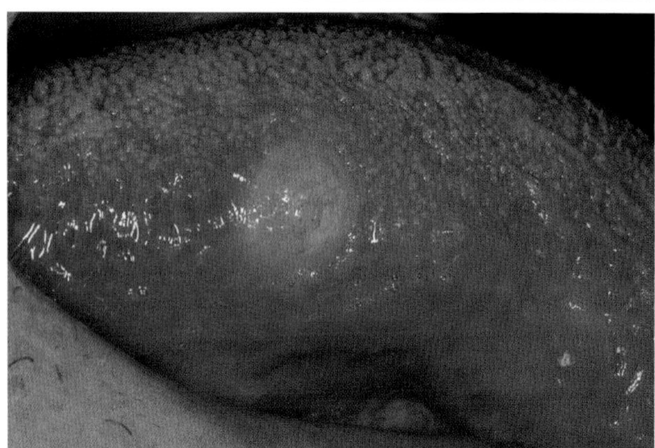

Figure 24.5

CO: A 42-year-old woman presented for an evaluation of a lump on the right lateral margin of her tongue that has been present over the last year.

HPC: The swelling was initially small but got slowly bigger reaching its present size of 1.5 × 1.0 cm. As for her medical record, previous trauma, local thermal or chemical irritation were not linked with the lesion development, while any past family history was not contributory.

OE: A well-circumscribed swelling of approximately 1.5 cm, in the lateral right margin of the tongue, opposite the first molar was found. The lesion was pinkish pale white in color, firm, adherent to the underlying structures, with a rough surface but covered with normal lingual papillae (Figure 24.5). Any case of regional lymphadenopathy was absent while no other similar lesions were found in her skin or other mucosae.

Q1 What is this lesion?

A Traumatic fibroma
B Xanthoma
C Oral carcinoma
D Schwannoma
E Granular cell tumor

Answers:

A No
B No
C No
D No
E Granular cell tumor is the correct answer. This tumor can appear everywhere in the body, but has a high predilection in the tongue (>70%) and especially of women rather than men. This lesion is presented as an asymptomatic, solitary, nodule on the anterior and sometimes on lateral margins of the tongue having a yellowish or pinkish color. This tumor is usually benign, of neural origin and from a histological point of view, it is composed of large polygonal, plump cells with eosinophilic granular cytoplasm within a fibrovascular corium

where the overlying epithelium shows a pseudoepithelial hyperplasia.

Comments: The slow growth of the tumor and absence of cervical lymphadenopathy is an indicator that the tumor is a benign lesion rather than a carcinoma. However, the diagnosis is based only on histological findings; xanthomas are characterized by numerous cholesterol laden histiocytes; fibromas by fibroblasts; schwannomas by uniformly spindled Schwann cells with Antoni A (cellular fascicular) and Antoni B (myxoid; vacuolated) regions; and carcinomas by neoplastic hyperchromatic epithelial cells.

Q2 What are the differences between congenital epulis and this lesion?

A Sex predilection
B Age predilection
C Location
D Immunocytochemical profile
E Malignant variant

Answers:

A No
B Congenital epulis is seen in newborns, while granular cell tumor is seen in adults.
C Granular cell tumors may occur everywhere in the body, but they do have a preference for the tongue, while congenital epulis tend to appear in the alveolar process of the maxilla and less in the mandible.
D Granular cell tumor has a positive immune histochemical reactivity to S-100 protein, neuron-specific enolase and myelin proteins, while congenital epulis has a negative one.
E Malignant congenital epulis has never been reported, but on the contrary, malignant granular tumor is rare and characterized by a necrotic, ulcerated overlying mucosa lesion, whose histological characteristics include numerous spindle and granular cells with vesicular nuclei and prominent nucleoli, increased mitotic activity and cellular and/or nuclear polymorphism.

Q3 Which of the histological characteristics below is/or are NOT indicator/s of the pathogenesis of this lesion?

A Proximity of the lesion with peripheral nerve fibers
B S-100 positive reaction
C Presence of myelin figures and axon like structures
D Positive reaction to myelin proteins and neuron specific enolases
E Pseudoepithelial hyperplasia

Answers:

A No
B No
C No
D No
E Pseudoepithelial hyperplasia is a reactive epithelial proliferation that is seen in response to a wide variety of conditions including infections, neoplasia, inflammation, and trauma. It is characterized by a hyperplasia of the oral mucosa due to hypergranulosis and ortho- or parakeratosis causing elongation and branching of rete ridges with scattered mitosis that sometimes mimics squamous cell carcinoma.

Comments: The granular cell tumors are now accepted to have a neural origin as these lesions are close to peripheral nerve fibers, demonstrate ultrastructural myelin figures and have a positive reaction to S100 proteins, neuron specific enolase and myelin proteins.

Section III

25

Normal Variations

During an oral examination, there are a plethora of anatomical variations that sometimes look peculiar and can be misdiagnosed by clinicians. These normal variations can be seen in any part of the oral mucosa and their understanding helps clinicians to evaluate various findings (normal vs. abnormal) and to take a decision about the appropriate course of management, if necessary (See Figure 25.0).

Some of these oral variations are listed according to their location in Table 25.

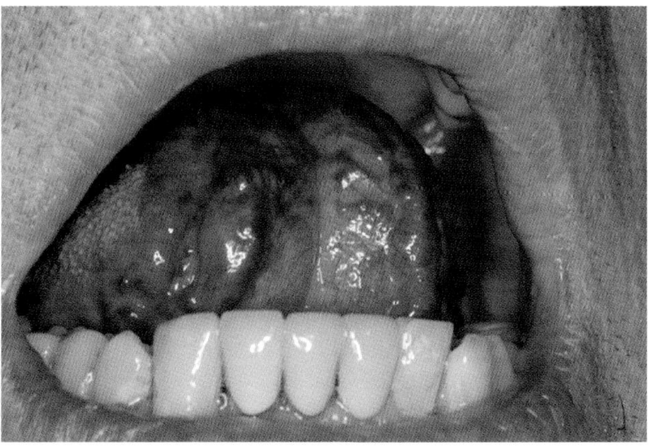

Figure 25.0 Varicose veins of the ventral surface of the tongue.

Table 25 Normal oral variations according to location.

- Lips
  - Fordyce spots
  - Leukoedema
  - Tooth imprints
  - Lip fissure/pits
- Buccal mucosae
  - Fordyce spots
  - Leukoedema
  - Linea alba
  - Stensen's papilla

Table 25 (Continued)

- Tongue
  - Median groove
  - Fissured tongue
  - Geographic tongue
  - Scalloped tongue
  - Papillae (folate/circumvallate)
  - Lingual tonsils
  - Plica fimbriata
  - Varicose veins
- Palate
  - Torus mandibularis
  - Median palatine raphe
  - Fovea palatina
  - Incisive papilla
- Floor of the mouth
  - Frenulum Tags
  - Salivary gland opening (sublingual/mandibular ducts)
- Gingivae
  - Racial pigmentation
- Jaws/teeth
  - Torus mandibularis
  - Exostoses
- Salivary glands
  - Accessory glands
- Neck
  - Vascular variations

Clinical Guide to Oral Diseases, First Edition. Dimitris Malamos and Crispian Scully.

Companion website: www.wiley.com/go/malamos/clinical_guide

Case 25.1

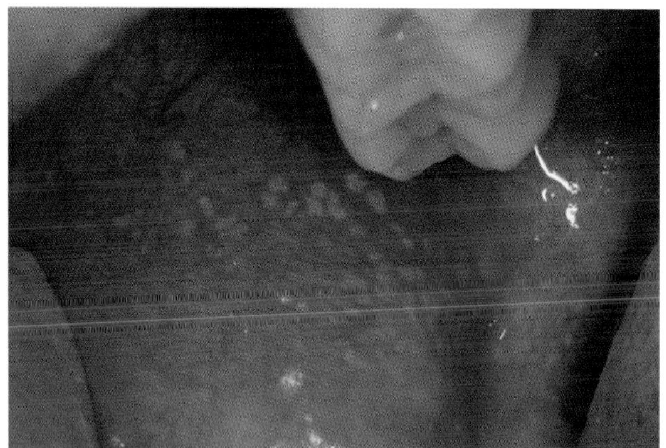

Figure 25.1a

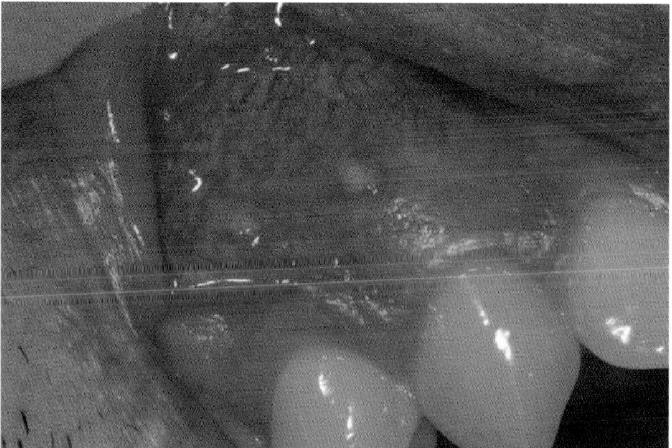

Figure 25.1b

CO: A 32-year-old man presented for evaluation of multiple yellow spots in both his buccal mucosae.

HPC: The lesions were first noticed by his dentist during a regular dental check-up last month.

PMH: He was a healthy young man with no serious medical problems and known allergies. He worked as a financial advisor and played soccer in his free time. He was a non-smoker but an occasional drinker of 2–3 glasses of beer at the weekends.

OE: The oral examination revealed multiple raised yellow spots on both his buccal mucosae (mainly opposite the molar areas) (Figure 25.1a) and at the vermilion border of his upper lips. These yellow lesions are painless spots with a smooth surface, fixed and not removed with a wooden spatula within a normal oral mucosa. These nodules are arranged either in groups of 10–20 (as seen in buccal mucosae and upper lip) or isolated 1–3 in number (in upper gingivae) (Figure 25.1b). No other similar lesions were seen on his skin or other mucosae.

Q1 What is the likely diagnosis?

A Lipomas
B Molluscum contagiosum
C Fibromas
D Xanthomas
E Fordyce spots

Answers:

A No
B No
C No
D No
E Fordyce spots are the diagnosis. Fordyce spots or granules are ectopic sebaceous glands, mostly found on male and female external genital organs and/or mouth and particularly on the vermilion border of the lips and buccal mucosae. Fordyce spots are not a kind of manifestation of a systemic disease, but sometimes cause severe concern in patients with anxiety or depression when they fear a venereal disease or malignancy.

Comments: Benign lesions such as reactive fibromas or lipomas are easily ruled out as both have normal or yellow color and consistency, but are usually single rather than multiple lesions and associated with previous chronic local trauma. Xanthomas are manifestations of hyperlipidemias and easily excluded from the diagnosis due to the young age and good health of the patient. Molluscum contagiosum are numerous infectious nodules with a characteristic central depression which was not seen in this young patient.

Q2 Fordyce spots are characterized by:

A Presence of hair follicles
B Seen exclusively in adults
C Higher risk of oral malignancy
D Tendency for development sebaceous hyperplasia
E Relation with hypercholesterinemia

Answers:

A No
B No
C No
D Multiple granules of sebaceous glands coalesce and form white-yellow cauliflower-like lesions, known as sebaceous hyperplasia mainly in the vermilion border of the lips and the facial skin.
E No

Comments: Hair follicles are closely located to the sebaceous glands (Fordyce spots) in the skin and genitals, but not in the oral mucosa. Fordyce spots appear at a very young age, and become more prominent during adulthood. Intra-oral ectopic sebaceous glands have been suspected of inducing sebaceous intra-oral carcinomas. These tumors are extremely rare in the oral mucosa despite the high incidence of Fordyce spots there.

Q3 What is the best treatment?

- **A** None
- **B** Antibiotics
- **C** Electrodessication
- **D** Cosmetic plastic surgery
- **E** Anti-cholesterol medicines

Answers:

- **A** Fordyce spots are harmless spots and require no treatment
- **B** No
- **C** No
- **D** No
- **E** No

Comments: The removal of Fordyce spots with electrodessication or plastic surgery is indicated only in patients with severe phobias, while reassurance and a six-month follow-up is the best treatment choice. Antibiotics and anti-cholesterol medicines are useless as the Fordyce spots are not the result of a bacterial infection or hyperlipidemia.

Case 25.2

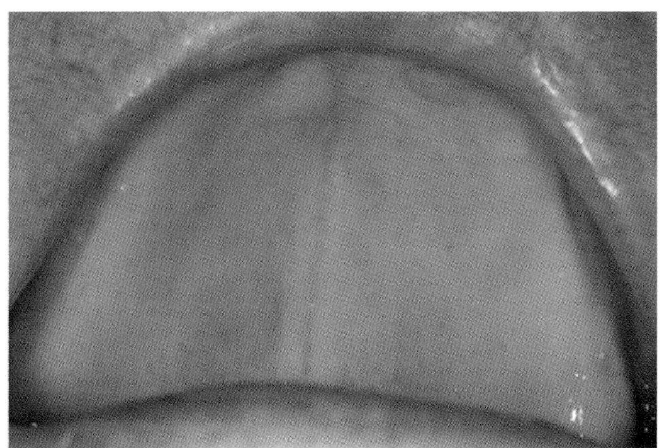

Figure 25.2

CO: A 62-year-old woman presented with pain in her palate.

HPC: The pain was not constant or sharp but was dull and appeared whenever the patient tried to wear her upper new denture.

PMH: This lady had suffered from late diabetes over the last five years, which was controlled with diet and metformin hydrochloride tablets, mild hypertension treated with amiopidine for nine years, and recently from severe osteoporosis for which she was on Vitamin D_3 and alendronate sodium tablets. No history of facial and local trauma or oral neuralgia had been reported.

OE: On examination, the patient was edentulous, but wearing full upper and lower dentures, well-fitted and with no ulcerations underneath. On palpation, a linear depressed area along the middle of her hard palate (Figure 25.2) was slightly more sensitive. This was the area from where a mild pain originated whenever the patient wore her upper new denture. The pain presented two months ago with her first attempt to try her new upper tight denture, but was not associated with facial numbness or other symptoms. Her upper denture was stable with no clinical signs of overpressure in the palate. Sinus and orthopantomogram (OPG) X-rays did not show any bony lesions or infection. A similar linear lesion was also found in the palate of her daughter.

Q1 What is the cause of her pain?

- **A** Trigeminal neuralgia
- **B** Ill-fitting denture
- **C** Median palatal raphe
- **D** Palatal cyst
- **E** Cleft palate

Answers:

- **A** No
- **B** No
- **C** Median palatal raphe was the cause for the pain and is the result of irritation of local nerve endings from the pressure of a very tight denture. This raphe joins the two palatine processes of the maxilla extending from the incisive papilla to the end of the hard palate, in the midline. It is characterized by a very thin mucosa overlying a thin but dense mucoperiosteum where superficial nerve endings are numerous.
- **D** No
- **E** No

Comments: The clinical and radiological findings easily exclude clefts and palatal cysts respectively while the symptomatology was irrelevant of trigeminal neuralgia, which is characterized by sharp, shooting pain.

Q2 Which other raphes apart from the palatine are familiar to dentists?

A Buccal
B Lingual
C Pterygomandibular
D Lateral palpebral
E Pharyngeal

Answers:

A Buccal raphe is found at the fusion of the maxillary with the mandibular process.
B Lingual raphe is found at the junction of two parts of the tongue and evidence of that is the lingual frenum.
C Pterygomandibular raphe is a ligament band of the buccopharyngeal fascia, and located superiorly to the pterygoid hamulus, inferior to the posterior end of the mylohyoid line of the mandible.
D No
E Pharyngeal raphe joints the right and left pharyngeal constrictors.

Comments: Lateral palpebral raphe involves the eyes and is attached to the frontosphenoidal process of the zygomatic bone, divided in two slips which are attached to the margins.

Q3 Which other lesions are associated with a palatine raphe?

A Epstein pearls
B Torus mandibularis
C Median palatal cyst
D Palatal abscess
E Pleomorphic adenoma

Answers:

A Epstein pearls are multiple benign cystic lesions along the palatal raphe, and appear as white nodules in nearly 50–85% of newborn infants. They arise either from the epithelium entrapped between the palatal shelves and the nasal process during palatal formation, or from epithelial remnants during development of minor palatal salivary glands after which they underwent cystic degeneration.
B No
C Median palatal cyst is a rare non-odontogenic fissural cyst that is located posterior to the palatine papillae, symmetrical to the middle line, with a cystic wall containing inflammatory cells but no cartilage or glandular tissues.
D No
E No

Comments: Torus palatinus and not mandibularis is associated with palatine raphe, while the palatal abscess and pleomorphic adenomas are commonly seen all over in the palate and not exclusively along the palatine raphe.

Case 25.3

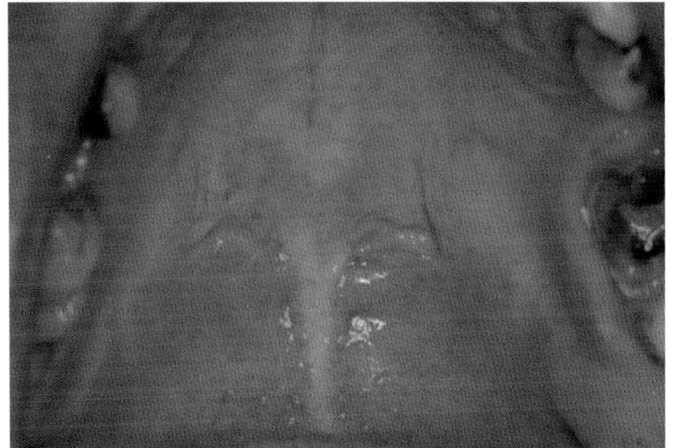

Figure 25.3

CO: A 37-year-old man presented for an evaluation of two pits on his hard palate.

HPC: These pits were first noticed by the patient two days ago during the brushing of his teeth.

PMH: This patient had suffered from depression over the last five years since his job loss, but was reluctant to take any medicine. He drank two beers daily and was a chronic smoker of two packets of cigarettes, despite that his father had died from an extensive cancer of rhinopharynx the previous month.

OE: His oral examination revealed two depressions of the posterior part of the palatal mucosa along the middle line (Figure 25.3). The palatal mucosa was normal apart from very mild inflammation of a few minor salivary glands ducts, due to smoking. His dentition was heavily restored with fillings and crowns, and his oral hygiene was inadequate.

Q1 What is the possible diagnosis of his palatal depressions?
- **A** Nicotinic stomatitis
- **B** Medial palatal raphe
- **C** Median palatal fistula
- **D** Fovea palatini
- **E** Incisive canal

Answers:
- **A** No
- **B** No
- **C** No
- **D** Yes. These are normal anatomical landmarks of the margins of the hard with the soft palate. Fovea palatini are two glandular openings in the palatal mucosa at the midline in an area rich with nerve endings. It does not have any particular function, but can be used by dentists as a guideline for the placement of the posterior palatal seal during a construction of full upper dentures.
- **E** No

Comments: Nicotinic stomatitis is characterized by a diffuse white patch intermingled with scattered numerous, erythematous, openings of minor salivary glands, while the mucosa in this patient was normal, with two salivary gland opening without severe inflammation along the middle line and close to the vibrating lines of the soft palate. The palatal raphe, fistula, or incisive canal have different clinical features and location, as they appear as a single linear depression (raphe) or opening in the middle of the palate (fistula) or an intraosseous canal through the anterior maxilla (incisive canal).

Q2 This anatomical variation is related to other anatomical landmarks for better upper denture retention:
- **A** Posterior vibrating line
- **B** Anterior vibrating lines
- **C** Uvula
- **D** Incisive papilla
- **E** Maxillary midline diastema

Answers:
- **A** The posterior vibrating line is significantly related to the fovea palatine of the soft palate, and is an indication of the posterior margins of the denture.
- **B** No
- **C** No
- **D** No
- **E** No

Comments: Other anatomical marks like the anterior vibrating lines, uvula and incisive canal and middle diastema seem to be unrelated to denture retention.

Q3 Which of the muscles of the soft palate are deficits after damage of the mandibular branch of the trigeminal nerve?
- **A** Tensor veli palatine
- **B** Palatoglossus
- **C** Palatopharyngeal
- **D** Levator veli palatine
- **E** Musculus uvulae

Answers:
- **A** Tensor veli palatine are the only muscles of the soft palate, and are innervated by the mandibular branch of the trigeminal nerve. Damage of this nerve causes deficits of these muscles.
- **B** No
- **C** No
- **D** No
- **E** No

Comments: Although the palatoglossus and levator veli palatine are involved with swallowing, the palatopharyngeus with breathing and musculus uvulae with the uvula, movement of all innervated with the pharyngeal plexus of the vagus nerve.

Case 25.4

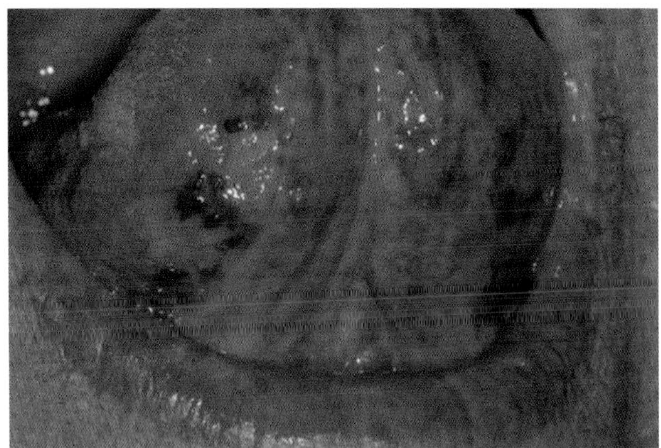

Figure 25.4

CO: A 69-year-old man presented with red and blue lesions on the inferior surface of his tongue.

HPC: The lesions had been noticed since adulthood, but remained unchanged since then and became rarely enlarged after the consumption of hot food or drinks, and only for a short period.

PMH: The patient suffered from hypercholesteremia, mild atrial fibrillation and prostate hypertrophy, and was under atorvastatin, atenolol and finasteride tablets respectively.

OE: A few scattered, asymptomatic, superficial red and blue swellings in the inferior tongue mucosa, following the branches of the lingual artery and veins which can easily bleach with constant pressure (Figure 25.4). No other lesions were detected within his oral and other mucosae and skin, or among his close relatives.

Q1 What is the cause of these lesions?

- **A** Osler-Weber-Rendu syndrome
- **B** Crest disease
- **C** Lymphangioma
- **D** Hemangioma
- **E** Varicose veins (Sublingual varices)

Answers:

- **A** No
- **B** No
- **C** No
- **D** No
- **E** Varicose veins of the tongue (sublingual varices), characterized by multiple purple or dark or black swellings (caviar tongue).These lesions are formed from small dilated veins which bleach with pressure and are easily seen underneath a thin mucosa of the ventral surface of the tongue. Varicose veins are usually asymptomatic, but sometimes cause concern in patients with anxiety or depression. These lesions are related to aging, smoking, or various cardiovascular diseases and become larger with aspirin or other anti-coagulant drugs, or hot food/drinks uptake.

Comments: The absence of nose or gut bleeding or similar lesions among his close relatives rules out Osler-Weber-Rendu syndrome. This is an autosomal genetic disorder causing abnormal vascular formation in the skin, mucous membranes (telangiectasia) and organs like the brain, liver, lungs and gut (arteriovenous malformations). The absence of calcinosis, Raynaud phenomenon, esophageal constriction, and scleroderma in this patient excludes Crest disease from the diagnosis. The late onset and the long, unchanged duration of these vascular lesions excludes hemangiomas or lymphangiomas as these lesions appear at a very young age and have a tendency of resolving over the years.

Q2 Tongue varicose veins are associated with:

- **A** Older age
- **B** Smoking
- **C** Hypertension
- **D** Ill-fitted denture wearing
- **E** Smoking

Answers:

- **A** Patients older than 50 years of age seem to have more detectable varicose veins due to vascular alterations seen underneath thinner oral mucosa during the aging process.
- **B** Smoking is a possible contributory factor and is closely related with cardio-pulmonary diseases in which coughing is predominant and vascular pressure is higher.
- **C** Hypertension alone or part of various cardiovascular diseases is common in older patients, and is always associated with tongue varicosities.
- **D** Ill-fitting dentures may contribute to the development of varicose veins by traumatizing the tongue causing local inflammation and neovascularization.
- **E** No

Comments: Smoking seems to be unrelated to varicose veins, as nicotine causes vasoconstriction rather than vasodilatation.

Q3 Which are the histological characteristics of tongue varicose vein walls?

- **A** Increased thinning of the muscle layers
- **B** Elastin fiber deficiency
- **C** Disproportional increase of fibrous tissues
- **D** Numerous Civatte bodies
- **E** Giant cell aggregation within the vascular wall

Answers:

- **A** Increased thinning of muscles layers is a characteristic finding due to reduced number of muscle cells.
- **B** Together with the muscle cells, elastin fiber deficiency is present.
- **C** Marked intimal hypertrophy due to fibrous tissue infiltration is easily detected.
- **D** No
- **E** No

Comments: Civatte bodies are often seen in skin diseases such as lichen planus, while accumulation of multinucleated giant cells together with inflammatory cells is characteristic of giant cell arthritis.

Case 25.5

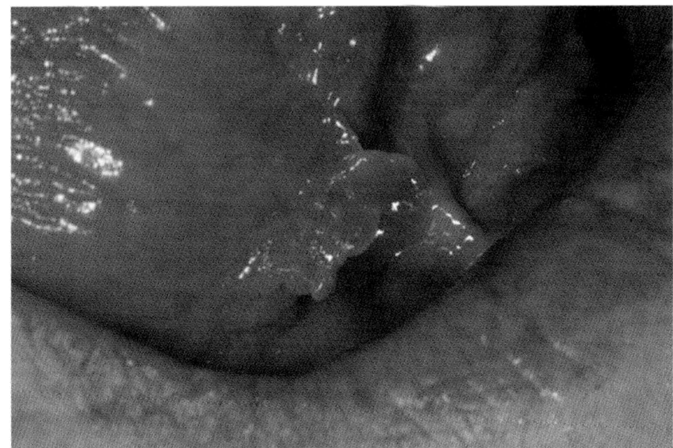

Figure 25.5

CO: A 28-year-old woman presented for an evaluation of a number of papillary lesions underneath her tongue mucosa.

HPC: The lesions were discovered accidentally by the patient during the brushing of her teeth last week. The patient was worried about the possibility of a sexually transmitted disease, as she had recently started a new relationship.

PMH: A healthy young woman who did not report of any serious medical problems or drugs uptake. She worked in a bank, spending her free time helping homeless people voluntarily. She was a rarely drinker of alcohol, but smoked one or two cigarettes per day.

OE: Her oral examination revealed a few papillary projections from the inferior surface of her tongue, with normal color and consistency, bilateral of the lingual frenulum (Figure 25.5). Her dentition was complete without fillings or orthodontic anomalies and her oral hygiene was very good. No skin, genital, or other mucosae lesions as well as cervical or systemic lymphadenopathy were seen.

Q1 What is the diagnosis?

- **A** Papilloma
- **B** Heck's disease
- **C** Condyloma acuminatum
- **D** Cowden syndrome
- **E** Hyperplastic plica fimbriata

Answers:

- **A** No
- **B** No
- **C** No
- **D** No
- **E** Plica fimbriata consists of sublingual mucosal fold, and are formed during the tongue's development and growth. Plica fimbriata are normal structures and consist of two or four mucosal folds of various

size, underneath the tongue, being close and parallel to lingual veins. These folds sometimes have papillary, fringe like endings and are often misdiagnosed as papillomas or condylomas.

Comments: Other conditions such as Cowden syndrome, Heck's disease, papilloma, or Condyloma acuminatum are characterized with papillomatous lesions, but differ in clinical features and family history. Cowden syndrome is an autosomal dominant condition characterized by multiple hamartomas including papillomatous lesions together with facial tricholemmoma, acral keratosis, and increased risk of breast, thyroid, and endometrial cancers, while condyloma acuminatum, Heck's disease or papilloma are acquired lesions and associated with an HPV infection.

Q2 Which of the structures below is/are NOT seen in the ventral surface of tongue?

- **A** Deep sublingual veins
- **B** Lingual frenulum
- **C** Plica fimbriata
- **D** Sublingual major salivary glands
- **E** Foliate papillae

Answers:

- **A** No
- **B** No
- **C** No
- **D** The sublingual major salivary glands are located within the floor of mouth and not in the ventral surface of the tongue where many minor salivary glands are located.
- **E** Foliate papillae are located at the lateral margins and not the ventral surface of the tongue.

Comments: The lingual frenulum connects the ventral surface of the tongue with the floor of the mouth. Lateral to the lingual frenulum, plica fimbriata structures are located and between them and the frenulum are seen the sublingual deep veins.

Q3 Which skin lesions resemble the plica fimbriata?

- **A** Skin tags
- **B** Neurofibromas (NF1)
- **C** Seborrheic keratosis
- **D** Cutaneous horns
- **E** Fibroepitheliomas

Answers:

- **A** Skin tags are benign soft pedunculated lesions, found in clusters in the neck, axillae, and skin folds particularly in obese patients.
- **B** Neurofibromatosis are characterized by numerous nodules in the skin together with café au lait pigmented lesions.
- **C** Seborrheic keratosis is seen in older people and characterized by numerous epithelial growths of variable clinical appearance within normal skin.
- **D** No
- **E** Fibroepithelioma of Pinkus is an unusual premalignant skin neoplasm with peculiar histological features, resembling seborrheic keratosis and basal cell carcinomas.

Comments: Cutaneous horns are usually single skin lesions and characterized by a conical projection of keratin above the skin, particularly in patients exposed to solar radiation while neurofibromatosis is characterized by numerous nodules with smooth but not papillary surface in the mouth and skin where café au lait pigmented lesions are present.

Case 25.6

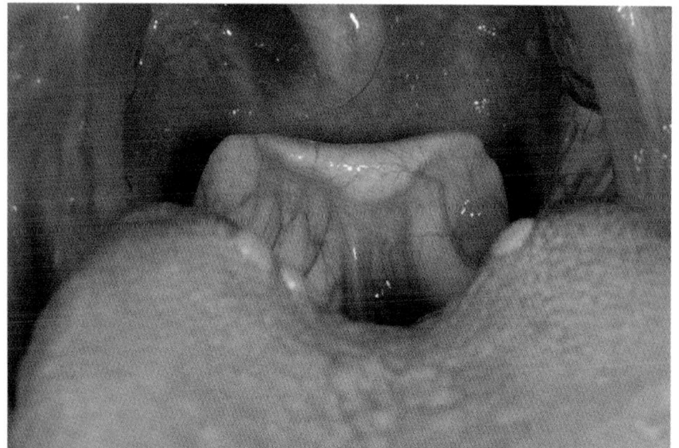

Figure 25.6

CO: A 22-year-old woman was referred by her dentist for a lump on the back of her throat.

HPC: The lump was discovered accidentally during a routine dental check-up by a young dentist whom the patient had visited for the first time.

PMH: This young undergraduate student had a clear medical history with no allergies or drugs intake. She spent her free time looking after babies and used to smoke 1 to 2 cigarettes daily only.

OE: The oral examination revealed a lump in front of the pharyngeal wall and backwards of the tongue. This lump looked like a yellow leaf and appeared whenever the patient widely opened her mouth or pronounced vowels (Figure 25.6). The lesion was asymptomatic and had an elastic cartilaginous consistency with a few blood vessels superficially, and did not cause any speaking, breathing, or eating problems. Cervical lymphadenopathy was absent. No other lesions were found in her mouth and no similar lesion was reported among her close relatives.

Q1 What is the diagnosis?

- **A** Tumor of rhinopharynx
- **B** Laryngomalacia
- **C** Pallister-Hall syndrome
- **D** Epiglottitis
- **E** High rising epiglottis

Answers:

- **A** No
- **B** No
- **C** No
- **D** No
- **E** High rising epiglottis is a rare normal anatomical variant that is seen in children rather than adults, mainly asymptomatic that may cause anxiety to the patients and their families.

Comments: The onset and duration and absent of combined symptomatology excludes epiglottitis, oropharyngeal tumors, laryngomalacia, or even Pallister-Hall syndrome from diagnosis. Epiglottitis is an acute swelling of the epiglottis due to inflammation causing a narrowing of the airway with breathing problems that require immediate antibiotic treatment or even laryngectomy. Oropharyngeal tumors are rare in young patients and usually accompanied with symptoms such as pain (local or referral), difficulties in swallowing or speaking and sometimes with cervical lymphadenopathy. Pallister-Hall syndrome is a rare condition characterized by polydactyly, syndactyly, hypothalamic hamartomas, bifid epiglottis, imperforate anus, and kidney abnormalities. Laryngomalacia is a congenital condition affecting the tissues above the vocal cords and causing inspiratory noises, cyanosis, choking feeding and poor weight gain from the very early age of 2.

Q2 Which is the best treatment of this asymptomatic lesion?

- **A** Only reassurance
- **B** Partial epiglossectomy
- **C** Epiglottopexy
- **D** Epiglottoplasty
- **E** Antibiotics

Answers:

- **A** As long as the rising epiglottis is asymptomatic, no treatment apart from the patient's or their family's reassurance is required.
- **B** No
- **C** No
- **D** No
- **E** No

Comments: The rising epiglottis is a normal variation and rarely causes severe symptoms such as speaking or breathing problems (apnea) and only then surgery like epiglossectomy, epiglottopexy, or epiglottopaxy may be required. Antibiotics are useful for epiglottitis and not for rising epiglottis.

Q3 Which other pathological conditions affect epiglottis?

- **A** Osteogenesis imperfecta
- **B** Pallister-Hall syndrome
- **C** Pierre Robin syndrome
- **D** Melkersson-Rosenthal syndrome
- **E** McCune-Albright syndrome

Answers:

- **A** Osteogenesis imperfecta may be related with laryngomalacia in some children.
- **B** Pallister-Hall syndrome presents with poly/syndactyly, hypothalamic hamartomas, bifid epiglottis, imperforate anus and kidney abnormalities.
- **C** Pierre Robin syndrome is characterized by micrognathia, glossoptosis, cleft palate, and rarely epiglottis anomalies.
- **D** No
- **E** No

Comments: McCune-Albright syndrome includes fibrous dysplasia, café au lait skin lesions, endocrine diseases such as precocious puberty, hyperthyroidism, pituitary, and testicular abnormalities while Melkersson-Rosenthal syndrome is characterized by facial paralysis, fissured tongue and granulomatous cheilitis. Abnormalities of epiglottis are not related with the above syndromes.

Case 25.7

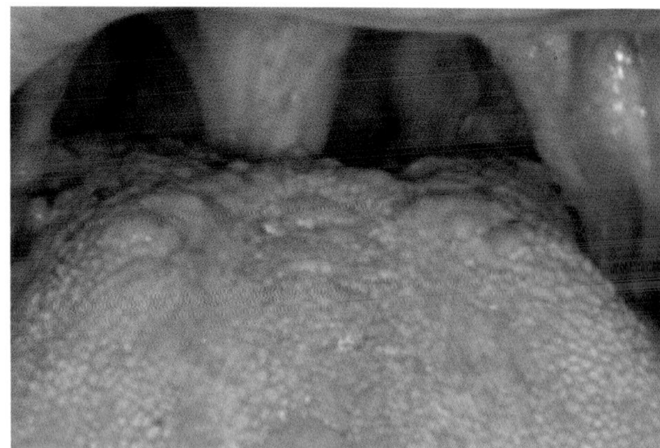

Figure 25.7a

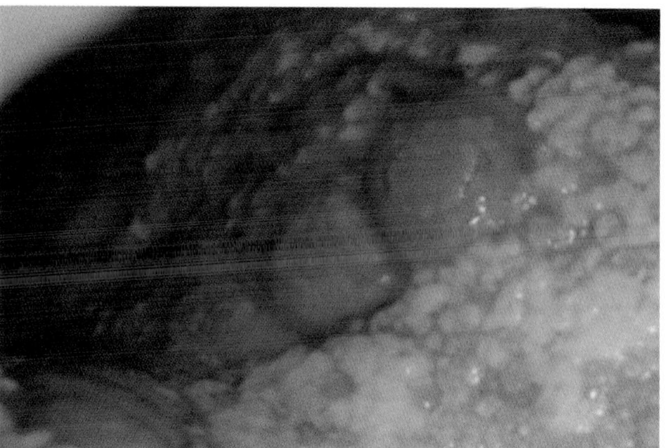

Figure 25.7b

CO: A 55-year-old woman complained about some nodules on the back of her tongue.

HPC: The lesions were discovered by the patient, accidentally, last week, during a self-examination of her sore throat and caused severe concern of its being cancer.

PMH: This middle-aged woman had suffered from chronic gastritis and an upper respiratory infection recently, for which she took a wide spectrum of antibiotics together with analgesic and antiseptic mouthwashes. She was a cancer-phobic patient as her younger sister was diagnosed with having breast cancer recently. Smoking or drinking habits were not recorded.

OE: The oral examination revealed normal oral mucosa apart from a mild erythema in her throat and whitish fur on her tongue, due to her recent respiratory infection. A few discrete pinkish colored dots were seen prominent at the back of her tongue, which were arranged in a reversed letter "v" structure, and caused the patient concern (Figure 25.7a and b). No other lesions were found in her mouth, skin, or other mucosae.

Q1 What is your diagnosis?
- **A** Molluscum contagiosum
- **B** Condylomas
- **C** Circumvallate papillae
- **D** Multiple fibromas
- **E** Lymphangioma

Answers:
- **A** No
- **B** No
- **C** Circumvallate papillae are 10–14 in number and located in front of the sulcus terminalis. The circumvallate papillae separate the anterior two-thirds, with the posterior one-third of the tongue and are mainly involved with a bitter taste and associated with the ducts of the von Ebner glands at their base. These papillae are innervated with the glossopharyngeal nerve and together with the foliate and fungiform papillae are the components of the gustatory system.
- **D** No
- **E** No

Comments: The distribution pattern of the circumvallate papillae and vascular pressure is higher like the reverse letter "v" easily excludes lymphangiomas, multiple fibromas, condylomas, and molluscum contagiosum from the diagnosis, as their lesions are different. In lymphangiomas a diffused pebbly swelling on the whole tongue is found, while in multiple fibromas, condylomas, and molluscum contagiosum the lesions are scattered on the dorsum of the tongue and other parts of the oral mucosa.

Q2 Which of the factors below is/or are NOT related with the enlargement of lingual papillae?
- **A** Heavy smoking
- **B** Hot, spicy foods
- **C** Food allergies
- **D** Iron deficiencies
- **E** Gut diseases

Answers:
- **A** No
- **B** No
- **C** No
- **D** Low iron levels are responsible for atrophy of the tongue mucosa with a significant reduction in number of all taste papillae (mainly the fungiform and circumvallate).
- **E** No

Comments: The location of circum vallate papillae at the back of the tongue easily allows their irritation and enlargement from a variety of stimulants like gastric acid, mouth allergens from foods, spices, and heavy smoking.

Q3 Which of the cells within the taste buds are responsible for the taste receptor renewal?

A Type I
B Type 2
C Type 3
D Type 4
E Supporting cells

Answers:

A No
B No
C No
D Type 4 or basal cells of the taste buds are not involved with taste reception per se, but participate in the renewal of taste buds every 10–14 days.
E No

Comments: The other taste cells play an important role in recognition and transmission of the tasteful stimulus from the taste buds to the brain. Type I are supporting glial-like cells controlling extracellular ion concentrations, while type II are the main receptor cells for sweet, bitter or umami taste, while the type III cells play an important role at the synapses, while the supporting cells may play a role in the integrity of the taste buds.

Case 25.8

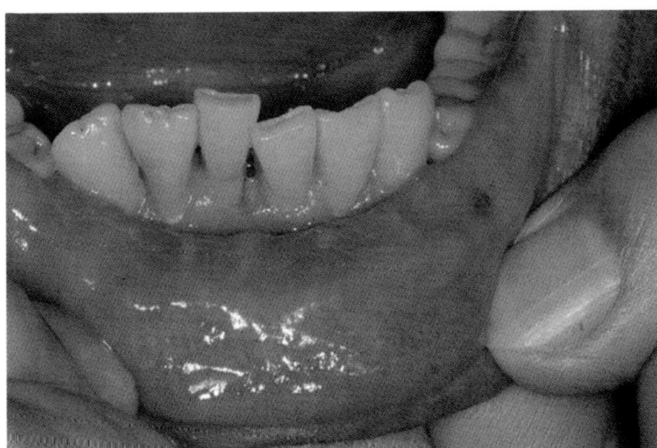

Figure 25.8a

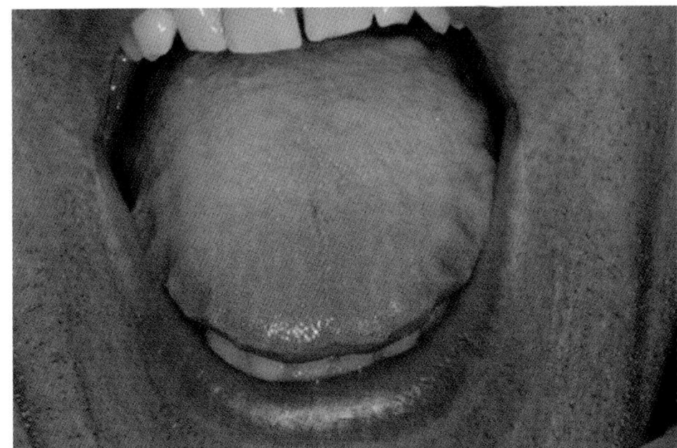

Figure 25.8b

CO: A 33 years old man presented for a regular oral and dental examination when the inner surface of his lower lip and lateral margins of tongue were found to be irregular.

HPC: The patient's lesions were discovered accidentally by his doctor and were asymptomatic with unknown duration.

PMH: A healthy but slight overweight man, with no serious medical problems or allergies. He smoked one packet of cigarettes daily and had the habit of playing his lower lip and tongue against his teeth. He ate extremely hot foods and used mint chewing gum regularly. He spent his free time on fishing.

OE: The oral examination revealed the inner surface of his lower lip to be slightly edematous due to trauma from lip biting, where a few raised and alternately depressed areas were seen. These lesions corresponded well to the morphology of the lower anterior teeth (Figure 25.8a). Similarly, the lateral margins of his tongue were corrugated following the adjacent teeth position and morphology (Figure 25.8b) while his buccal mucosae showed a diffused white opalescence which disappeared with stretching.

Q1 Which of the lesions below can be seen both in his lower lip and tongue?

A Teeth imprints
B Leukoedema
C Frictional keratosis
D Traumatic ulceration
E Focal epithelial hyperplasia

Answers:

- **A** Teeth imprints are commonly seen in overweight patients as well as in patients with the habit of biting their lips, tongue, or buccal mucosae. This parafunctional habit causes a reactive mucosal hyperplasia that follows teeth morphology with minimal inflammation underneath.
- **B** No
- **C** No
- **D** No
- **E** No

Comments: Leukoedema and traumatic ulceration were seen on the inner surface of his lower, lip but not on his tongue, while the reactive lesions such as frictional keratosis and focal epithelial hyperplasia were not found at both sites.

Q2 Which of the irritants below are responsible for patient's lesions?

- **A** Chemical
- **B** Mechanical
- **C** Thermal
- **D** Solar radiation
- **E** Allergens

Answers:

- **A** No
- **B** The compression of tongue and lips against adjacent teeth cause chronic mechanical irritation and swelling locally, leading to teeth imprints on the oral mucosa.
- **C** No
- **D** No
- **E** No

Comments: All the other irritants were easily excluded, as there was no history or clinical evidence of allergies from food or chewing gum, burns from hot food or spice consumption, and from solar radiation exposure during fishing to participate in the development of these mucosal lesions. Solar radiation induced oral lesions are always restricted on lips and never inside patient's mouth.

Q3 Which of the diseases below is/are presented with scalloping tongue and lips?

- **A** Down syndrome
- **B** Angioneurotic edema
- **C** Hypothyroidism
- **D** Sarcoidosis
- **E** Vitamin B deficiencies

Answers:

- **A** Down syndrome is characterized by hypotonia, neurological and cardiological pathologies, and dental-orofacial abnormalities. The latter cause mouth breathing, open bite, and an enlarged and protruding tongue that has numerous fissures, and is compressed against adjacent teeth leaving their imprints.
- **B** Angioedema presents as an acute swelling of the oral tissues sometimes causing edematous tongue and lips with marked teeth imprints on them.
- **C** Hypothyroidism causes a puffy face and sometimes lips and tongue enlargement which show scalloping on their surface.
- **D** Sarcoidosis is a chronic granulomatous disease sometimes causing persistent enlargement of the tongue and lips, leading to scalloping.
- **E** Vitamin B deficiency, particularly B12 or B2, causes a swollen, erythematous, depapillated, and corrugated tongue.

Case 25.9

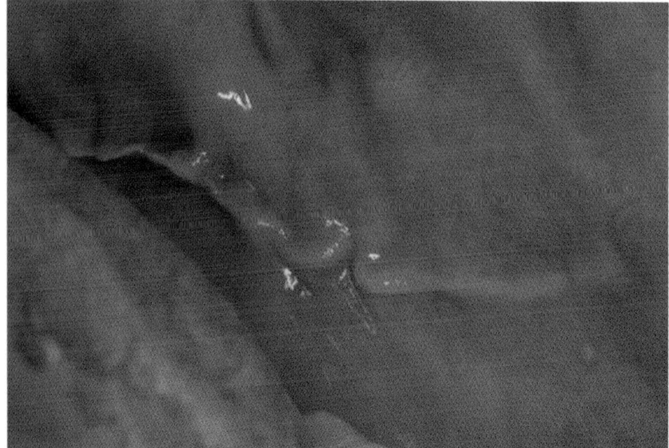

Figure 25.9

CO: A 42-year-old trumpet player presented for an evaluation of the lesions on both his buccal mucosae.

HPC: The lesions were first noticed by the patient during an oral examination following an accident of tongue biting. The lesions were asymptomatic for many years, but seemed to be slightly sensitive after playing the trumpet.

PMH: This man had no serious health problems apart from vitiligo on the skin of his face, hands, and genitals as well as an allergy to pollen for which he took antihistamines whenever necessary. He was a non-smoker or drinker.

OE: The oral examination revealed two symmetrical mucosal linear elevations on both buccal mucosae adjacent to the occlusion line. These elevations had a normal color and were more prominent at the molar areas following the occlusion margins of adjacent teeth (Figure 25.9). No other lesions were seen, and no signs of infection on his periodontium or other parts of his mouth, skin, or other mucosae. His oral hygiene was very good and his dentition was complete without any fillings.

Q1 What is the diagnosis?

- **A** Frictional keratosis
- **B** Leukoplakia
- **C** Linea alba
- **D** Lichen planus
- **E** Submucous fibrosis

Answers:

- **A** No
- **B** No
- **C** Linea alba is the answer. It is characterized by a horizontal mucosal linear of hyperplastic fibrous streaks on the buccal mucosa from the molar area to the commissures. These lesions are the result of a chronic friction of the mucosa against the occlusion surface of the adjacent teeth. These lesions are asymptomatic, do not have a tendency for malignant transformation and sometimes fade with the removal of the causative teeth.
- **D** No
- **E** No

Comments: The frictional keratosis, leukoplakias, lichen planus and submucous fibrosis are more extensive white oral lesions with various clinical pictures and symptomatology in contrary to the linear with a normal color lesion that was seen in this patient.

Q2 Which is the best treatment for this lesion?

- **A** Plastic surgery
- **B** Intra-lesional injection of steroids
- **C** None
- **D** Tooth capping
- **E** Anti-anxiety drugs

Answers:

- **A** No
- **B** No
- **C** As the lesion does not cause any serious problems, treatment is not required. Reassurance of the anxious patient is sometimes necessary.
- **D** No
- **E** No

Comments: Tooth capping and anti-anxiety drugs may be helpful only for patients with irregular teeth morphology and strong parafunctional habits, while plastic surgery or intra-lesional injections of steroids are of no use.

Q3 Which of the conditions below is/are associated with buccal fibrosis?

- **A** Scleroderma
- **B** Superficial burns
- **C** Minor aphthous stomatitis
- **D** Mucous membrane pemphigoid
- **E** Fibrous dysplasia

Answers:

- **A** Scleroderma is characterized by altering the underling of mucosa connective tissue by increasing collagen synthesis, leading to diffuse fibrosis and finally to sclerosis.
- **B** No
- **C** No
- **D** Mucous membrane pemphigoid is a chronic subepithelial bullous disease which sometimes causes oral scarring in the areas where ulcerations constantly reappear.
- **E** No

Comments: The effect of superficial burns or minor aphthae stomatitis on the submucosa connective tissue is minimal and therefore fibrosis is minimal. Fibrous dysplasia involves the bones including jaws, but not the oral mucosa.

Case 25.10

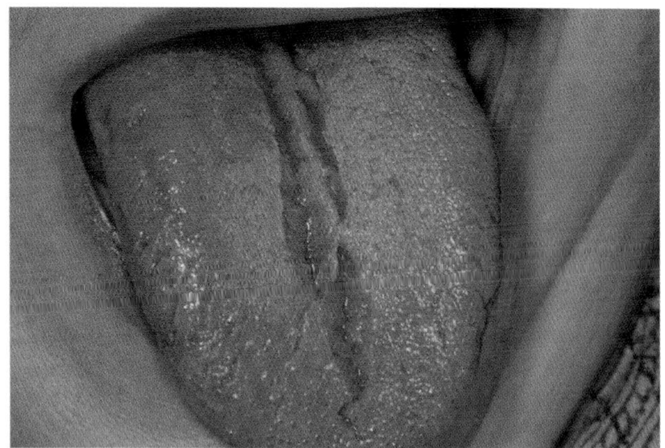

Figure 25.10

CO: A 47-year-old woman was worried about a deep groove in the middle of the dorsum of her tongue.

HPC: This groove had been there since childhood, but seemed to become deeper during the last two years causing her a slight burning sensation with spicy foods.

PMH: This patient suffered from chronic asthma and took steroids in crisis. No other close relatives had a similar lesion. She was non-smoker and non-drinker.

OE: The oral examination revealed a deep fissure in the middle of the dorsum which separated the tongue incompletely in two parts, leaving normal mucosa underneath (Figure 25.10). The rest of her oral mucosa, face, and skin were normal.

Q1 What is the diagnosis of this groove?

A Median groove of tongue
B Fissured tongue
C Geographic tongue
D Traumatic cut
E Bifid tongue

Answers:

A The median groove of the tongue is a longitudinal depression of the dorsum of the tongue that is extended from the tip to the foramen cecum of the tongue. The epithelium adjacent and underneath the fissure is normal and is not associated with a previous trauma, infections, or neoplasias.
B No
C No
D No
E No

Comments: The groove begins from the tip and completely separates the tongue into two parts in bifid tongue, while in the middle groove type the split is incomplete. Numerous, shallow grooves radiating from the central groove to the lateral margins are characteristic of fissured tongue, while in geographic tongue irregular denuded patches surrounded by thickened epithelium are seen. History of serious tongue injury at childhood was not reported and therefore old was excluded.

Q2 Fissures are commonly seen in:

A Angular cheilitis
B Down syndrome
C Plasma cell cheilitis
D Pustular psoriasis
E Lip fissures

Answers:

A Angular cheilitis is an inflammation of one or both commissures, due to local infection from bacteria like *Staphylococcus* and fungi like *Candida*; or due to local irritation from drooling, malnutrition, or immunodeficiency. It appears with erythema, swelling, or even ulcerations, cracking or deep fissures and crusting extended from the inner surface of the lip to its perioral skin.
B Down syndrome presents a number of facial abnormalities such as a flat face and nose, almond-shaped eyes, and an enlarged fissured tongue protruding out of the mouth.
C No
D Among the manifestations of psoriasis is the fissured tongue.
E Lip fissures are persistent linear ulcerations in the sagittal plane of the upper or lower lip, possibly due to the fusion's weakness of the embryonic plates of the brachial 1st arch. Contributory factors are the patient's exposure in cold weather, smoking or alcohol consumption, infections and parafunctional habits.

Comments: Plasma cell cheilitis is presented as erosive edematous erythematous patches but not fissures on lower lip mainly

Q3 Which of the syndromes below includes a median tongue groove among their manifestations?

A Down syndrome
B Marfan syndrome
C Treacher Collins syndrome
D Cleft tongue syndrome
E Simpson Golabi-Behmel syndrome

Answers:

A No

B No

C No

D No

E Simpson-Golabi-Behmel syndrome is characterized by macrosomia, hyperterolism, macroglossia with a deep groove in the middle, hepatosplenomegaly, and heart disease, and occurs primarily in males.

Comments: The tongue is enlarged and has numerous fissures in Down syndrome while is completely split (bifid) in cleft tongue syndrome. The Treacher Collins and Marfan syndromes have numerous facial deformities and dental anomalies, but do not have a median groove in the dorsum of the tongue.

26

Oral Lesions According to Patient's Age

Oral diseases are globally the most common, non-prevalent diseases causing pain, discomfort, disfigurement, and reducing quality of life with serious social and economic impacts or even death. These diseases are derived from the intersection of the oral microbiome, environmental issues, behavior, and lifestyle, as well as genetic factors. The most common oral diseases are dental caries (tooth decay), periodontal diseases causing tooth loss, and cancers of the lips and oral cavity. Oral diseases affect people throughout their lifetime, but some of them have a higher prevalence, like caries, in children and teenagers and periodontal diseases in adults, while cancer is mostly seen among middle-aged and older patients, especially in low and middle-income countries (Figure 26.0a–e). Some of the oral diseases are preventable, affect local or distant tissues, and can be either spontaneously healed or require special care.

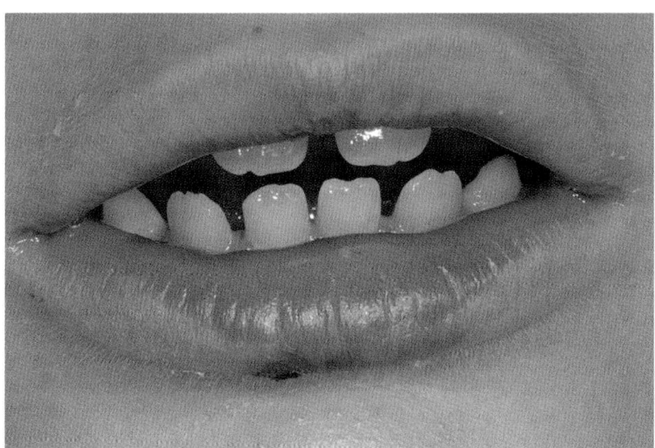

Figure 26.0a Licking cheilitis in a baby.

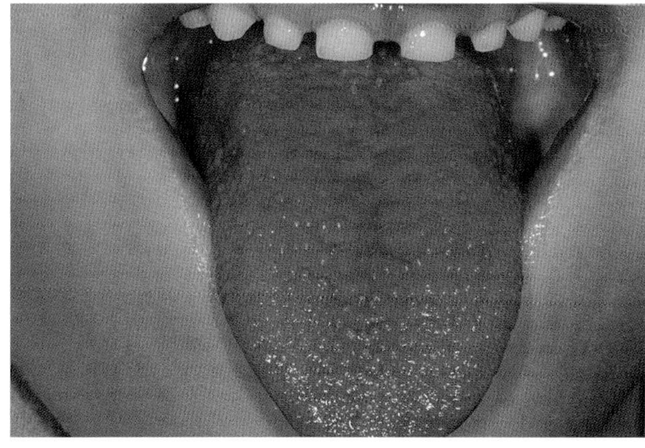

Figure 26.0b Tongue papillitis due to a viral infection in a child.

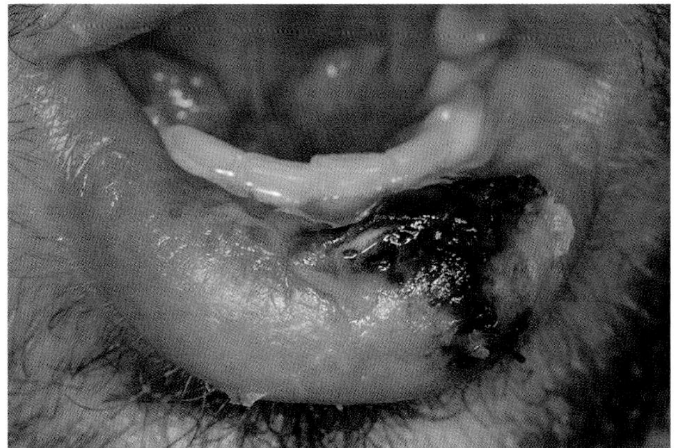

Figure 26.0c Traumatic lip ulceration in a teenager.

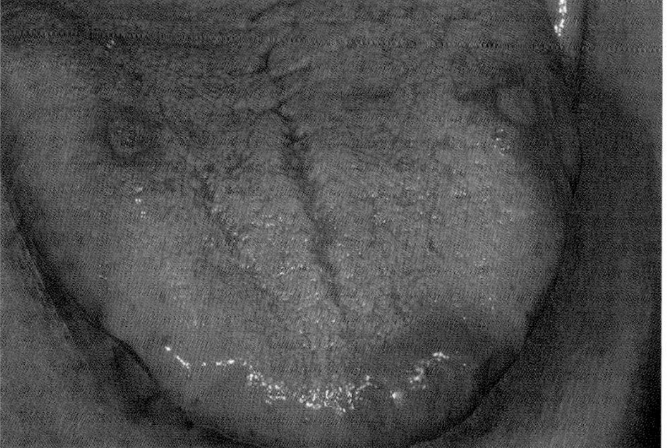

Figure 26.0d Multiple tongue aphthae in a lady with iron anemia.

Clinical Guide to Oral Diseases, First Edition. Dimitris Malamos and Crispian Scully.

Companion website: www.wiley.com/go/malamos/clinical_guide

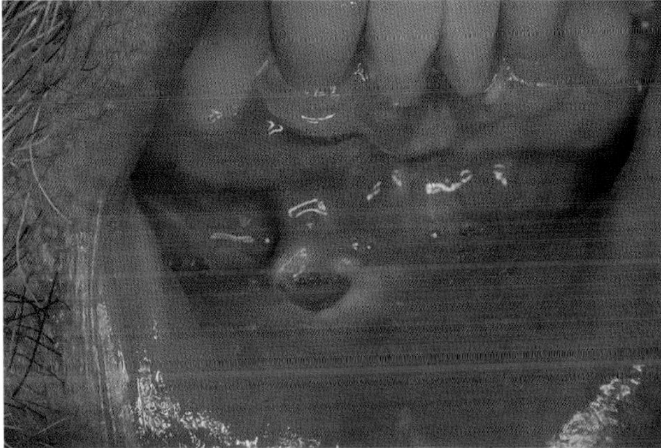

Figure 26.0e Traumatic aphthous like ulceration of the lower anterior sulcus caused by the hook of a loose denture.

Table 26 lists the more common and important oral lesions/diseases according to the patient's age. Table 26a is about lesions which are seen in babies up to 1-year-old; Table 26b lists lesions in children; Table 26c lesions in teenagers; while Table 26d lists lesions in adults; and finally Table 26e lists lesions in older patients. The most common lesions in each group are highlighted with bold letters.

Table 26 Common and important lesions according to patient's age.

(a) Infancy (up to 1 year)

- Congenital
  - Clefts
    - **Lips**
    - In association with syndromes
  - Cysts
    - Thyroglossal cyst
    - Dermoid
    - Epidermoid
  - Developmental
    - Bifid tongue
  - Bifid papillae
  - Teeth anomalies
    - Anodontia
      - Total
      - Partial
      - Natal and prenatal teeth
  - Teeth alterations
      - Size
      - Shape
      - Color
      - Number
      - Composition
      - Mineralization
  - Tongue variations
      - Fissured
      - Scaffold
      - Geographic
      - Ankyloglossia

Table 26 (Continued)

  - Vascular malformations
    - **Hemangiomas**
    - Lymphangiomas
- Acquired
  - Trauma
    - Riga-Fede ulcerations
    - Mucoceles
    - Ranulas
    - Facial injuries
  - Cysts
    - **Eruption cyst**
    - Epstein pearls
    - Bohn's nodules
    - Gingival cysts
  - Infections
    - Bacterial
      - Staphylococcal
      - Streptococcal
      - Congenital syphilis
    - **Viral**
      - Primary herpetic stomatitis
    - **Fungal**
      - Candidiasis
        - **Acute**
        - Chronic
    - Neoplasms
    - Benign
      - **Congenital epulis**
    - Malignant
      - Langerhans histiocytosis
      - Sarcomas
      - Melanomas
    - Autoimmune
    - Neonatal bullous disorders
      - Pemphigus

(b) Childhood (up to 12 years)

- Congenital
  - Similar to those seen in infancy
    - Fordyce spots
- Acquired
  - **Caries**
  - Trauma
    - Mechanical
      - Ulcerations
      - Frictional cheek-biting
    - Burns
      - Electrical
      - Chemical
      - Thermal
  - Cysts
    - Gingival
    - Eruption
    - Periapical
    - Mucoceles
    - Ranula

Table 26 (Continued)

- Infections
  - Bacterial
    - Streptococcal pharyngitis
  - Viral
    - Herpetic
      - **Primary**
      - Secondary
  - Fungal
    - Candidiasis
      - **Acute**
      - Chronic
- Inflammatory
  - **Recurrent oral ulcerations**
    - Minor
    - Major
    - Herpetic
    - Associated with syndromes
  - **Cheilitis**
    - Licking
    - Exfoliated
- Neoplasms
  - **Benign**
    - Fibromas
    - Papillomas
  - **Malignant**
    - Sarcomas

(c) Adolescence (from 13 up to 19 years)

- Congenital
  - Similar to those seen in infancy or childhood
  - Fordyce spots
- Acquired
  - **Caries**
  - Trauma
    - Mechanical
      - Ulcerations
      - Friction cheek-biting
    - Burns
      - Electrical
      - Chemical
      - Thermal
    - Cysts
    - Gingival
    - Eruption
    - Periapical
    - Mucoceles
    - Ranula
  - Infections
    - Bacterial
      - Streptococcal pharyngitis
      - **Gingivitis**

Table 26 (Continued)

      - Necrotizing
      - Pericoronitis
    - Viral
      - Herpetic
        - **Primary**
        - Secondary
      - Verruca vulgaris
      - Molluscum contagiosum
    - Fungal
      - Candidiasis
        - Acute
        - Chronic
    - Inflammatory
    - **Recurrent oral ulcerations**
      - Minor
      - Major
      - Herpetic
      - Associated with syndromes
    - Cheilitis
      - Licking
      - Exfoliated
      - Drug-induced (i.e. for acne)
    - Reactive
    - Pyogenic granuloma
    - Immune-related
    - Erythema multiforme
    - Neoplasms
    - Benign
      - Fibromas
      - Papillomas
    - Malignant
      - Mucoepidermoid carcinomas
      - Lymphomas
      - Sarcomas

(d) Adulthood (from 20 to 65 years)

- Congenital
  - Similar to those seen in infancy (in remission)
- Acquired
  - Trauma
    - **Mechanical**
      - Ulcerations
      - Friction cheek-biting
    - Burns
      - Chemical
      - Thermal
  - Cysts
    - Gingival
    - Periapical
    - **Mucoceles**

Table 26 (Continued)

- Infections
  - Bacterial
    - Streptococcal pharyngitis
    - Gingivitis
    - Periodontitis
      - Necrotizing
      - Pericoronitis
    - Venereal diseases
      - Syphilis
      - Gonorrhea
      - Others
  - Viral
    - **Infectious mononucleosis (young adults)**
    - Herpetic stomatitis
      - Primary
      - Secondary
    - Verruca vulgaris
    - Molluscum contagiosum
  - Fungal
    - Candidiasis
      - Acute
      - Chronic
- Inflammatory
  - Recurrent oral ulcerations (resolving by the time)
    - Minor
    - Major
    - Herpetic
    - Associated with syndromes
  - Cheilitis
    - Licking
    - Exfoliated
    - Actinic
- Immune-related
  - **Erythema multiforme (young age)**
  - **Lichen planus (middle age)**
- Autoimmune disorders
  - Bullous diseases
  - Sjogren's syndrome
- Potentially malignant lesions
  - Leukoplakia
  - Erythroplakia
- Neoplasms
  - Benign
    - Fibromas
  - Malignant
    - Oral carcinomas
    - Sarcomas
    - Melanomas

Table 26 (Continued)

- Oral manifestations of systemic diseases
  - Gut
    - Deficiencies of vitamins/minerals
  - Blood
  - Skin
  - Others
- Drug-induced
  - Xerostomia
  - Ulcerations
  - Secondary infections

(e) Maturity (above 65 years)

- Congenital
  - Similar to those seen in infancy (in remission)
- Acquired
  - Trauma
    - Mechanical
      - Ulcerations induced by dentures
      - Friction cheek-biting
    - Burns
      - Chemical
    - Thermal
  - Cysts
    - Gingival
    - Periapical
  - Infections
    - Bacterial
      - Periodontitis
        - Associated with tooth loss
      - Tuberculosis
    - Viral
      - **Herpes zoster**
      - Herpetic stomatitis
        - Primary
        - Secondary
    - Fungal
      - **Candidiasis**
        - Acute
        - Chronic
      - Deep mycoses
  - Inflammatory
    - Cheilitis
      - Licking
      - Exfoliated
      - Angular cheilitis
      - **Actinic**
  - Immune-related
    - Lichen planus
  - Autoimmune disorders

Table 26 (Continued)

- **Bullous diseases**
- Sjogren's syndrome
- Potentially lesions
  - Leukoplakia
  - Erythroplakia
- Neoplasms
  - Benign
    - Fibromas
    - Denture-induced hyperplasia
  - Malignant
    - **Oral carcinomas**
    - Sarcomas
    - Melanomas

Table 26 (Continued)

- Oral manifestations of systemic diseases
  - Gut
    - Deficiencies of vitamins/minerals
  - Blood
  - Skin
  - Others
- **Drug-induced**
  - Xerostomia
  - Ulcerations
  - Secondary infections

Case 26.1

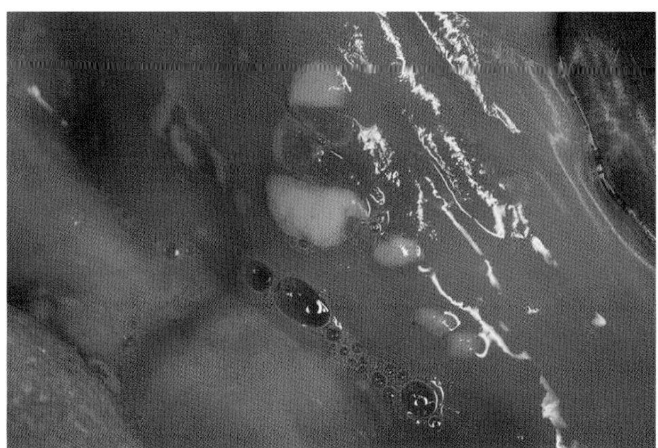

Figure 26.1

CO: A 10-month-old, male, healthy baby was referred by his mother for an examination of white deposits on the right and left buccal mucosae.

HPC: The white lesions had been present over the last two weeks without any suggestion of sensitivity, pain, fever or general symptomatology.

PMH: His medical, family, and dental history was irrelevant. This baby was born normally but prematurely, and kept for three weeks in an incubator. He was breastfed until the day of oral examination. His mother was a young, 27-year-old woman with no serious medical problems apart from a recent fungal infection of her nipples caused by an irritation from the baby's teeth.

OE: The intra-oral examination revealed whitish curd-like loosely adherent patches seen on both buccal mucosae, dorsum of the tongue, inner surface of the lower lip and soft palate (Figure 26.1). Despite his lack of cooperation during the examination, the white lesions were easily scrapable, leaving the erythematous area underneath. No other lesions were found inside his mouth or skin and his pediatrician's examination did not reveal any systemic diseases.

Q1 What is the diagnosis?

A White sponge nevus
B Acute pseudomembranous candidiasis
C Uremic stomatitis
D Milk remnants
E Chronic mucocutaneous candidiasis

Answers:

A No
B Acute pseudomembranous candidiasis is a common infection of babies, children, and older patients with systemic diseases. It is more common in males and is characterized by numerous white creamy sloughs which are easily removable with a wooden spatula, leaving erythematous and sometimes painful mucosa underneath.
C No
D No
E No

Comments: The acute onset of oral lesions and lack of nail, skin, and other mucosae involvement in this baby and among his close relatives excludes both chronic mucocutaneous candidiasis and white sponge nevus from diagnosis. The baby's good health and the scrapable white lesions also rule out the uremic stomatitis which is accompanied with well-fixed lesions and halitosis in chronic renal failure patients. Moreover, food and milk fragments are easily removable by rinsing the baby's mouth with water, but in contrast with the patient's lesions, they leave normal mucosa.

Q2 What was the cause of this baby's lesions?

- **A** Previous medications
- **B** Immune deficiencies
- **C** Parenteral nutrition
- **D** Mother's nipple infection
- **E** Vaginal delivery

Answers:

- **A** No
- **B** No
- **C** No
- **D** The infection of the baby's mother's nipples is the possible cause of *Candida* sp. transmission. The reason for this is that both the mother's nipple thrush and her baby's thrush occurred at the same time and his nutrition was based on breastfeeding and not on parenteral nutrition.
- **E** No

Comments: The type of delivery (vaginal) has been implicated in the transmission of *Candida* sp. from an infected mother to her newborn baby, but this is not the case as a fungal genital infection was not reported in his mother and his oral thrush should have appeared soon after birth. The lack of previous medications in the baby or his mother and the breastfeeding nutrition excludes medication and long parenteral nutrition as the possible causes of his thrush. The lack of other bacterial infections and good health status of the baby also exclude various congenital or acquired immunodeficiencies which can be easily identified with routine blood tests.

Q3 Which is the best treatment for this baby?

- **A** None
- **B** Gentian violet
- **C** Nystatin oral suspension
- **D** Fluconazole oral suspension
- **E** Ketoconazole tablets

Answers:

- **A** No
- **B** No
- **C** Nystatin oral suspension is the best treatment with minimal complications and interactions with other medications. It is useful for treating superficial oral and not blood-borne fungal infections, and it should be given in 2 ml of 100 000 units four times daily, for babies and infants, avoiding feeding for 5–10 minutes. When it comes to children and adults, the dose must be double and it should be also retained in the mouth as long as possible before swallowing.
- **D** No
- **E** No

Comments: The two weeks duration of the lesions require additional treatment for the baby and his mother and pediatrician. Gentian violet was used in the past to treat oral and nipple thrush, but it is avoided nowadays as it is toxic to the oral mucosa causing occasionally ulcerations and allergies. Fluconazole is the preferable drug in the cases of prevention and treatment of invasive candidal infections in high-risk babies (e.g. <28 weeks gestation or <1000 g weight) and is therefore the second choice for this baby, while ketoconazole use is contraindicated due to its severe hepatotoxicity.

Case 26.2

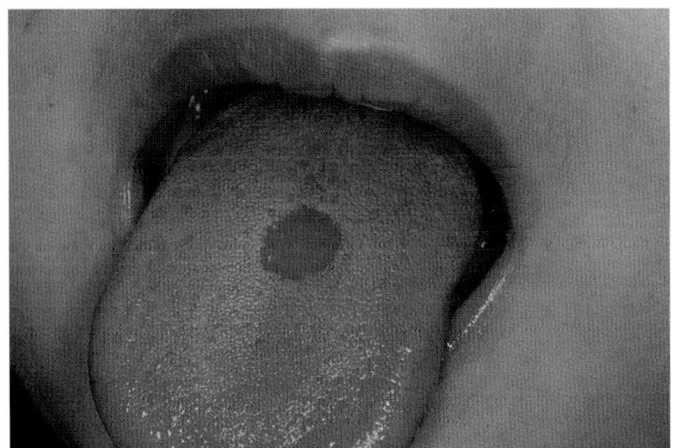

Figure 26.2

CO: A 12-month-old baby was referred by her pediatrician regarding of a red spot on the dorsum of her tongue.

HPC: The lesion was asymptomatic and discovered accidentally by her mother one day ago.

PMH: Her medical record and family was clear from any serious diseases. The baby was delivered on time with a Cesarean section and was breastfed up to six months, and she had recently started to chew chilled teething rings in order to relieve the pain caused from the eruption of her upper lateral incisors. Her mother had a normal pregnancy and the cesarean delivery was planned due to her very high myopia.

OE: The intra-oral examination revealed a round red area in the middle of the dorsum of tongue and in front of the geustic lambda. This red area showed a temporal loss of filiform papillae centrally with irregular white margins at the periphery. Its maximum diameter was almost 1 cm and did not bleed or cause pain and discomfort on examination. No other similar lesions were found in any other part of her mouth and other mucosa. Within the following five days, the lesion disappeared as it was covered with normal papillae.

Q1 What is the possible cause of baby's tongue lesion?
- **A** Trauma from chilled rings
- **B** Erythematous candidiasis
- **C** Median rhomboid glossitis
- **D** Geographic tongue
- **E** Atrophic glossitis induced by anemia

Answers:
- **A** No
- **B** No
- **C** Geographic tongue is the possible cause and characterized by erythematous atrophic areas with a loss of filiform papillae, being surrounded by the white circinate borders and by a tendency to change their size and shape and disappearing within the next hours or days.
- **D** No
- **E** No

Comments: Chilled rings can sometimes cause the loss of lingual papillae, but later on, this loss is restricted to the application area such as the anterior one and not in the back of tongue. Candidiasis causes pseudomembranous rather than erythematous, diffuse, infection in the baby's tongue, while the median rhomboid glossitis shows a more permanent rhomboid, lobular, red looking depapillated lesion; therefore, they should be excluded from diagnosis. On the other hand, anemia in babies rarely causes atrophy of lingual papillae, but is always accompanied with pale skin, poor feeding, and fast heart rate, features that are not seen in this baby.

Q2 Which is/are the clinical pattern(s) of this condition in infants?
- **A** Linear
- **B** Circulate
- **C** Rhomboid
- **D** Wavy
- **E** Spiral

Answers:
- **A** No
- **B** In a circulate pattern, the shape of the lesions remains the same and the tongue is gradually affected and subsequently heals over time.
- **C** No
- **D** In a wavy pattern, the loss of lingual papilla initially appears from a small area and is gradually extended like waves into the whole tongue.
- **E** In a spiral pattern, the lesions tend to be self-sustaining and will linger for a longer duration of time.

Comments: The lesions of geographic tongue never have a linear or rhomboid pattern.

Q3 What is/are the difference/s of a lingual papillitis from this condition?
- **A** Location of lesions
- **B** Clinical appearance of lesions
- **C** Type of lingual papillae involved
- **D** Onset
- **E** Symptomatology

Answers:
- **A** No
- **B** The lesions in geographic tongue are characterized by atrophic areas which are surrounded by hypertrophic white margins, while in papillitis they are characterized by localized or systemic nodules representing hyperplastic lingual papillae.
- **C** In geographic tongue, the main lingual papillae involved are filiform papillae while in papillomatosis, are fungiform papillae. Secondly, in geographic stomatitis, the red areas represent some local loss while the white margins show some hypertrophy of filiform papillae. While In lingual papillitis, the fungiform papillae are hyperplastic and appear in three variants; the localized, systemic, and papillokeratotic.
- **D** No
- **E** Lingual tonsillitis is accompanied with pain or burning sensation to such a degree that it affects eating, while the majority of geographic tongue lesions are asymptomatic.

Comments: Both conditions affect the dorsum of the tongue in patients, regardless their age or sex and have an acute transient onset.

Case 26.3

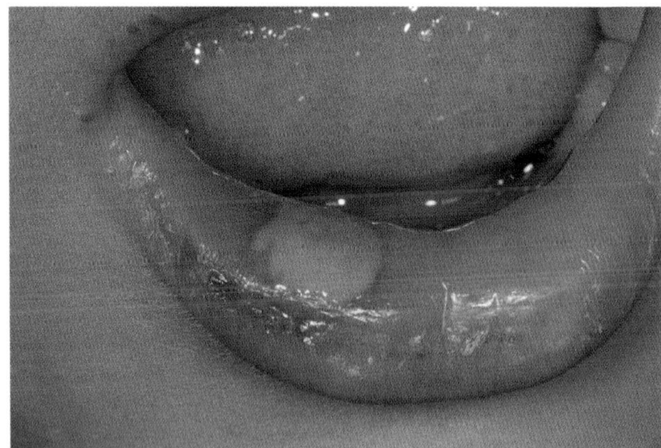

Figure 26.3

CO: A six-year-old, healthy boy showed up with a painful ulceration at the vermilion border of his lower lip.

HPC: The lesion appeared suddenly five days ago and reached its biggest size two days ago. A burning sensation preceded the ulcer appearance for two days.

PMH: His medical history did not reveal any blood, gut, and skin diseases or allergies, while recent trauma and drug use were not recorded. His father also reported similar mouth ulceration during his childhood that was completely gone at the age of 18 when he started smoking.

OE: A healthy young boy with a painful ulceration at the lower vermilion border close to the upper right lateral incisor and canine. The lesion was oval in shape, superficial, with a necrotic center and covered with fibrin with an erythematous zone at its periphery and measured 1 cm maximum diameter (Figure 26.3). No other similar lesions were found inside his mouth, skin, genitals or other mucosae. Cervical lymphadenopathy, general malaise or fever were not recorded. A similar episode of three small ulcerations, were reported by his parents, five months ago, but had healed within one week without any treatment.

Q1 What is the diagnosis?

- **A** Traumatic ulcer
- **B** Aphtha (minor)
- **C** Hand, foot and mouth (HFMD) disease
- **D** PFAPA syndrome (periodic fever, aphthous stomatitis, pharyngitis, adenitis)
- **E** Crohn's disease

Answers:

- **A** No
- **B** A single aphtha is the correct diagnosis and characterized by an oval superficial, painful ulceration covered with fibrinous slough and surrounded with soft, flat erythematous margins (halo), located on the vermilion border of the lower lip, having the possibility of recurrence and spontaneous healing over time.
- **C** No
- **D** No
- **E** No

Comments: The absence of a recent trauma in the area excludes traumatic ulcerations while the clinical characteristics of the lesion such as its place at the vermilion border and not on soft palate, the lack of periodic fever and general symptomatology, or the presence of other skin and not gut lesions exclude herpangina, PFAPA, and Crohn's disease from the diagnosis.

Q2 What is the best treatment for this child?

- **A** General measures (diet/toothpaste)
- **B** Systemic steroids
- **C** Local anesthetic
- **D** Local cauterization
- **E** Antiseptic/anti-inflammatory mouthwash

Answers:

- **A** Certain foods, nuts, chocolate, and fruits should be avoided as they may be implicated in prolonging the course of old aphthae and trigger the eruption of new ones. Dental care products containing sodium lauryl sulfate should be avoided as well.
- **B** No
- **C** Pain relief is very important and can be obtained using topical lidocaine as 2 per cent gel rather than spray or any solutions that can be applied on the lesion.
- **D** No
- **E** No

Comments: Systemic steroids are not used for the treatment of a single, short-lasting aphtha, but are mostly used for the rescue treatment of multiple, long-lasting ulcerations which inadequately respond to other therapies like colchicines, pentoxifylline, or dapsone. Mouthwashes with antiseptic, anti-inflammatory and analgesic effects are useful in the treatment of intra-oral aphthae but they have minimal effects on lip lesions. Additionally, local cauterization with hydrogen peroxide 0.5 per cent or silver nitrate 1–2 per cent solutions were widely used in the past, but have been withdrawn nowadays due to their risk of burning healthy tissues around the lesions.

Q3 Which of the clinical characteristics below differentiate other oral ulcerations from the patient's lesion?

- **A** Shape
- **B** Margins
- **C** Symptomatology
- **D** Course
- **E** Preceding lesions

Answers:

- **A** Oral aphthae like viral (herpetic) ulcerations have an oval, round symmetric shape in contrast with erythema multiforme, pemphigus or pemphigoid ulcerations that are irregular with a tension of expansion at the periphery.
- **B** In the majority of aphthae (minor; herpetiform), the margins are flat, soft and surrounded with an erythematous halo, but they can be indurated in long-lasting large aphthae and the aphthae like ulcerations of Crohn's disease. The erythematous halo is characteristically seen in oral aphthae, but not in other blood or skin lesions.
- **C** Mild pain or burning sensation is reported with minor aphthae and aphtae like ulcerations of various blood dyscrasias, more pain with larger aphthae and herpangina, while severe pain is characteristic of herpetiform aphthae, herpetic ulcerations and atypical lesions of HIV+ patients. None or minimal pain is reported in bacterial ulcerations like syphilis (chancre) or tuberculosis.
- **D** All aphthae, regardless of their type, can spontaneously heal and after a variable period of remission, they might recur with the same or worse severity. Herpetic ulcerations also recur, but with less severity while erythema multiforme appear again later but with the same severity. Malignant ulcerations do not heal or recur, but become worse and extend to the surrounding tissues or distant organs over time.
- **E** A mild burning or itching sensation precedes the aphthae, while vesicles or bullae appear before various viral infections and bullous disorders.

Case 26.4

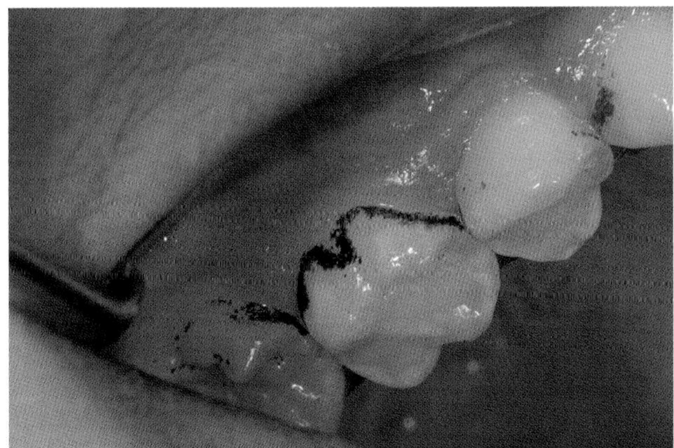

Figure 26.4

CO: A 7-year-old, healthy, boy was brought by his father for an evaluation of black discoloration of his teeth.

HPC: The discoloration was discovered three months ago and remained unchanged despite the intense toothbrushing by his parents.

PMH: His medical history did not reveal any serious diseases or drug use while his diet was high in sugar. He consumed colored candies or sweets on a daily basis but no presence of caries were reported.

OE: A black linear discoloration was found along the third cervical line of the buccal surface of his posterior teeth (upper > lower) of both sides and on the lingual surface of the anterior teeth (Figure 26.4). This discoloration was hard to wipe off by tooth brushing and was only removed with scaling, as it was not associated with caries and soft tissue discolorations inside his mouth, skin, and other mucosa. Oral hygiene was adequate too.

Q1 What is the cause of his teeth discoloration?

- **A** Cervical caries
- **B** Excessive use of chlorhexidine mouthwash
- **C** Medications
- **D** Pulp necrosis
- **E** Black stain

Answers:

- **A** No
- **B** No
- **C** No
- **D** No
- **E** Black tooth stain is the characteristic extrinsic black discoloration that occurs along the third cervical line of the buccal and/or lingual surfaces of primary

teeth mainly. These stains appear early on the tooth enamel at the age of two or three, causing parents' esthetic concerns and low confidence of the child.

Comments: Having in mind the negative medical and family history of this child and the fact that his teeth staining was external as it was easily removed with scaling, other internal staining can be easily excluded from the diagnosis. Pulp necrosis and severe thalassemia requiring chronic use of iron medications or regular blood transfusion lead to a diffuse rather than linear, non-removable, iron staining into hard dental tissues, are easily excluded too. The lack of cervical cavities or regular use of chlorhexidine mouth washes by the child rule these causes out from the diagnosis.

Q2 Which are the components of this black staining?
- **A** Food debris
- **B** Chromogenic bacteria
- **C** Iron salts
- **D** Dental plaque poor in calcium and phosphate
- **E** Fungal colonies

Answers:
- **A** No
- **B** Chromogenic bacteria like *Prevotella melaninogenica*, *P. intermedia* and *P. nigrescens*, together with *Porphyromonas gingivalis* and *Actinomycetes* play an important role in black stain.
- **C** Iron salts, mainly ferric sulfate, arise from the interaction of hydrogen sulfide produced by chromogenic bacteria, with iron found in salivary and gingival exudates.
- **D** No
- **E** No

Comments: Black staining is a special plaque stain where food debris and fungi do not play a special role.

Q3 Which is/are the cause/s of low susceptibility to caries of black teeth?
- **A** Low concentration of *Streptococcus mutans*
- **B** High concentration of *Lactobacillus acidophilus*
- **C** Diet poor in sugars
- **D** Adequate oral hygiene
- **E** High concentration of calcium and phosphorus in saliva and plaque of patients with black teeth

Answers:
- **A** No
- **B** No
- **C** No
- **D** Patients with black teeth try to remove the black staining from the surface of their teeth by rigorously brushing their teeth and eventually eliminating the accumulation of the pathogenic for caries bacteria there.
- **E** The black stain is a special plaque containing a high concentration of calcium and phosphorus minerals that play an important role in tooth remineralization.

Comments: The diet and saliva concentration of fluoride seem to be irrelevant with a low risk of caries in children with black teeth, as other factors such as the plaque composition of pathogenic bacteria play the crucial role. However, *Streptococcus* mutants and *Lactobacillus acidophilus* are Gram-positive bacteria that participate in tooth decay, but their concentration in the patients' oral cavity with black teeth is variable.

Case 26.5

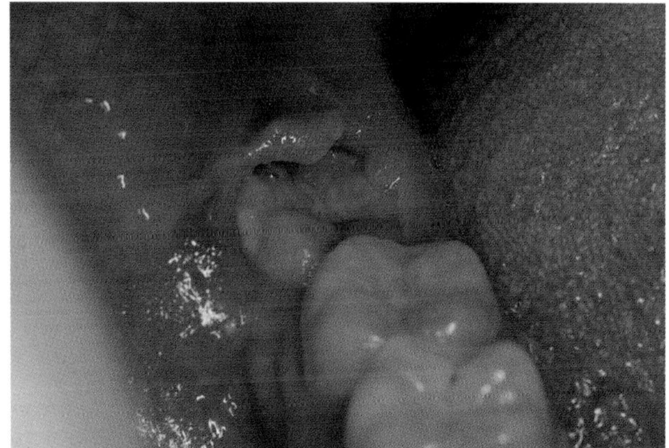

Figure 26.5

CO: A 17-year-old high school student presented with swelling and pain at the right side of his face and neck.

HPC: The pain was a dull and constant, arising from the lower right molars and reflected toward his right, ear but worsened with biting his teeth during eating. The pain started five days ago and was associated with trismus, facial swelling at the area of the angle of the mandibles, fever, and malaise.

PMH: His medical history was unremarkable and his diet was normal as he lives with his parents.

OE: The intra-oral examination revealed swollen, erythematous, painful gingivae around the crown of the partially erupted lower right third molar and pus was coming out with probing causing malodor (Figure 26.5). The adjacent molars were caries-free and his mouth opening was limited; inter-incisal distance was only about 20 mm (trismus). A facial swelling below and around the lower border and angle of the mandible was noted and was hot, soft with a red area centrally, but did not interfere with swallowing or breathing. Halitosis and an ipsilateral cervical lymphadenopathy was detected as well.

Q1 What is the cause of the pain?

- **A** Necrotizing gingivitis
- **B** Periapical infection of 3rd molar
- **C** Scurvy
- **D** Pericoronitis
- **E** Ludwig's angina

Answers:

- **A** No
- **B** No
- **C** No
- **D** Pericoronitis is an inflammation of the gingivae surrounding the crown of partially erupted or impacted third molars. This inflammation is caused by the accumulation of bacteria and food debris beneath the operculum leading to its enlargement to such a degree that it meets with the crowns of the opposite molars and becomes traumatized.
- **E** No

Comments: Halitosis is also found in necrotizing gingivitis and periapical abscess, but these diseases are easily excluded as the interdental papillae or pulp necrosis were not involved. Given that the inflammation was not so severe to affect swallowing or breathing and not extended to the floor of his mouth and upper neck, the risk of its being Ludwig's angina is rather minimized. His diet, high in vegetables and fruit, immediately excludes scurvy from the diagnosis.

Q2 Which of the factors below contribute to pericoronitis induced by an impacted third molar?

- **A** Poor oral hygiene
- **B** Immunodeficiencies
- **C** Uncontrolled diabetes mellitus
- **D** Trauma by opposing teeth
- **E** Eruption disturbance of impacted molar

Answers:

- **A** Poor oral hygiene allows the growth of a number of pathogenic bacteria that easily enter and grow within the gingivae around the crown of an impacted molar, thus causing pericoronitis.
- **B** Various immunodeficiencies cause a series of bacterial infections in the mouth and skin leading to pericoronitis, that is sometimes one of the first manifestations of these diseases.
- **C** Uncontrolled diabetes mellitus patients appear to be more susceptible to pericoronitis, facial cellulitis and deep neck infections developed from odontogenic infections from the impacted wisdom teeth.
- **D** Opposing teeth cause local trauma of the gingivae surrounding the wisdom teeth, the gingivae of which become inflamed and swollen as well as bleeding on probing.
- **E** The mesial, distal, buccal, or lingual orientation of the third wisdom teeth allows the accumulation of food debris and dental plaque, providing a suitable environment for the growth of various anaerobic bacteria, capable of inducing pericoronitis.

Q3 What is/are the most serious complication/s of this condition?

- **A** Osteomyelitis of the mandible
- **B** Periodontal abscess
- **C** Bacteremia
- **D** Trismus
- **E** Caries

Answers:

- **A** No
- **B** No
- **C** Dental procedures like scaling and cleaning the infected operculum or even extraction of the inflamed wisdom tooth causes immediate bacteremia from anaerobic bacteria like *Prevotella*, *Mycobacterium* and *Peptostreptococcus*, as well as aerobic *Streptococcus* and *Staphylococcus* species that are capable of being transferred to distant organs like the heart, lungs, and spine, causing a secondary infection. Infective endocarditis is the most characteristic complication of bacteremia.
- **D** No
- **E** No. Extensive.

Comments: Extensive caries induce caries, acute or chronic inflammation of peri-apical and odontal tissues leading into trismus and sometimes in severe infection of the alveolar bone (Osteomyelitis) but none of them could jeopardize patient's life. Trismus or jawlock is characterized by inflammation of the masticatory muscles arising from wisdom tooth infection. This inflammation causes muscle contraction and mouth opening restriction, with serious eating, swallowing or speaking problems. Osteomyelitis is an infection of the extremities, spine and pelvis and rarely of the jaws. Chronic osteomyelitis or Garré's osteomyelitis is a chronic non-suppurative sclerotic bone inflammation, but is seen in the area of the first rather than the third molar, with a characteristic onion skin appearance on X-ray.

Case 26.6

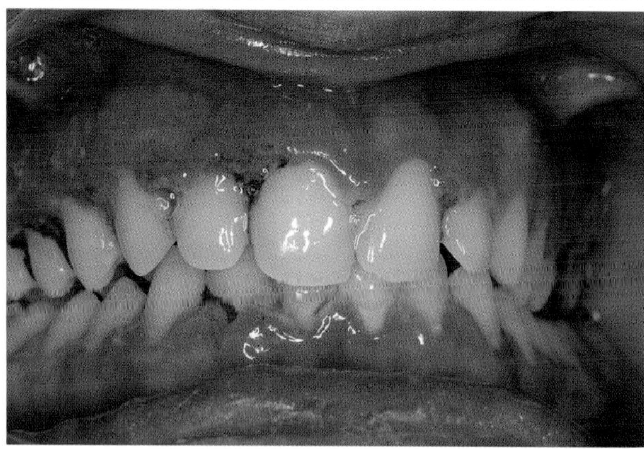

Figure 26.6

CO: A 18-year-old girl was presented with some pain from her gingivae.

HPC: The problem started one week ago with an acute, sharp, throbbing pain arising from the lower anterior gingivae, but was gradually extended to all her gingivae, causing her general upset and problems during brushing her teeth or eating.

PMH: Her medical and family history were clear from any serious diseases, allergies or drug use. Her diet was poor in vegetables and fruits but rich in fats, and her smoking was up to 10 cigarettes per day.

OE: The intra-oral examination revealed erythematous, swollen gingivae with necrosis of the inter-dental papillae, especially at the anterior upper and lower teeth. The gingivae were very sensitive and easily bled with probing, while their necrotic interdental papillae were covered with white-yellowish fibrinous slough (Figure 26.6). Her oral hygiene was poor due to the patient's difficulty to brush her teeth properly, thus leading to marked malodor. A mild erythema with a few superficial ulcerations on the buccal mucosae close to the infected gingivae was recorded while cervical lymphadenopathy was detected and associated with general symptoms like malaise, fever ($<38^{\circ}$C). A similar condition was recorded in her boyfriend's mouth three weeks ago, which responded well to a broad range of antibiotic uptake.

Q1 What is her gingival problem?

- **A** Gingivitis
- **B** Desquamative gingivitis due to lichen planus
- **C** Necrotizing gingivitis
- **D** Primary herpetic stomatitis
- **E** Necrotizing stomatitis

Answers:

- **A** No
- **B** No
- **C** No
- **D** No
- **E** Necrotizing stomatitis is the answer. This condition is characterized by acute gingival inflammation with necrotic inter-dental papillae being associated with superficial ulcerations, severe halitosis and general yet mild symptomatology. It is an infection from anaerobic bacteria, particularly fusobacteria and spirochetes, in patients with poor oral hygiene, smoking habits, poor nutrition, stress or a weak immune system.

Comments: Gingivitis is a common infection of the gingivae which is mostly found among young people, but is not associated with interdental necrosis, pain and halitosis as it is seen in this patient. Desquamative gingivitis is not the cause, as it affects older patients and is characterized by desquamation, erythema involving free and attached gingivae, and not restricted to interdental papillae. This desquamation associated with white striated lesions in lichen planus or with bullae in bullous disorders. The presence of superficial oral ulcerations together with interdental necrosis allows the diagnosis of necrotizing stomatitis rather than gingiviitis.

Q2 Which is the most common necrotizing lesion in the mouth?

- **A** Giant cell arteritis
- **B** Noma (cancrum oris)
- **C** Gangrenous leukemic ulceration
- **D** Sialometaplasia
- **E** Actinomycosis

Answers:

- **A** No
- **B** No
- **C** No
- **D** Necrotizing sialometaplasia is the most common oral necrotizing lesion in humans, and is mainly seen at the junction of the hard and soft palate. Local trauma, anesthesia, alcohol overuse or smoking and vascular diseases play a causative role. Initially the ischemic necrosis of the lobules of the affected minor salivary glands leads to an erythematous swelling which eventually centrally ulcerated, and can spontaneously heal within four to six weeks.
- **E** No

Comments: All the other necrotizing ulcerations are also seen in human mouth but are rather rare, as they are only seen in certain groups such as in patients with vasculitis (giant cell arteritis); malignancies (leukemic gangrenous ulceration) and immunodeficiencies (noma and actinomycosis).

Q3 What is/are the differences between this gingival condition and cancrum oris?

- **A** Incidence
- **B** Geographic distribution
- **C** Oral involvement
- **D** Disease complications
- **E** Prevention

Answers:

- **A** Necrotizing gingivitis (NG) appears in a number of young smokers with poor oral hygiene and an unhealthy diet, while noma is less common and noticed in patients with malnutrition, poor oral hygiene and severe immunodeficiencies.
- **B** Noma is mainly found in Africa countries, while NG can be seen all over the world.
- **C** The NG lesions are restricted to gingivae causing necrosis of the tip of interdental papillae, while noma is a devastating disease that leads to severe tissue massive necrosis, moving from the inside to the outside, often involving major portions of the face and not only the gingivae.
- **D** Untreated NG can initially lead to a progressive loss of alveolar bone known as necrotizing periodontitis or in more severe cases, orofacial destruction as is seen in noma. Noma can lead to facial disfiguration or even death.
- **E** No

Comments: Both diseases are preventable by educating the young patients into improving their oral hygiene, reducing or stopping hazardous habits like smoking or drinking, as well as reducing the risk of various diseases with vaccination like measles, and HIV by following safe sex instructions.

Case 26.7

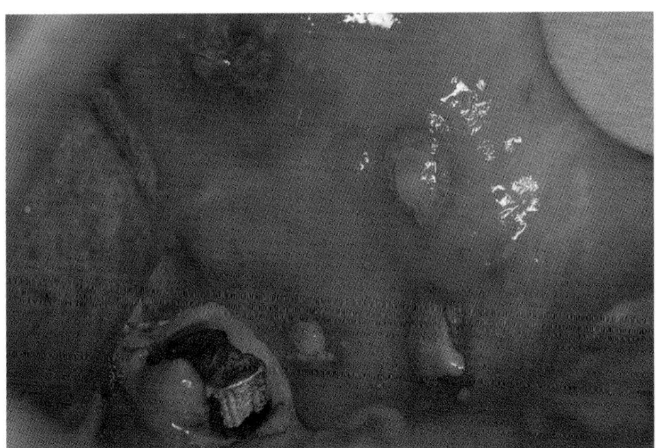

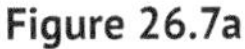

Figure 26.7a

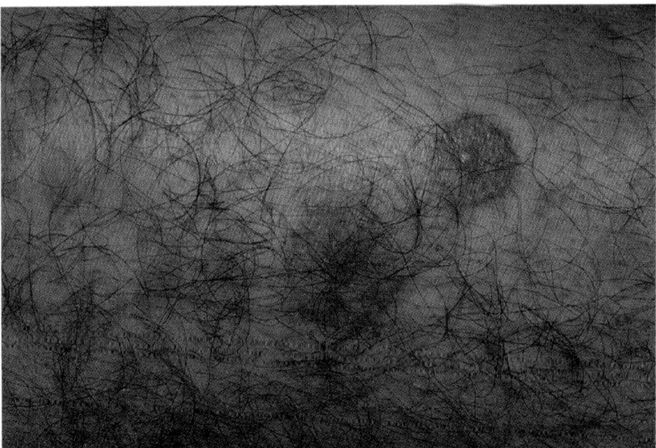

Figure 26.7b

CO: A 19 year old man presented with multiple oral lesions and skin exanthema which had occurred over the last week.

HPC: The lesions initially appeared as an itchy red skin rash with a purple-gray center, target like lesions which were symmetrically located on his legs preceding the oral and genital ulcerations.

PMH: His medical history was clear from any serious diseases apart from a few recurrent episodes of herpes labialis, the frequency of which was increased over the last year. Two other episodes with similar oral and genital ulcerations were recorded over the last year, but were less severe and spontaneously resolved within 10–12 days. Both episodes happened after a flu-like infection with sore throat.

OE: The intra-oral examination revealed numerous, superficial erythematous plaques intermingled with painful superficial bullae and erosions (Figure 26.7a). The lesions were more prominent on buccal and tongue mucosae and less on the floor of his mouth, palate and vermilion borders of the lips. Numerous target like-lesions were found on the skin of his legs where pigmented marks from previous healing ulcers were seen (Figure 26.7b). An erythema with superficial erosion on the tip of his penis was found, but disappeared within the next three days after the examination. Finally, cervical lymphadenopathy, fever and other general symptomatology were not recorded.

Q1 What is the possible diagnosis?

- **A** Herpetic stomatitis
- **B** Actinic prurigo
- **C** Erythema multiforme
- **D** Syphilis (second stage)
- **E** Adamantiades-Behcet's syndrome

Answers:

- **A** No
- **B** No
- **C** Erythema multiforme (major) is the correct diagnosis. This condition is characterized by an acute, self-limited, recurrent episode of oral, genital, and skin ulcerations due to an IV hypersensitive reaction associated with certain bacterial, viral, fungal infections, medications and other various trigger factors like diseases, vaccinations, contactants, and flavors.
- **D** No
- **E** No

Comments: The presence of general symptomatology such as fever, general malaise and cervical lymphadenopathy is a characteristic finding of primary herpetic stomatitis and not of erythema multiforme. In erythema multiforme and Adamantiades Behcet's disease, the lesions appear with the same severity in contrast to the secondary herpetic infections, the lesions of which have less severity being restricted to the lips or inside of the mouth. As opposed to the erythema multiforme, the ulcerations of Adamantiades Behcet are similar in severity but surrounded by an erythematous halo involving of a number of organs. What is more, the secondary lesions of syphilis sometimes resemble those of multiple erythema, but differ as they are usually asymptomatic and always associated with local or systemic lymphadenopathy. The itchy and ulcerated lesions of the patient's legs resemble actinic prurigo, but in the latter the lesions are always associated with solar exposure along with serious lip involvement.

Q2 Which of the pathogenic viruses below is the most common trigger factor for erythema multiforme?

- **A** Herpes 1 or 2
- **B** Adenoviruses
- **C** Epstein-Barr virus
- **D** Coxsackie virus B5
- **E** Measles virus

Answers:

- **A** Human herpes simplex virus 1 (HSV-1) and to a lesser extent herpes 2 (HSV-2) are factors that are implicated in the development in the majority of erythema multiforme, via a mechanism of autoimmune cross-reactivity in which a major role of 180 kDa bullous pemphigoid antigen is suspected.
- **B** No
- **C** No
- **D** No
- **E** No

Comments: All the above viruses have been implicated in the pathogenesis of erythema multiforme, but to a less degree.

Q3 Although Stevens Johnson syndrome (SJS) and toxic epidermal necrolysis (TEN) are both types of the same condition, they differ in:

- **A** Frequency
- **B** Prodromal signs
- **C** Pathogenesis
- **D** Body distribution
- **E** Treatment response

Answers:

- **A** SJS seems to be more common than TEN, as 1.2 to 6.0 cases in million people per year suffer from SJS, while 0.4 to 1.2 cases suffer from TEN.
- **B** No
- **C** Although both conditions are the result of a hypersensitivity reaction to various drugs, SJS is additionally triggered by viruses like herpes 1 or 2 and bacteria like *Mycoplasma*.
- **D** The SJS affects only the 10 per cent of the body surface, while the TEN is more serious and affects more than 30 per cent of the body.
- **E** No

Comments: Both conditions start with persistent fever and flu-like symptoms, before skin and oral mucosa lesions appear. These lesions respond well to cyclosporine, early pulse corticosteroid therapy, and plasma exchange as well as immune globulin application.

Case 26.8

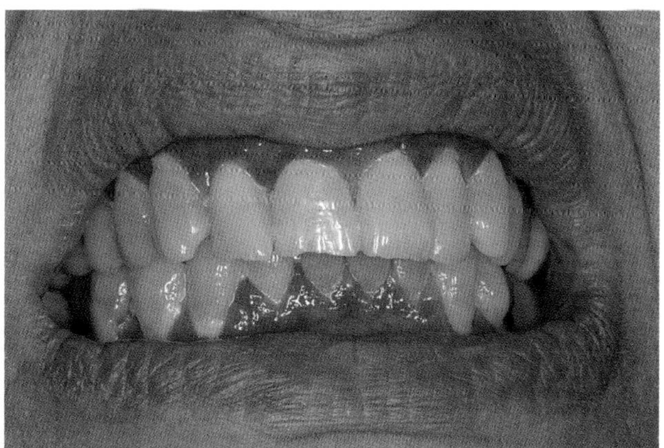

Figure 26.8

CO: A 56-year-old woman was presented with erythematous gingivae.

HPC: Her gingivae had been swollen and erythematous over the last six months. In the beginning, the anterior upper and lower gingivae were fragile and showed evidence of small areas of desquamation which were finally extended to the whole free and attached gingivae, with periods of exacerbation and remission.

PMH: Her medical and personal history did not reveal any serious diseases, drug use or habits like smoking or self-induced gingival picking.

OE: The intra-oral examination revealed diffuse erythema and desquamation of both free and attached gingivae, mainly of her anterior teeth (Figure 26.8). The affected gingivae had lost their stripping, but had a granular surface, were fragile and with some slight pressure they tended to exfoliate (Nikolsky phenomenon positive) regardless or not of plaque accumulation. No other lesions were found apart from a few superficial ulcerations on both buccal mucosae, causing her a burning sensation with the intake of acids foods/drinks. Other mucosae (eyes and genitals) and skin were unaffected. Finally, the gingival biopsy revealed a subepithelial clefting with scattered mixed chronic inflammatory reaction to the underlying corium, and deposition of granular IgG immunoglobulin along the basement membrane with indirect immunofluorescence (IDIF).

Q1 What is the cause of gingival desquamation?

- **A** Strawberry gingivitis
- **B** Periodontitis
- **C** Plasma cell gingivitis
- **D** Erythroplakia
- **E** Benign mucous membrane pemphigoid

Answers:

- **A** No
- **B** No
- **C** No
- **D** No
- **E** Benign mucous membrane pemphigoid is a rare autoimmune blistering disease that is characterized by desquamative gingivitis, erosions and superficial blisters in the oral mucosae, eyes, genitals and anus rather than skin. Moreover, a repeated corneal involvement may cause scarring that finally leads to blindness.

Comments: The clinical characteristics such as the location of erythema on free and attached gingivae excludes gingivitis and periodontitis from the diagnosis. The histological characteristics such as the presence of subepithelial clefting and not epithelial dysplasia, as well as the presence of a diffuse and not a perivascular infiltration of mixed chronic inflammatory cells, and not plasma cells, rules out a diagnosis of erythroplakia or strawberry gingivitis respectively.

Q2 Which of the bullous diseases below do not or rarely affect the oral mucosa?

- **A** Pemphigus foliaceus
- **B** Paraneoplastic pemphigus
- **C** Bullous pemphigoid
- **D** Hailey-Hailey disease
- **E** Linear IgA dermatosis

Answers:

- **A** Pemphigus foliaceus is characterized by crusty sores on the scalp, chest back, and face, but never inside the mouth.
- **B** No
- **C** Bullous pemphigoid is characterized by large bullae on the flexor surfaces of the skin, like the upper abdomen, thighs or armpits, and rarely oral and other mucosae (<30–40%).
- **D** Hailey disease is a rare genetic familiar pemphigus characterized by blisters and erosions on the neck, skin folds and genitals, but rarely on the oral mucosa.
- **E** No

Comments: Paraneoplastic pemphigus and linear IgA dermatosis are two different bullous disorders with different pathogenesis, but both affect the oral mucosa in the majority of their cases.

Q3 Which other diseases have IgG depositions along the basement membrane zone in IDIF?
- **A** Pemphigus vulgaris
- **B** Bullous pemphigoid
- **C** Epidermolysis bullosa acquisita
- **D** Dermatitis herpetiformis
- **E** Linear IgA dermatosis

Answers:
- **A** No
- **B** Bullous pemphigoid is characterized by deposition of C3 or IgG or both along the basement membrane zone where C3 is superior to IgG in intensity.
- **C** In epidermolysis bullosa acquisita, an intense deposition of IgG rather than IgA or C3 complement is consistently present.
- **D** No
- **E** No

Comments: In dermatitis herpetiformis and linear IgA diseases, the immunoglobulin deposition along the basement membrane zone is IgA and not IgG, while in pemphigus vulgaris, the deposition of IgG and C3 was intercellular and mainly in the lower epithelial layers and not along the basement membrane zone.

Case 26.9

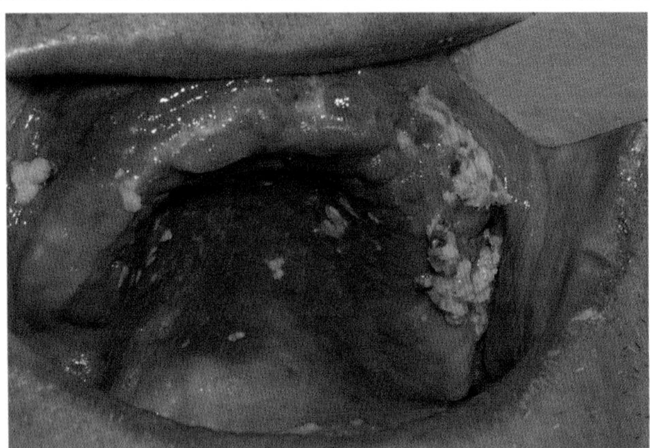

Figure 26.9

CO: A 62-year-old, overweight woman was complaining about a burning sensation in her mouth.

HPC: Her burning sensation had been present over the last four years, but had worsened over the last month after a course of antibiotic uptake for a respiratory infection.

PMH: Her medical history revealed diabetes insipidus which was partially controlled with metformin and hypercholesterolemia with statin tablets. Her diet was inappropriate and her smoking habit was stable up to a packet of cigarettes daily.

OE: The physical examination revealed an overweight woman with a diffuse erythema on her palatal mucosa. The erythema was diffuse and in places granular and sensitive in touching; it was also restricted to the area underneath her upper denture (Figure 26.9). The denture was old, dirty from smoking and food stains and did not fit properly, leaving a great number of food remnants underneath. The corners of her mouth were cracked and inflamed, but no other lesions were found despite her poor oral hygiene.

Q1 What is the diagnosis?
- **A** B12 deficiency
- **B** Denture-induced stomatitis
- **C** Allergic stomatitis
- **D** Nicotinic stomatitis
- **E** Thrombocytopenic purpura

Answers:
- **A** No
- **B** Denture-induced stomatitis is a common oral condition characterized by a mild inflammation and redness of the oral mucosa that mostly occurs in elderly people who constantly wear a full upper denture. *Candida* species are involved in about 90 per cent of the cases, and may be clinically seen as pinpoint hyperemia, diffuse erythematous, granular or papillary lesions on palatal surface.
- **C** No
- **D** No
- **E** No

Comments: Other diseases may cause diffuse or discrete palatal erythema, but have different clinical manifestations like numerous small single or multiple erythematous hemorrhagic lesions like petechiae, ecchymosis, blisters (thrombocytopenic purpura) or diffuse erythema and superficial ulcerations (allergic stomatitis) together with atrophic glossitis (B12 deficiency) or even a combination of red spots with white plaque lesions (nicotinic stomatitis).

Q2 Which of the factors below play a significant role in the development of this condition in this lady?
- **A** Affinity of *Candida* to acrylic dentures
- **B** Saliva underneath dentures
- **C** Inadequate oral hygiene
- **D** Smoking
- **E** Steroid inhaler use

Answers:
- **A** *Candida albicans* has a high affinity to attach and grow in acrylic dentures. The number of *Candida* seems to be dependent on the presence of roughness or instability of old ill fitted dentures, and the type of acrylic resin used for their construction.
- **B** The accumulated saliva underneath an upper denture allows the growth of various pathogenic bacteria and fungi responsible for inflammation there. This inflammation is reinforced by the lack of saliva cleaning (flushing) action of food debris from the area, and the lack of palatal microflora exposure to various salivary antimicrobial enzymes due to denture cover.
- **C** Inadequate oral hygiene permits the accumulation of dental plaque and food debris underneath the dentures. During eating procedures and when food debris is hard in consistency, it can traumatize the palatal mucosa where debris can easily degrade and release minerals and substances necessary for the growth of pathogenic microflora. These germs are responsible for the palatal inflammation seen in patients who wear ill-fitting dentures.
- **D** No
- **E** No

Comments: Although the local application of drugs like steroids in creams or inhalers alter the local immunity and microflora, and smoking causes xerostomia and vasoconstriction, exacerbation of pathogenic immune responses and in attenuation of defensive immunity, their participation in denture-induced stomatitis is doubtful as the palatal mucosa is covered with the denture and is therefore protected from smoking or steroids inhaler side-effects.

Q3 The antifungal action of fluconazole is based on:
- **A** Inhibition of nucleic acid synthesis of fungi
- **B** Inhibition of ergosterol pathways on the fungal membrane
- **C** Disrupting membrane integrity by binding to ergosterol
- **D** Altering membrane integrity by binding to non-sterol lipids
- **E** Inhibiting glucan–biosynthesis pathways

Answers:
- **A** No
- **B** Azoles like fluconazole inhibit the synthesis of ergosterol in the endoplasmic reticulum of the fungal cell.
- **C** No
- **D** No
- **E** No

Comments: Some antifungal drugs act by altering the structure of the fungal cell membrane by binding with ergosterol (like nystatin) or with non-sterol lipids (like sertaconazole), or they inhibit the glucan biosynthesis (like endocardins), while in others, flucytosine is converted within the fungal cell to 5-fluorouracil, that inhibits fungal DNA synthesis.

Case 26.10

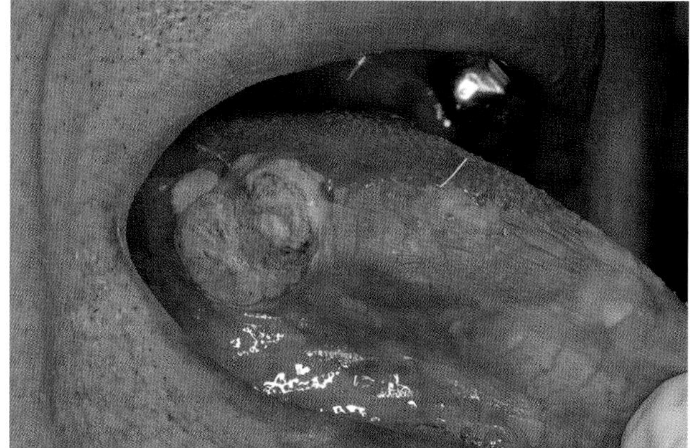

Figure 26.10

CO: A 72-year-old man presented with an asymptomatic lump on the right lateral border of his tongue.

HPC: The lump was discovered accidentally by the patient one month ago in an attempt to wear his lower partial denture. As the lesion was asymptomatic, it did not cause him any concern, despite the fact that there was an extensive white plaque covering the lateral tongue border which showed a mild dysplasia in a biopsy taken four years ago.

PMH: His medical and family history was unremarkable in relation to the lesion, but his personal history revealed daily smoking of one packet of cigarettes for more than forty years and drinking of wine and other heavy spirits on a regular basis.

OE: The oral examination revealed a white plaque on the whole right border of his tongue. The white plaque was in places superficial and smooth, while some furrows had a rough surface and an overgrowth with irregular margins at the posterior part, close to the lingual tonsils (Figure 26.10). The growth was an exophytic, hard in consistency, painless lesion with a maximum diameter of 2.5 cm and well-fixed into the underlying muscles, causing mild restrictions of tongue movements. The lesion was found close to a broken clasp of his lower denture. No other lesions were found apart from a large ipsilateral submandibular lymph node which was well-fixed into the surrounding neck tissues.

Q1 What is the lesion?

- **A** Chronic traumatic ulcer from a broken cusp
- **B** Large aphtha
- **C** Oral carcinoma
- **D** Tongue abscess
- **E** Verrucous leukoplakia

Answers:

- **A** No
- **B** No
- **C** Oral carcinoma is the lesion. It is the most common oral malignant neoplasm among chronic smokers and/or drinkers, and appears as a chronic ulceration with irregular margins, white or red plaques or even growths, which are well-fixed with the underlying tissues and often associated with lymph node metastasis. The tumor is initially asymptomatic, but gradually extends to the surrounding tissues, especially the nerves and blood vessels, causing paresthesia, pain, and bleeding respectively, finally resulting in local or distant metastasis.
- **D** No
- **E** No

Comments: Other tongue lesions like large aphthae, traumatic hyperplastic ulcers, and soft tissues abscesses are easily excluded from the diagnosis based on the patient's age, lack of pain and hard or fluctuant consistency of the lesion. Aphthae of all types are common in young patients; pain accompanies traumatic and aphthous ulcerations and in soft tissues abscesses, the consistency is soft or fluctuant while in verrucous leucoplakia neck metastasis is extremely.

Q2 Which is the best first choice treatment for this patient?

- **A** Surgical excision of the tongue lesion only
- **B** Chemotherapy
- **C** Immunotherapy
- **D** Cyber knife radiotherapy
- **E** Partial glossectomy and neck dissection

Answers:

- **A** No.
- **B** No
- **C** No
- **D** No
- **E** Partial glossectomy is the removal of part of the tongue, in order for the margins of the excised tumor to become clear of at least 1 cm at all directions. This surgery should be followed by the removal of the neck lymph nodes (neck dissection). The type of dissection such as a radical, modified or selective one, is dependent on the clinical and CT or MRI neck findings.

Comments: Simple tumor excision is not adequate as it does not deal with his neck metastasis, while chemotherapy or immunotherapy alone are not as effective for oral cancer as surgery. Cyber knife radiotherapy is effective but very expensive and should be only recommended for the tumors that are not accessible for surgery or as second choice treatment where other previous treatments have failed.

Q3 Which of the complications below have been associated with partial glossectomy?

- **A** Lingual nerve injury
- **B** Tongue bleeding
- **C** Bell's palsy
- **D** Loss of taste
- **E** Xerostomia

Answers:

- **A** This surgery can injure the lingual nerve during the tumor removal and appear as a temporal numbness of the ipsilateral lingual surface of gingivae tongue, and lip.

B Trauma of the lingual artery during or within the first week of glossectomy is common. Mild bleeding is normally seen in patients within the first days of surgery and controlled with local procedures, but excessive bleeding causes tongue swelling, and breathing difficulties. Therefore, the patient should be admitted immediately to hospital in order to get the hematomas removed and control hemorrhage.

C No

D No

E No

Comments: Bell's palsy is a common complication of surgery for the removal a tumor from the parotid gland and not from the tongue, that results in an inability to control the facial muscles of the affected side. Xerostomia and loss of taste are not reported after glossectomy as there are a great number of remaining normal salivary glands and taste buds. Chemotherapy and radiotherapy for head and neck cancer increase the apoptotic rate of taste buds and the atrophy of salivary gland acini, leading to a loss of taste and xerostomia for many months.

27

Clinical Tests, Signs and Phenomena

Clinicians must have an adequate knowledge of medical phenomena and clinical tests in order to understand various diseases and provide their best possible treatment.

Medical phenomena are defined by any sign or objective symptom; any observable occurrence or fact. In the field of oral medicine and dermatology, this term has been applied to several peculiar clinical occurrences or laboratory observations. The phenomena are described in three broad categories, namely, those based on clinical, laboratory, and histopathological observations. On the other hand, signs only refer to important physical findings on observation made by the clinician during his patient's examination, while the clinical tests are designed to identify all patients with the disease or those who are disease free (See Figure 27.0a–c).

Table 27 lists the most important clinical tests that can be used to confirm various objective symptoms and signs of oral/skin diseases, giving emphasis on characteristic clinical phenomena.

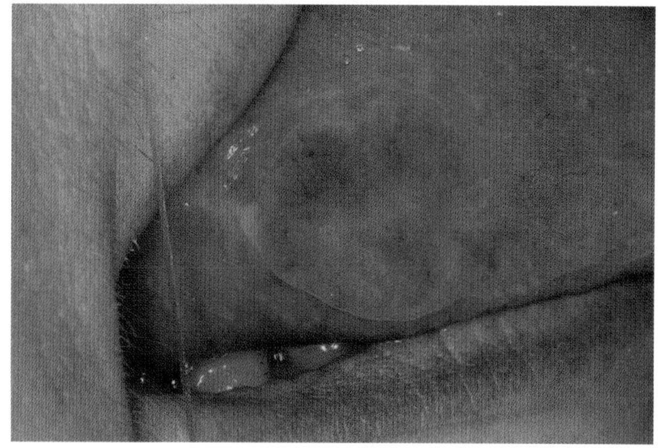

Figure 27.0b Clinical (bleaching) test to confirm a vascular lesion.

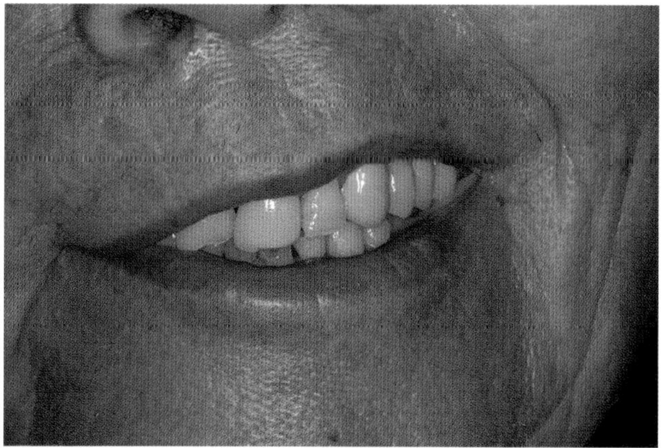

Figure 27.0a Clinical sign of facial muscle palsy (incomplete smile).

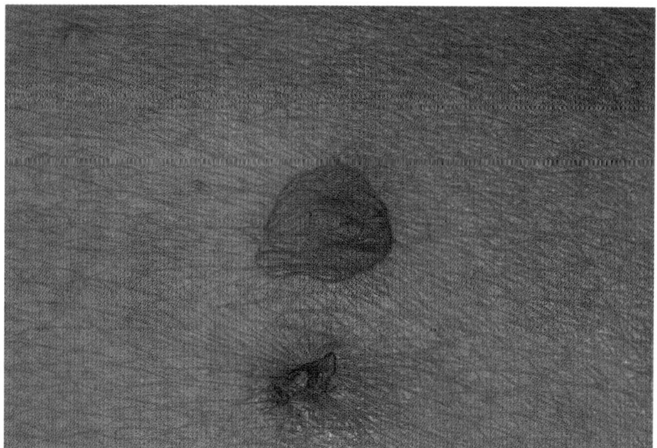

Figure 27.0c Koebner phenomenon in bullous dermatoses.

Clinical Guide to Oral Diseases, First Edition. Dimitris Malamos and Crispian Scully.

Companion website: www.wiley.com/go/malamos/clinical_guide

Table 27 Clinical tests, signs, and phenomena commonly seen in oral medicine patients.

Clinical tests		
Tests to confirm or not a sign of	**Clinical findings**	**Diseases**
Dryness	Sticky mucosa Frothy saliva Lobulated tongue	Sjogren's syndrome Drug-induced
Halitosis	Breathing patient's expired air	Necrotizing gingivitis (NG) Neglected mouth
Lesions – white	Removal or not with scrubbing	Candidiasis vs. leukoplakia
Lesions – pigmented	Bleach or not with glass slide	Vascular vs. pigmented lesions
Oroantral communication	Frothy saliva from the socket Characteristic noise induced by inflating patient's cheeks	Complications with antrum after upper molar surgery
Paralysis of facial muscles	Inability to: close both eyes smile whistle wrinkle forhead	Facial palsy
Localized sweating	Iodine positive stain of the starch applied on the affected skin	Frey's syndrome

Clinical signs		
Name	**Clinical findings**	**Diseases**
Asboe-Hansen sign	Blister spreading with pressure	Pemphigus, bullous pemphigoid
Auspitz sign	Pin-point bleeding after removal of scales	Psoriasis
Barnett's sign	Ridging and tightening of neck	Scleroderma
Buttonhole sign	Invagination of neurofibromas with pressure	Neurofibromatosis-NF1
Crowe's sign	Axillary freckles	Neurofibromatosis-NF1
Forchheimer's sign	Petechiae or enanthema on soft palate	Infectious mononucleosis; rubella
Gorlin's sign	Tongue touching the nose	Ehlers-Danlos syndrome
Meffert's sign	Ectopic sebaceous glands on lips causing a lipstick-like mark left on the rim of a glass mug after consuming a hot beverage	Fordyce disease
Nikolsky's sign	Peeling and new bullae formation with rubbing off the unaffected skin or oral mucosa	Pemphigus
Reverse Nikolsky's sign	Pseudoepithelial peeling	Toxic epidermal necrolysis; staphylococcal scaled skin
Osler's sign	Blue-black sclera	Alkaptonuria
Stafne's sign	Widening of the periodontal ligament space	Systemic sclerosis

Table 27 (Continued)

Clinical phenomena		
Name	**Clinical findings**	**Diseases**
Bell's phenomenon	Inability to close the affected eye	Facial nerve palsy
Brocq's phenomenon	Subepidermal hemorrhage, which occurs on careful scraping of a classical lesion of skin disease	Lichen planus
Isotopic phenomenon	Occurrence of a different or unrelated dermatological disease at the site of the healed disease (commonly herpes zoster)	Herpes zoster
Kasabach-Merrit phenomenon	Triad of vascular tumors, thrombocytopenia, and bleeding diathesis.	Infantile hemangiomas, Blue rubber bleb nevus
Koebner phenomenon	Development a new similar lesions along lines of trauma	Psoriasis, lichen planus, vitiligo
Koebner inverse phenomenon	A skin condition which inhibits the development of another autoimmune disease	Psoriasis and alopecia areata
Koebner remote reverse phenomenon	Spontaneous repigmentation is seen in distant patches after autologous skin graft surgery	Vitiligo
Koebner reverse phenomenon	Clearance of an area of skin disease after trauma	Psoriasis
Pathergy phenomenon	An erythematous papule of more than 2 mm at the site of a non-specific trauma like pricking with a 20–22-gauge needle	Behcet's disease, Sweet's syndrome
Raynaud's phenomenon	Episodic changes in blood flow in the cutaneous vasculature in cold weather	Connective tissue diseases, Sjogren's syndrome
Rebound phenomenon	Reappearance of a skin disease after stopping steroid treatment	Various dermatosis

Case 27.1

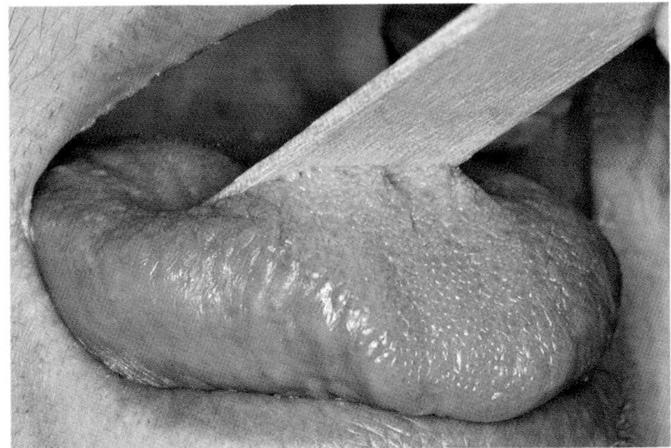

Figure 27.1a

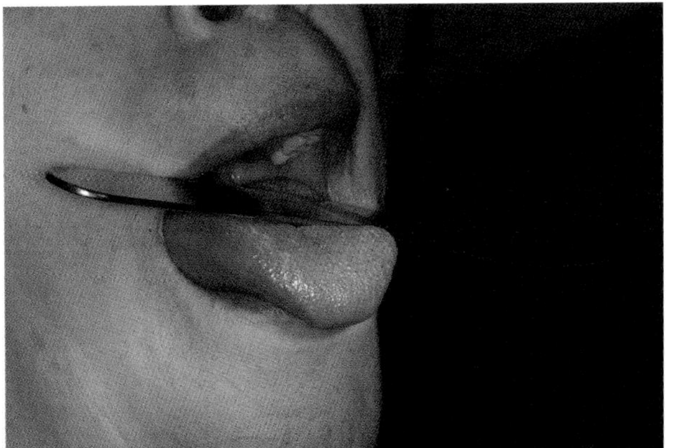

Figure 27.1b

CO: A 72-year-old woman presented with severe xerostomia over a couple of months' duration.

HPC: Her xerostomia was more prominent at night and early mornings, but was improved gradually during the daytime by drinking more than 10 glasses of water.

PMH: From her medical records, a mild hypertension and hypercholesterolemia were reported and controlled with irbesartan and statins while on the other hand, a cervical cancer was also diagnosed when she was 70 years old. She had a total hysterectomy and since then, she has been complaining about urine incontinence problems which were partially improved with a muscarin antagonistic (solifenacin). Other serious diseases including respiratory, endocrinal, and connective tissues were not reported.

OE: The oral examination did not reveal any oral lesions apart from severe xerostomia. This was demonstrated by the difficult detachment of a wood spatula of the dorsum of the tongue (Figure 27.1a) and by the balance of a heavy metallic spatula there (Figure 27.1b). The xerostomia caused difficulties to the patient in keeping in her old upper and lower dentures. Xerophthalmia, skin dryness and cervical lymphadenopathy were not detected.

Q1 What is the cause of her xerostomia?

- **A** Dehydration
- **B** Mouth breathing
- **C** Hypercholesterolemia
- **D** Hysterectomy
- **E** Drug-induced

Answers:

- **A** No
- **B** No
- **C** No
- **D** No
- **E** Drugs like muscarin antagonistic which were taken to control urinary incontinence were responsible for the patient's xerostomia. Statins and irbesartan did not affect salivary production and secretion.

Comments: Mouth breathing could be the cause, but in that case, xerostomia should only appear during the waking hours and disappear during the day. Dehydration always comes with fluid imbalance, but that is not the case here, as the patient used to drink more than 10 glasses of water daily, and did not seem to lose fluids either through episodes of vomiting, respiration, or excessive bleeding. Finally, hysterectomy and hypercholesterinemia do not directly affect saliva production or secretion.

Q2 What are the oral indicators of xerostomia mainly seen in this patient?

- **A** Loss of teeth
- **B** Sticky mucosa
- **C** Rampant caries
- **D** Difficulties in holding in dentures
- **E** Gingival bleeding

Answers:

- **A** No
- **B** The saliva is thick and causes a wooden or metallic spatula to stick to the oral mucosa.
- **C** No
- **D** Severe xerostomia causes instability of dentures, leading to problems in holding them in.
- **E** No

Comments: The loss of teeth, presence of rampant caries and gingival problems have not been associated with the patient's xerostomia, as this saliva dysfunction appeared only recently (two years ago only).

Q3 Which of the drugs below are related to xerostomia?

- **A** Clozapine
- **B** 5-Hydroxyzine
- **C** Dihydrocodeine
- **D** H_2-receptor antagonists
- **E** Protease inhibitors

Answers:

- **A** No
- **B** Hydroxyzine is an antihistamine widely used for relieving chronic pruritus, and allergies, but it can cause a dry mouth.
- **C** Dihydrocodeine is widely used for muscle and joint pain, fibromyalgia and endometriosis, but is associated with serious side-effects such as constipation, auditory hallucinations, itching, and dry mouth.
- **D** H_2-receptor antagonists are used to treat gastritis, or inflamed stomach and peptic ulcers causing constipation, dry mouth and skin, headaches, ear problems and trouble urinating.
- **E** Protease inhibitors are used widely for the treatment of HIV +ve patients, but cause parotid lipomatosis, taste disturbances, perioral paresthesia and sometimes xerostomia.

Comments: Clozapine increases saliva secretion despite its strong alpha-2 antagonistic and M4-muscarinic activities.

Case 27.2

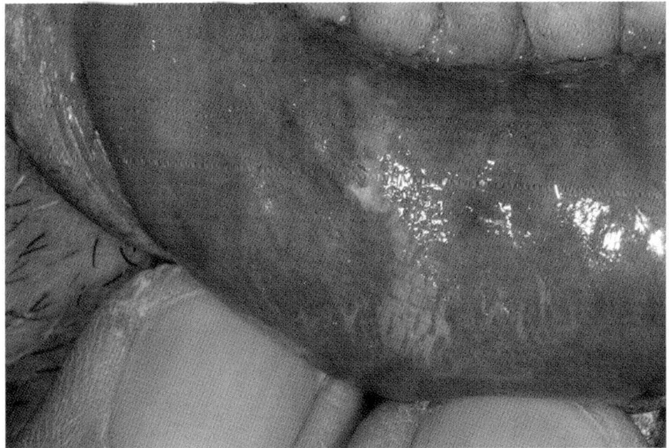

Figure 27.2a

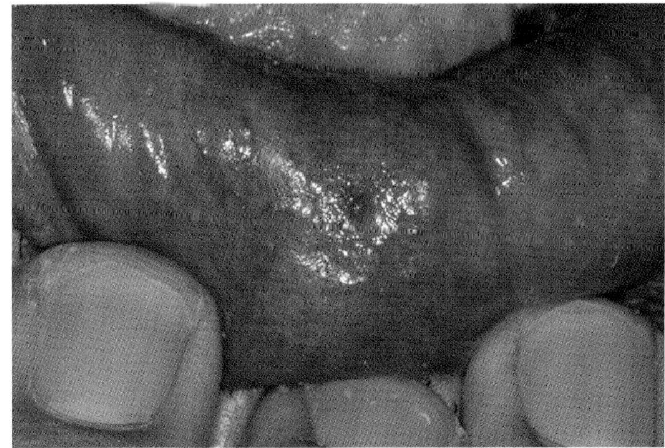

Figure 27.2c

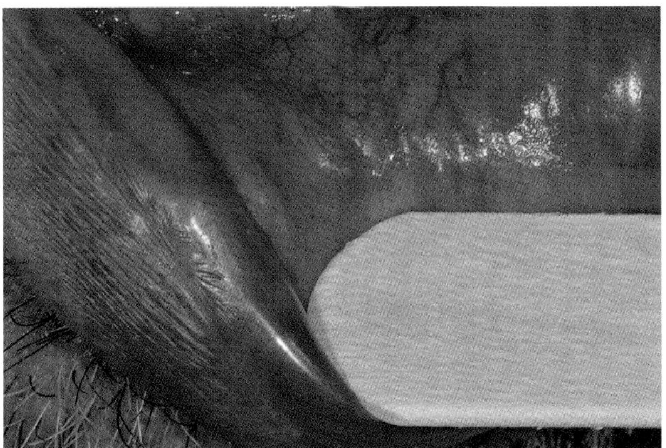

Figure 27.2b

CO: A 42-year-old man was presented with white slough from the inner surface of his lower lip and both buccal mucosae.

HPC: The white slough appeared soon after the beginning of a long course of antibiotics that was given for the eradication of *Helicobacter pylori* found during a gastroscopy one month ago.

PMH: Chronic gastritis and esophageal reflux were his main medical problems, and relieved with cimetidine and fruit-flavored chewing gum on a daily basis. A recent gastroscopy revealed an erythematous esophagus and a small, asymptomatic, healing ulcer in his stomach. For this reason, a sample was taken from the area which confirmed the presence of *Helicobacter*, and therefore the patient started a triple antibiotic course of clarithromycin, amoxicillin, and metronidazole together with omeprazole for 14 days.

OE: The oral examination did not reveal any oral lesions apart from a white slough covering the inner surface of his lower lip, both buccal mucosae and soft palate (Figure 27.2a) This slough was easily removed with a wooden spatula (Figure 27.2b) leaving an erythematous area underneath which was very sensitive to touch (Figure 27.2c). No evidence of a similar slough on his teeth or gingivae was noted as the patient had good oral hygiene and his dentition was clear from caries or fillings. No local or systemic lymphadenopathy, or skin or other mucosae lesions were recorded.

Q1 What is the origin of patient's oral slough?

A Materia alba
B Pseudomembranous candidosis
C Friction keratosis
D Cinnamon-induced stomatitis
E Uremic stomatitis

Answers:

A No
B Pseudomembranous candidiasis is the cause as it is an acute fungal overgrowth infection induced by the use of antibiotics for eradication of *H. pylori* from the patient's gut. The white creamy slough

consists of a mixture of *Candida* hyphae, desquamated epithelial cells, fibrin, inflammatory cells, and food debris.

C No

D No

E No

Comments: Uremic stomatitis and frictional keratosis are not the cause, as both come as well-fixed lesions that are associated with kidney problems and friction habits respectively. Materia alba is easily excluded as it is often seen in patients with neglected oral hygiene and when it is removed, it leaves normal mucosa underneath, features that are not seen in this patient. Cinnamon-induced stomatitis is often associated with erythematous lesions mainly on both buccal mucosae and lateral margins of the tongue, and is a local reaction to cinnamon from the constant use of chewing gum with mint or cinnamon flavor and not with fruit flavor.

Q2 This white lesion can be diagnosed clinically by its:

A Location

B Symptomatology

C History

D Fixation or not with adjacent tissues

E Duration

Answers:

A No

B Pseudomembranous candidiasis appears with a mild symptomatology like burning sensation, itching, or sensitivity on touching while other white lesions are asymptomatic or cause a roughness feeling.

C His previous medical history may confirm serious disease and drug uptakes that are liable to cause local or systemic immunodeficiency, altering oral biofilms and therefore provoking the growth of *Candida* species.

D The easy removal of this white slough with scrubbing with a wooden spatula differentiates this type of candidiasis from other well-fixed white lesions such as frictional keratosis, leukoplakia, or submucous fibrosis.

E The pseudomembranous candidiasis is a classical example of an acute fungal infection and appears within the first 10 days, while the chronic type (erythematous or hyperplastic) appears after two weeks and lasts longer.

Comments: Acute pseudomembranous candidiasis affects any part of the oral mucosa, but is more obvious in certain parts like the soft palate and buccal sulcus, where the slough is unlikely to be wiped off with chewing movements.

Q3 Which of the congenital conditions below predispose directly to *Candida* infections?

A DiGeorge syndrome

B Chédiak-Higashi syndrome

C Autoimmune polyendocrinopathy-candidiasis-ectodermal dystrophy (APECED) syndrome

D PLCG2-associated antibody deficiency and immune dysregulation (PLAID) syndrome

E Kostmann disease

Answers:

A DiGeorge's syndrome is a primary immunodeficiency that causes the abnormal development of certain tissues including the thymus gland during fetal development, leading to a T-lymphocyte impairment as well as frequent bacterial and fungal infections.

B Chédiak-Higashi syndrome (CHS) is a rare severe genetic disorder which is characterized by partial oculocutaneous albinism, mild bleeding, neurological dysfunction, and severe immunodeficiency leading to bacterial and fungal infections.

C APECED syndrome is characterized by the triad of chronic mucocutaneous candidiasis, hypoparathyroidism, and Addison's disease.

D PLAID syndrome is an inherited condition characterized by antibody deficiency and cold-induced urticaria, autoimmunity, atopy, and humoral immune deficiencies which lead to recurrent infections including candidiasis.

E No

Comments: Kostmann disease is an autosomal recessive disease characterized by neutropenia and predisposition of bacterial but rarely with fungal infections from an early age. Fungal infections appear only with severe neutropenia or extended antibiotic use.

Case 27.3

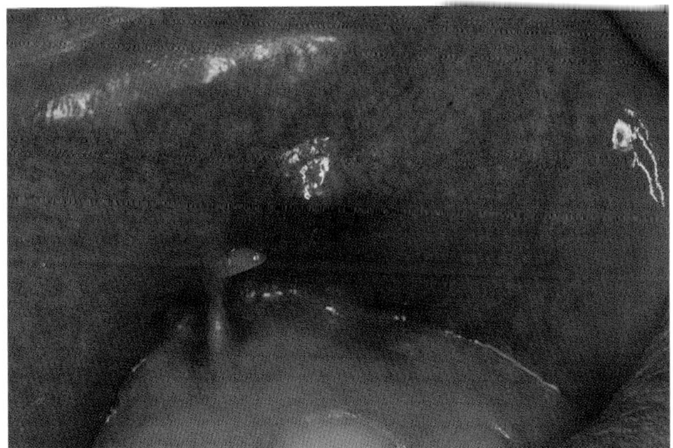

Figure 27.3a

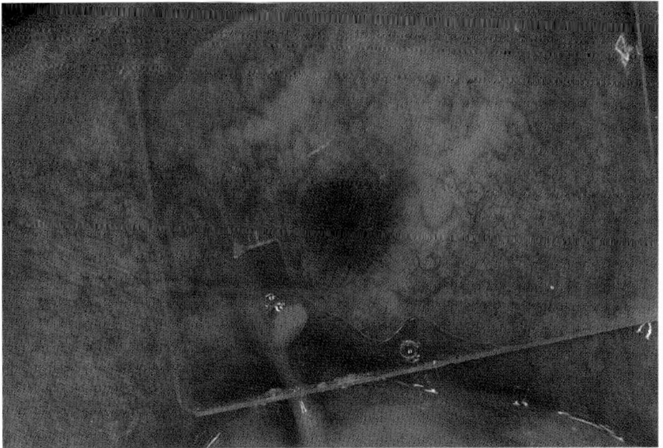

Figure 27.3b

CO: A 35-year-old man presented with an asymptomatic blue lump in the inner surface of his upper lip.

HPC: The lesion had been present since childhood, and reached its biggest size during puberty, remaining stable since then.

PMH: His medical and family history was unremarkable. Habits like smoking 10 cigarettes and drinking of a bottle of beer per meal on a daily basis were not related to the lesion.

OE: The intra-oral examination revealed a nodule in the labial mucosa of the upper lip close to the central labial frenulum. The lesion was soft and slightly fluctuant in palpation, and covered with intact oral mucosa. The lesion was measured and was approximately 1.2 cm maximum in diameter, while its color was dark blue (Figure 27.3a). It bleached slightly with the pressure of a microscopic slide (Figure 27.3b). According to the patient, the lesion reduced its size with cold drinks or foods and increased with the consumption of hot, spicy foods or drinks. No other similar lesions were found inside the patient's mouth, skin, and other mucosae.

Q1 What is this lesion?

- **A** Nevus
- **B** Deep mucocele
- **C** Hemangioma
- **D** Hematoma
- **E** Kaposi's sarcoma

Answers:

- **A** No
- **B** No
- **C** Hemangioma is the diagnosis and characterized by a proliferation of vascular endothelial cells thus forming a soft, benign lesion. This lesion is usually manifested within the first month of life and follows a rapid proliferative and finally a resolution phase. It is histologically classified into capillary, cavernous, or mixed.
- **D** No
- **E** No

Comments: The long duration of the lesion excludes other lesions with a short duration like hematoma, sarcoma, and deep mucoceles, while simple pressure empties the blood and changes the color of hemangioma, but not nevus lesions.

Q2 Which is the simplest clinical test to distinguish a vascular lesion from other pigmented lesions?

- **A** Photography
- **B** Color changes (bleaching) with pressure
- **C** Aspiration
- **D** Diascope
- **E** Ultrasonography (Doppler)

Answers:

- **A** No
- **B** Manual pressure compresses the vascular lesion that easily empties of blood, causing a size reduction and color bleaching. This is a very easy way for a clinician to distinguish whether a superficial pigmented lesion is vascular or melanocytic.
- **C** No
- **D** No
- **E** No

Comments: Full body photography and a diascope are very useful for the examination and follow-up of various types of nevi and melanomas rather than oral hemangiomas. Fine needle aspiration confirms that the lesion contains blood, but in inexpert hands can cause uncontrolled bleeding and should be avoided, while Doppler ultrasonography is not a clinical test.

Q3 Which is/are the recommended treatment/s for this lesion?

- **A** Antifibrinolytic therapy
- **B** Cryotherapy
- **C** Surgery
- **D** Embolization
- **E** Interferon-2A

Answers:

- **A** No
- **B** Cryotherapy can be used for this vascular lesion effectively by in situ destruction of the tissues by the application of extremely low temperatures.
- **C** Surgical excision is considered as a primary treatment of small, localized superficial hemangiomas and visceral or ocular hemangiomas which are unresponsive to drugs like steroids. It is also used for cosmetic removal of the excess skin usually remaining after the involution of deeper lesions.
- **D** No
- **E** No

Comments: Embolization, interferon-2A and antifibrinolytic therapy have been successfully used for the treatment of inoperable lesions that do not respond to corticosteroids, but having a high risk of cerebrovascular accident or renal insufficiency.

Case 27.4

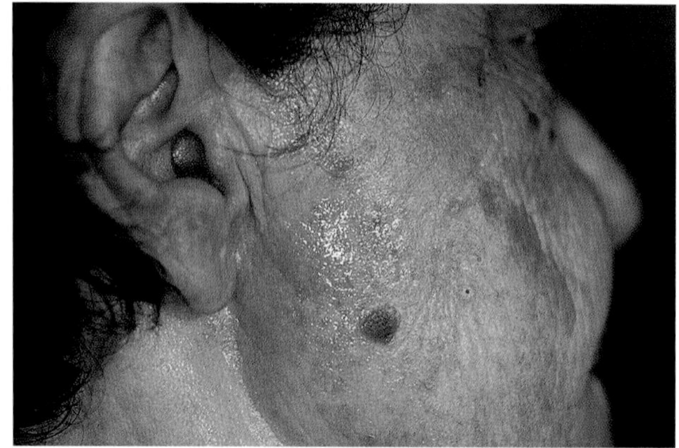

Figure 27.4a

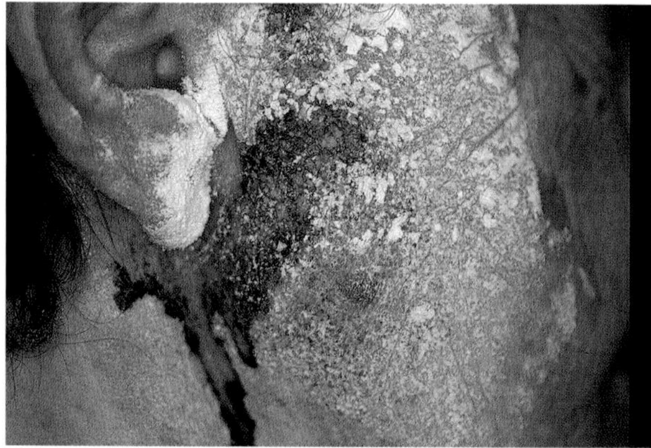

Figure 27.4b

CO: A 77-year-old-woman was referred for an examination for a sweating episode on her right cheek associated with eating.

HPC: The problem started five years ago and appeared whenever the patient tried to eat acidic foods or drinks. It appeared initially as an erythema on the right preauricular skin that gradually faded and was accompanied with sweating. The sweating came with transient anosmia which gradually disappeared over the last year, while the sweating remained and increased in quantity.

PMH: Her medical history was unremarkable in relation to the problem except for a partial parotidectomy for the removal of a mixed salivary gland tumor from her right parotid gland 14 years ago. Allergies or skin diseases were not reported and irbesartan was the only drug taken by the patient to control her mild hypertension.

OE: A healthy, good looking lady with no serious systemic abnormalities, sensory, or motor deficits presented a periauricular erythema within seconds after eating lemons, candies, and biscuits. The facial flushing was extended from the temple to the corner of her mouth and faded within a few minutes and accompanied with sweating and a mild burning sensation and swelling as well (Figure 27.4a). The presence of sweating was restricted to the area of face where her parotid tumor was removed and confirmed by a positive Minor's test (Figure 27.4b). Fistulae arising from dental tissues, oral mucosa and parotid or tongue or lip swelling were not found.

Q1 What is the possible cause?

- **A** Orocutaneous fistula
- **B** Hyperhidrosis
- **C** Food allergy
- **D** Frey syndrome
- **E** Harlequin syndrome

Answers:

- **A** No
- **B** No
- **C** No
- **D** Frey syndrome is the cause and characterized by a flushing and sweating of one part of the face during eating acid foods or drinking strong-flavored drinks. This syndrome is caused by the reinnervation of postganglionic parasympathetic neurons to nearly denervated sweat glands and cutaneous blood vessels. It mostly occurs as a surgery complication involving the ipsilateral parotid gland, following neck dissection, facelift procedures or local trauma.
- **E** No

Comments: The restricted area of facial sweating and its association with previous parotid surgery excludes other sweating disorders like hyperhidrosis, Harlequin syndrome and food allergies. In the diffuse hyperhidrosis, the sweating affects many body areas, while in Harlequin syndrome, the flushing and sweating occur in half of the face and chest, and appear after some exercise. On the other hand, in the case of food allergy, it is associated with some diffuse facial flushing and intra-oral erythema, but occurs in many parts of the patient's mouth and skin, provoked by certain foods and not by eating procedures. Fistula was not found on clinical examination, and it was therefore easily excluded from the diagnosis.

Q2 Which is the best clinical diagnostic test for this condition?

- **A** Starch iodine test
- **B** Skin prick test
- **C** Sweat test
- **D** Nikolsky test
- **E** Ball-point pen test

Answers:

- **A** The starch iodine test, also known Minor's test, is useful to confirm Frey syndrome. This can be implemented by painting the affected area of the face with iodine, allowing it to dry and finally applying corn starch while the patient tries to eat something acid like lemon-flavored candies. Sweating appears causing the starch to become dark blue, during the exposure to iodine.
- **B** No
- **C** No
- **D** No
- **E** No

Comments: Nikolsky's test is useful to confirm a bullous skin disorder by rubbing normal mucosa and thus provoking bulla formation; the prick test to detect any food or cosmetic allergy by detecting skin reaction to certain food, drugs, or cosmetic allergens; the sweat test by measuring chloride concentration in the sweat for cystic fibrosis; while the ball-point pen test may induce dermographism in chronic urticaria.

Q3 What is /are the best treatment/s for this condition?

- **A** Auriculotemporal nerve transection
- **B** Scopolamine ointment
- **C** Botulinum toxin A
- **D** Antiperspirants
- **E** Oral anticholinergics systematically

Answers:

- **A** No
- **B** Scopolamine ointment has a local anticholinergic action with good yet temporal results.
- **C** Injections of Botulinum toxin A (Botox) in the affected area improves several symptoms and the patient's life quality for 9 to 12 months, but requires repeated injections.
- **D** No
- **E** No

Comments: Systemic use of antidepressants or anticholinergics causes significant complications like skin irritation, dry mouth, blurred vision and urine retention. Nerve transaction improves Frey's symptoms, but its results are temporary and require extremely skilled surgeons in special care centers.

Case 27.5

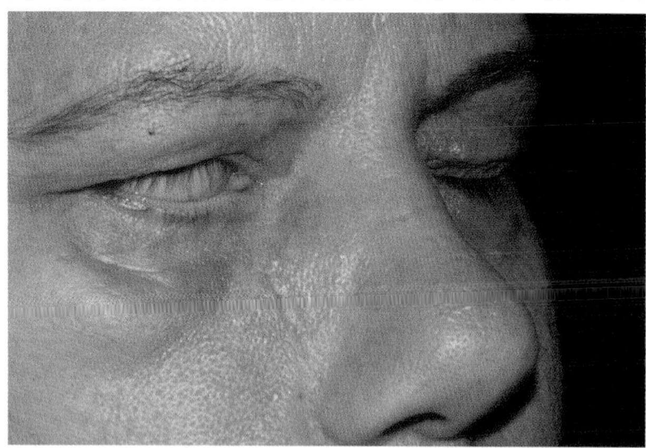

Figure 27.5

CO: A 53-year-old woman presented for a dental check-up and during her examination a facial muscle paralysis of the right part of her face was recorded.

HPC: Her muscle paralysis appeared immediately after her birth and had remained unchanged since then. According to the patient's mother, her labor was a very difficult one and was executed with forceps that caused facial injuries to the baby.

PMH: Her medical history did not reveal any allergies or serious diseases apart from chronic depression due to her facial paralysis. This paralysis caused her low self-esteem due to some cosmetic disfiguration and bullying at school.

OE: The extra-oral examination revealed weakness (paralysis) of all facial muscles on the right side of her face causing drooping of the corner of her mouth, disappearance of ipsilateral nasolabial folds, wrinkles of the temple and difficulty in smiling, blinking, whistling, and eating or drinking. In an attempt to firmly close both her eyes, the affected eye moved outwards and upwards (Figure 27.5). On the other hand, the intra-oral examination did not reveal any teeth or jaw abnormalities or mucosal lesions.

Q1 What is the cause of the patient's facial muscle paralysis?

- **A** Congenital facial paralysis
- **B** Bell's palsy
- **C** Melkersson-Rosenthal syndrome
- **D** Ramsay Hunt syndrome
- **E** Intracranial hemorrhage during labor

Answers:

- **A** Congenital facial paralysis is a very uncommon (8–14% of all pediatric) facial paralysis that can be classified into traumatic or developmental; unilateral or bilateral; and complete or incomplete. The most frequent cause of unilateral congenital facial palsy is birth trauma related to a difficult delivery. The pressure for the forceps at the stylomastoid foramen could traumatize the facial nerve, causing some transient facial neurapraxia or complete transection of the nerve as happened in this lady
- **B** No
- **C** No
- **D** No
- **E** No

Comments: The paralysis of the facial muscles in Bell's palsy are also ipsilateral, but are temporary and relayed by a swelling and inflammation, while they might be a reaction to a viral infection. The absence of painful shingles rash excludes Ramsay-Hunt syndrome, while the lack of fissured tongue, granulomatous cheilitis together with recurrent facial palsies exclude Melkersson-Rosenthal syndrome from the diagnosis. What is more, intracranial hemorrhage is a serious complication of trauma in infants, but is accompanied with a series of symptoms like lethargy, seizures, apnea, and abnormal tone apart from facial deficits that were not recorded in this patient.

Q2 Which of the functions below could not be tested in this patient like?

- **A** Smile
- **B** Whistle
- **C** Wrinkle her temple
- **D** Close both eyes
- **E** Protrude her tongue

Answers:

- **A** No
- **B** No
- **C** No
- **D** No
- **E** Tongue movements are controlled with the hypoglossal nerve (XII cranial nerve) while branches of facial nerve (VII cranial nerve) provide only the taste of the anterior part of the tongue.

Comments: The lower motor nerve paralysis causes weakness of the ipsilateral facial muscles, leading to a failure of smiling or whistling. The lack of contraction of the muscles below the forehead skin causes difficulty in wrinkling ipsilaterally, while paralysis of orbicularis oculi causes an upward and outward movement in an attempt to close the ipsilateral eye, a case which is known as Bell's phenomenon.

Q3 Which of the specialized tests below is/or are useful in the diagnosis of this paralysis?

- **A** Skull MRI
- **B** Electromyography
- **C** Electroneurography
- **D** Blood tests
- **E** Biopsy

Answers:

- **A** Skull MRI is used to rule out brain tumors, intracranial hemorrhages, skull fractures and infections as the possible etiology of the patient's paralysis.
- **B** Electromyography measures muscle electrical activity when the muscles are stimulated, and how fast the muscle responds, while it is also used to detect any nerve damage and determine its severity by checking the possibility of facial paralysis recovery.
- **C** No
- **D** No
- **E** No

Comments: Electroneurography is a test used to evaluate the function of peripheral nerves such as the facial nerve, but this test is useless in this patient as ideally, it must be performed within the first 14 days of the onset of paralysis. Blood tests are rarely used to determine if a virus or an infection could be the cause of the facial nerve paralysis. Finally, the biopsy of facial nerve is seldom used to distinguish whether the paralysis has vascular, inflammatory, or degenerative etiology.

Case 27.6

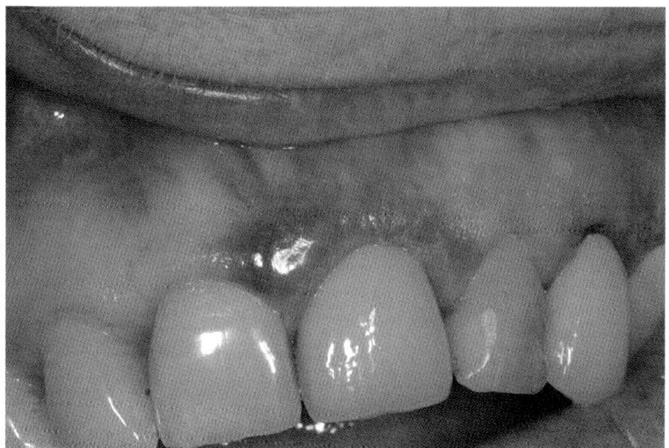

Figure 27.6a

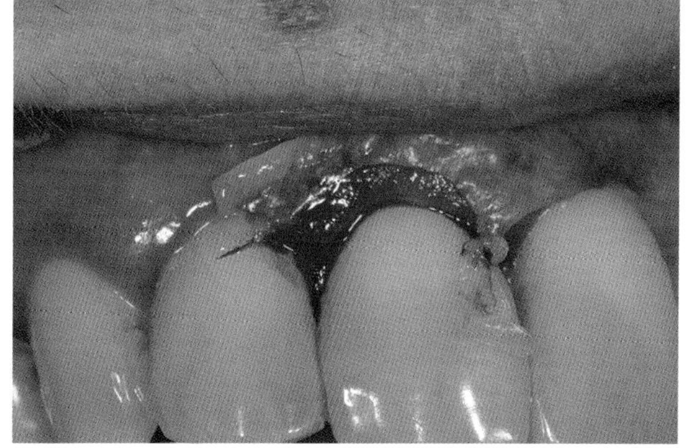

Figure 27.6b

CO: A 42-year-old woman presented with a complaint of multiple ulcerations in her mouth and body as well as a burning sensation when taking spicy hard foods.

HPC: Her ulcerations appeared two years ago and showed a temporary healing with a short duration of corticosteroid treatment. The ulcers developed after the breakage of superficial bullae that were seen on the skin of her abdomen, extremities, genitals, and mouth.

PMH: Her medical and family history was not contributory to her skin problem.

OE: Extra-orally, a few small fragile bullae that were easily broken with friction of the skin of her hands, while intra-orally, a few superficial ulcerations with irregular margins in the buccal mucosae, floor of the mouth and soft palate were noticed. Her dentition was free of caries and her oral hygiene was adequate despite the fact that her gingivae were sensitive, erythematous and edematous in places and bled with probing (Figure 27.6a). Rubbing her normal-appearing gingivae with a cotton, made the gingival mucosa dislodge, leaving a superficial painful ulceration (Figure 27.6b). The gingival biopsy revealed an intraepithelial bulla close to the suprabasal layer.

Q1 What is the causative disease?

- **A** Desquamative gingivitis
- **B** Pemphigus vulgaris
- **C** Bullous pemphigoid
- **D** Strawberry gingivitis
- **E** Gingivitis

Answers:

A No

B Pemphigus is a chronic blistering disease of oral and other mucosae of conjunctiva, nose, esophagus, penis or vagina, anus and skin. It is characterized by the presence of fragile blisters that easily break, leaving painful ulcerations. These blisters are found in histological sections at the lower epithelial layers due to acantholysis, or breaking away from intercellular connections through an autoantibody-mediated response to the desmoglein-1 and -3 components of the desmosomes.

C No

D No

E No

Comments: Gingivitis is characterized by inflammatory infiltrates that are confined to the connective tissue adjacent to the pocket epithelium, while in strawberry gingivitis, a granulomatous response of mixed inflammatory cells of neutrophils, mostly eosinophils, plasma cells and Langerhans type giant cells are seen. The inflammation of the underlying connective tissue is the predominant element of both forms of gingivitis, while the presence of subepithelial bullae is characteristic of bullous pemphigoid. Desquamative gingivitis is a describing term, and is a symptom of a number of diseases apart from pemphigus.

Q2 Which of the clinical characteristics below are seen in this disease?

A Transient oral ulcerations

B Skin ulcerations preceding oral lesions

C Fragile bullae more often seen in the mouth rather than the skin

D The floor of the mouth, soft palate and oropharynx are the predilection sites of this disease

E Pressure on the roof of an oral bulla causes peripheral extension

Answers:

A No

B No

C No

D The floor of the mouth, soft palate and oro-pharynx are more prevalent to diffuse oral ulcerations as their mucosa is vulnerable to friction during mastication and breakage of flaccid oral bullae.

E No

Comments: In pemphigus vulgaris, the bullae are more often seen in the patient's skin rather than the mouth, as the oral bullae break easily with mastication, leaving persistent irregular ulcerations. Oral bullae precede skin lesions and break with minimum pressure on their roof, in contrast to the skin bullae that extend peripherally.

Q3 Which of the clinical signs below characterize this disease?

A Battle's sign

B Nikolsky's sign

C Crowe's sign

D Darier's sign

E Asboe-Hansen sign

Answers:

A No

B Nikolsky's sign is characterized by the shearing of the normal-looking oral mucosa or skin on applying tangential pressure or rubbing with gauze or cotton, and it is mostly seen in pemphigus, toxic epidermal necrolysis and staphylococcal scalded skin syndrome.

C No

D No

E Asboe-Hansen sign characterizes the extension of a blister to adjacent unblistered skin when a pressure is applied on the roof of the blister. This sign is also called Nikolsky II sign, and takes places in the skin and not in the oral mucosa of patients with pemphigus.

Comments: The other signs are manifestations of other diseases such as skin writing (dermatographia) in dermatographic urticaria (Darier's sign); freckling in neurofibromatosis (Crowe's sign) or mastoid ecchymoses in basal skull fractures (Battle's sign).

Case 27.7

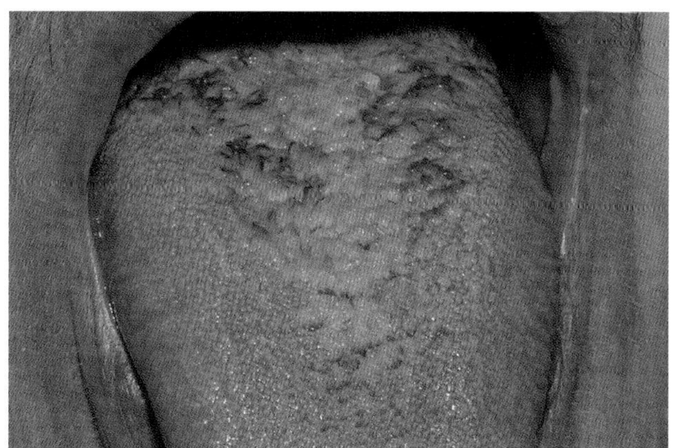

Figure 27.7a

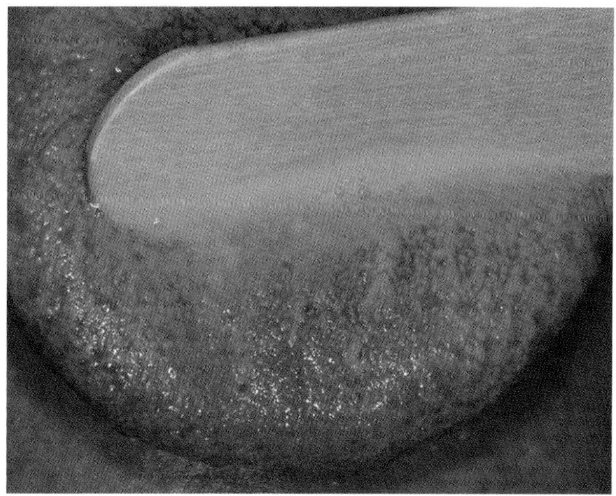

Figure 27.7b

CO: A 28-year-old woman complained about having bad breath over the last two to three months.

HPC: Her bad breath was first noticed by her boyfriend and was more obvious when she was waking up, but reduced during the day.

PMH: Her medical history was clear apart from an episode of acute sinusitis three months ago that was treated with antibiotics and nasal sprays. Her sinusitis exacerbated her problems with chronic mouth breathing habits due to nasal septum deviation. Her personal habits revealed smoking of 10–15 cigarettes daily for more than nine years.

OE: The oral examination revealed a furred, partially discolored yellowish-brown tongue (Figure 27.7a). According to the patient, her tongue became more furred after the use of antibiotics for the treatment of her sinusitis three months ago, but scrubbing with a wooden spatula produced a mixture of dead epithelial cells, debris of food, and bacteria in saliva (Figure 27.7b) with bad odor. No other oral lesions were found apart from a mild nicotinic stomatitis in her palate due to chronic smoking, and chronic gingivitis due to inadequate oral hygiene.

Q1 Which of the factors below contribute to the patient's halitosis?

- **A** Smoking
- **B** Gingivitis
- **C** Sinusitis
- **D** Mouth breathing
- **E** Hairy tongue

Answers:

- **A** Smoking is an extrinsic factor of halitosis and is directly attributed to chemicals released from the tobacco burning and to induced xerostomia; the latter indirectly allows the growth of pathogenic bacteria that are responsible for halitosis.
- **B** Gingivitis is characterized by an acute or chronic inflammation of the gingivae where a plethora of pathogenic bacteria is located, capable of releasing volatile sulfur compounds which contribute to halitosis. All forms of gingivitis and particularly, it's necrotizing type, can cause notable halitosis.
- **C** No
- **D** Mouth breathing is responsible for the majority of morning halitosis as the mouth is open most of the time, thus causing the evaporation of the water in saliva and leading to xerostomia. The latter is a condition which, along with the growth of anaerobic bacteria, is responsible for malodor.
- **E** Hairy tongue is characterized by the elongation of filiform papillae that retain large amounts of desquamated cells, leucocytes, and microorganisms. The germs produce malodorous gasses like indole, skatole, polyamines, hydrogen sulfide, methyl mercaptan, allyl methyl sulfide, and dimethyl sulfide.

Comments: Inflammation of the nose, throat, and paranasal cavities has been implicated with halitosis. Bad breath is however, a temporary symptom that lasts as long as the inflammation does. Therefore, it cannot be attributed to the patient's halitosis, as her sinusitis appeared three months ago, and was treated successfully with antibiotics while her halitosis recently.

Q2 How can you diagnose malodor subjectively?

- **A** Organoleptic measurement
- **B** Gas chromatography
- **C** Dark field microscopy
- **D** Polymerase chain reaction
- **E** Portable detectors

Answers:

- **A** An subjective detection of halitosis is by smelling the exhaled air through the patient's mouth or nose or by smelling the material obtained by scrubbing patient's tongue. When the odor is detectable from the mouth but not from the nose, there is a greater chance of coming from oral or pharyngeal area, while in the case of the nose alone, it is likely to be coming from the nose or sinuses. However, in rare cases, when the odor from the nose and mouth are of a similar intensity, a systemic cause of the malodor may be possible.
- **B** No
- **C** No
- **D** No
- **E** No

Comments: All the other measurements are rarely used, as they require special skills and are very expensive and time-consuming. The dark field microscopy and polymerase chain reaction (PCR) techniques confirm the presence of pathogenic germs being responsible for halitosis, while gas chromatography remains the precise technique of preference. It is used for separating various volatile gases that are responsible for halitosis, some of which are detected with portable detectors.

Q3 Which of the disease(s) below is/ are not directly associated with halitosis?

- **A** Lung cancer
- **B** Kidney failure
- **C** Pemphigus
- **D** Acute ulcerative necrotizing gingivitis
- **E** Rheumatoid arthritis

Answers:

- **A** No
- **B** No
- **C** No
- **D** No
- **E** Rheumatoid arthritis is not related to halitosis, but in some patients with this disease, halitosis might be secondarily attributed to either xerostomia or drugs taken like penicillamine. The degradation of this drug raises the pH level favoring the growth of Gram-negative bacteria in the oral cavity and thus producing halitosis.

Comments: Acute diseases like necrotizing area gingivitis or chronic diseases like bullous diseases (i.e. pemphigus); tumors (oral and lung cancers); and kidney and liver failure, release a plethora of malodorous substances that are responsible for extra-oral halitosis.

Case 27.8

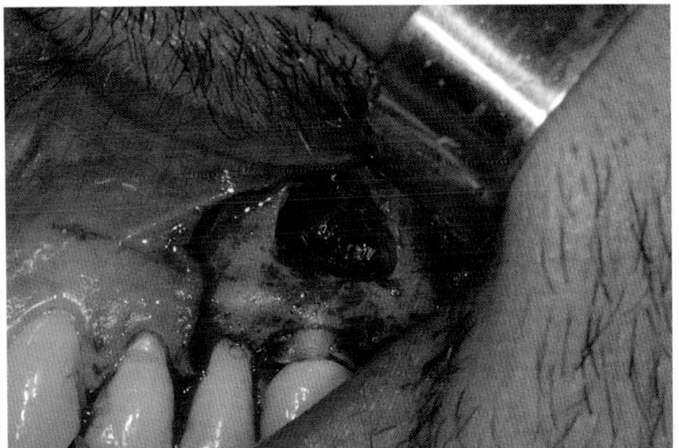

Figure 27.8

CO: A 32-year-old man presented for an apicectomy of his first upper left molar.

HPC: His upper first molar had a root canal treatment six years ago and was asymptomatic. Swelling and pain which had arisen from a periapical, inflamed, cyst from the same tooth appeared one month ago and symptoms disappeared within one week's antibiotic treatment.

PMH: His medical history was unremarkable.

OE: After the apicectomy of his upper left first molar, a large defect was left surrounded with bone, while its roof was lined with partially intact antral mucosa. A bloody and frothy fluid was coming from the defect, when the patient tried to exhale the inspired air through his closed nose (Figure 27.8).

Q1 What is the cause of his bloody secretion from the area of apicectomy?

- **A** Oroantral fistula
- **B** Antral polyp
- **C** Oroantral communication
- **D** Sinusitis
- **E** Periapical cyst

Answers:

- **A** No
- **B** No
- **C** The oroantral communication is an abnormal communication between the maxillary sinus and the oral cavity. It was the result of the removal of his periapical cyst following apicectomy. It is visualized by the dark opening of the sinus, the presence of frothy blood and the characteristic noise produced by the rushing of air through the communication when the patient is trying to breathe or blow his nose.
- **D** No
- **E** No

Comments: Although a periapical cyst close to the antrum can cause an irritation of the adjacent antral mucosa leading finally to sinusitis or antral polyp formation, these lesions present with different symptomatology from oroantral communication, like running or stuffy nose, facial pain or pressure and fever. Oroantral fistula has common symptomatology with the oroantral communication, but tends to appear later if the communication is left untreated.

Q2 What is/are the clinical test(s) that can be used by clinicians to diagnose this defect?

- **A** Valsalva maneuver
- **B** Cheek blowing test
- **C** Probing the defect
- **D** Checking for halitosis
- **E** Antral radiopacity

Answers:

- **A** The Valsalva maneuver is a useful clinical test as the patient is instructed to exhale through a blocked nasal airway, producing a noise and frothy bloody saliva arising from the communication area.
- **B** Blowing air into the cheeks against a closed mouth increases the air pressure in the antrum, finally causing the leakage of blood through the patient's nostrils. This test can cause the spread of the microorganisms from the oral cavity into the maxillary sinus.
- **C** Probing the defect with a periodontal probe allows clinicians to estimate the length of oroantral communication, but incorrect manipulations can lacerate the antral membrane and increase its defects.
- **D** No
- **E** No

Comments: Radiopacity of the maxillary antrum is a common radiographic and not a clinical finding of sinusitis, induced by an oroantral communication. This defect is often accompanied with halitosis, the causes of which are many apart from oral-antrum communication.

Q3 Which is the most popular technique for closure of this defect?

- **A** Local soft tissue flaps
- **B** Distal soft tissue flaps
- **C** Bony grafts
- **D** Xenografts
- **E** Acrylic surgical splint

Answers:

- **A** The local soft tissue flap from the adjacent buccal mucosa is most commonly used for the closure of small to moderate size oroantral defects. The second choice, is the flap coming from the palatal gingival at the premolar area and is applied in cases where clinicians want to retain the depth of the buccal vestibular; the height remains in the original position for future prosthesis.
- **B** No
- **C** No
- **D** No
- **E** No

Comments: Distant flaps from the tongue, auricular cartilage or masseter muscles and bone grafts can be used for the closure of large defects and in previous failures of oroantral communication. Xenografts with synthetic materials like collagen, gelatin films or BioOss® bone substitute are rarely used alone, while in combination with soft tissues, flaps can show promising results. Acrylic splints are rarely used in patients with immunosuppression and oroantral communication when a surgical intervention is contraindicated.

Case 27.9

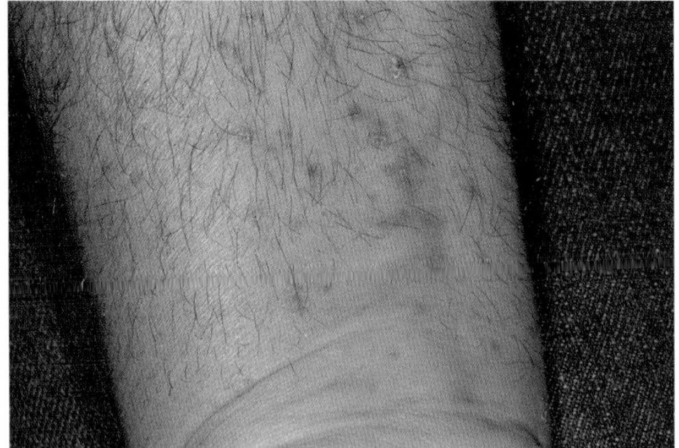

Figure 27.9a

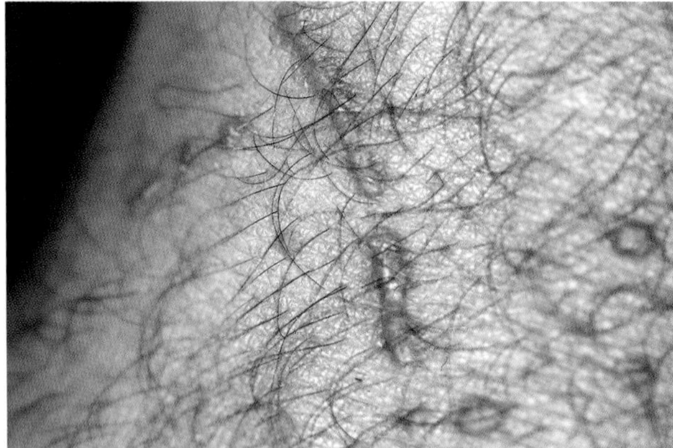

Figure 27.9b

CO: A 42-year-old man presented with an erythematous skin rash and a group of oral white lesions on his oral mucosa.

HPC: His skin lesions appeared six months ago and became associated with itching, while his mouth lesions were asymptomatic and incidentally discovered during a dental check-up the previous month.

PMH: His medical and family history was unremarkable. Chronic gastritis and penicillin allergy were his main medical problems and the patient was not on any drugs. Smoking of 10–15 cigarettes daily was recorded from the age of 18.

OE: The extra-oral examination revealed an itchy rash made up of clusters, slightly raised pink papules with fine white streaks on their surface. This rash affected the insides of his wrists, shins, and lower back (Figure 27.9a). A red line of papules on the skin of his left wrist was found as the patient used to scratch this area (Figure 27.9b). Intra-orally small white papules in a reticular pattern were seen symmetrically on both buccal mucosae and the dorsum of his tongue (Figure 27.9c).

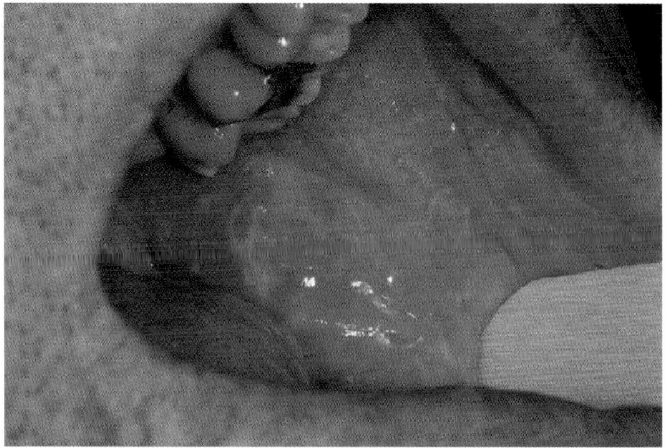

Figure 27.9c

Q1 What is the clinical diagnosis?

- **A** Drug lichenoid reaction
- **B** Chronic graft host disease
- **C** Psoriasis
- **D** Eczema
- **E** Lichen planus

Answers:

- **A** No
- **B** No
- **C** No
- **D** No
- **E** Lichen planus is the cause of the patient's skin rash. Lichen planus is a chronic skin disease characterized by a variety of lesions made up from discrete purple-colored, itchy, flat-topped papules with interspersed lacy white lines (Wickham striae). Skin lesions appear in lines of trauma and especially in areas of skin friction alone or in combination with oral lesions. The oral lesions often precede skin lesions and appear in the reticula, erosive or ulcerative, papular or plaque, atrophic and rarely as hyper-pigmentosum or a bullous pattern.

Comments: The negative patient's history either of drug use such as anti-hypertensive, antidepressants, diuretics and NSAIDS, or having transplantation, both exclude the possibility of a lichenoid drug reaction or chronic graft versus host disease from the diagnosis. The distribution of the lesions in both skin and mouth excludes eczema and psoriasis too; the latter can appear anywhere in the patient's skin and in younger patients.

Q2 Which of the diseases below, apart from this condition, is/or are characterized by a similar linear distribution of new lesions induced by trauma?

- **A** Psoriasis
- **B** Warts
- **C** Molluscum contagiosum
- **D** Halo nevus
- **E** Vitiligo

Answers:

- **A** In the case of psoriasis, new skin lesions appear in areas in which the skin had been previously traumatized. This is known as an isomorphic response or Koebner phenomenon, among dermatologists.
- **B** No
- **C** No
- **D** Halo nevi may follow the Koebner phenomenon, arising when a skin mole has been injured.
- **E** Koebner phenomenon has been observed in a number of skin diseases, including vitiligo. In vitiligo, this phenomenon occurs in 22 to 62 per cent of the patients and the new post-traumatic depigmented lesions are clinically and histologically indistinguishable from the initial vitiligo lesions.

Comments: A pseudo-Koebner response occurs with infective lesions like warts or molluscum contagiosum, as the Koebner phenomenon develops at sites of cutaneous injury (such as a scratch), in previously healthy skin and have the same clinical and histological features as lesions of the patient's original skin disease. What is more, they are not due to an allergic reaction or due to an infectious agent like HPV or molluscum contagiosum viruses respectively.

Q3 The linear arrangement of itchy papulae is characteristic of a:

- **A** Reverse Koebner phenomenon
- **B** Remote reverse Koebner phenomenon
- **C** Koebner phenomenon
- **D** Inverse Koebner phenomenon
- **E** Pseudo-Koebner phenomenon

Answers:

- **A** No
- **B** No
- **C** Koebner phenomenon is characterized by the formation of new lesions in a linear pattern within the next 10–20 days after an injury.
- **D** No
- **E** No

Comments: A pseudo-Koebner response occurs with infections arising in an area of trauma in contrast with the Koebner phenomenon, where a local injury makes the existing lesion disappear. Remote reverse Koebner phenomenon is seen in vitiligo patients, in which spontaneous repigmentation is seen in distant patches after autologous skin graft surgery. Inverse Koebner is seen in patients with two autoimmune diseases simultaneously.

Case 27.10

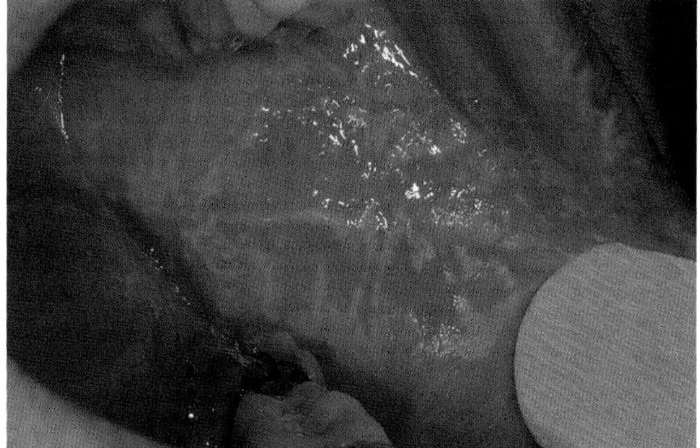

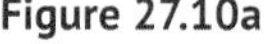

Figure 27.10a

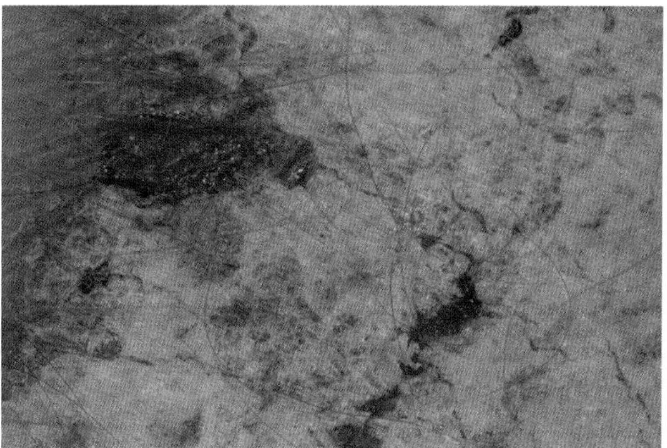

Figure 27.10b

CO: A 52-year-old woman presented for evaluation of white lesions on her buccal mucosae.

HPC: The lesions were first noticed by her dentist during a routine dental check-up last year and remained unchanged since then, despite a course of antifungal treatment, causing her a roughness and mild burning sensation with spicy foods.

PMH: Her medical history did not reveal any serious diseases apart from a mild hypertension and predisposition for diabetes type II which were controlled with diet. Any history of allergies was not reported, but there was a chronic skin irritation with white scaling lesions on her knees and scalp.

OE: Extra-oral examination revealed multiple white-silver scaly plaques on both her knees, elbows, and back. The lesions are scattered and in some places are itchy or painful and sometimes crack and bleed with scratching (Figure 27.10a). Scaly erythematous plaques were found on her scalp causing alopecia. Intra-orally white, well-fixed lesions forming a network were seen on her buccal mucosae (Figure 27.10b) and associated with areas of migratory-fissured glossitis. Her oral hygiene was adequate and her dentition was restored with amalgam fillings and porcelain crowns on the molars. Cervical lymphadenopathy was absent.

Q1 What is the cause of the patient's lesions?

- **A** Lichen planus
- **B** Leucoplakia
- **C** Chronic hyperplastic candidiasis
- **D** Psoriasis
- **E** White sponge nevus

Answers:

- **A** No
- **B** No
- **C** No
- **D** Psoriasis is a chronic autoimmune, but common skin disease characterized by patches of red, itchy, scaly skin. The skin plaques are silver, white scales surrounded with erythematous areas and can be isolated or cover the whole body. Oral psoriasis lesions are not rare, and come together with skin plaques, sometimes associated with geographic tongue.
- **E** No

Comments: The presence of skin lesions excludes leucoplakia, while the late onset of oral and skin lesions excludes white sponge nevus from the diagnosis. The negative response of the patient's oral lesions to previous antifungal treatment, the distribution and the type of skin lesions exclude chronic candidiasis and lichen planus too.

Q2 Which of the clinical types below are exclusively to this skin condition?

- **A** Vesiculobullous
- **B** Pustular
- **C** Plaque
- **D** Inverse
- **E** Pigmented

Answers:

- **A** No
- **B** Pustular type is characterized by numerous pustules filled with pus that can be seen localized to the hands and feet or generalized to the whole body.
- **C** Plaque type is the commonest type and is composed of silvery, white scales on the elbows, knees, scalp, and back. This type is seen in this patient.
- **D** The inverse type appears in the skin folds around the genitals, overweight abdomen and under the breasts after an infection, local trauma or heat.
- **E** No

Comments: The vesicular type is the characteristic of various bullous disorders in which the bullae contain a clear fluid in contrast with the pustular type where the vesicles are filled with pus. The post-inflammatory hyperpigmentation is not only a characteristic of psoriasis, but it can be also seen in a number of skin conditions in which inflammation dominates.

Q3 Which of the signs/phenomena below is/or are characteristic of this condition?

- **A** Brocq's phenomenon
- **B** Auspitz sign
- **C** Koebner phenomenon
- **D** Sandpaper sign
- **E** Carpet tack sign

Answers:

- **A** No
- **B** Auspitz sign is found when pinpoint bleeding is detected on the removal of silvery scales from psoriatic skin.
- **C** Koebner phenomenon is characterized by the development of new psoriatic lesions after a local trauma or irritation.
- **D** No
- **E** No

Comments: Brocq's phenomenon refers to a subepidermal hemorrhage which occurs on a careful scraping of a classical lesion of lichen planus, and not in the case of psoriasis. The carpet tack sign refers to the horny plugs which are seen to occupy follicles after the removal of scales in discoid lupus erythematosus (DLE), while the sandpaper feeling is noticed in palpation of solar keratosis lesions.

Abbreviations

AIDS	acquired immunodefeciency syndrome
a PTT	activated partial thromboplastin time
ALK-1	Activinn receptor like kinase
ACTH	adrenocortricorthrophic hormone
ALT	alanine transferase
ABH	Angina bullosa hemorrhagica
ACE	Angoitensin converting enzyme
SSB Abs	anti -Sjogren's syndrome beta
ANA	antinuclear antibodies
SSA Abs	anti-Sjogren 's syndrome alpha
ATKIN	arabidopsis kinesin gene
AST	aspartate transaminase
AFP	atypical facial pain
PAS II	Autoimmiune polyendocrine syndrome
APECED syndrome	autoimmune polyendocrinopathy, Candidiasis and ectodermal syndrome
BMZ	Basal membrane zone
BMMP	benign mucous membrane pemphigoid
BRBNs	Blue rubber bleb nevus syndrome
CNS	central nervous system
CSF	Cerebrospinal fluid
CHS	Chediak-Higashi syndrome
CKDs	chronic kidney diseases
CLL	Chronic lymphocytic leukemia
CRF	chronic renal failure
COL1AI	Collagen type I alpha 1chain
CT	computer tomography
CMV	cytomegalovirus
DSSP	Dentin sialophosphoprotein
DMSO	dimethylsulfoxide
DI	direct immunofluorescenc
DLE	discoid lupus erythematosus
EBV	ebstein barr virus
ENG	Endoglin gene
EM	Erythema multiforme
ESR	Erythrocyte sedimentation rate
FA	Fanconi anaemia
FGFR3	Fibroblast growh factor receptor 3
GERD	gastroesopharyngeal reflex disease
GDP	general dental practitioner
GPCRs	G-protein coupled receptors
GVHSDs	graft versus host skin diseases
G-CSF	growt -grannulocyte stimulating factor
HFMDs	hand, footh, mouth diseases
HHT	Hereditary hemorrhagic telangectasias
HSV	herpes simplex virus
HIV	human immunodeficiency virus
HPV	human papilloma virus
IDIF	indirect immunoflourescence
LCH	Langerhans histiocytosis
LOK	leymphocyte oriented kinase
LP	lichen planus
MRI	magnetic
MRSA infection	methicillin-resistant Staph.aureus infection
MAGIC	mouth and genital ulcerations together with inflammed cartilages
MMP	mucous membrane pemphigoid
NF	neurofibromatosis
NSAIDs	Non steroid antimflammatory drugs
PV	Pemphigus vulgaris
PFAPA	periodic fever,aphthous stomatitis, pharyngitis and adenitis
PJS	Peutz- jeghers syndrome
PTEN	phosphatase and tensin homolog
PCL	phospholipase
PHAs	polycyclic aromatic hydrocarbons
PCR	polymerase chain reaction
PET scan	position emission ntomography
PHACE syndrome	posterior fossa anomalies,facial hemangiomas,arterial and cardiac anomalies; eyes problems
PWS	Prader-Willi syndrome
RUNX	Runt-related transcription factor
SGPT	serum glutamic pyruvic transaminase
SGOT	serum glutamic oxalocatic transaminase
SJS	Steven Johnson syndrome
SLE	Systemic lupus erythematosus
TSH	Thyroid stimulating hormone
TEN	toxicepidermal necrolysis
TMJ	Ttemporomandibular joint
TB	tuberculosis
U/S	ultrasonography
VZV	Varicella zoster virus

Clinical Guide to Oral Diseases, First Edition. Dimitris Malamos and Crispian Scully.

Companion website: www.wiley.com/go/malamos/clinical_guide

Diagnostic Flow Charts According to the Location of Oral Lesions

Flow Chart 15a

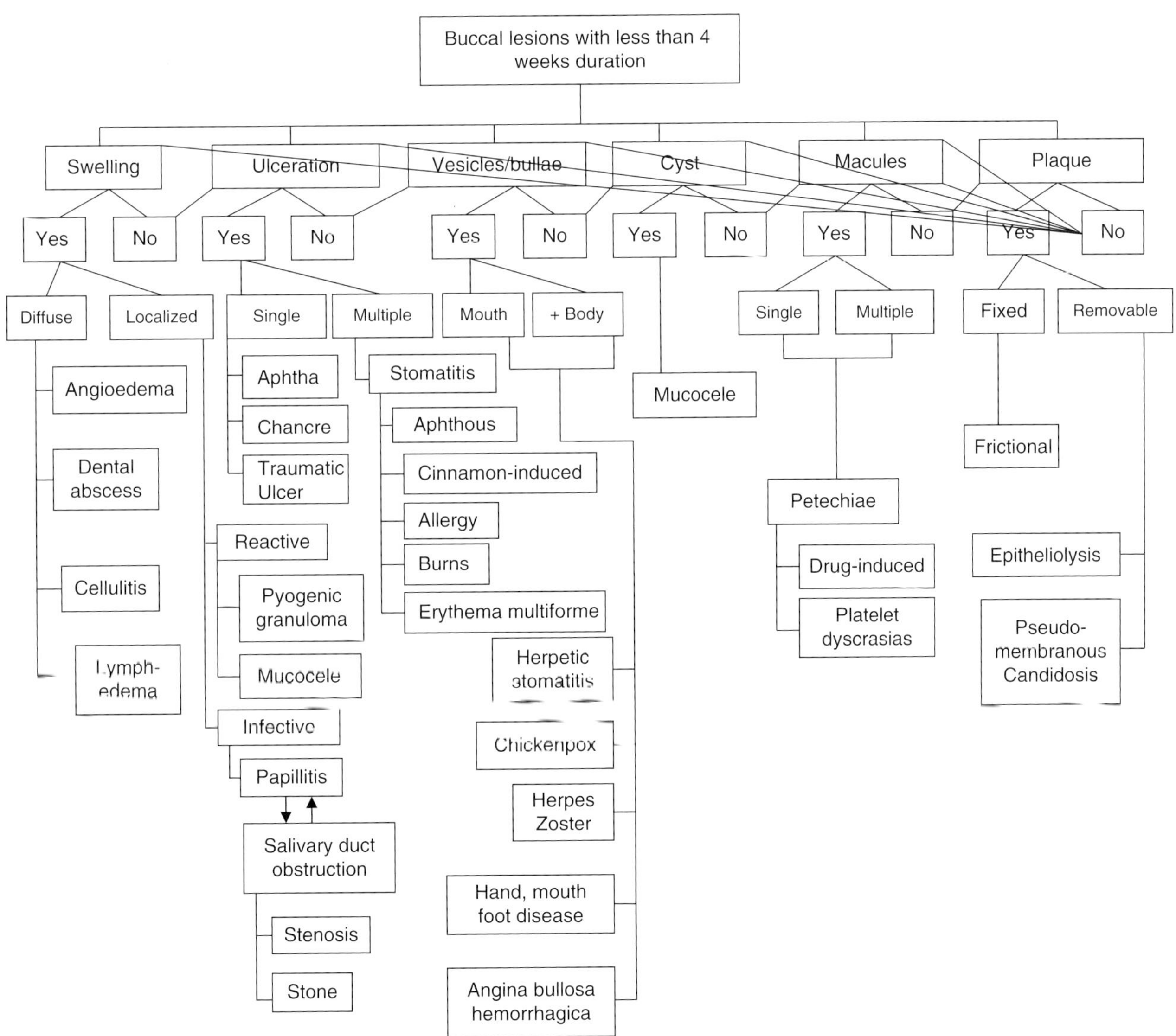

Clinical Guide to Oral Diseases, First Edition. Dimitris Malamos and Crispian Scully.

Companion website: www.wiley.com/go/malamos/clinical_guide

Flow Chart 15b

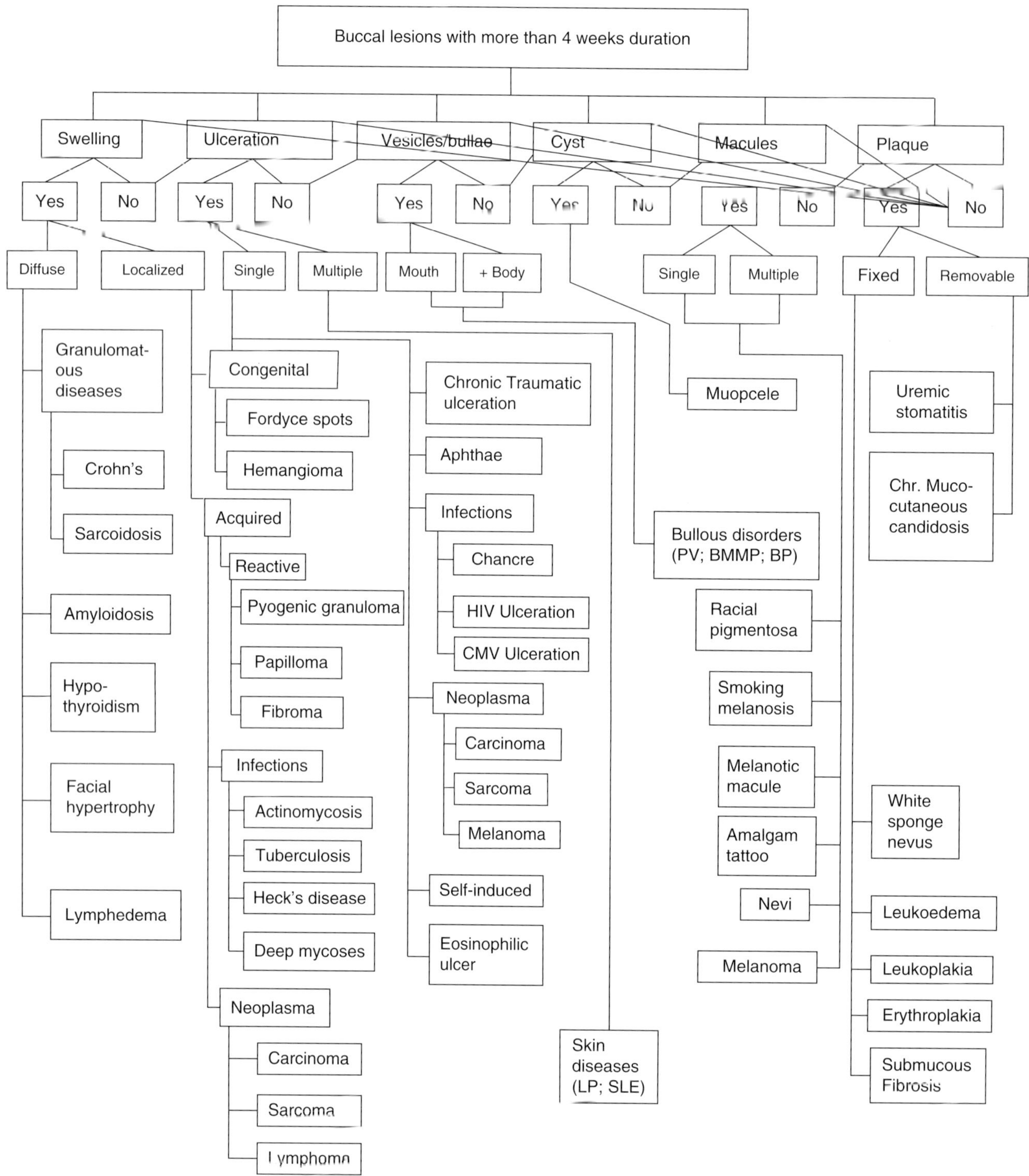

Flow Chart 16a

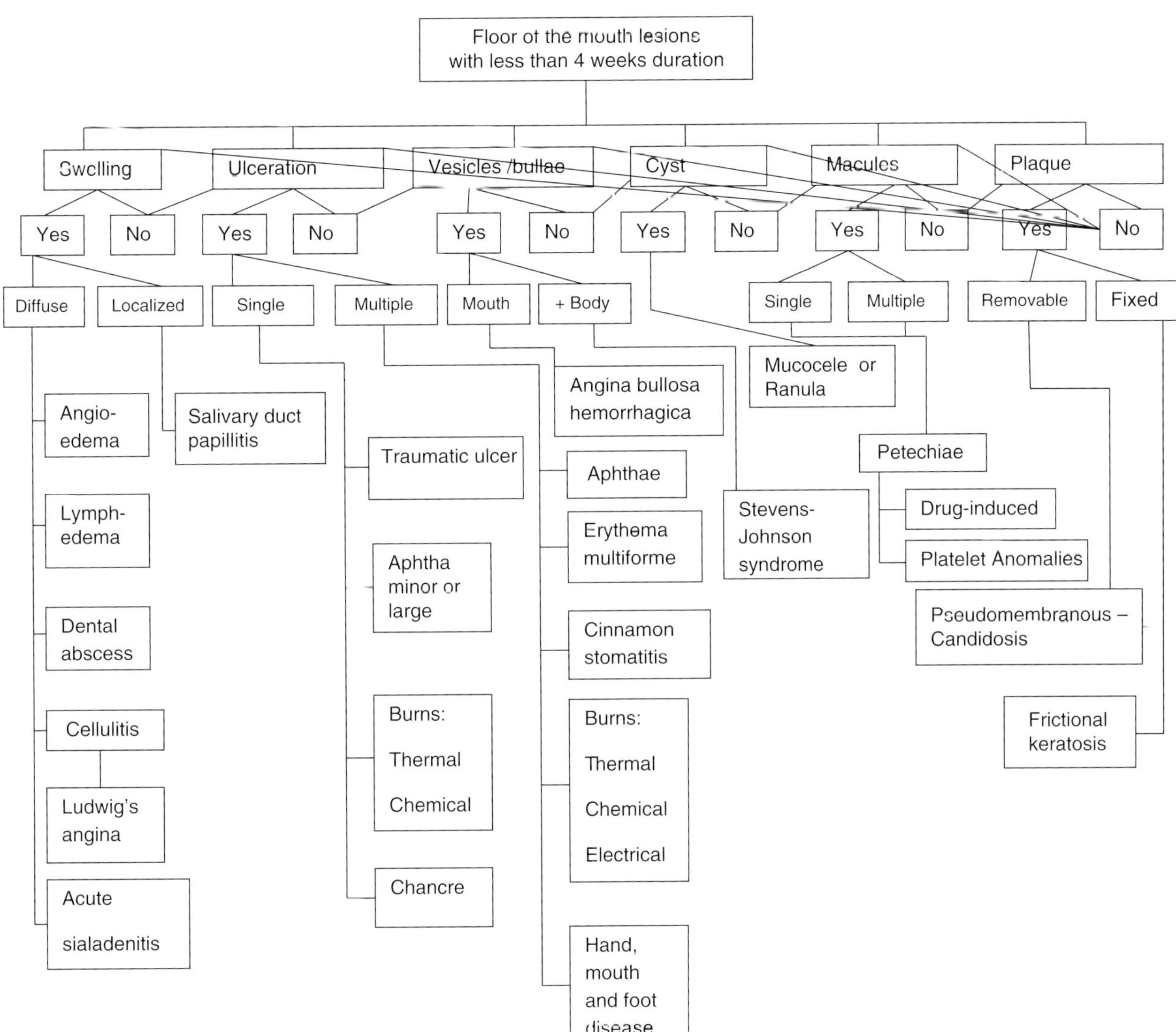

Flow Chart 16b

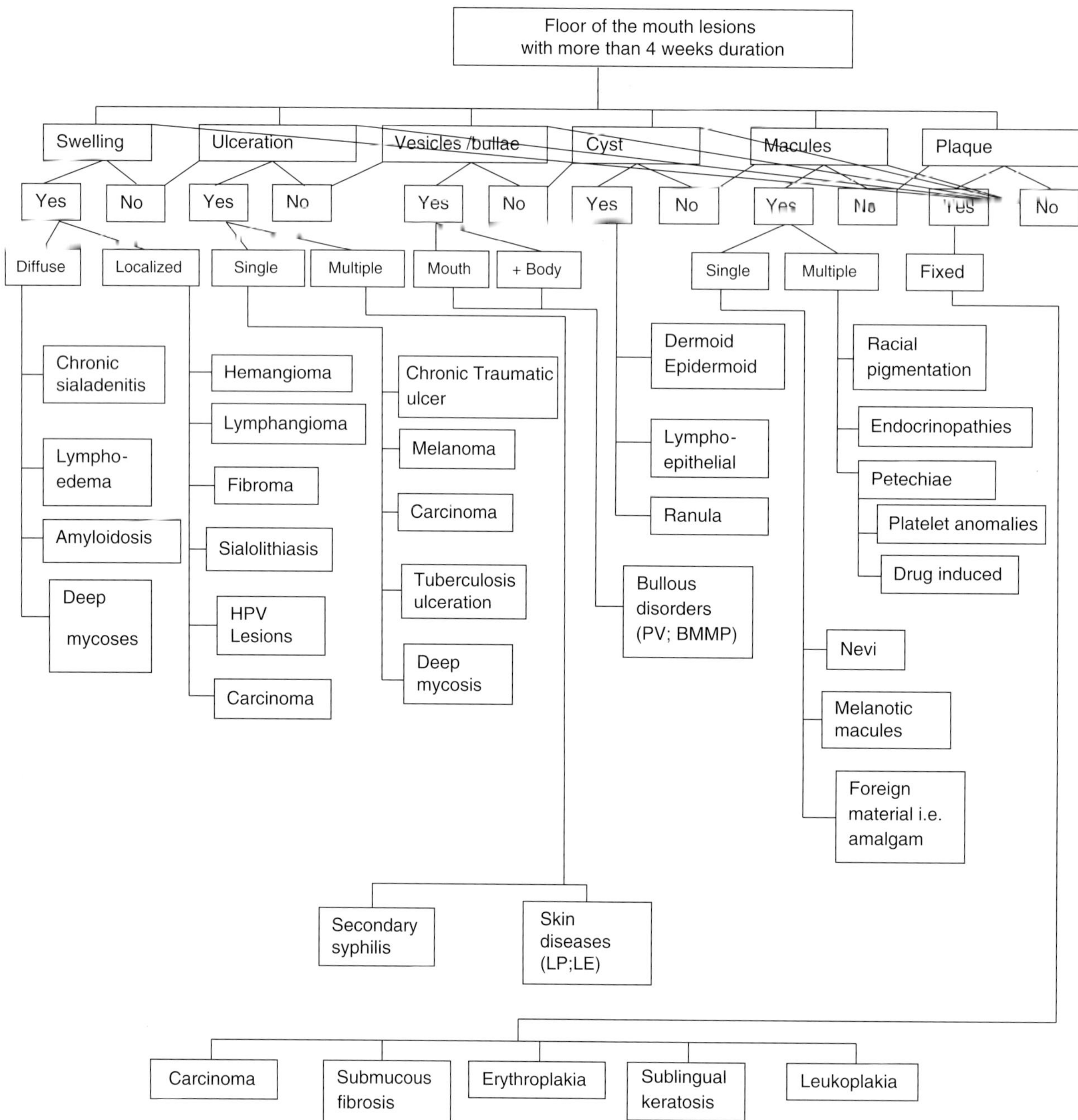

Flow Chart 17

Gingival lesions: according to their cause
(A): Acute.< 4 weeks duration
(C): Chronic: > 4 weeks duration
Acquired:
Regardless patient's age
Traumatic
Neoplastic
Infective
Malnutrition
Medications (C)
Immune-related
Tr.Ulcer (A ,C)
Epulis
Fissuratum (C)
Pyogenic (A,C)
Giant cell (C)
Smoking gingival melanosis
Benign
Keratosis (C)
Malignant (C)
Sarcoma
Melanoma
Lymphoma
Carcinoma
Bacterial
Fungal
Viral
Gingivitis (A,C)
Necrotizing Gingivitis (A)
Periodontitis (C)
Necrotizing Periodontitis (A,C)
Deep mycoses (C)
Primary Herpetic Gingivitis (A)
Linear gingival erythema (A)
Scurvy (C)
Anti-convulsants
Ca-channel blockers
Immuno-suppressivee
Granulomatous – Gingivitis (C)
Desquamative-Gingivitis due to LP; SLE, PV, BMMP. (C)
Congenital:
From birth to childhood (C)
Gingival:
Racial gingival pigmentation
Familiar-hyperplasia
Hemangiomas
White sponge nevus
Granular cell tumor
Familiar bullous disorders

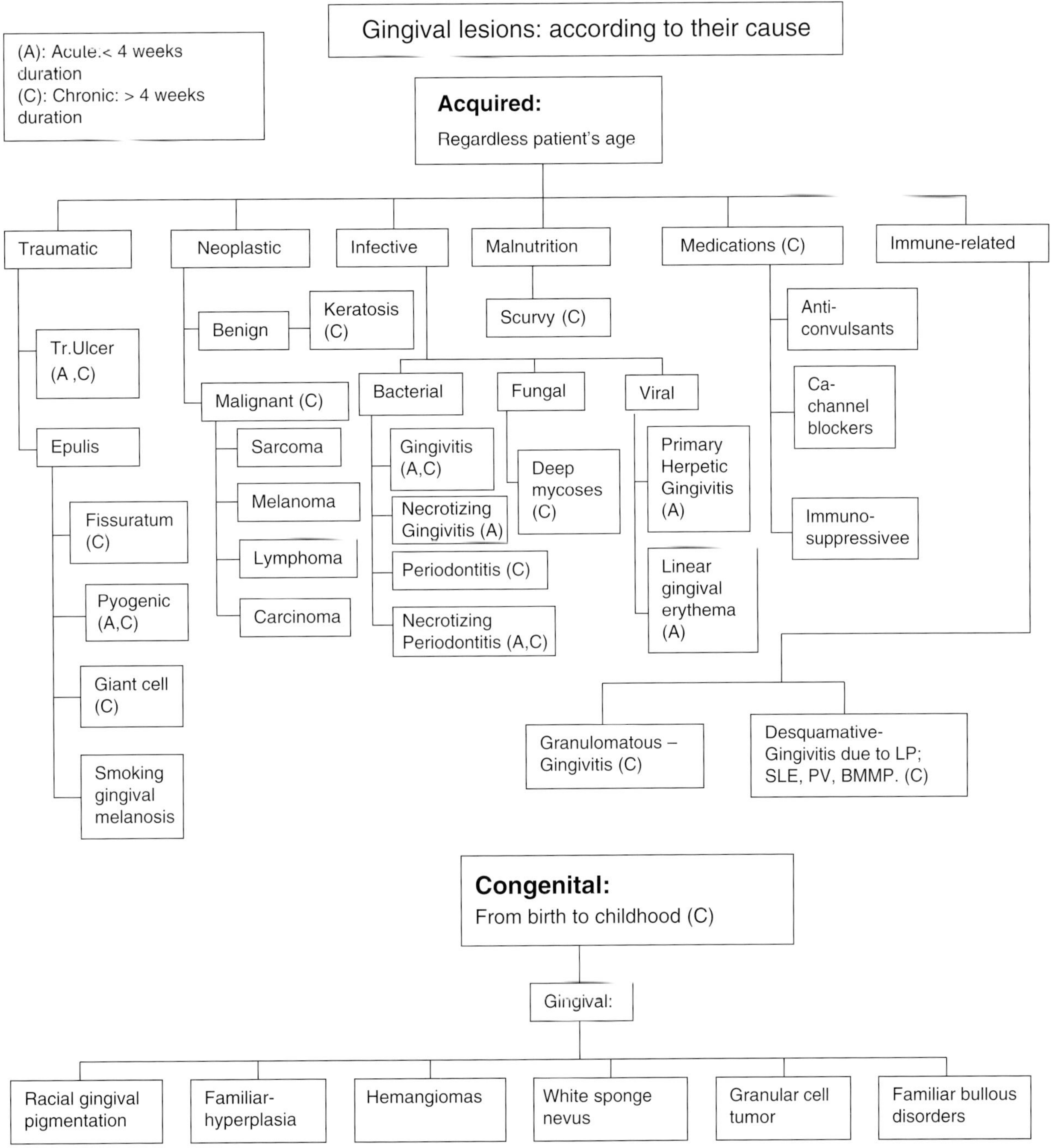

Flow Chart 18a

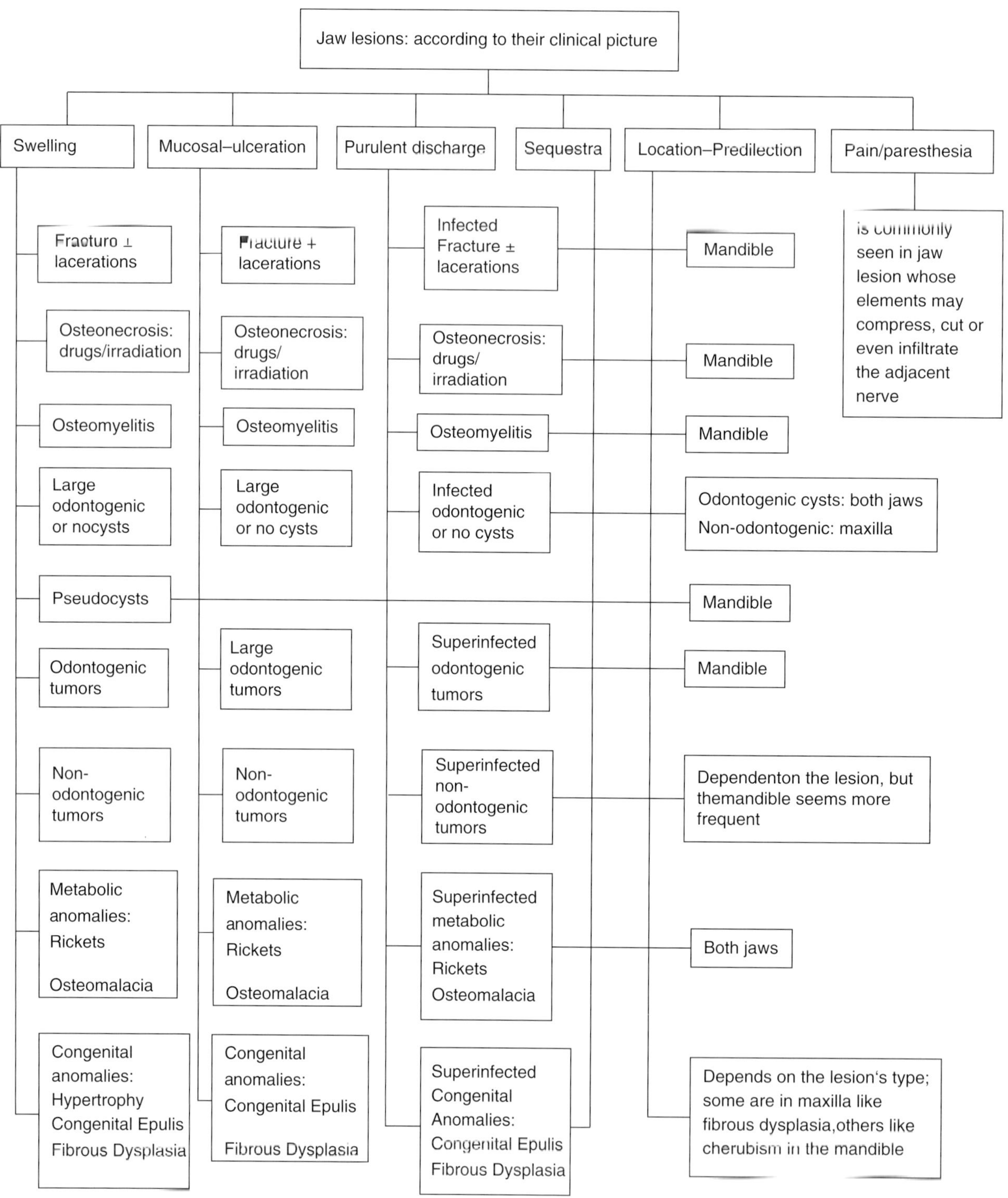

Flow Chart 18b

Jaw lesions: according to their causes
Congenital
Aplasia
Atrophy
Hypertrophy
Congenital epulis
Fib. dysplasia
Osteopetrosis
Acquired
Trauma
Fracture
Fracture + soft tissue lacerations
Infections
Fungal
Mucormycosis
Bacterial
Osteomyelitis
Acute
Chronic
Osteonecrosis
Irradiation -induced
Drug-induced
Cysts
Odontogenic
Radicular
Residual
Lateral periodontal
Dentigerous
Keratinocyst
Gingival
Non-odontogenic
Nasopalatine-duct
Nasolabial
Pseudocysts
Solitary bone
Aneurysmal
Latent (Stafne bone cavity)
Tumors
Odontogenic
Ameloblastoma
Ameloblastic fibroma
Myxoma
Non-odontogenic
Benign
Osteomas
Malignant
Osteosarcoma
Metastatic
Anomalies
Endocrinal
Rickets
Hypofunction – Thyroid-Parathyroid-Pituitary
Metabolic
Osteopenia
Osteoporosis
Paget
Osteomalacia

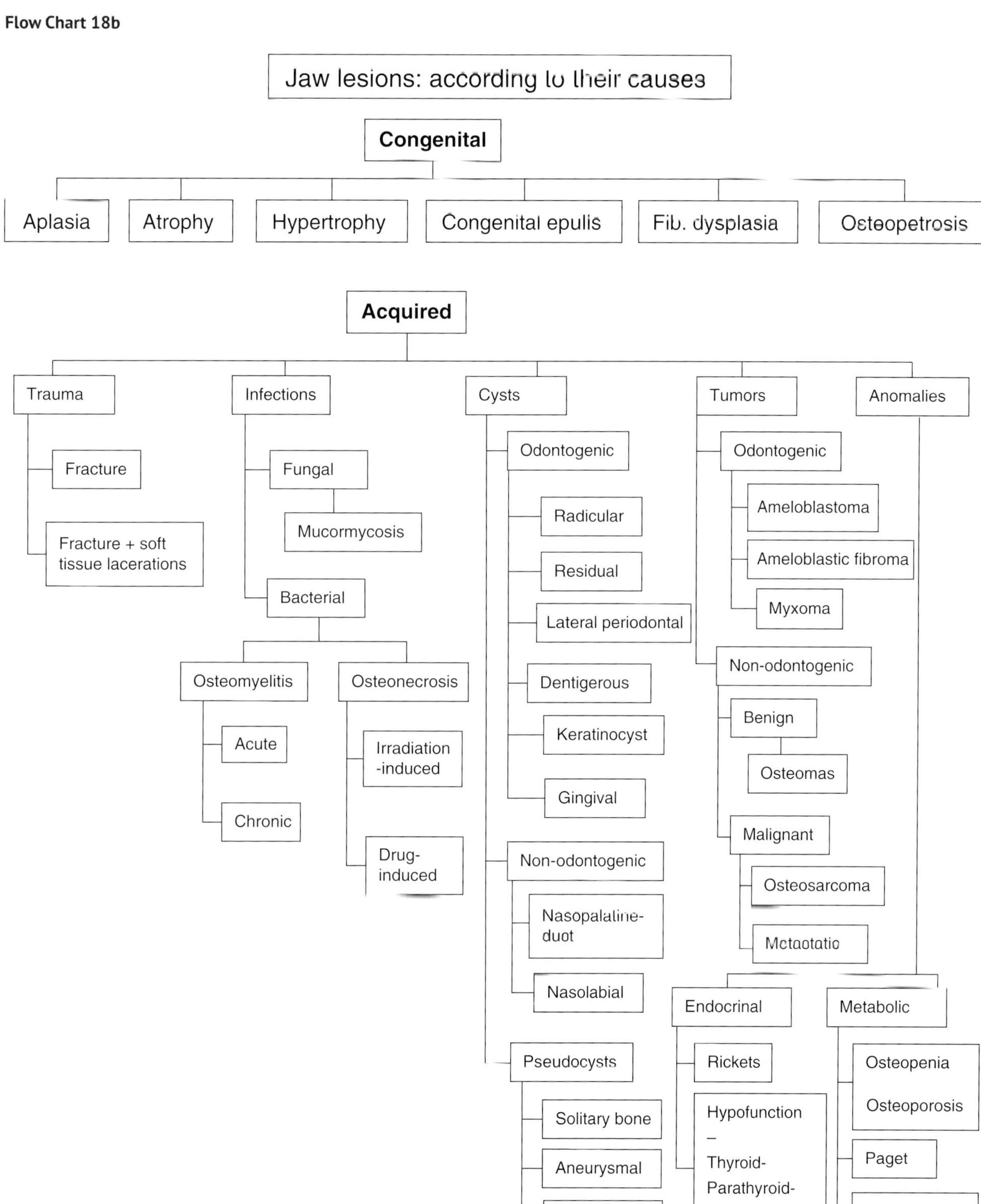

Flow Chart 19a

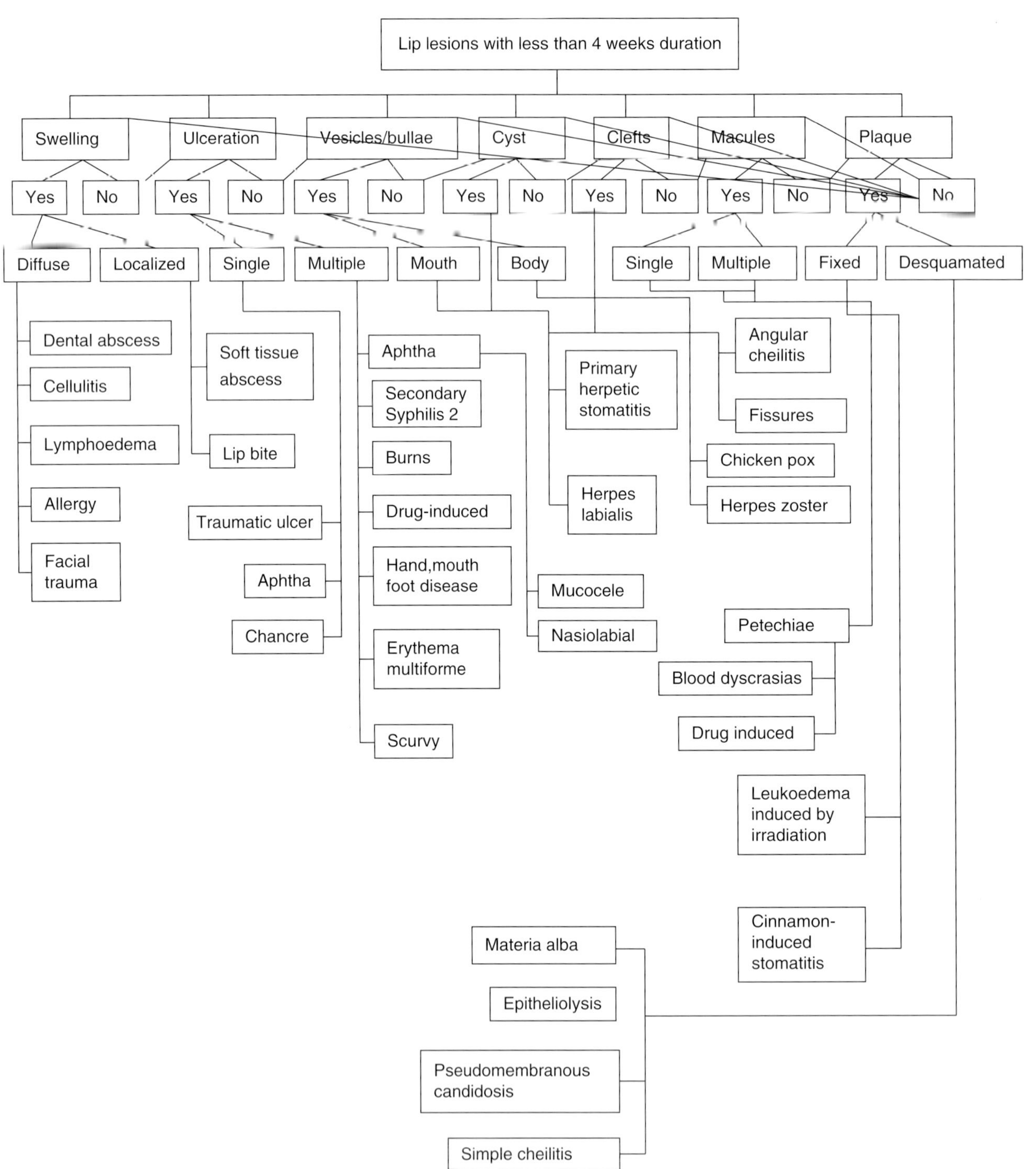

Flow Chart 19b

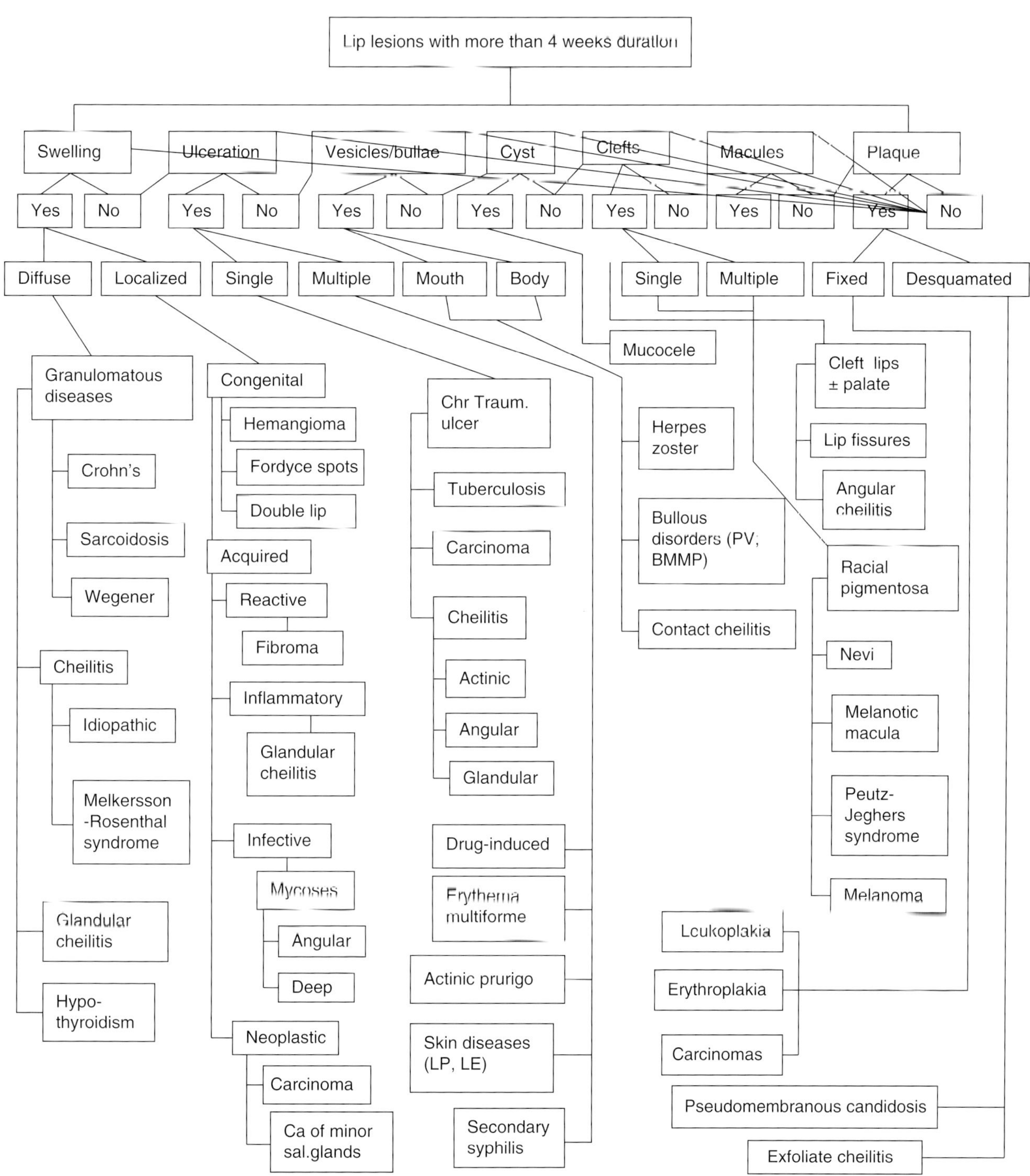

Flow Chart 20a

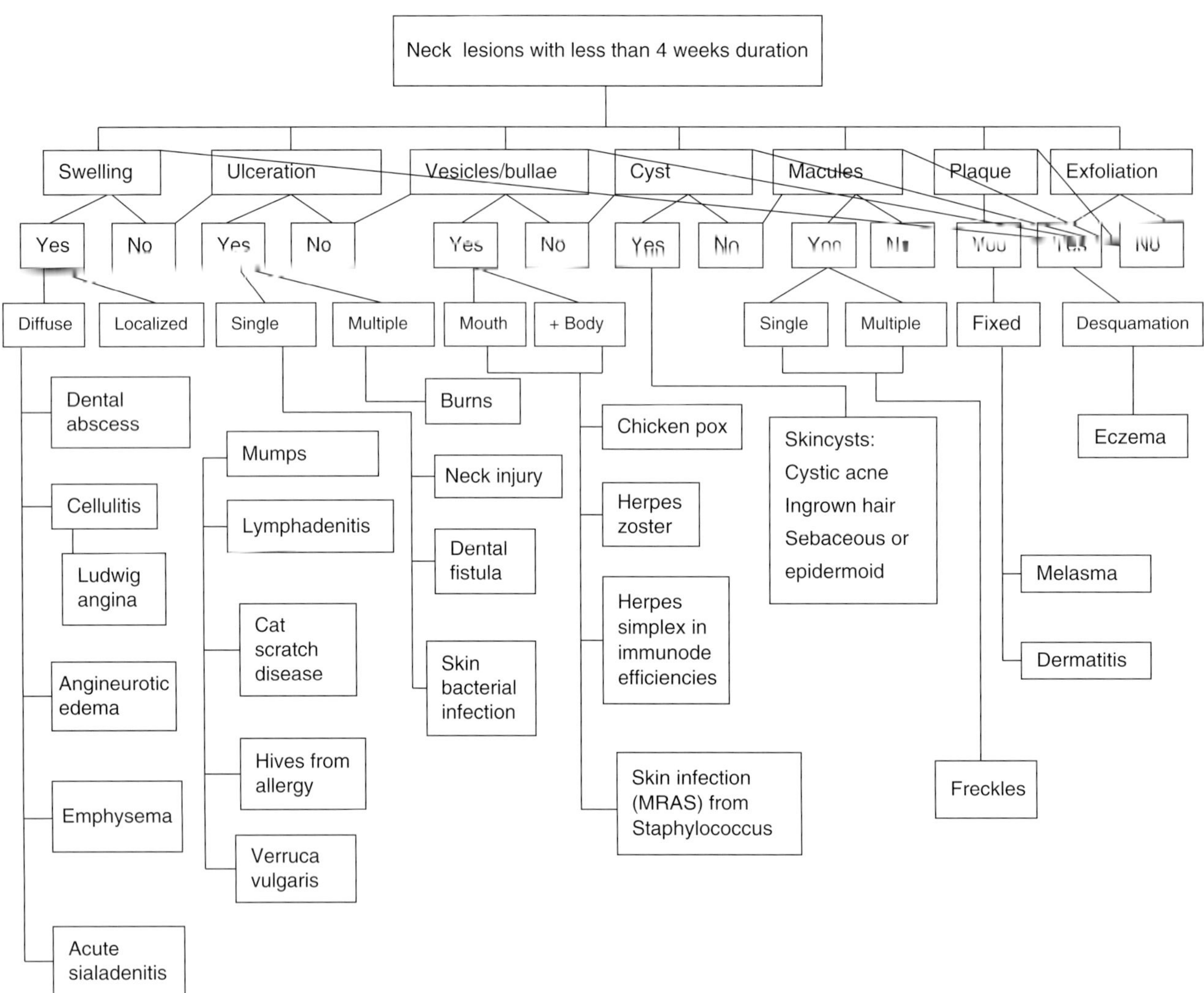

Flow Chart 20b

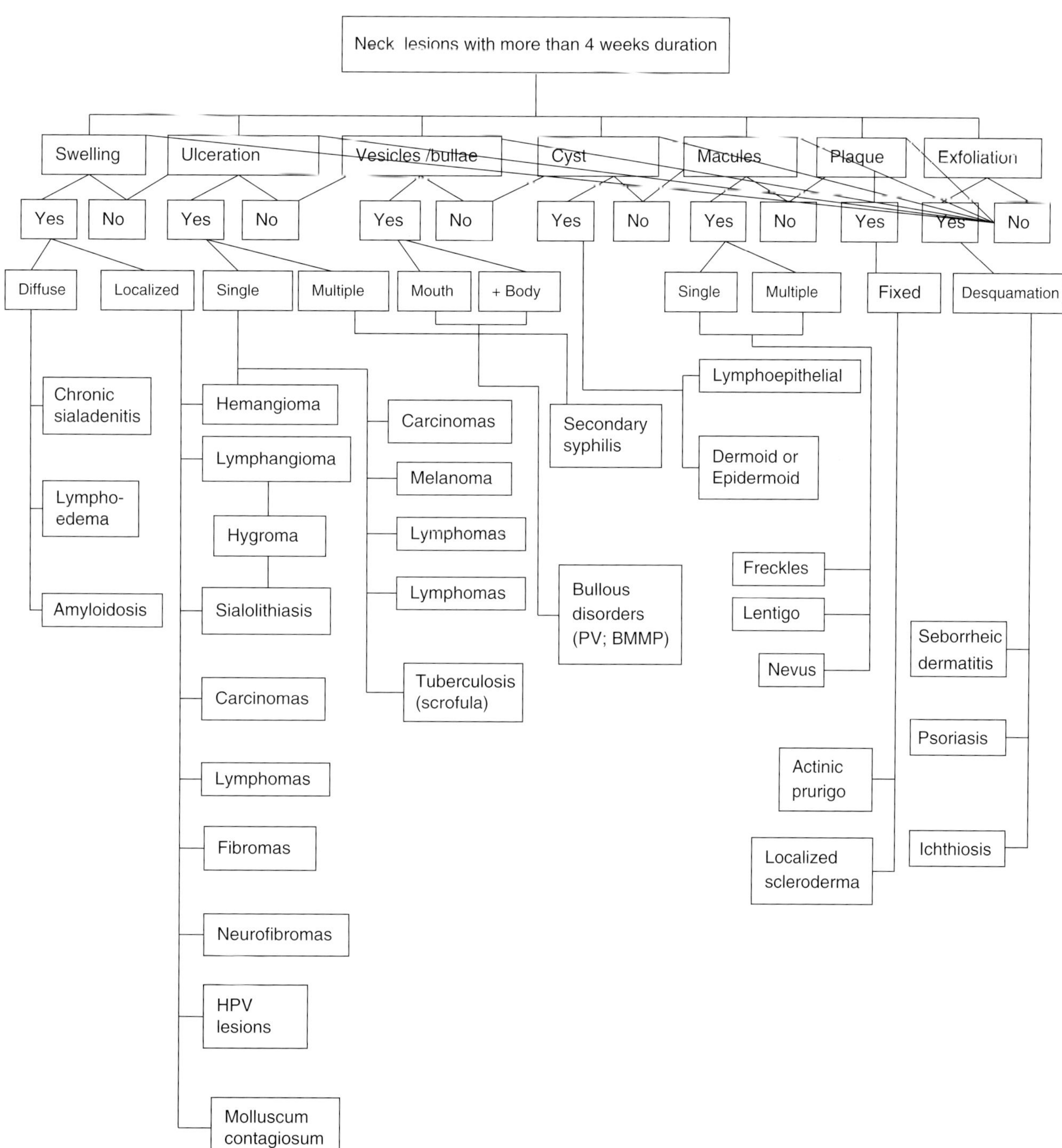

Flow Chart 21a

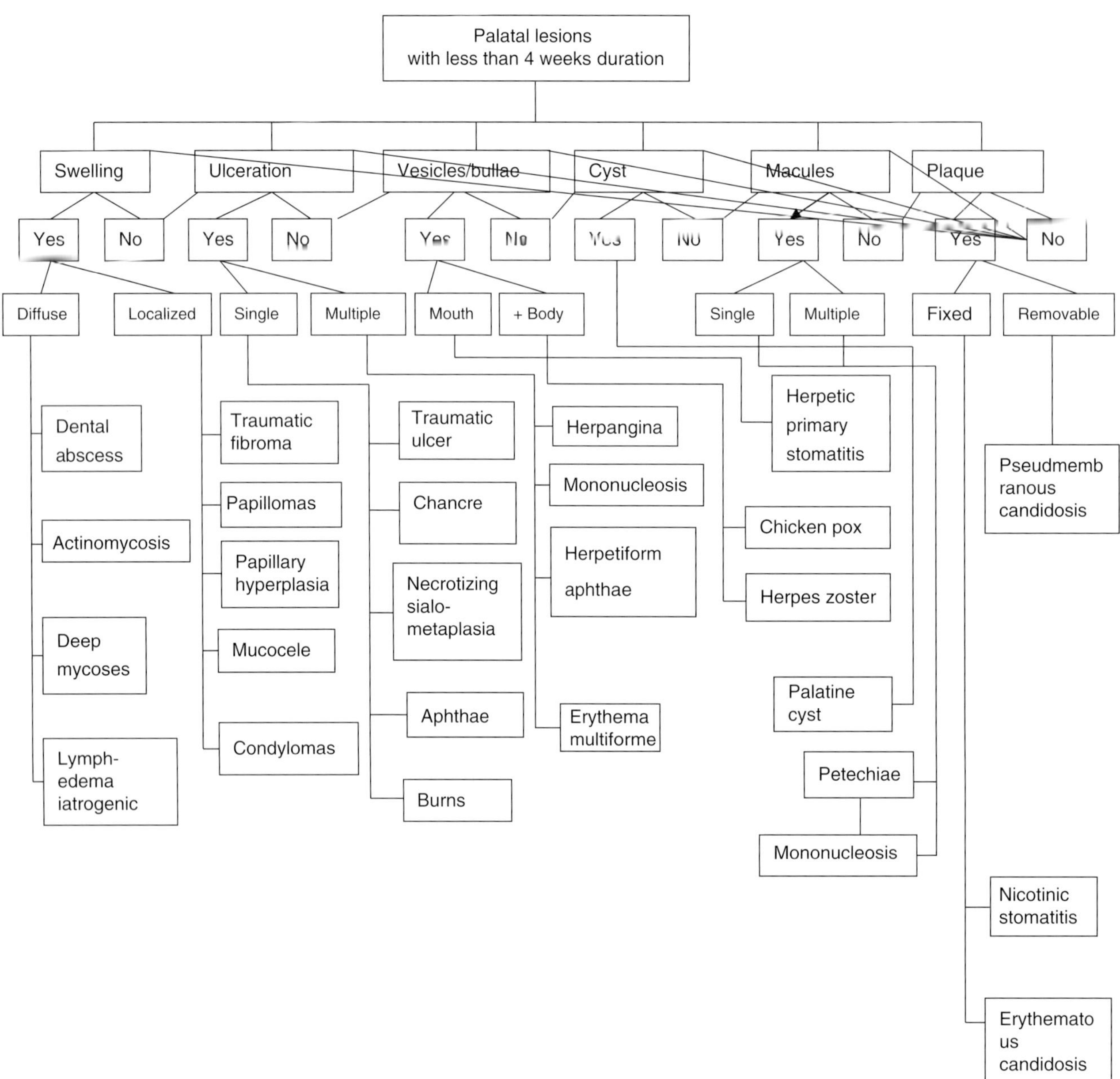

Flow Chart 21a

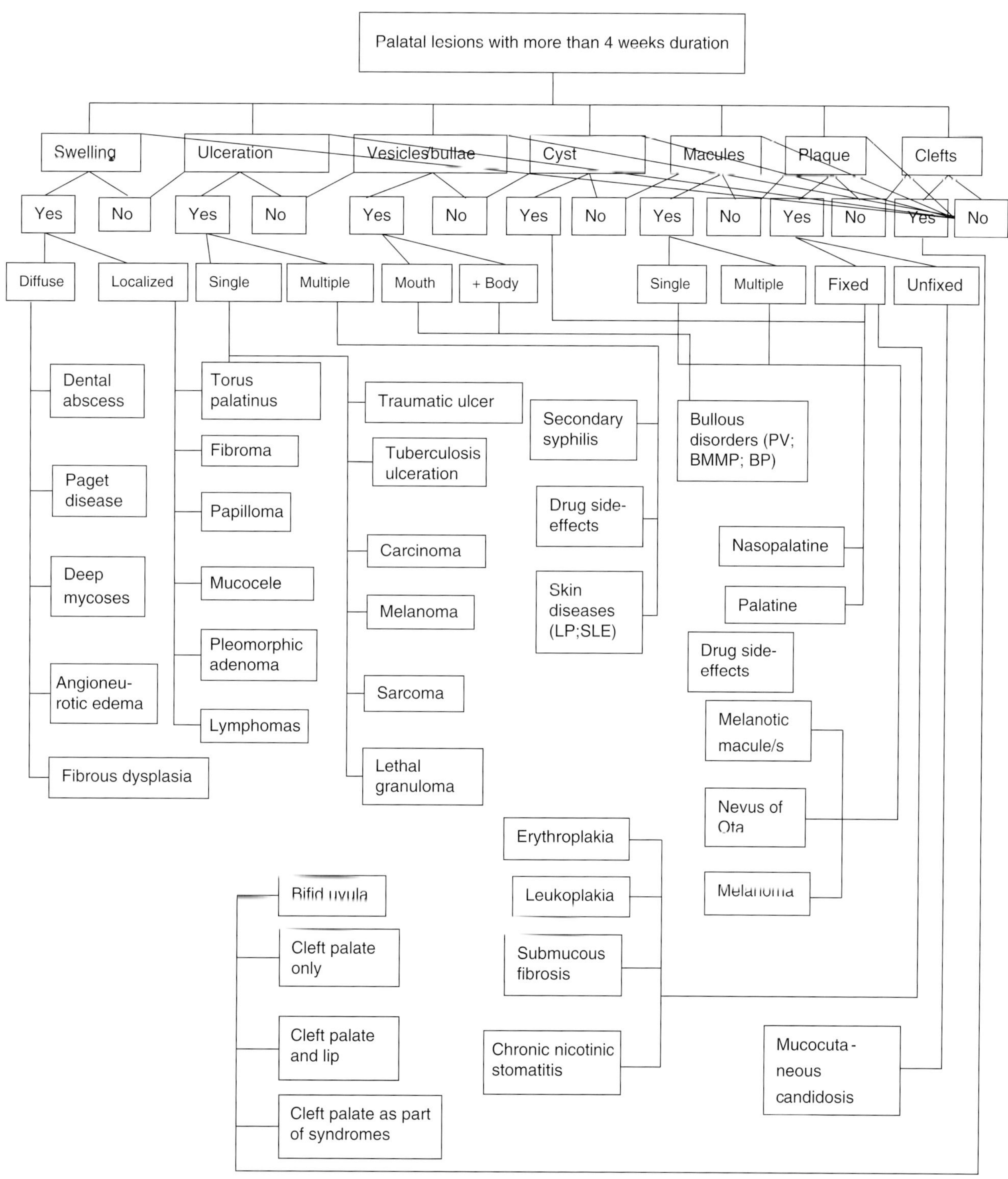

Flow Chart 22a

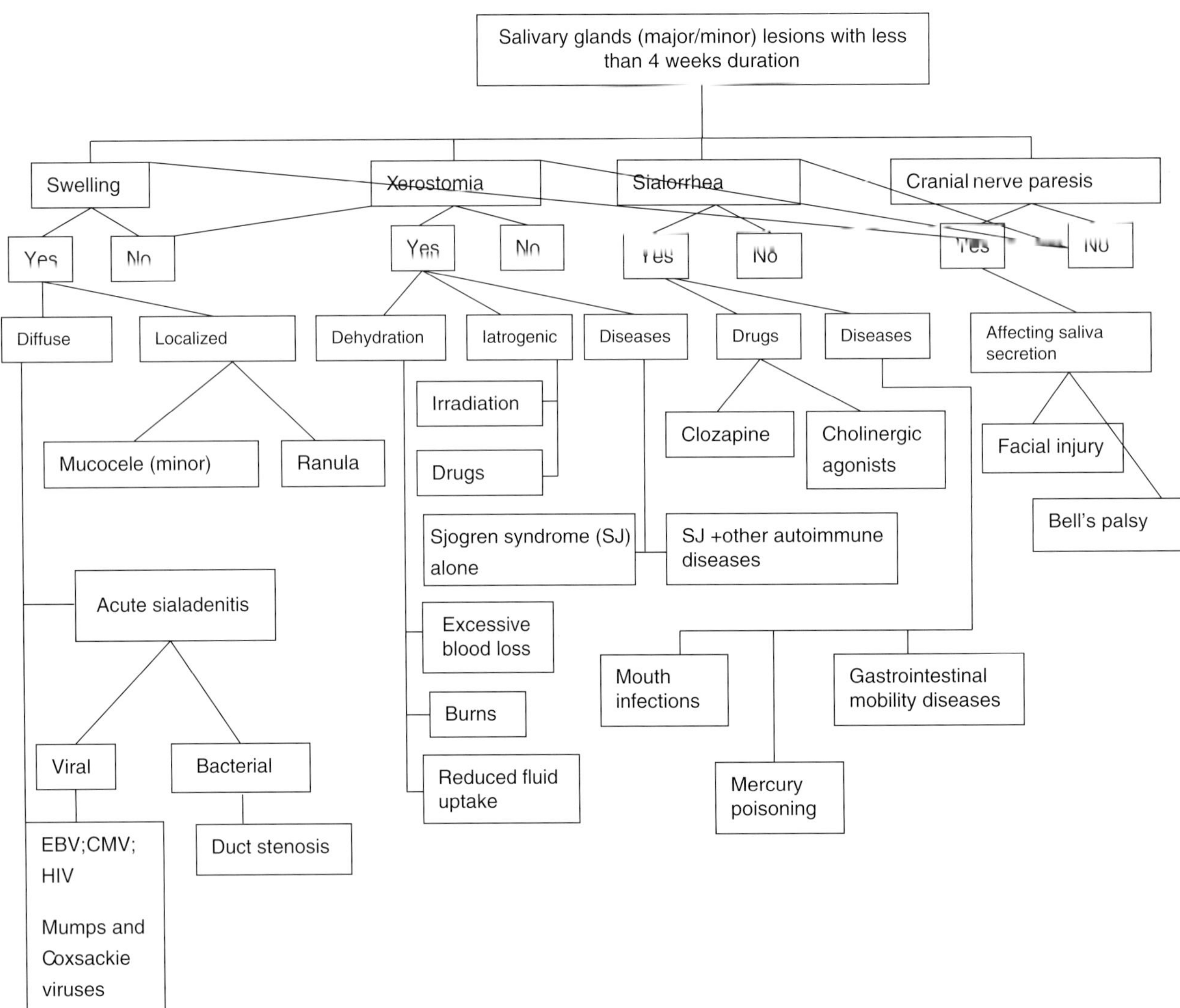

Flow Chart 22b

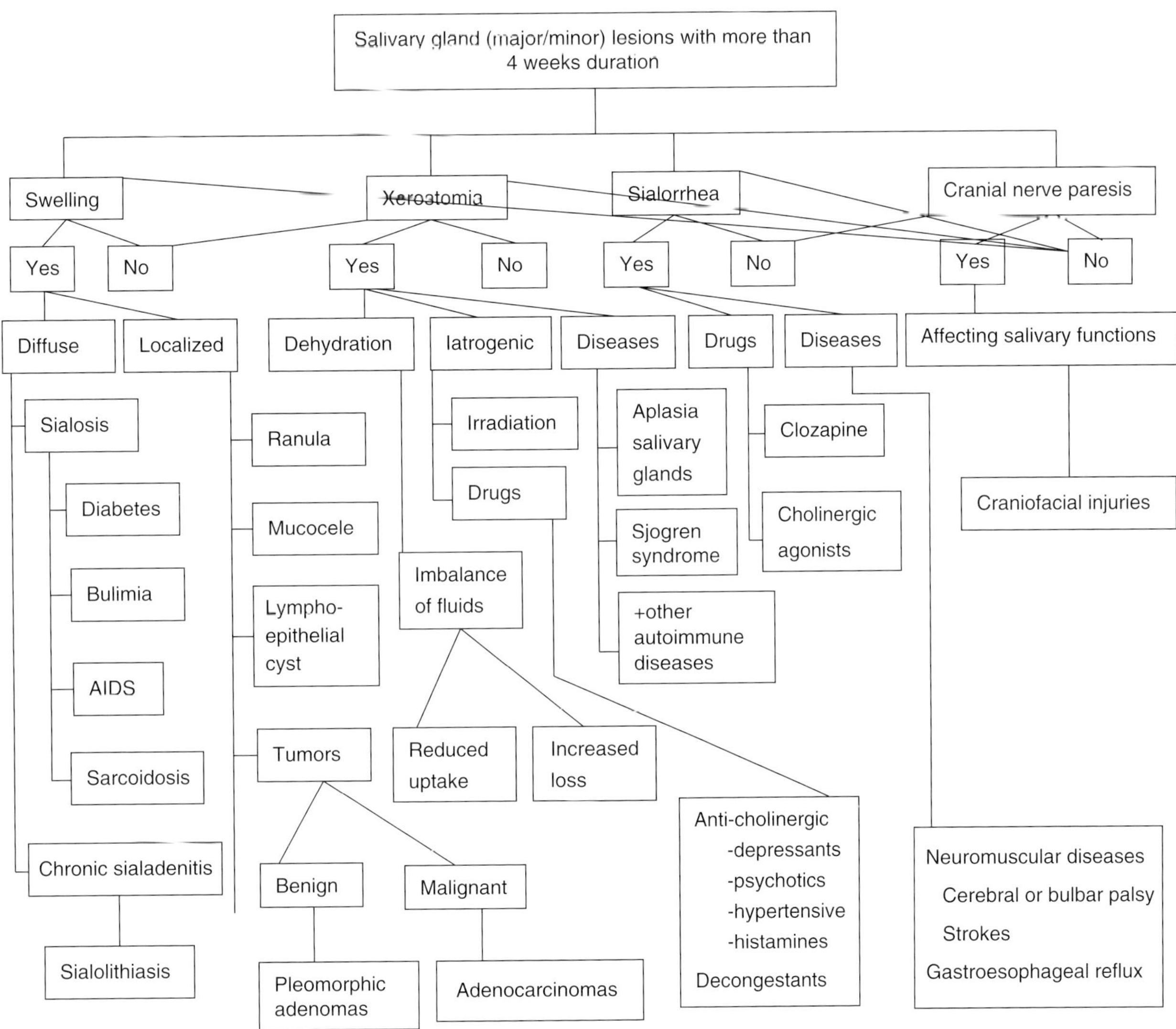

Flow Chart 23a

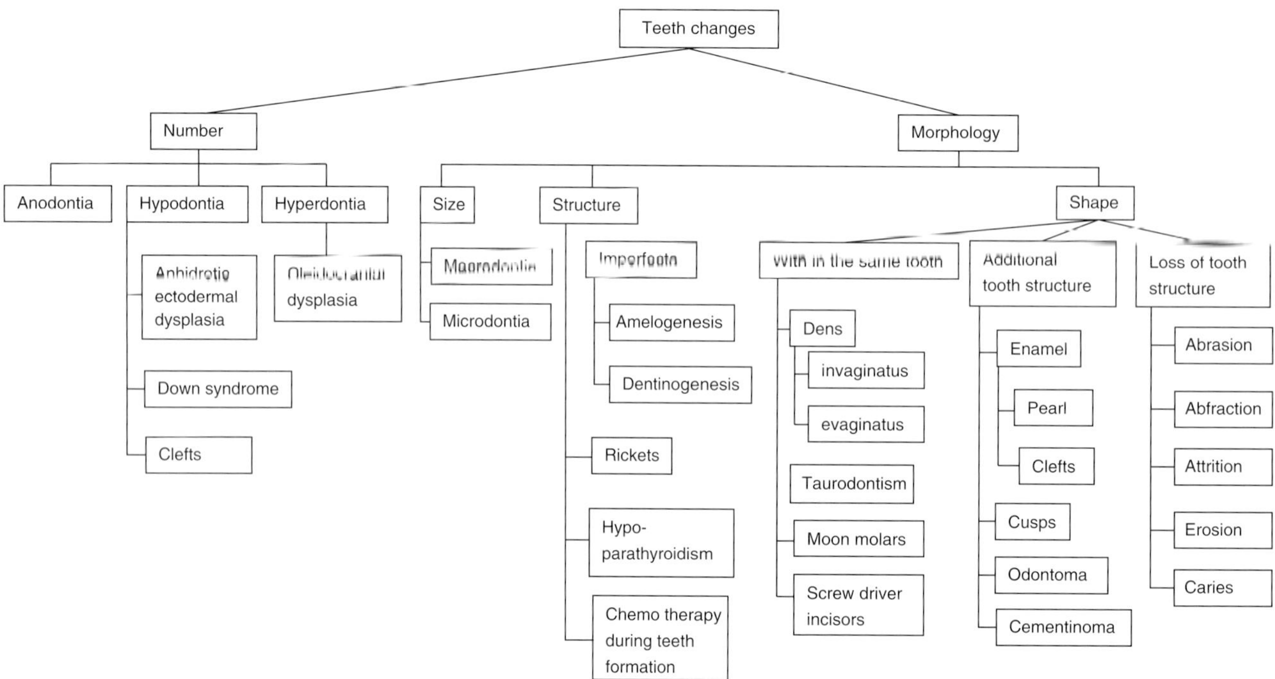

Flow Chart 23b

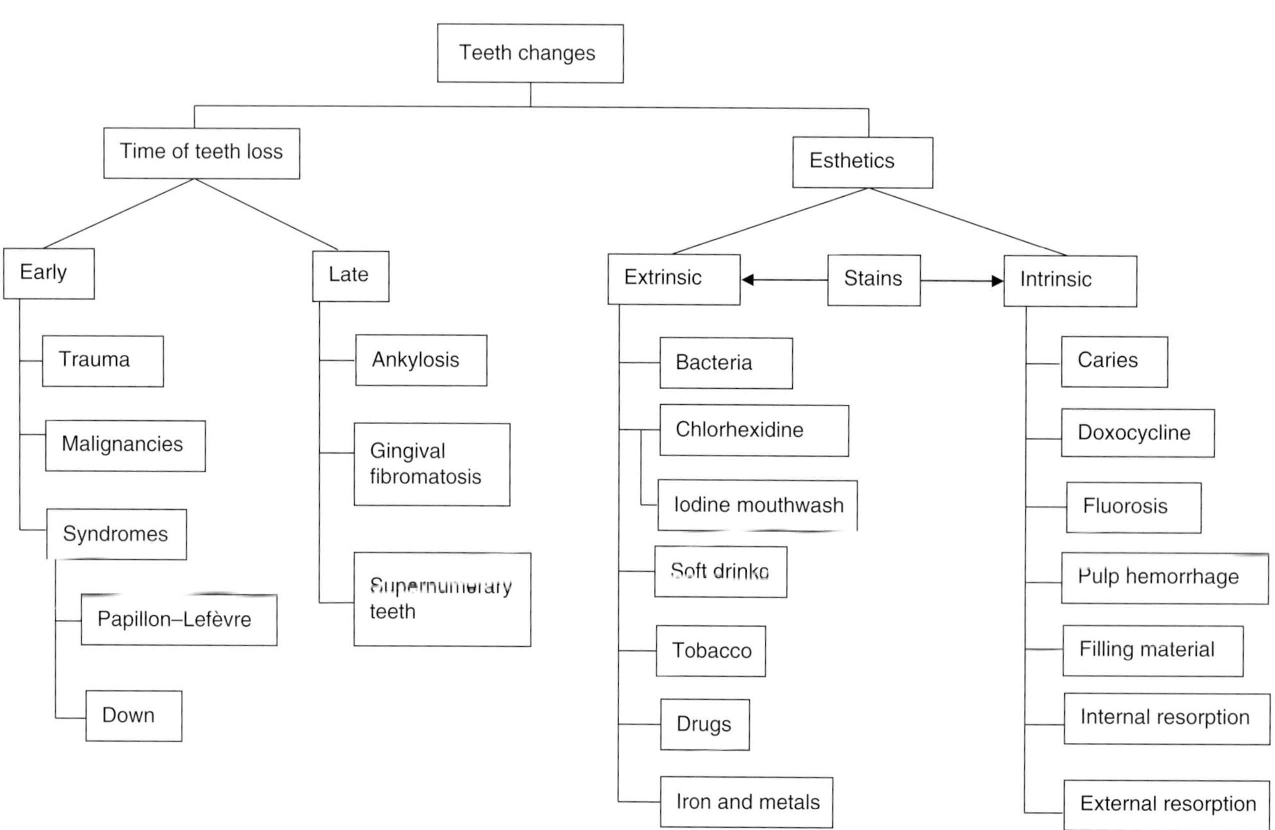

Flow Chart 24a

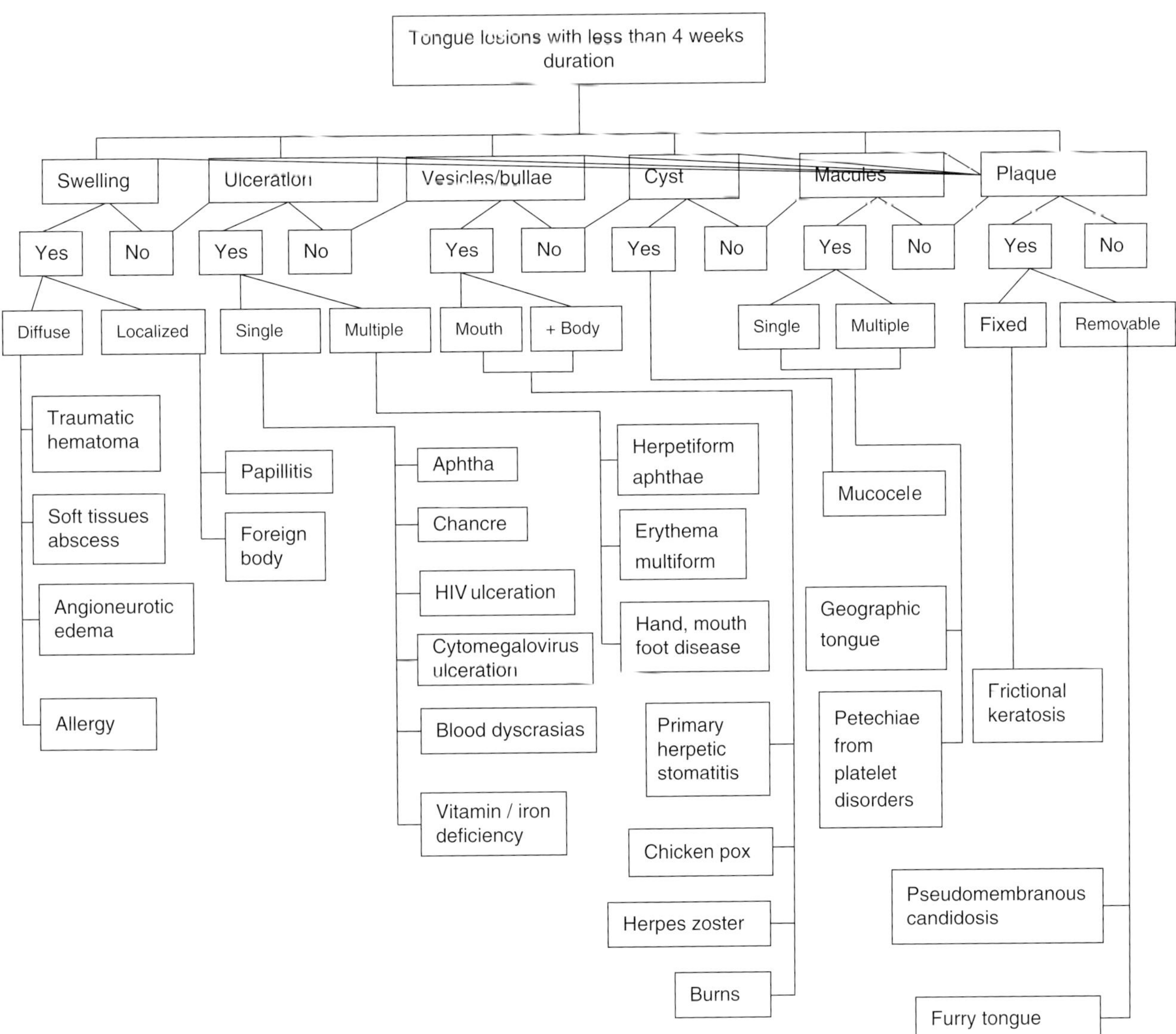

Flow Chart 24b

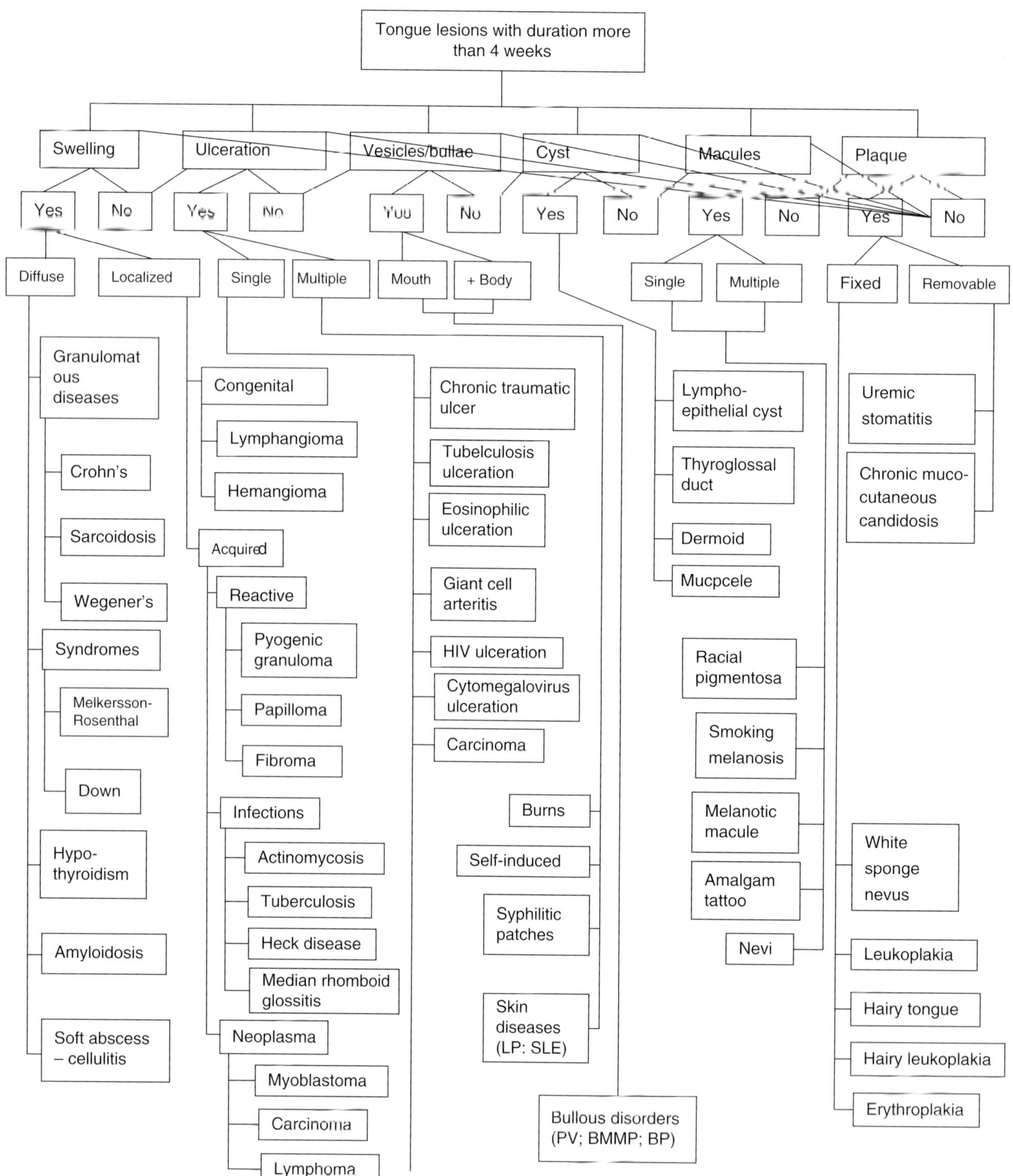

Appendix

ICD-10 Codes of Oral Diseases/Lesions

Oral disease	ICD-10
A	
Abscess-oral soft tissue	K12.2
- periodontal	K04.7
Acanthosis nigricans – benign	L83
- malignant	L83
Acinic cell tumor	C08.9
Acquired immune deficiency syndrome (AIDS)	B23.0 and B24.0
Acrodermatitis enteropathica	E83.2
Actinomycosis	A42.9
Adamantinoma	C41.4
Adenocarcinoma	C06.9
Adenoid cystic carcinoma	C08.9
- squamous cell carcinoma	C07
Adenoma – pleomorphic	D11.0
- malignant	C08.9
- sebaceous	D23.9
Agranulocytosis	D70.1
Alba linea	K13.1
Allergic stomatitis	K12.1
Amalgam tattoo	K13.79
Ameloblastoma	D16.5 and C41.4
Amelogenesis imperfecta	K00.5
Amyloidosis	E85.9
Anemia – aplastic	D61.9
- iron deficiency	D50.9
- thalassemia	D56.9
- pernicious	D51.9
Angioneurotic edema	T78.3
Ankyloglossia	Q38.3
Aphthae – herpetiform	K12.0

Oral disease	ICD-10
- major	K12.0
- minor	K12.0
- others/syndromes	M04.8
B	
Bacterial infections	A49.9
Biting	X83–X71
Bullous epidermolysis	Q81.39
- acquisita	L12.32
Burkitt's lymphoma	C83.7
Burns – chemical	T30.0
- thermal	T30.0
- irradiation	L55–L59
- electrical	T30.0
C	
Cancrum oris	A69.0
Candida endocrinopathy syndrome	E31.0
Candidosis – atrophic	B37.0
- erythematous	B37.0
- hyperplastic	B37.9
- mucocutaneous	B37.9
- multifocal	B37.9
- pseudomembranous	B37.0
Carcinoma – adenoid cystic	C08.0
- basal cell	C44.91
- lymphoepithelial	C30.0
- minor salivary gland	C08.9
- spindle cell	C26.1
- squamous	C06.9
- verrucous	C06.9
Causalgia	G56.40

Clinical Guide to Oral Diseases, First Edition. Dimitris Malamos and Crispian Scully.

Companion website: www.wiley.com/go/malamos/clinical_guide

Oral disease	ICD-10
Cellulitis	K12.2
Cementoma	K09.0
Cemento-ossifying fibroma	M27.9
Chancroid	A57
Cheilitis – actinic	K13.0
- angular	K13.0 and B37.83
- contact	L23.9 and C25.9
- exfoliate	K13.0
- glandularis	K13.0
- plasma cells	K13.0
- drug-induced	K13.0
Cherubism	M27.8
Chondroectodermal dysplasia	Q77.6
Cleft-lip	Q36.9
- palate	Q35.9
- lip and palate	Q35–Q37
Cleidocranial dysplasia	Q74.0
Coccidiodomycosis	B38.9
Conduloma acuminatum	A63.3
- lata	A53.3
Congenital dyskeratosis	Q82.8
- epulis of newborn	K06.8
- nail dystrophy	Q84.5
Cowden's disease	Q85.8
Crohn's disease	K50–K52
Cystadenoma papillary lymphomatosum	D11.3
Cyst – aneurismal bone	M85.50
Non odontogenic	K09.0
- aneurismatic	M85.50
- branchial cleft	Q18.0
- dermoid/ epidermoid	L72.0
- cystic hygroma	D18.1
- lymphoepithelial	K09.8
- mucocele	K09.8
- nasolabial	K09.1
- nasopalatine	K09.1
- ranula	K11.6
- retention cyst	K11.6
- solitary bone	N60,09
Odontogenic	K09.1
- calcified	K09.0
- dentigerous	K09.0
- eruption	K09.0
- gingival	K11.6

Oral disease	ICD-10
- glandular	K09.8
- keratocust	K09.0
- lat.periodontal	K04.8
paradental	K09.0
- periapical	K04.8
- primordial	K09.0
- residual	K04.8
Cystic fibrosis	E84.9
- hygroma	D18.1
D	
Dentinogenesis imperfecta	K00.5
Denture stomatitis	K12.1
Deposits – metals	Z18.10
Dermatitis herpetiformis	L13.0
Developmental anomalies	Q89.7
Diabetes mellitus	E11.9 (type II) and E10.9 (type I)
Drug-induced oral lesions	K13.79
Dyskeratoma, warty	L85.8
E	
Ectodermal hypohidrotic dysplasia	Q82.4
Eosinophilic ulcer	L98.3
Epidermolysis – bullosa aquisita	L12.30 and L12.31
Epulis fissuratum	K06.8
- newborn congenital	Q38.6 and K06.8
Erysipelas	K12.2 and A46
Erythema multiforme	L51.9
Erythroplasia	K13.29
Exostoses	M27.8
F	
Facial palsy	G51.0
Fellatio-induced petechiae	R23.3
Fibroma – giant cell	K06.8 and M27.1
- peripheral ossifying	D10.39
- traumatic	K13.79
Fibrous dysplasia	M85.00
Fistula – granuloma	K04.7
- periodontal	K05.6
Fluorosis	K00.3
Focal epithelial hyperplasia	K13.29
Fordyce's granules	K13.29
Freckles	L81.2

Oral disease	ICD-10
G	
Gingival enlargement	K06.01–13
- fibromatosis	K06.1
- recession	K06.1
Gingivitis	
- acute	K05.0
- chronic	K05.10
- acute necrotizing ulcerative	A69.1
- desquamative	K06
- mouth breathing, induced	K06
- plasma cell	K06 and E88.9
Gingivostomatitis – herpetic primary	B00.2
- streptococcal	B95.0
Glossitis – atrophic	K14.4
- intertiary syphilis	K14.0
- interstitial	K14.0
- plasma cell	K14.0
- rhomboid	K14.2
Glossodynia	K14.6
Gonorrhea	A54.9
Granular cell tumor	D10.1
Granuloma – fistula	L29.9
- giant cell peripheral	M27.1
- middle-line lethal	M31.2
- post-extraction	K06.8
- pregnancy	K13.4 and L98.0
- pyogenic	L98.0
Gumma	A52.3
H	
Hairy leukoplakia	K13
Hairy tongue	K13.4
Hand, foot and mouth disease	B08.4
Heck's disease	K13.29
Heerfordt syndrome	D86.89
Hemangioma	D18.09
Hematoma – traumatic	T79.2XXA
Hemochromatosis	E83.119
Hereditary hemorrhagic telangiectasia	I78.0
Herpangina	B05.0 and 074.0
Herpes labialis	B00.1
- zoster	B02.9

Oral disease	ICD-10
Herpetic secondary stomatitis	K12.1 and B00.2
Histiocytosis X	C96.6
Histoplasmosis	B38.9
Hodgkin's disease	C81.90
Horn – cutaneous	L85.5
- oral	L85.5 and K13.5
Hypoglossal nerve paralysis	G52.3
I	
Incontinentia pigmenti	Q82.3
Infections – bacterial	A49.9
- fungal	B49
- others	A07.9
- viral	B34.9
Infective mononucleosis	B27.90
Injuries – mechanical	T14.8 and W19
- radiation induced	T66
J	
Jaw fractures	S02
K	
Kaposi sarcoma	C46.7
Keratoacanthoma	L85.8
L	
Leiomyoma	D25.9
Leishmaniasis – cutaneous	B55.9
Lentigo – maligna	C43.9
- simplex	L81.4
Leprosy	A30
Leukemia – acute	C95.00
- chronic	C91.10 and C95.10
Leukoedema	K13.29
Leukoplakia – simple	K13.21
- associated with *Candida*	B37. and K13.21
Lichen planus	L43.9
Lips – double	Q38.0 and K13.0
- pits	Q38.0 and K13.0
Lipoid proteinosis	E78.8
Lipoma	D17.0
Ludwig's angina	K12.2
Lupus erythematosus – discoid	L93.0
- systemic	M32.9
Lupus vulgaris	A18.4
Lymphangioma	D18.1

Oral disease	ICD-10
Lymphatic malignancies	C96.9
Lymphoepithelial -carcinoma	C00–C006
- cyst	K09.8
- lesion	K11.8
Lymphoma – Burkitt's	C83.7
- non-Hodgkin's	C85.9
- Hodgkin's	C81.90
Lymphonodular pharyngitis	J02.8
M	
Macroglobulinemia	C88.0
Macular syphilides	A51.39
Marble bone disease	Q78.2
Masseter hypertrophy	M62.89
Measles	B05.2
Melanoma	C43.0
Melanotic neuroectodermal tumor of infancy	D48.1 and Z85.831
Medicamentosa stomatitis	K12.1 and K12.30
Metastatic tumors	C79.89
Methotrexate ulcerations	K12.30
Mucocutaneous candidosis chronic	B37.9
Mucoepidermoid tumor	C07
Mucormycosis	B46.5
Mucous patches	K13
Multiple exostoses	Q76.8
Multiple myeloma	C90
Mycosis fungoides	C84.09
Myxoma	D21.9
N	
Necrotizing sialometaplasia	K11.8
Neurofibroma	D36.10
Neurofibromatosis	Q85.00
Neuroma traumatic	T78.30
Nevus – blue	D23.9
- compound	D22.9
- intramucosal	D10.30
- junctional	D22.9
- ota	D22.39
Nicotinic stomatitis	K12.1
Noma	A69.0
Normal oral pigmentation	L81.9
Nutritional disorders	E63.9

Oral disease	ICD-10
O	
Odontoma – complex	D16.4
- compound	D16.4
Operculitis	K05.3
Orofacial digital syndrome	Q87.0
Osteitis alveolar (dry socket)	M27.3
Osteoarthritis of TMJ	M26.9
Osteogenesis imperfecta	Q78.0
Osteoma	D16.9
Osteopetrosis	Q78.2
Osteomyelitis	M86
Osteosarcoma	C41.1
P	
Papillae hypertrophy of – circumvallate	K14.3
- follate	k14.3
- fungiform	K14.3
Papillary hyperplasia of the palate	K13.6
Papilloma	D10.30
Parotitis	K91.89 and K11.20
Pellagra	E52
Pemphigoid – bullous	L12.0
- cicatricial	L12.1
- childhood	L12
Pemphigus – erythematosus	L10.4
- familial	L10.9 and Q82.8
- foliaceous	L10.2
- vegetans	L10.1
- vulgaris	L10.0
Periodontitis	K05.6
Perioral dermatitis	L71.0
Peripheral – giant cell granuloma	M27.1
- ossifying granuloma	K06.8
Plasmacytoma	C9.30
Polycythemia vera	D45
Porphyriae	E80.20
Protein deficiency	D53.0
Psoriasis	L40
Pyostomatis vegetans	L08.81
R	
Radiation-induced lesions	L55-L59
Ranula	K 11.6

Oral disease	ICD-10
S	
Salivary gland diseases	K 11.8
- abscess	K11.3
- atrophy	K11.0
- disturbance of secretion	K11.7
- fistula	K11.4
- hypertrophy	K11.1
- sialolithiasis	K11.5
Sarcoidosis	D86.9
Sarcoma of soft tissues	C49
Scarlet fever	A38.9
Schwannoma	D36.10
Scleroderma	M34
Scurvy	E54
Sebaceous adenoma	D23.9
Sialadenitis – acute	K11.21
- chronic	K11.23
Sialolithiasis	K11.5
Sublingual varices	I86.0
Submucous fibrosis	K13.5
Suppurate parotitis	K11.0
Syndromes – Acquired immune deficiency	B20
- Behcet	M35.2
- Candida endocrinopathy	E31 and B37
- Ehlers-Danlos	Q79.6
- Frey	G50.8
- Goltz	Q82.8
- Heerfordt	D86.89
- Focal palmoplantar and oral hyperkeratosis	Q82.8
- Klippel-Trènaunay-Weber	Q82.7
- Maffucci	Q78.4
- Melkersson-Rosenthal	G51.2
- Mikulicz	K11.8
- Mucocutaneous lymph node	M30.3
- Oro-facial digital	Q87.0
- Papillon-Lefèvre	Q82.8
- Peutz-Jeghers	Q85.8
- Plummer-Vinson	Q85.8
- Reiter	M02.30
- Sjogren	M35.0
- Stevens-Johnson	L15.1
- Sturge-Weber	Q85.8
Syphilis – congenital	A50
- late	A59.0
- primary	A51.2
- secondary	A51.3
- tertiary	A52.3
T	
Tattoo amalgam	L81.8
Teeth caries	K02
- arrested	K02.3
- on smooth surfaces	K02.5
- on roots	K02.7
- unspecified	K02.9
Teeth – disorders of development and eruption	
- abnormality of size or form	K00.2
- anodontia	K00.0
- disturbances in tooth eruption	K00.6
- formation	K00.4
- structure	K00.5
- mottled teeth	K00.3
- supernumerary	K00.1
- teething syndrome	K00.7
Teeth – embedded	K01.0
- impacted	K01.1
Teeth – diseases of hard tissues	KO3
- abrasion	K03.1
- ankylosis	K03.5
- attrition	K03.1
- cracked tooth	K03.81
- deposits	K03.6
- erosion	K03.2
- hypercementosis	K03.4
- posteruptive teeth staining	K03.7
- resorption	K03.3
Teeth – pulpitis	K04
- reversible	K04.01
- irreversible	K04.02
- pulp necrosis	K04.1
- degeneration	K04.2
- hard tissue formation	K04.3
- apical periodontitis – acute	K04.4
- chronic	K04.5
- periapical abscess – with sinus	K04.6

Oral disease	ICD-10
- without	K04.7
- Radicular cyst	K04.8
Teeth and supporting tissues – other disorders	K08
- Loss of teeth due to	
- caries	K08.13
periodontal diseases	K08.12
- systematic diseases	K08.0
- trauma	K08.11
- unspecified causes	K08.10
Thrombocytopenic purpura	D69.3
Tongue – bifid	K14.8
- crenated	K14.8
- fissured	K14.5
- geographic	K14.1
- hairy	K14.3
Torus – mandibularis	M27.0
- palatinus	M27.0
Toxic epidermal necrolysis	L51.2
Trigeminal neuralgia	G50.0
Tuberculosis	A15–A19

Oral disease	ICD-10
Tuberous sclerosis	Q85.1
Tumors	C00-D49
U	
Ulcer	L81.99
V	
Varicella	a1–B02
Verruca vulgaris	B07.9
Verrucum xanthoma	K13.4
Verrucous hyperplasia	K13.6
Vitiligo	L80
W	
Wegener granulomatosis	M31.30
White sponge nevus	Q38.6
X	
Xanthoma verruciform	K13.4
Xeroderma pigmentosum	L81.8
Xerostomia	K11.7 and R68.2
Z	
Zoster	B02.9

Index

Page locators in **bold** indicate tables. Page locators in *italics* indicate figures. This index uses letter-by-letter alphabetization.

Clinical Guide to Oral Diseases, First Edition. Dimitris Malamos and Crispian Scully.

Companion website: www.wiley.com/go/malamos/clinical_guide

b

C

d

e

p

r